Mario Parisi

Operative
DENTISTRY

Operative
DENTISTRY

H. WILLIAM GILMORE, D.D.S., M.S.D.

Professor of Operative Dentistry,
Indiana University School of Dentistry, Purdue University,
Indianapolis, Indiana

MELVIN R. LUND, D.M.D., M.S.

Professor and Chairman, Department of Operative Dentistry,
Indiana University School of Dentistry, Purdue University,
Indianapolis, Indiana

with 675 illustrations

SECOND EDITION

THE C. V. MOSBY COMPANY

SAINT LOUIS   1973

SECOND EDITION

Copyright © 1973 by The C. V. Mosby Company

All rights reserved. No part of this book may be reproduced in any manner without written permission of the publisher.

Previous edition copyrighted 1967

Printed in the United States of America

Distributed in Great Britain by Henry Kimpton, London

Library of Congress Cataloging in Publication Data

Gilmore, Homer William.
    Operative dentistry.

    First ed., by H. W. Gilmore, published in 1967 under title: Textbook of operative dentistry.
    1. Dentistry, Operative.   I.   Lund, Melvin R.,
1922-   joint author. II. Title. [DNLM: .
1. Dentistry, Operative.   WU 300 G486t   1973]
RK501.G5   1973   617.6   72-14447
ISBN 0-8016-1821-5

This book is affectionately dedicated to our wives and children

SHARON LEE GILMORE   MARG LUND
GREGORY WILLIAM   MARK SANDER
MICHAEL AUSTIN   KRISTINE KAY
MATTHEW EDWARD   KELLY SUE
CAROLEE

Foreword

TO FIRST EDITION

The ultimate goal in all of the health professions is the elimination of disease. As the incidence of dental caries decreases, the dentist will be able to focus more of his attention upon the diagnosis and treatment of other dyscrasias of the oral cavity. While it is appropriate that in dentistry increasing emphasis is now being placed upon research in preventive measures, for the immediate future there is every indication that the restoration of the carious lesion or the replacement of tooth structure lost as a result of caries will continue to command a major share of the time of the general practitioner. Furthermore, it is now recognized that restorative dentistry is a major component of a total dental care program that is designed to prevent dental caries and periodontal disease. Restorations that are correctly planned and inserted will arrest the propagation of caries and instill within the patient a desire to maintain the dentition through proper oral hygiene. For these and other reasons operative dentistry will remain an area of great significance in the practice of dentistry and in the curriculum of the dental school.

Although the importance of operative dentistry will not likely decrease, the concepts and methods of treatment will certainly be revised in the light of research findings and the changing pattern of dental caries. Even a cursory survey of the literature or of current therapy clearly indicates that the basic philosophy of operative dentistry has already undergone a major transition during the past 10 to 15 years.

Traditionally, operative procedures were largely founded upon empiricisms. The design of the prepared cavity and the techniques for manipulating and placing the restorative material evolved principally from trial and error. Little effort was expended to relate fundamental biologic and physical phenomena to the behavior of the restoration in situ.

Fortunately, in every era throughout the history of restorative dentistry there has been a nucleus of highly motivated dentists who have utilized their well-controlled practices as vehicles for research. Many meaningful observations have been made relative to the parameters that influence the clinical success or failure of the restorative treatment. It is remarkable how frequently the fundamental principles of operative dentistry, which were established by these clinical observations, have withstood the test of time when subsequently evaluated by modern sophisticated laboratory experimentation. The dental profession should indeed be grateful to these dedicated individuals who used their operatory and laboratory as tools for research. Many of their contributions are cited in the chapters that follow.

Through these same years dental research itself was characterized by distinct barriers between the scientific disciplines. For example, the oral pathologist displayed little or no interest in studying the effects of materials and instrumentation upon dental tissues. On the other hand, the researcher in the science of dental materials remained divorced from biologic considerations as he developed newer materials and techniques in order to provide superior physical properties. The greatest void was the total lack of communication between the investigator and the clinician. Their interests and pursuits followed divergent paths.

Thus it was to be expected that the technology of operative dentistry and the course content in the dental school curriculum would be identified with mechanical skills and their concepts based upon a tenuous foundation of empiricisms.

This type of research and academic environment no longer prevails. Dental science has come of age. The cross-fertilization of disciplines and the realization that laboratory and clinical research are interdependent have resulted in a scientific and systemic approach to the treatment of oral diseases in all of the clinical areas. It is within this framework of reference that a new concept of operative dentistry has materialized. This philosophy has brought a refreshing lure and challenge to the field.

Endless examples might be cited to illustrate the nature of this transformation. The engineering sciences are contributing knowledge on the forces of mastication and the stress distribution on oral structures and appliances. These data are altering certain of the classic principles of cavity design that were previously believed to be irrevocable. The present-day operative dentist takes into consideration the biologic effects of instrumentation and materials. As research on dental materials is producing an avalanche of new products with an accompanying panorama of chemical and physical properties, the dentist now assumes a a certain responsibility in understanding these properties and in relating them to the clinical restoration.

The use of accepted methods in preventive dental therapy is essential if the anticipated lifetime of the restoration is to be realized. Thus the practitioner must be conversant with the current status of anticariogenic measures. He must attain a workable appreciation of occlusion and the etiology of the diseases of the soft tissues so that he may equilibrate restorations correctly and provide proper contour and contact for the restored tooth.

Yet a great portion of the actual time allocation in operative dentistry is devoted to the manual tasks of removing caries, preparing the cavity, manipulating and placing the material, and finishing the restoration. There are those who would depreciate this activity as a pedestrian one and would belittle its importance to the present and future role of the operative dentist.

Such an attitude is unrealistic and to be deplored. The eventual success or failure of the operative procedure rests to a considerable extent upon the technical abilities of the dentist to perform the operations in such a manner that the optimal characteristics necessary for success will be assured. It is to be acknowledged that the perfect restoration has never been made. However, the dentist continually strives for that perfection, not only by the use of scientific principles but also by the attainment of exceptional mechanical skills. It is obligatory that subject matter in texts such as this be properly distributed between the sciences and the details that will nurture technical competence. As it has been time-honored in the past, operative dentistry will always represent a unique blending of science and creative art. Excellence is attained only by an appreciation and acquisition of both.

Such then is the changing complexion of this field of dentistry, with its own particular values and rewards. This book was written with these concepts in mind.

Ralph W. Phillips

Foreword

TO SECOND EDITION

A considered review of the foreword written for the first edition and a reading of the manuscript for this revision make it readily apparent that the structure, objectives, and content of the two editions are indeed parallel. Since that foreword was written in the hope that it would capture the philosophy of the book, it would be superfluous to reword it. Rather it is appropriate that it be carried again in this edition of a text that has enjoyed wide acceptance by both dental educators and practitioners.

The challenges associated with operative dentistry have compounded during the past 5 years. These include an increased armamentarium available for the restoration of the carious lesion, renewed emphasis upon preventive dentistry, a further awareness of biologic considerations in instrumentation and the biocompatability of dental materials, and a more serious look at the role of auxiliary personnel. As was emphasized in the original foreword, it is that type of conceptual thinking that offers intrigue to the author who is writing a text for modern-day operative dentistry, while at the same time it cultivates an ever-critical and demanding audience.

A review of the manuscript for this edition has not found it lacking in accuracy, timeliness, or clarity. The presentation of the techniques described is logical and based upon an up-to-date appreciation of the accepted knowledge in the basic and applied sciences related to restorative dentistry. The book has been further enhanced by the addition of a co-author of recognized stature.

Careful adherence to the principles that are emphasized should make the reader even more appreciative of the satisfaction and rewards to be derived from the practice of operative dentistry, and they are considerable. The contents have been wisely altered to reflect the changes that have occurred during this time interval and are sufficiently abreast of the changing concepts in the field that the text should remain current for the lifetime of this edition. One could ask little more.

Ralph W. Phillips

Preface

Clinical dentistry has continued to advance and has provided many diagnostic and treatment procedures that make this the all-time high era for patient service. Early recognition of disease, preventive measures, and restorative procedures remain as the cornerstones of dental practice. In this second edition we have developed a text that again includes the recognized procedures of comprehensive dental care. The book has been updated by including new, currently accepted routines. In many cases the technical procedures utilize a similar approach, but the treatment objectives are more conveniently attained by employing the developments of research. The procedures naturally include many concepts from the biologic, materials, and instrumentation fields.

The dental profession is concerned with the delivery of more dental care and in maintaining the high quality of service for which the United States is recognized; therefore, the text was written to be helpful for the practitioner, beginning student, and the auxiliaries who are included on the practice team. The chapters are referenced for additional study to maintain the forward and scientific theme of the textbook.

In addition to the new concepts, a chapter has been added on porcelain restorations. Line drawings have been developed to supplement the recommendations for cavity preparation design. The manipulation of materials has been expanded and simplified to include the interests of the auxiliaries. Essentially the same format has been maintained to permit a continuing revision as better and improved procedures are developed.

Special citation is given to Dr. Joao Galan for the line drawings and suggestions given in illustrating the second edition. An active group of departmental graduate students assisted with the manuscript. Appreciation is given to Dr. David Bales, Dr. Jerome Rudolph, Dr. Ronald Harris, Dr. Thomas Wilson, Dr. Fidel Marquez, Dr. Dean Schloyer, Dr. Richard Harper, and Dr. Sigfuss Eliasson.

Dr. Ralph Phillips supported the revision by acting as constant counsel and by reviewing the manuscript. His enthusiasm and insight are reflected again in the revised foreword. Other members of the Dental Materials staff that were helpful were Professor Marjorie Swartz and Dr. Richard Norman.

Special gratitude is given also to Dean Ralph McDonald for making the available time to complete the project. Excellent assistance was provided by the illustrations staff of the Indiana University School of Dentistry.

Operative departmental support was given by Dr. Drexell Boyd, Dr. Fredrick Hohlt, and Dr. Norris Richmond. The typing was accomplished by Miss Kay Raikos and Mrs. Betty Hardesty.

Again material was used from many colleagues with special thanks being given to Dr. Lloyd Baum, Dr. Robert Kinzer, Dr. Kenneth Mertz, Dr. Harold Schnepper, and Dr. Daniel Gordon. The information was included mainly in the chapters on porcelain, cohesive gold, and gold castings and provided valuable additions to the text. Some of the line drawings for direct gold were submitted by Ellis R. Jones.

Continuing education is one of the privileges of being a member of the dental profession. Personal actions and attitudes are reflected by the importance given to and eventual involvement in scholarship. It is the purpose of this book to contribute to professional development and, hopefully, to the level of dental care that is practiced by the reader.

H. William Gilmore
Melvin R. Lund

Contents

Operative
DENTISTRY

chapter 1

Scope of operative dentistry

Operative dentisty can be defined as the prevention and treatment of defects in natural teeth. Because of the lack of biologic research, the dental profession has been concerned mainly with treatment. Because of the size of the field and the area it occupies in the dental curriculum, the practice of operative dentistry remains one of the most popular aspects of the profession. Originally operative dentistry comprised the entire profession, and the term was synonymous with patient services. Examination of early textbooks will demonstrate that many of the subjects now considered specialty areas were originally included in operative dentistry.[1-3] The books that were first used were voluminous and contained everything that was known at the time regarding treatment of the patient. Subjects such as pedodontics, orthodontics, oral surgery, and oral pathology were considered to be categories within the field of operative dentistry because they were practiced in the dental operatory. The field of operative dentistry is now considered by the Federal Dental Services to be general dental practice.

The scope of operative dentistry has in a sense been reduced. The American Dental Association now recognizes eight specialty groups, all of which require additional study beyond the regular dental degree and have strict requirements for qualification.

Beginning in 1950 there was a tremendous increase in research and publication of scientific data in all professions. Most of the scientific publications have appeared in the last 20 years. Although a relatively small percentage of these publications was concerned with dentistry, all have had a profound influence on the profession. Data have accumulated in all areas of dentistry to such a degree that it is now evident that in the future it will be difficult to stay abreast of information in even one specialty. The amount of material relating to some specialty groups published in just the last few years is comparable to all of the original books on operative dentistry, and it places demands for scholarship in all areas of the profession.

With the division of the subject matter area, operative dentistry now consists of the highly mechanical and exacting methods of restoring natural teeth. This process involves cavity preparation of the affected tooth and a subsequent restoration to replace the missing parts. The concepts being advocated are founded either on scientific data or on the experiences of predecessors in the field. Although established scientific procedures are used, empirical clinical procedures still serve the unknown. Many accepted procedures are being further studied and improved.

The practice of operative dentistry has changed in that it is more refined and precise in its function of maintaining the natural dentition. Highly refined motor skills are needed to perform today's tooth operations. This refinement in technique is made possible by better working conditions, expansion of knowledge through research, and development of new instruments. Despite the reduced subject coverage, the total field of operative dentistry is approximately the same as it was in its early days because of new techniques and materials. Many techniques that have been developed are associated with the refinement of dental materials. The need for continued education is much greater because of this new information. The field of instrumentation has also continued to expand. New cutting instruments and methods have been produced and are commonplace in the dental office. Speed ranges have been greatly increased. The treatments produce a higher level of dentistry. Moreover, the newly refined operative dentistry produces more permanent restorations that allow for longer and more reachable goals for maintaining the natural dentition.

HERITAGE OF OPERATIVE DENTISTRY

At the beginning of the nineteenth century dentists were regarded as operative dentists. Dentists came to the United States from Europe, mainly from France and Germany. In the eastern cities new men were trained as apprentices until they were well enough established to open their own practices. Dentistry at this time was considered to be more of a trade than a profession. Most services were aimed at the relief of pain, and restorative dentistry was a limited concern at this stage of development.

The way in which amalgam was introduced into the country created an issue.[4] Two French dentists brought an alloy product called "Royal Mineral Succidaneum" into the country as a mineral paste. This compound was definitely a departure from that being used, and its advocates suggested that it be wiped into existing caries and precarious areas of the tooth to restore the affected tooth as well as prevent future caries. Some of the pioneers felt that this amalgam paste should not be used to treat patients. A political issue developed and soon the "amalgam war" developed. There were, of course, dentists representing both sides of the issue, but for a short period of time is was considered malpractice and unethical to use amalgam for the restoration of teeth. There were many publications on the subject and creeds developed that were used as a code of ethics for dental societies in respective areas of the country.

The cities involved in the amalgam war were New York, Philadelphia, St.

Louis, and Chicago. There were one or two leaders in each of the cities who managed to prolong the amalgam war for several years. This controversy inspired one of the amalgam antagonists, Chapin A. Harris from New York, to open the first dental school in the United States in Baltimore in 1841. This was the Baltimore College of Dental Surgery, which is presently part of the University of Maryland. Harris was also instrumental at this time in starting the first national dental society in New York City. Thus it can be said that amalgam, because of the controversy it raised, served as an incentive for the establishment of dentistry as a profession in the United States.

Some of the techniques and materials being used in operative dentistry helped to create and develop interest in the field and to further unite it. When the rubber dam was developed by Robert C. Barnum in 1864 in New York City,[5] many articles were published concerning its use as well as the feasibility of certain men being able to patent the rubber material and technique. Many debates developed in the dental societies over its application. Although it was not realized at the time, invention of the rubber dam by Barnum remains one of the greatest developments in the field of operative dentistry. It became possible to develop a surgical environment for placing different types of dental restorations. The development of the rubber dam made contoured restorations possible. Gold foil was very popular in the early days of dentistry but is was not used then as it is today. The material was noncohesive and was simply packed into a tooth to fill up the crater. This technique was responsible for the origin of the term "filling."

In many cases the pioneers became the original investigators. By 1875 there were numerous dentists doing research with technical procedures. Although their work was elemental and done by trial and error, it was very useful as a guide. Some of this early research is still quoted in academic circles because it formed the foundation of modern research. Further interest in research soon developed; some of the early investigators had a profound influence on the practice of operative dentistry, and in most sections of the country their principles are still being used. Investigators developed special interests and confined themselves to certain areas. This resulted in writing and publishing in their respective regions, giving dentistry a geographic recognition in the United States. Certain areas of the United States were recognized as better in one procedure than in another, but as the profession and the country have progressed, this has changed.

The father of modern operative dentistry is G. V. Black. He practiced in Jacksonville, Illinois, and held both dental and medical degrees.[6] He became associated with Northwestern University as professor of operative dentistry and dean of the school of dentistry. Black's writings were novel and extensive and remain unequaled to this time. They developed the foundation of the profession and caused the field of operative dentistry to be placed on an organized and scientific basis. The early writings of G. V. Black were concerned mainly with caries, erosion, and oral pathology. Much attention was given to diseases of the pulp and tissue degeneration that occurred in clinical conditions. Black established principles of cavity preparation, classified caries and cavity preparations, set up nomenclature, and identified attributes of the various restorative materials. Today the practice of operative dentistry cannot be successfully accomplished unless Black's work is understood and applied to the variables that exist in oral disease. Other outstanding contributions of G. V. Black include the original work on annealing amalgam and the mercury alloy ratio and formulation of the first silver amalgams used in the profession. Black also exhibited biologic interest in stains of the teeth and did a great deal of work on staining and the problems produced by oral bacteria.

Arthur D. Black, son of G. V. Black, followed closely in his father's footsteps. It has been stated that "Dr. Arthur Black added glory to the reputation of his illustrious father who was the most beloved as well as the most distinguished man in the dental profession."[6] He had the habit of working late hours, and this dedication and motivation were probably due to his close association with his father.

Arthur Black developed many of the instruments and techniques advocated by his father and used them in teaching, which was his greatest interest. He developed a model organizational plan for the Illinois State Dental Society that is still being used and that has been copied by many states. The connection of the Blacks with the Northwestern Dental School extended over an uninterrupted period of 40 years. The impact these two gentlemen had on the dental profession at the beginning of the twentieth century is still felt and their work remains alive today. The card catalog system for dental books used daily in libraries is one of Arthur Black's contributions.

Leadership in the profession soon began to extend to different areas of the country as new urban centers developed. The Blacks' reputation was instrumental in inspiring Charles E. Woodbury, who practiced in Council Buffs, Iowa. Woodbury not only practiced in Council Bluffs but traveled across the river to teach in Omaha, Nebraska. He greatly influenced dental education in this area and started a gold foil study club that remains active and meets regularly twice a year. He started study clubs in other states and traveled to give instruction in many other cities. Some of the clubs functioned for a while, but none has remained as active as the original Woodbury Club in Omaha, Nebraska. Woodbury is mainly noted for his work in gold foil and was one of the first to modify Black's principles.[7] The Class III Woodbury preparation was designed to produce a more esthetic outline form for proximal anterior gold foil restorations. Woodbury also designed a set of hand instruments that he advocated for use in the Class III cavity preparation. This set of instruments, thirty-nine in number, became known as the Woodbury kit and is probably the most universally used set of hand instruments. In addition to these instruments and different foil preparations, Woodbury designed different types of condensing points to be used for building the gold foil restoration. Through his work he did much to raise the level of dentistry in the Great Plains states, and his name is still heard in many places.

A colorful pioneer in operative dentistry was E. K. Wedelstaedt of St. Paul, Minnesota. He was strongly influenced by the Blacks and visited them many times, discussing research topics and the requirements of cavity preparation. Wedelstaedt started the G. V. Black study clubs in the Midwest and persuaded Black to travel around the states of Iowa and Minnesota teaching the members postgraduate courses. Today the most active club is the original G. V. Black Club in Minneapolis, which at one time was larger than the Minnesota State Dental Association. Wedelstaedt became associated with Dr. Searl of Minneapolis and the two traveled through the United States giving courses on operative dentistry and starting study clubs. Because of the lack of dental schools and the popularity of these men, the courses were very successful. The information received in these courses was practically the only training in modern techniques of tooth restoration available to dentists at the time. Publications and communications did not keep dentists adequately informed. Wedelstaedt's outstanding contribution was the system he developed for measuring dental instruments. This system is still being used. He also developed new hand instruments that could be used in the techniques being taught in the study clubs. The most popular of these intruments was the Wedelstaedt chisel, the most universally used chisel today. The Wedelstaedt chisel has a mesial and distal cutting edge and is advocated for use in most anterior gold foil preparations. This instrument and the system of measurements he developed are the outstanding marks left by Wedelstaedt.

One of the most outstanding pioneers in the field of operative dentistry was Waldon I. Ferrier of Seattle, Washington.[8] In the 1920's he was taught by Wedelstaedt and Searl and was noted for his outstanding work in their course. Because of the distance and complications involved in teaching their courses throughout the United States, Dr. Ferrier was appointed by Wedelstaedt and Searl to teach postgraduate courses in the Pacific Northwest. Soon he developed a study club and taught its members all the techniques being used in operative dentistry at that time. Today there are more active study clubs in the state of Washington than in any other place in the United States and the credit for them is given to Ferrier. Ferrier again modified the gold foil procedures being used and developed new outline forms to correspond with the techniques. Ferrier is considered to be the father of modern gold foil procedures. To be capable of performing these procedures today the dentist must first understand and be able to apply Ferrier's principles. This involves studying his original publications and the techniques he taught throughout his career.

This outstanding teacher also developed a set of new instruments that are called the Ferrier set. These instruments are more refined than others and have a uniform thickness on the cutting edge as well as other dimensions that are more precise. More precise cavity preparation, which is the forte of the Ferrier method, can be accomplished with the use of these instruments. A group of separators was also designed by Ferrier. These devices are the most universally used today and are modifications of the original group designed by Perry. The separators come in a group of six and can be applied to all types and sizes of teeth in the oral cavity. The design of the separators makes it possible to secure them with compound and stabilize all the teeth in the field of operation to enhance the operative procedure. To aid in modern gold foil preparations, Ferrier designed a set of condensers. These instruments are used to condense gold foil and they fit the angles of his preparation quite accurately. They can be used to apply the proper lines of force needed in building up the gold foil restoration. Ferrier stated that the greatest thing he accomplished to improve the practice of operative dentistry was to advocate the use of the lingual-gingival shoulder in the Class III gold foil preparation.

Another pioneer in operative dentistry deserving mention is George Hollenback. Upon graduation he moved west and for 60 years has been outstanding in the practice, teaching, and research aspects of operative dentistry. Hollenback has published many articles on operative dentistry and his most important contribution is considered to be his work on the physical properties of gold foil[9] and the shrinkage of gold during the casting process.[10] Much work has been done by this investigator on the science and technique of the cast restoration, and he has written numerous other articles associated with individual tooth restoration (Fig. 1-1). During many years of dedicated service he has done much to improve the theory of dental practice. Hollenback's research has been enhanced by his ability to design and build research tools. When a research

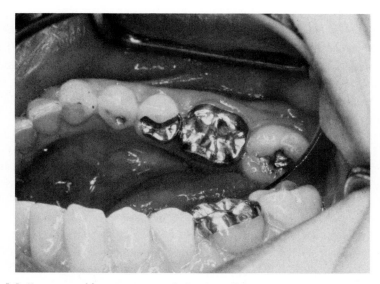

Fig. 1-1. Two cast gold restorations made by the indirect method studied by Hollenback.

project is suggested, Hollenback is able to construct different types of instruments that can be used to measure physical and chemical changes within the laboratory. Certainly the operative dentist can benefit greatly by reading Hollenback's collected reprints and taking his postgraduate courses.

Many outstanding people have contributed and are working in the field of operative dentistry. Although they are too numerous to mention here, their work is evident in the literature and textbooks that have been published. They will always be respected for their laborious efforts to increase the understanding of general practice. The field of operative dentistry can be credited with the development of the dental profession in both the United States and the world.

THE CHALLENGE OF CLINICAL PROBLEMS

In all cases the objective of treatment is to correct the deficiency or defect that exists in the teeth. Treatment then comprises the major part of the actual service performed by operative dentists, with preventive dentistry making rapid gains.

A survey conducted by the U. S. Public Health Service[11] in 1962 shows that a large portion of the population of the United States needs some kind of dental treatment. The survey states that (1) 98% of the population has either had or will have dental caries, (2) two thirds of all adults eventually have periodontal problems, (3) one fifth of the population of children has orthodontic problems, and (4) to further complicate the situation, 20 million adults in the United States are edentulous. Another recent survey stated that there are 4 million new untreated cavities per year in the United States.[12] By simply providing treatment and nothing else it would be impossible to completely eliminate dental caries in the United States. These figures were helpful in creating interest in preventive dentistry.

The latest figures on dental need in the United States show[13]:

1. There are 23,000 victims of oral cancer each year.
2. One in every 700 children is born with a cleft lip or palate.
3. Twenty percent of the children have deforming orthodontic problems.
4. Sixty percent of the young adults, 80% of the middle aged, and 90% of the older population have periodontal disease.
5. Ninety-five percent of the population has caries.

The work load for restorative problems is overwhelming and is not close to being solved by the dental profession, either the private or the governmental sector.

Deficiencies in the materials being used in tooth restoration affect the amount of treatment needed. Although restorative materials serve a useful and critical health purpose, they are far from being perfect. An ideal restoration would be one that would never need to be replaced, and at the present time we have no compound that can be considered entirely permanent. Numerous surveys concerned with the efficiency of dental restorations and the failures that exist in

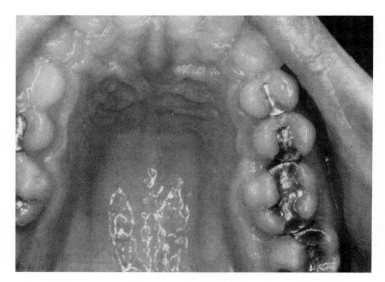

Fig. 1-2. Amalgam restoration on the first molar that required replacement.

clinical treatment have provided alarming statistics.[14] From the data it appears that dentists will spend a large portion of their time replacing restorations that have been unable to withstand the conditions in the oral cavity (Fig. 1-2). The fault is not the dentist's or patient's but rather the weaknesses that exist in some of the restorative materials themselves. D. L. Moore surveyed operative services and reported that defective materials produced a major need for restorative treatment.[15] Replacements could conceivably become the major role of the practitioner rather than the elimination of primary disease.

Patients are usually unaware of the need for dental treatment, and patient education is needed. Such education can be offered by the dentist, who understands the importance of dental health and the procedures involved in tooth rehabilitation. Most patients come to the dentist because they have symptoms of pain. It is a responsibility of the dentist to relieve the pain by correcting the problem that has caused the discomfort (Fig. 1-3). Dental health education is best accomplished by professionals who address schools, industries, and lay groups. Demand for care is sharply increasing and has surpassed the profession's ability to develop delivery systems.

A significant amount of time is needed to place an individual tooth restoration. It becomes necessary for the dentist to divide his practice into categories of diagnosis, treatment, and maintenance. Because of the alarming amount of work that needs to be done, the greatest portion of the dentist's time will be spent in treatment. The dentist's services are enhanced by employing an efficient and thorough routine and offering the best type of operative dentistry possible. The time factor in treatment is critical because of the exacting procedure re-

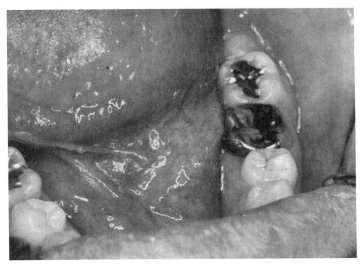

Fig. 1-3. Lower first molar that was previously mutilated by caries and produced painful symptoms following meals. A pin-retained amalgam restoration was used to restore the tooth.

quired. The pressure of details is often fatiguing. Although this phase of the dental service often becomes the primary burden of a dental practice, it should be remembered that the patient does not achieve optimum dental health until treatment is completed.

The aspects of preventive dentistry are the effective mechanisms in which the backlog of treatment can be controlled. If the occurrence of carious lesions is reduced, the dentist's work load becomes lighter. Factors working against this possibility are population growth and the insufficient number of dentists being trained in our schools. Whereas the dentist per population ratio is decreasing, the demand for dental care continues to increase rapidly. This indicates that optimum dental health care depends upon preventive measures.[16] Diagnosis and maintenance are the two primary preventive measures in an operative program. Preventive measures should be kept in mind at all times while providing service to the patient. Because of the importance of preventive dentistry, it probably will soon occupy as large an area and demand as much time as patient treatment.

Preventive dentistry has many applications in a practice, and it has recently "mushroomed" as a result of the impact of biologic research. It is difficult to stay abreast of all recent refinements, but the careful dentist can measure and evaluate the adjuncts offered by research and fit most of them into the individual routines of his practice. Preventive dentistry has become increasingly popular, and surveys indicate that dentists increase their incomes by integrating preventive services with treatment. With combined therapy it is possible to prevent over 90% of the expected carious lesions in the permanent dentition.[17] Combined therapy includes the proper use of communal fluoridation, topical fluorides, and dentifrices and adequate home care. The fluorides serve to strengthen the tooth in the oral environment and home care serves to keep the teeth clean. It is important to eliminate from the diet the types of food that cause enamel decalcification and caries.

The cost of combined services is quite low and this lends additional encouragement to the use of practical preventive measures. In the firmly established preventive practice the type of treatment that is given changes rapidly. In some ways more need for operative dentistry is created because patients retain their teeth longer. Yet the great reduction in the occurrence of smooth surface caries will lower the operative dentist's work load in this area. However, the caries in enamel defects and occlusal surfaces will usually still occur. This is especially true in the lingual and buccal pits of the teeth as well as in the poorly coalesced grooves on the occlusal surfaces of the posterior teeth. The pit and fissure lesions that tend to develop in such areas dictate the use of conservative restorative procedures. The use of fluoride appears to limit the size of the carious lesion, requiring a different outline form. In this way the work load is increased and the demand for operative dentistry becomes more apparent.

Trends in government and education are being made to extend the services of paradental personnel.[18] Licensure is being written and training programs are being developed to permit more treatment being accomplished by the trained dental auxiliary. It is the purpose of these programs to give more treatment and reduce the dental needs of the population. It is obvious that the demand for dental care is changing the philosophy, education, and practice of dentistry.

Prevention should be an integral part of dental practice and utilized at all times. Certainly it is the greatest adjunct that can be used to support a sound program of treatment. Combined, the factors of prevention and treatment are the most effective means by which a dentist can protect and preserve the natural dentitions of his patients, which is now called a "control program."

OBJECTIVES OF OPERATIVE DENTISTRY

Maintaining the natural dentition in an optimum state of health, function, and esthetics is the main objective of general practice. This objective is comparable to that of other health-related fields since, by definition, the tooth can be considered an organ. During cavity preparation, enamel and dentinal tissue are removed mechanically, and since the excision of vital tissue is involved, cavity preparation is considered a surgical procedure. The restoration that is placed in the prepared cavity must satisfy the preceding objective and produce no unfavorable reactions in the tooth. As a result of the operation the tooth should be in as good a state as it was prior to the cavity preparation. These are general objectives and they are included in nearly all fields of the health professions.

A discussion concerning the maintenance of the natural dentition certainly should be initiated by considering the health of the dental pulp. Tooth vitality

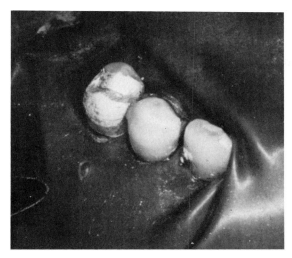

Fig. 1-4. Pin-retained amalgam to be used as a bridge retainer core. Pulp vitality has been preserved.

is derived from the pulp, which is a highly vascular and innervated piece of connective tissue. The pulp must be kept alive and healthy to allow the tooth to age normally in the oral cavity (Fig. 1-4). This tissue receives blood, which means it is oxygenated and nourished by the systemic circulation. Circulation is essential to all tissue life and it appears to be very critical in the pulp. The nerve tissue responds to pain and other types of stimuli. The pulp protects the tooth throughout its clinical life and functions adequately only when it is healthy.

When the pulp is injured, there is a mechanism that serves to give added protection to the tissue. Inflammation and reparative dentin usually result from injury. If the pulp is severely injured or openly contaminated, the tissue usually degenerates. Once this occurs the tooth can be retained by endodontic procedures or extracted. Pulpal degeneration is ordinarily caused by severe trauma produced by caries, accidents, or cavity preparation. After endodontic treatment the restorative dentist must restore the tooth for it to function. It is safe to say the tooth cannot be retained under ideal conditions unless the health of the pulp is maintained. Pulp protection receives much consideration in operative dentistry and is automatically considered before attempting an operating procedure.[19]

Health of the supporting tissues is of equal importance in the life of a tooth. A healthy gingival tissue is one that adapts tightly to the necks of the teeth. Usually the epithelial borders cover the cementum and rest freely against the enamel at the cervical surface. The gingival tissue is described as light pink in color and exhibiting an orange-peel consistency. The gingival tissue is festooned around the necks of the teeth. Its prominence is a result of the thickness of the lamina dura, and it is observed around the root portions of the most prominent teeth in the arch. Proper toothbrushing maintains healthy tissues. The epithelial sulcus should be stimulated and cleaned regularly to enhance the adaptation of the tissue to the teeth. Recession of well-cared-for gingival tissues is slight and that which occurs later in life is mainly attributed to the physiologic attrition caused by aging.

Gingival tissue can be affected by restorative materials. From the standpoint of health it is best for gingival tissues to rest on sound enamel. Many histologic studies have been conducted to determine the reaction of gingival tissue when resting on restorations. Gingival tissue is seen to react differently to each restorative material and displays some degree of irritation to all. Restorations made of polished gold and glazed porcelain most nearly approximate the relationship of sound enamel.[20]

The gingival tissue is usually the first to be affected when the supporting structures are damaged. The tissue becomes tumified and inflamed, which produces food impaction. The food in the crevice creates additional bacteria and forms materia alba, which serves as an irritant to the underlying supporting structures. Eventually a periodontal pocket is formed around the tooth and the additional food impaction and resulting irritation involve the connective tissues. If this condition is allowed to continue, it can cause periodontal disease. The sequelae of these conditions occur if proper care is not taken of gingival tissue during the restorative techniques. The use of materials capable of providing good margins, smooth surfaces, and adequate contour is necessary when the restoration is below gingival tissue. A clinical study reported that inflammation of gingival tissue is initiated by bacteria, making faulty restorations more of a problem in controlling gingival health.[21]

The health of the gingiva in the interproximal space must be considered. Food must not be allowed to remain in contact with these tissues for long periods of time or similar breakdown will occur. The proximal contact of the teeth must be tight enough to resist the forces of the food during chewing and not allow material to be pushed into the interproximal space. The shape of the contact point and the flare of the proximal enamel walls radiating from the embrasure will influence the protection of the interproximal gingiva. These structures create an interproximal space that should be filled with healthy tissue at all times.

The interproximal restoration must not only prevent mechanical damage but it should also promote health by being in direct contact with the tissue. The material next to the tissue must be smooth and nonirritating, as in accessible gingival areas. The margins of the restoration should be closely adapted to tooth structure, avoiding a discrepancy in areas that cannot be cleaned. The proximal surface of the restoration should be suitably contoured to protect the gingival tissues. The contour should also allow the tissue to be cleansed and stimulated during the brushing procedure and should present a smooth surface for the adjacent tissues. If a condition of health is maintained in the periodontium, the

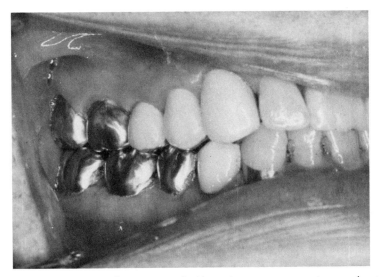

Fig. 1-5. Tooth function being restored with castings on two opposing quadrants.

tooth can be retained indefinitely. Home care that includes proper brushing, cleaning, and diet eliminates regression except that caused by physiologic processes.

The restoration must restore function to the tooth. In mastication the teeth work as individuals as well as a group, and function is usually restored by replacing the anatomic structure of the tooth that has been destroyed by the defect (Fig. 1-5). The arch should be stabilized and an acceptable arrangement of the teeth preserved to allow normal movement of the periodontal membranes. This is made possible by maintaining the mesial-distal diameter of the tooth and by equalizing pressures on the teeth as they come together in mastication.[22] The size and shape of the restoration will influence the success of these functional factors. Adverse pressures can be produced when the teeth are interdigitated or during mastication and can contribute to breakdown of the supporting structures. Care should be taken not to produce a contour that will cause the tooth to function prematurely. The replaced tooth anatomy is usually the element in a dental restoration that restores function, and excessive contours can cause damage.

Many factors influence the stability of the teeth in the arch. In addition to muscular forces the dimension of the tooth is very important. The mesial-distal diameter of the tooth influences the angulation of the tooth and the relationship of the adjacent tooth at the contact point. To replace the proximal surface of a tooth, materials should be used that have qualities of stability and permanence. In most cases metallic restorations are used because they do not shrink, expand, or dissolve in the oral cavity. Although such restorations wear slightly with attrition, they preserve the dimension of the tooth, which is needed to restore function.

The maintenance of proximal dimension is very critical in anterior teeth. Unless the entire contact point is replaced or protected, the teeth will drift and cause damage to the epithelial tissue. It is difficult for the patient to clean around teeth that become rotated, causing subsequent bone damage. To prevent anterior tooth movement, most cavity preparations try to preserve the contact point. This means that only enough tooth structure is removed in the preparation to provide access needed for the procedure. To enhance esthetics and to conserve tooth structure the labial plate is maintained in upper anterior teeth and the lingual plate in lower anterior teeth. This procedure supports the contact point of the teeth being restored and it is the best way in which to preserve proximal dimension.

In mastication the teeth work on a 1:1 or 1:2 ratio. One tooth usually occludes with either one or two opposing teeth. The teeth in occlusion should be restored so that the cusps have contacts in fossae, primary grooves, or occlusal embrasures of the opposing teeth. An attempt should also be made to produce equalized pressure between the arches and parallel to the axial lines of the tooth. When possible the working cusps should be located in opposing fossae in order to hold the tooth in its proper arch relationship.[23]

During movement of the lower jaw no abnormal forces should be produced on the occlusal surfaces, which means that none of the restored parts should

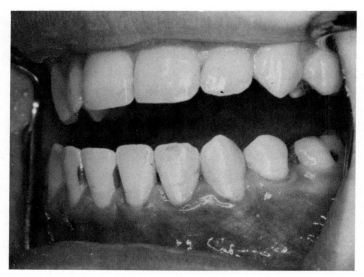

Fig. 1-6. Proximal surface of the lower central incisor restored with a conservative gold foil restoration. The bulk of tooth structure around the contact point has been preserved.

collide during function. An ideal natural occlusion has been described as one having complete disengagement of the teeth as they leave centric relation and no posterior contacts in lateral and protrusive excursions. Balancing contacts on natural teeth or restorations are thought to produce abnormal forces.[24]

The main functions of anterior teeth are the incising and tearing of food. The restorative dentist must protect the incisal edges, and this is aided by conserving the contact point. The proximal carious lesion should be restored by conservative measures whenever possible (Fig. 1-6). The incisal edges of anterior teeth are supported by the contact point, and these structures are lost or weakened when the decayed area is enlarged and the cavity preparation extended.

The physiologic role of the cuspid has been described in many ways, indicating that restoring the function of the tooth could involve many techniques.[25] From a restorative standpoint the cuspid is the key to both arches and is considered the most important tooth in the mouth. Both root structure and bone support make it possible for the canine to absorb a great amount of stress without deleterious effects. This strength makes the cuspid the keystone of the arch for mastication and the support of prosthetic appliances. At all times the cuspid tooth must be protected and maintained in a healthy state in order to preserve the other components of the dentition. Because this tooth is so essential, it is popular for root canal treatment. All measures should be taken to retain the cuspid in a good state of health and function.

The dispute concerning the cuspid involves its role in occlusion. The consensus seems to be that the cuspids must not collide in the chewing cycle as do other teeth. Some dentists feel that the lingual contour should allow no contact of the cuspids in the chewing cycle but serve to separate the jaws in border mandibular movements. This jaw separation prevents abnormal contacts in the posterior teeth, which minimizes bone destruction and wear patterns in the enamel. The anterior teeth are protected in the same way by the cuspid, and this relationship is called mutually protected occlusion.[26] These functions point out the importance of good cuspid teeth in supporting restorative care. Many occlusal schemes are recommended and strived for by altering the teeth by equilibration or restoration.[27] Their success must be attributed to the distribution of forces in all mandibular positions.

The demand for esthetics is very prominent in operative dentistry. Most patients are concerned about the appearance of their teeth after they are restored. Recently there has been much emphasis on esthetics, and some authors feel that this factor is a primary consideration in the selection of restorative materials. The demand for esthetics might dictate the type of preparation to be used with different types of restorative materials. Appearance is improved by conserving tooth structure, but caries-immune boundaries are required for all types of restorations. A major plight of the profession has been the development of a suitable tooth restorative that has the same color as enamel and dentin.[28]

Tooth-colored materials available at the present time have undesirable properties and limit the clinical life of the restoration.[29]

The area demanding esthetics is anterior to the mesial surfaces of the first molars. Full coverage can be used to improve appearance, although this does not really solve the problem. There are many factors associated with full-coverage restorations that limit their use in dental practice, i.e., the size of the pulp, age of the patient, economic problems, and available time. There are cases in which the full crown is the only way to achieve good esthetics and function, but other methods should be explored first.

Large extended preparations in bicuspids have always been a problem. Gold inlays have been indicated for these cavity preparations because the color is not as objectionable as that of silver amalgam restorations. Discoloration has been a problem with amalgam restorations. Silver and tin ions migrate from the amalgam restoration into dentin and cause the tooth to be darkened. There are methods that protect the tooth against ion migration, and it is necessary to follow these procedures in order to maintain an esthetic tooth.[30]

The incisor teeth have always presented a problem in esthetics. They are the most visible and receive the critical observation of others. Minimizing the outline of the restoration has been used to hide the restorative material.[31] Small cavities create problems of retention because of the limitations placed on access and tooth structure. Mechanical separators can be used to produce more room interproximally. Separation is sometimes employed to restrict the outline form of the cavity preparation and display even less restorative material, thus combating the esthetics problem.

In anterior teeth the lingual approach technique is recommended to completely hide restorative materials.[32] This means that all the instrumentation and insertion of the restoration are accomplished from the lingual surface. In this type of operation most of the labial enamel wall is preserved, which means that the technique is not indicated in restoration of large carious lesions. Contra-angle instruments, both rotary and hand, are used. All work is done indirectly and requires a highly disciplined operator. Success can be achieved in this case by using a careful and exacting approach. The lingual approach has application in both metallic and tooth-colored materials and must be mastered if complete patient service is to be offered.

Generally a neat-appearing outline will enhance the esthetic results of the dental restoration. The neat, well-formed margin looks much better than a jagged, rounded, or scalloped restoration that has been placed in a slipshod manner. The profession still needs a tooth-colored material that bonds to tooth structure, but until this is discovered, refinement of the preparation is necessary. The neat-appearing restoration produces great patient satisfaction and is a mark of operative skill. Patients still place emphasis on a restoration that complements the appearance of the tooth, and achievement of this objective develops rapport and respect in the dental office. Permanent esthetics can only be developed with ceramic restorations. Fused porcelain has vastly improved and has enjoyed a drastic increase in dental practice.[33]

These basic objectives should be fully understood before attempting to master the field of operative dentistry. Principles and techniques used for individual tooth restoration must be selected to fulfill the objectives. Again, the major goal of operative dentistry should be to maintain the tooth in a state of optimum health, function, and esthetics. This being the case, it will be necessary to employ at one time or another all of the accepted procedures, mechanical, biologic, and preventive, that are used in the field of restorative dentistry.

ESSENTIAL FACTORS IN OPERATIVE DENTISTRY

Certain factors are accepted as essential for the successful dental practice. It is not possible to include these factors in every case, but they should be kept in mind. Application of the rules will become second nature as experience is gained. An attempt should be made to understand the essential factors, and the following are the conditions that should exist.

Professional attitude

A profession is characterized by additional study over that which is ordinarily required. For an area of knowledge to be called a profession requires continuous study and learning. The dental profession is worthy of such status and consequently should be regarded on the same level as other professional groups. It is the attitude of those in a profession that determines the success or failure of the group, and certainly one should strive for the highest goals that can possibly be attained by a profession.

Motivation and learning in the profession have been discussed for many years. Because of the great amount of knowledge that must be acquired and the manual skills that must be mastered, there is a great need for motivation in the study of dentistry. The dentist must be willing to put in long hours in the library and in practice. It is also necessary to have a desire to serve others since dentists, as members of a health profession, must put the patient's welfare first. High quality and efficiency are the guideposts in health-oriented professions.

A receptiveness to learning creates a favorable attitude. A professional person should have a thirst for knowledge and should strive to learn new and different things at all times. Being informed about dental subjects is necessary, as well as being conversant in other subject matters. The influence of research on treatment makes it necessary to be open-minded and accept change. The best treatment procedure should always be used when it can be defined. Continuous education is the key to a successful practice of dentistry. Since lifetime learning is considered a necessity in professions, it is necessary for the dentist to follow organized postgraduate activities.

A great deal of practice is required to practice operative dentistry. The nature of the subject makes it necessary, because tooth restoration is highly sequential and precise. Each step in procedure must be done ideally before proceeding to the next. If the expected result is not obtained, the exercise must be repeated until the work is satisfactory. Repeating work or performing refined operations requires patience and a constructive attitude.

Proper dress and cleanliness must be maintained at all times to display an attitude that is characteristic of a profession. It is necessary for the student and practicing dentist to make public appearances, and the impression they make on others is lasting and is a reflection on the profession. Close patient contact makes dentistry a personal service that requires a neat appearance and aseptic instrumentation.

There are many extracurricular activities that should be supported for the welfare of both the individual and the profession. An active part should be taken in dental organizations. Other allied organizations in the community need to be supported, and professional people usually assume many civic responsibilities. The role of the professional man becomes widened when all these responsibilities are considered.

Subject knowledge

During undergraduate training it is necessary to learn all that is presented in the curriculum. Dental education is well planned and time-consuming. All the time available in the classroom and clinic must be utilized, because after graduation it is impossible to learn under the same conditions. The information presented in the dental curriculum produces knowledge and develops judgment in each student. The basic doctrines taught will be used for treating patients or conducting research throughout the candidate's lifetime. In the undergraduate program the student usually has little choice between the biologic and clinical courses and those of special interest to him. To develop complete and fundamental knowledge, all areas presented in the curriculum must be studied. Dentistry is based on science and even to provide mechanical therapy the biologic processes must be understood. The mechanical principles are commonly accepted and promote research findings and new types of treatment that improve the profession.

A planned program of continued education should be organized for each graduate. This could involve collecting a personal library and attending postgraduate courses. Regular weekly time should be allotted for these purposes in order to remain informed of current development in the profession. The dentist who does not participate in planned programs of continued education soon becomes outdated and is dissatisfied with the way he is practicing.

Study clubs are useful and sometimes the only answer in continuing education. Successful clubs meet on a regular basis and can be either clinical groups or groups that involve discussion and scientific presentations. At any rate it is possible to discuss problems with associates in the field and evaluate the results of other dentists. A valuable appraisal of skill can occur when one subjects himself to the criticism of associates. The clinical study club is more helpful in this regard in that clinical procedures are observed by dentists and evaluated for the way in which they are handled.

The study of operative dentistry develops a structured learning that is utilized throughout the dental curriculum. This type of learning involves the recognition of a group of principles that work together. Operative dentistry first teaches working positions, posture, attitudes, and habits and then how they are related to clinical procedures. Being structured, the learning process can be transferred to other fields such as periodontics and crown and bridge prosthodontics, thus providing a foundation that can be used in learning other subjects. Therefore operative dentistry is helpful in the total teaching program because it acquaints students with other areas of the curriculum by the transfer of basic skills and principles.

Vision

To perform dental operations, access to the surgical field must be provided. It is a burden to work in the oral cavity when the patient's lips, cheek, or tongue are in the path of the work and the operator's vision. Retraction of these tissues must be provided and the teeth made available to the light source. The light can be applied directly or reflected, and the tissues can be retracted with different types of instruments. The devices that can be used are the mirror, rubber dam, cotton holders, retractors, and bite blocks. Access must be provided at all times because restorations cannot be placed by tactile senses.

Of equal importance is the type of illumination that is directed on the teeth. The light source should come from the dental unit and illuminate the dental field. A direct path must be provided or the light can be reflected by a mirror onto the surgical field. The light from the dental unit should be of great enough intensity to fully illuminate the tooth being restored and at the same time blend into the lighting used in the operatory. Eye damage can result from too much contrast in the illuminations.

The visual acuity of the operator is another important consideration. Vision must either be naturally good or be corrected by glasses. For safety reasons, glasses should be worn at all times in the operatory. They are necessary to deflect fragments of tooth and debris that are removed in cavity preparation and other procedures. A factor related to acuity is depth perception, and the two factors must be coordinated to furnish the proper image.

Surgical environment

The condition of the operating field contributes to the results of the procedure. Cavity preparation is considered a surgical procedure and an aseptic environment should be established when working on the teeth. An ideal dental field is one that maintains the teeth in a dry condition and that is free from bacteria and debris. It is necessary to completely isolate the teeth from saliva to produce such a condition.

The best method of producing an aseptic dental field is with the rubber dam. Regular latex rubber sheets are used for this purpose. Holes are punched in the rubber sheet and placed around the teeth. The rubber dam, once it is tucked, holds back saliva and produces a relatively aseptic surgical environment for operative procedures. When the dark-colored rubber dam is used, vision is also improved because of the color contrast with the teeth. An ideal surgical environment is necessary to obtain good results in operative dentistry.

Instrumentation

The proper type of rotary and hand instruments must be employed for operative procedures. Instruments are designed for specific purposes, hence the reason for their different shapes and sizes. Access and efficiency are provided by design and aid in producing the cavity preparation; thus the location and type of lesion dictate the use of one instrument over another. An orderly, sequential procedure is advocated for most instrumentations. Tooth structure is very hard and brittle, making it necessary to maintain sharp cutting edges. Dental instruments are carefully manufactured and alloyed for the purpose of cutting tooth tissues, but periodic sharpening in the operatory is still a necessity for the hand instruments.

The rotary cutting devices can be classified as milling or grinding tools. Diamond and carborundum abrasives are used for grinding, primarily to finish the walls of tooth structure for different types of preparations. The burs are more commonly used for the excision of tooth structure, and they work by a milling process. Burs are characteristically used for the extension, excavation, and refining of the cavity preparation. Gross reductions are usually accomplished with a bur; however, some finishing and refining can be accomplished with the fissure type of burs.

There are numerous hand instruments that are used for the final refinement of the cavity preparation. Hand instruments are needed for the exacting dimensions required. The use of hand instruments must be mastered as well as the understanding of where they should be used. For the sake of efficiency and order hand instruments should ideally be used only once during the cavity preparation. After each instrument is utilized completely, it is discarded and another one is selected for the next task. The instruments are best used with light, delicate strokes to allow the cutting edge to work effectively.

Posture and stability

The time involved in appointments makes posture important to both the dentist and the patient. The patient's posture is easier to adjust since he is confined to the dental chair during the appointment. The chair should be adjusted to eliminate strained positions and placed at a level that makes the work convenient. The angulation of the chair and light should be adjusted to provide good illumination. Contoured chairs are being used more commonly and are more comfortable for the patient. Since the trend in the profession is to work in longer appointments, the contoured chair is useful.

The posture of the dentist is very important to his health and livelihood. Many hours are spent in an operating position. An unstrained position should be assumed in order to prevent skeletal changes over a period of years. It is possible to work in a standing or sitting position and not cause curvature of the spine. The surgical field should be 12 to 14 inches from the dentist's eyes to allow for adequate vision in the working area. For balance the weight should be distributed evenly on the feet. The forearms should be parallel to the floor and the elbows held close to the sides. This position will not be tiresome and will give stability to the operator. The working conditions in the office should not cause the dentist to be fatigued at the end of the day.

Proper posture will enhance stability in the dental operation. Stability is also increased by the proper grasp of the instruments. The instruments must be held firmly and applied with definite and delicate strokes. This is especially true of the hand instruments, in which an accurate thrust is needed for cutting. Proper application of the hand instruments establishes confidence in the patient.

Operator ability

Successful restoration of the teeth is partly related to the psychomotor ability of the dentist. This facility is sometimes claimed to be inherent, but most psychologists feel that motor skills can be developed. Part of the intrigue and some of the disappointments of restorative dentistry result from the highly refined skills it requires. Dental education is characterized by the challenge to develop these skills, hence the reason for the many laboratory and clinical assignments. The conscientious operator should always strive to improve his ability. Many factors promote motor skills. Repetition of a given task is beneficial because the more a certain type of work is performed, the better the result. Following definite directions and maintaining an orderly procedure also improve ability. Practice sessions and a desire to become better trained are helpful in improving operative ability.

Ability can be evaluated by comparing the work of one dentist with that of another and by obtaining criticisms from colleagues. Study clubs are useful for this purpose and they serve to continue the development of individual abilities. The pressure and constructive criticism involved in subjecting oneself to study club work are valuable parts of postgraduate evaluation. Ideally each operator should feel that his dentistry has improved from year to year, and this improvement might be in part a measure of the improvement and refinement of his individual motor abilities.

Patient control

The attitude of the patient is a very important factor in achieving a successful treatment. The patient should understand the importance of dental health and its relationship to the systemic functions of the body. Patient attitude will be improved by an understanding of the functional and esthetic value of natural teeth. The well-kept dentition does not involve the expense that one requiring an extensive amount of restorative care does. An additional means of improving patient attitude is to explain that a natural dentition makes other problems in life less complicated. Common geriatric problems involving digestive and nutritional disorders would be minimized by having the natural teeth or suitable replacements.

Cooperation during treatment is achieved by explaining to the patient in simple terms precisely what is being done to the teeth. The patient should understand the treatment and why it is being performed. The value of restorative care should be emphasized repeatedly. The expenses should also be presented at each appointment so that no misunderstanding occurs. As soon as the patient realizes that an actual health service is being provided, understanding is developed and a proper attitude established. Then the dentist need be concerned only with the work load involved in the case and with appointment book mechanics.

After the proper patient attitude is established and the dentist begins working in a dedicated manner, the patient soon becomes motivated. At this time he is receptive to suggestions that are related to dental care. Patients will not only appreciate having their teeth restored but they will desire to maintain their dentition in a healthy condition. It is only the motivated patient who will exercise adequate home care and maintain a sound diet. This type of patient is also faithful in keeping the recall appointment. All patients should be motivated to develop the attitude necessary for a sound program of restorative care.

• • •

Restorative dentistry has had a colorful development. Many principles advocated in the past are still applicable today. The heritage that exists is the result of the influence that operative dentistry has had in the development of the profession and of the work of many dedicated and talented men. As the profession ages, the field should grow in stature because of the continued improvement in patient care and the demands and needs imposed by patients.

REFERENCES

1. Black, G. V.: Operative dentistry, ed. 3, Chicago, 1917, Medico-Dental Publishing Co., vol. 2.
2. Ward, M. L.: The American textbook of operative dentistry, ed. 7, Philadelphia, 1940, Lea & Febiger.
3. Johnson, C. N.: A textbook of operative dentistry, ed. 4, Philadelphia, 1923, P. Blakiston's Son & Co.
4. McCluggage, R. W.: A history of the American Dental Association, Chicago, 1959, American Dental Association.
5. Barnum, S. C.: Inventor of the rubber dam, Dent. Cosmos **12:**260, 1870.

6. Black, C. E., and Black, B. M.: From pioneer to scientist, St. Paul, Minn., 1940, The Bruce Publishing Co.
7. Woodbury, C. E.: The making and filling of cavities in the proximal surface of the front teeth with gold foil, Iowa Dent. Bull. **15**:3, 1929.
8. Ferrier, W. I.: Gold foil operations, Seattle, 1959, University of Washington Press.
9. Hollenback, G. M.: An evaluation of the physical properties of cohesive gold, J. So. Calif. Dent. Assoc. **29**:280, 1961.
10. Hollenback, G. M., and Skinner, E. W.: Shrinkage during casting of gold and gold alloys, J.A.D.A. **33**:1391, 1946.
11. Selected dental findings in adults by age, race and sex, United States 1960-1962, Publication No. 1000, Washington, D. C., 1962, U. S. Department of Health, Education, and Welfare.
12. Hollinshead, B. S., director: The survey of dentistry; final report, Washington, D. C., 1961, American Council on Education.
13. Dimensions of unmet dental needs in the U. S., Dent. Abstract **16**:385, 1971.
14. Brekhus, P. J., and Armstrong, W. D.: Civilization—a disease, J.A.D.A. **23**:1459, 1936.
15. Moore, D. L., and Stewart, J. L.: Prevalence of defective dental restorations, J. Prosth. Dent. **17**:376, 1967.
16. Bernier, J. L., and Muhler, J. C., editors: Improving practice through preventive measures, ed. 2, St. Louis, 1970, The C. V. Mosby Co.
17. Bixler, D., and Muhler, J. C.: Combined use of three agents containing stannous fluoride: a prophylactic paste, a solution and a dentifrice, J.A.D.A. **68**:792, 1964.
18. Report of the inter-agency committee on dental auxiliaries, J. Dent. Educ. **36**:41, 1972.
19. Stanley, H. R., Swerdlow, H., Stanwich, L., and Suarez, C. L.: A comparison of the biologic effects of filling materials with recommendations for pulp protection, J. Am. Acad. Gold Foil Operators **12**:56, 1969.
20. Waerhaug, J.: Histologic considerations which govern where the margins of restorations should be located in relation to the gingiva, Dent. Clin. N. Am., Mar., 1960, pp. 161-176.
21. Sortes, S. L., Van Huysen, G. V., and Gilmore, H. W.: A histologic study of gingival tissue response to amalgam, silicate and resin restorations, J. Periodont. **40**:543-546, 1969.
22. Hollenback, G. M.: Most important dimension, J. So. Calif. Dent. Assoc. **29**:46, 1961.
23. Stuart, C. E., and Stallard, H.: A syllabus on oral rehabilitation and occlusion. II. Post graduate education, San Francisco, 1965, School of Dentistry, University of California.
24. Stuart, C. E.: Good occlusion for natural teeth, J. Prosth. Dent. **14**:716, 1964.
25. D'Amico, A.: The ideal functional relation of the natural teeth of man, J. So. Calif. Dent. Assoc. **26**:194, 1958.
26. Stallard, H., and Stuart, C. E.: Concepts of occlusion. What kind of occlusion should recusped teeth be given? Dent. Clin. N. Am., Nov., 1963, pp. 591-606.
27. Huffman, R. W., Regenos, J. W., and Taylor, R. R.: Principles of occlusion. Columbus, Ohio, 1969, H and R Press.
28. Phillips, R. W., and Ryge, G., editors: Adhesive restorative dental materials, proceedings of a workshop, Indianapolis, 1961, Indiana University School of Dentistry.
29. Gilmore, H. W.: Restorative materials and cavity preparation design, Dent. Clin. N. Am. **15**:99-114, 1971.
30. Massler, M., and Nansukhani, N.: Testing liners under cements in vitro, J. Prosth. Dent. **10**:964, 1960.
31. Ellsperman, G. A.: Refinement of the gold foil restoration, J.A.D.A. **27**:342, 1940.
32. Jeffery, A.: Invisible Class III gold foil restorations, J.A.D.A. **54**:1, 1957.
33. Johnston, J. F., Mumford, G., and Dykema, R. W.: Modern practice in dental ceramics, Philadelphia, 1967, W. B. Saunders Co.

chapter 2

Caries classification, control, and diagnosis and treatment planning

As mentioned previously, restorative dentistry is divided into preventive and mechanical methods of treatment.[1] Restoration of the individual tooth by mechanical means is concerned with repairing the carious lesion. This type of treatment constitutes a major portion of the practice. Caries is defined as "a disease of the calcified tissues of the teeth, characterized by a demineralization of the inorganic portion and a destruction of the organic substance of the tooth." Dental caries is the most prevalent chronic disease affecting the modern human race.[2] A number of factors are involved in the decay process and this can best be explained by the following formula[3]:

Refined carbohydrate + Bacteria = Acid plaque
Acid plaque + Susceptible tooth surface = Dental caries

Dental caries is widespread, affecting 98% of the population at one time or another, and it is characterized by many contributing factors.[4] Decay is observed in all age groups, both sexes, and all economic classes. A person is susceptible as soon as the tooth erupts in the oral cavity. The problem of caries is further complicated by factors such as the diet and personal habits of the patient.

The work load of the restorative dentist was revealed in a survey of Maryland schoolchildren between the ages of 6 and 15 years.[5] It was found that 50% of the boys and 56% of the girls had caries in their permanent teeth by the time they were 8 years old. By the time the children reached the age of 14 the caries rate had increased to 95% in boys and 96% in girls. The decayed, missing, or filled tooth rate (DMF) for the combined group was 5.23. These data were collected in an area where fluoridated water was not used.

Caries incidence appears to be increasing in some areas where people consume a more refined diet with greater amounts of sugar. The American Dental

Association revealed that an average of 3.17 dental restorations were required for each individual in 1953.[6] The estimated unfilled cavities in the United States is one-half billion, a number that would make an impossible work load for operative dentists if suddenly everyone demanded treatment. However, statistics reveal that only 45% of the population seeks regular dental care.[7] The statistics also show that 40% of the dentist's income is derived from placing dental restorations.

The beneficial results of preventive therapy in dental practice will further alter the work load. Communal fluoridation, regular dental care, and increased motivation of the patient to save his teeth have caused a change in the size, location, and incidence of carious lesions.[8] Formerly the proximal lesion was prevalent, but now developmental groove defects are most frequent. Moreover, the size of the carious lesion is now being limited by fluoride compounds, permitting use of an ideal preparation for preserving tooth structure, and the incidence of decay is also decreasing. In the past, surveys conducted among schoolchildren found the greatest evidence of decay in the permanent first molars, which resulted in many of these teeth being lost. Now, however, the patient who has matured in a fluoridated area can expect to have sound teeth and conservative outlines in the restorations needed (Fig. 2-1).

The changes occurring in dental practice can be seen in the more idealistic operative service being offered. Now plans for financing dental care make service available to more people. The reduction in the number of carious lesions will not cause the dentist to be idle because more people are beginning to seek

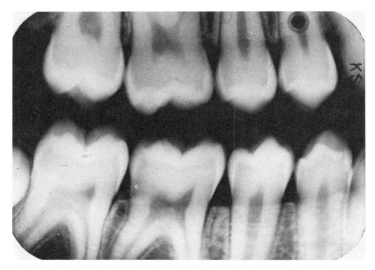

Fig. 2-1. A typical dentition in which caries is lacking, showing a 17-year-old patient who has lived in a city with a fluoridated water supply and has received other preventive dental care.

regular care plans. The modern treatment of caries is more feasible for all. In some cases preventive methods can be delegated to the hygienist or control therapist.[9]

The communal preventive programs have made it possible for more patients to have sound dentitions and ostensibly healthy mouths.[10] The treatment in such cases involves maintenance and examination. In time some corrective treatment might be necessary to eliminate or allay a pathologic condition that may be prevalent in specific age groups. Treatment methods destined to occupy a large area of the dental practice of the future include control of physiologic changes in the periodontium, tooth movement, and occlusal reshaping.

ETIOLOGY

It is not the purpose of this book to cite the voluminous literature dealing with dental caries but to explain the salient factors that support the indicated type of treatment. Theories concerning the etiology of dental caries have been divided into three groups—acidogenic, proteolytic, and proteolysis-chelation. They differ mainly in predicting the type of bacteria that cause dissolution of the tooth or the type of mechanism by which mineral salts are removed. Caries development is studied to support the concepts of cavity preparation.

The acidogenic theory of Miller and Black appears to have been the most widely accepted of the three, and it was used as the basis for caries research.[11,12] This theory suggests that certain bacteria produce acid in or near the surface of the tooth that decalcifies the inorganic portion. The caries process, however, is proposed to start with the breakdown of the organic cementing substance, penetration of the enamel, the destruction of the dentin by numerous organisms. Miller conducted research with different types of bacteria and food materials in incubated saliva and teeth and was first to develop the acidogenic theory. He concluded that caries was a chemoparasitic process, with the first stage being decalcification of the enamel and dentin, followed by the dissolution of the softened residue. He believed damage to result primarily from the action of lactic acid formed by the breakdown of carbohydrates and starches. He also stated that probably more than one microorganism was involved in developing the lesion.

A workshop was conducted at the University of Michigan to study the mechanism and control of caries.[3] Following is a list of the indirect factors, as formulated by the group, that could influence the etiology of caries:

    A. Tooth
        1. Composition
        2. Morphologic characteristics
        3. Position
    B. Saliva
        1. Composition
            a. Inorganic
            b. Organic

    2. pH
    3. Quantity
    4. Viscosity
    5. Antibacterial factors
C. Diet
    1. Physical factor
      a. Quality of the diet
    2. Local factors
      a. Carbohydrate content
      b. Vitamin content
      c. Fluorine content

The tooth. The variations in morphology and position are listed because they influence the degree of caries as well as the chemical composition of the tooth. Teeth have areas of caries susceptibility where lesions usually occur, and these are divided into pit and fissure areas and smooth surface areas. The boundaries between these areas on the tooth surfaces make up the cavity wall and are used to judge its location.

The pit and fissure areas are caused by the development of pits and grooves that result from poor coalescence between the enamel lobes.[1] The undesirable grooves are usually fissured and have a small amount of enamel or none at all at the bottom of the opening. These areas are undercut and cause food entrapment that accelerates the development of caries. Adequate brushing and rinsing will not remove the impacted food, and this condition is responsible for practically the same incidence of caries on the occlusal surfaces of posterior teeth as in the lingual pits of the maxillary incisors. In a fluoridated area the defective grooves are more darkly stained and they are sometimes mistaken for caries. The groove defect will always be a nidus for caries regardless of how effectively the surface is protected. Fissure sealants are being employed to seal these areas to prevent or arrest lesion development.

The smooth surface lesions of the proximal and facial areas are attributed to neglect. In poorly cleaned adjacent teeth the lesion develops just below the contact area. The gingival lesions begin next to the epithelial tissue and are the result of inadequate toothbrushing. The tooth is decalcified by the apposition of food material and the subsequent formation of acid. Areas that are difficult to clean rapidly accumulate plaque even when sound hygienic measures are followed, and this also contributes to the development of smooth surface caries. The occurrence of this type of lesion is dramatically reduced in the general practice by using a topically applied fluoride solution.

The position of the tooth in the arch is a factor in the development of caries. Crowded areas caused by inadequate growth or bone support cause rotation and supereruption associated with poor proximal relationships of the teeth. This condition is conducive to food impaction and results in lesions similar to those caused by neglect. This type of caries is reduced by the use of dental floss and other methods that can reach the impacted material and dislodge it. Orthodontic treatment and the use of periodontic water devices are helpful in reducing caries in malposed teeth.

Studies have been conducted on "individual tooth" susceptibility.[1] Lesions seem to occur most frequently on surfaces that are exposed for the longest period of time to the oral fluids, and they can be complicated by eruptive patterns. For example, the first molar is the most susceptible tooth in the mouth, its occlusal surfaces being most liable to caries, followed by the mesial and then distal surfaces. Exposure time is the common variable in these occurrences. Surveys show that maxillary teeth are more susceptible to caries than mandibular teeth, a fact attributed to the force of gravity acting to coat the lower teeth with salvia.

Hypoplasic areas on the teeth were originally thought to be incipient carious lesions. The same local finding associated with other defects is related to these areas—the integrity of the enamel surface. Hypoplasia from inadequate formation is usually smooth and should not be restored except for esthetic purposes. Larger hypoplastic defects and hypoplasia occurring on surfaces that receive excessive toothbrushing should be repaired if the enamel is missing and the dentin exposed. The intact defect is thought to become more concentrated when fluoride solutions are used; therefore it should be treated conservatively.

The occurrence of certain types of lesions are common in different age groups, again indicating that eruption and gingival protection are important factors. Occlusal caries occurs between the ages of 7 and 12, while proximal caries in molars occurs in the early teen years. Anterior proximal lesions and gingival cavities are discovered more often in early adulthood.

Some studies concerning the trends in caries development are interesting but should not be relied upon solely in making an examination. These studies attempt to explain the difference in location either by pointing out that caries is not unilateral or that it follows the same pattern in families with similar living conditions. The detection of caries is accomplished by a thorough, systematic examination of all the clinical crowns of the teeth.

Saliva. The nature and amount of saliva influence the development of caries. Approximately 1 ml. of saliva is produced each minute in order to keep structures in the oral cavity lubricated.[13] An insufficient or inadequate flow of saliva can cause caries by not washing the teeth during mastication, with the result that food is impacted and materia alba formed. Cases of rampant caries develop when there is an inadequate amount of saliva.

The viscosity of the saliva also affects the type of cleaning the teeth receive during mastication. The salivary mucous glands are responsible for viscous or "ropy" saliva by the secretion of mucopolysaccharides. Again the result is food impaction, and patients with this problem develop characteristic lesions that develop beyond the line angles of the posterior teeth. This condition is difficult to treat because the full-coverage restoration needed to correct it involves a risk, and stress is still apt to occur in the patient with ropy saliva. Acute cases result in "patchwork" treatment because no known preventive measure can arrest the extensive decalcification. Methods are needed to alter the character of saliva.

The pH, carbon dioxide–combing power, and buffer capacity of saliva are properties of saliva that can retard decalcification of the tooth.[14] The pH of saliva does not vary extensively, but it is above the value necessary to decalcify the enamel. The pH does not differ greatly in caries-immune and caries-active patients and it normally ranges from 5.2 to 5.5. The buffer capacity of saliva acts to neutralize acids that are formed in the plaque or ingested in the diet. The effect of the buffer capacity on the plaque is much less than on food because plaque is not easily penetrated. To study the difference in salivary capacity the titratable alkalinity is measured; it is conceivable that this property accounts for differences in caries incidence when the pH and flow rate are the same. The studies conducted show conflicting data on buffer capacity in groups having high and low caries experience, which further confuses the student on the real value of this property. It is reasonable to state that the property that neutralizes acid would act in favor of the saliva for preventing caries.

Many other types of properties, functions, and components of saliva are listed by Afonsky.[15] His book should be consulted for a thorough understanding of saliva because it is a compilation of pertinent data. At this time no specific constituent promoting or preventing dental caries has been isolated from saliva.

Diet. This aspect of caries etiology has been studied but not to the same extent as saliva and fluoride. Since diets are difficult to regulate and in some cases cannot be changed, other factors to strengthen the tooth have been explored. It is evident, however, that the composition of food and its physical characteristics are influential in the development and progress of caries.[16] The main problem is the intake of refined carbohydrates, which are reduced in the mouth to lactic, butyric, and pyruvic acids that are held in contact with the enamel surface by the plaque, causing tooth decalcification.

The intake of carbohydrates is correlative with the concentration of acid-producing bacteria and dental caries. The role of the *Lactobacillus acidophilus* has been studied in this regard, and this microorganism has been found to be prevalent in the caries-susceptible patient.[17] When the intake of carbohydrates, especially mono- and polysaccharides, is restricted, a reduction in the concentration of these microorganisms is observed. As a result the *L. acidophilus* has been used as an indicator of caries susceptibility for analysis of the effectiveness of preventive measures. *Streptococcus* is said to also produce plaque and acid on tooth structure.

The acidity of saliva and plaque has been studied by using glucose rinses and the consumption of other carbohydrates. The extent of the damage is related to the pH in the plaque, which is lower than that of saliva, and to the contact time of the acid with the tooth.[16] These two factors have developed values for the cariogenicity of foodstuffs and have resulted in the organization of diets that are minimal in caries potential. The reason for a lower pH concentration in dental plaque is found in the high concentration of acid-producing streptococci. They are present in higher concentrations than other microorganisms and produce the acid only minutes after receiving the substrate.

The physical characteristic of food is considered to be a factor in preventing dental caries. Fibrous and tough foods that are available should be eaten at the end of a meal to naturally scrub the teeth and gingival tissue during mastication. An example of such foods is celery; much of the debris that collects in the teeth after eating is removed when this is chewed. Modern dietary trends depart from this principle by using soft foods that are sweetened, and this further encourages food impaction. The amount of sugar consumed in the United States has been seen to reflect the incidence of caries in the nation.[18]

The influence of diet on caries has been studied from the tooth surface and systemic aspects in both developing and formed teeth. Preventive factors urgently demanded of the dentist concern erupted teeth and advice about the proper selection of foods. When speaking with parents, the dentist should emphasize nutritional factors and vitamin and mineral supplements so as to encourage good tooth development. Caries control diets are available.

Plaque. Studies have been conducted to determine the composition of dental plaque. It is described as a nitrogenous network of mucin, desquamated cells, and microorganisms.[19] The plaque is resistant to oral fluids, difficult to remove, and quickly formed on areas of the tooth that are difficult to reach in cleaning. The apposition of the plaque with the enamel is the site of actual damage to the tooth because the plaque holds the acids in contact with the enamel. The pH of the plaque solution is usually different from that of saliva because the surface of plaque is not easily penetrated. The plaque deposit acts as a semipermeable membrane on the tooth and is identified as the medium responsible for the initiation of caries.

The relationship between plaque removal, toothbrushing, and caries experience has been studied. The argument that a clean tooth is less susceptible to decay has never been resolved.[20] Although good brushing and other hygienic measures reduce the amount of caries, the process cannot be eliminated. One problem is that plaque is reformed quickly after removal from the susceptible area of the tooth. Toothbrushing serves as a method of control but it cannot remove all the conditions conducive to plaque formation. The deposits are removed by the abrasive action of toothbrushing, if it is done properly. It has been stated that toothbrushing helps to maintain esthetics and to stimulate the periodontal tissues but that it will not eradicate caries.

A complicating factor associated with plaque is the formation of acid immediately following the ingestion of food. Delaying the toothbrushing by a matter of minutes is too late to stop the actual damage. It is helpful, although not in the interest of etiquette, to rinse the mouth with water following the meal. The process of acid formation will be retarded by dilution and rinsing away food particles. "Swish and swallow" is a sound method of removing debris following the meal.

To reiterate, there are many contributing factors in the development of dental caries. The dentist should understand the contributing factors, be ac-

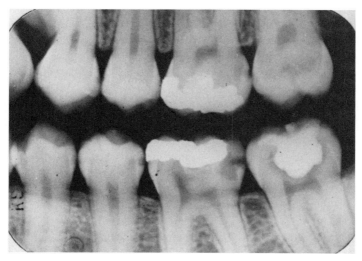

Fig. 2-2. Example of acute caries with lesions deeply penetrating the dentin in the distal surface of the first molar, lower second bicuspid, and buccal surface of the second molars. (Courtesy Dr. Jack D. Carr.)

quainted with research on the subject, and be able to employ control measures in his practice. Both mechanical and preventive methods are still advocated in the treatment and control of caries.

TERMINOLOGY AND CLASSIFICATION

The type of caries is determined by the severity or the location of the lesion.[21]

Acute caries (rampant). Acute caries is a rapid process involving a large number of teeth (Fig. 2-2). The acute lesions are lighter colored than other lesions, being light brown or gray, and their caseous consistency makes the excavation difficult. Pulp exposures are often observed in patients with acute caries.

Chronic caries. These lesions are usually of long-standing involvement, affect a fewer number of teeth, and are smaller in size than acute caries (Fig. 2-3). The decalcified dentin is dark brown in color and leathery in consistency. Pulp prognosis is hopeful in that the deepest of lesions usually requires only prophylactic capping and protective bases. The lesions range in depth, including those that have just penetrated the enamel.

Primary caries (initial). A primary caries is one in which the lesion constitutes an initial attack on the tooth surface. It is designated as primary because of the initial location of the lesion on the surface rather than the extent of damage.

Secondary caries (recurrent). This type of caries is observed around the edges of restorations (Fig. 2-4). The common causes of secondary involvement are the

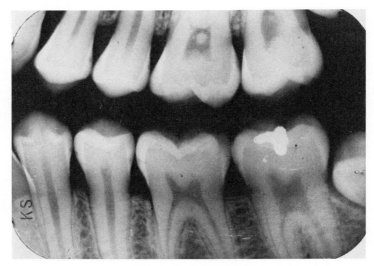

Fig. 2-3. Chronic caries, as observed by the enamel etchings on the interproximal surfaces of the molars and bicuspids. (Courtesy Dr. Jack D. Carr.)

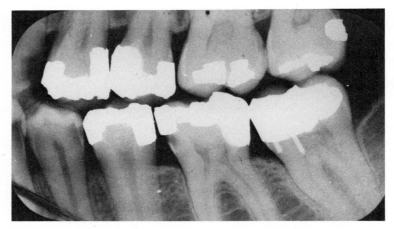

Fig. 2-4. Recurrent caries on the mesial surface of the mandibular first molar beneath the amalgam restoration. An acute carious lesion is on the distal surface of the mandibular first bicuspid.

rough or overhanging margin and fracture on surfaces in the posterior teeth that are naturally prone to caries because of difficulty in cleaning.

The carious lesions are designated as surfacelike occlusal caries on the molar, proximal caries on the bicuspid, or cementum caries. In the charting system the location of the tooth is given by number, and when examining and recording in the office, this system is the most practical.

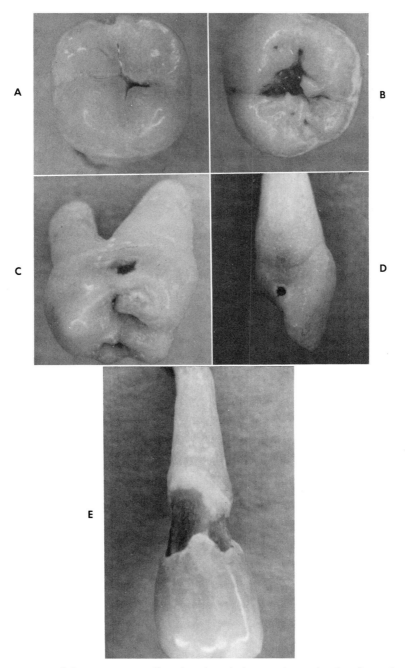

Fig. 2-5. A, Pit and fissure incipient Class I carious lesion on the occlusal surface of a molar. **B,** Extensive carious lesion on the occlusal surface of the molar. **C,** Typical Class II carious lesion on the mesial surface of the maxillary molar. **D,** Class III smooth surface carious lesion on the incisor. **E,** Caries on the incisor tooth of an elderly patient. This condition is often untreatable.

The classification of caries outlined by Black[1] is useful in describing techniques in the literature or in discussing cases with students. The lesions are named for the cavity classification used to restore the tooth (Fig. 2-5).

Class   I   Occlusal surface caries in the molars and bicuspids
Class   II   Proximal surface caries in the molars and bicuspids
Class III   Proximal surface caries in the anterior teeth
Class   IV   Proximal surface caries in the anterior teeth that involve the loss of
              the angle
Class   V   Carious lesions that occur on the gingival aspect of the labial, buccal,
              and lingual surfaces of all the teeth
Class   VI   Occasionally used to describe caries located above the height of con-
              tour on anterior teeth

CARIES DETECTION

There are a number of ways to detect a carious lesion during the oral examination.[22] The examination method should be thorough and organized, beginning and ending in one place. The necessary examination materials include the mouth mirror, small, sharp explorer, radiographs, dental floss, and occasionally a separator. An assistant does the charting while the examination is performed at the dental unit, where adequate lighting is available. The exploration should include all surfaces; some lesions will be overlooked if only the explorer or radiographs are used.

To begin, a cursory examination should be made of the radiographs. If this is this first evaluation of the patient, a complete set of periapical and bitewing films are made. For the recall prophylactic appointment only bitewing radiographs are used but the same general plan of organization is employed. The films provide a quick appraisal of the number and location of the teeth and the contact size and contour on the proximal surfaces. The embrasure size and alveolar bone crests will be noticed around all the teeth when making a rapid early appraisal of proximal caries. The lesions should be noted and marked at this time and the films should be dried and mounted.

The examination begins with the maxillary right third molar and progresses through every tooth. The teeth are thoroughly dried in the quadrant before beginning the section or the assistant follows the operator with the air syringe until the examination is completed. Cotton rolls and the saliva ejector are useful at this time because, if saliva covers the enamel surfaces, the evaluation cannot be done. The color contrast of the teeth with the gingival tissue is not as apparent as when using the rubber dam, but part of the frustration can be removed by using loupes during the examination.

The occlusal surface is the first part of the tooth to be explored. A small, sharp explorer is placed in the main pits and fossae of the tooth or in areas of discoloration if they are present. The point is then placed in the grooves that radiate from the fossae to see if any of the areas are soft and cannot support the weight of the explorer. The tooth should be restored if the susceptible site can be punctured and if soft tooth tissue that is usually accompanied by chalky enamel and stain surrounding the area is found.

The defective pits or hypoplastic areas of the tooth should be examined in the same way as the main pits and fossae to determine whether the enamel is broken. The tine of the explorer can be turned on its side to see if the surface of the hypoplasia is smooth. The sharp point of the explorer is used to examine the buccal and lingual grooves of the tooth to see if there are involvements or communications with the occlusal surface. The same rule governing the need for a restoration also applies to these areas.

Examination of the proximal surface of the tooth is more difficult because the lesions are hidden. The radiographs are magnified and observed on the view box to see if there are proximal involvements. Because of the angulation of the x-ray beam and the overlapping of teeth, it might be necessary to use other methods of examining the proximal surface. The explorer can be used in the gingival embrasure to locate most large lesions; however, the incipient involvement just below the contact area cannot be reached.

The use of waxed dental floss is helpful in determining the smoothness of the surface in question. A 12-inch length is wrapped around the index fingers and it is gently slipped through the contact area on the bias. The examination is made by slowly moving the floss from the buccal to the lingual surface until the bottom of the free margin is reached. This enables the gingival embrasure to be polished, and if caries is present the string will catch or be torn on removal. Caries should not be confused with calculus deposits for it is assumed that a thorough prophylaxis will be given before each examination.

If the condition of the proximal surface cannot be determined by the methods just described, the separator should be utilized. The teeth are parted to allow direct vision of the area in question, or the increased space can be used for a better examination with the dental floss or explorer. This method is time-consuming and is used only as a last resort.

The dentition is examined in the manner described by inspecting each surface. The teeth are systematically examined to detect all pathologic conditions that need to be restored or recorded, and the caries or defects that need restoration are recorded on the chart. This information is used later to formulate the treatment plan.

CONTROL AND TREATMENT

Caries can be treated in a number of ways. The overall plan in chronic or acute treatment is determined by the number and depth of the lesions. The information gathered from the examination is used in developing the treatment plan. Existing caries must be removed, defective restorations explored, and new cavity preparations and restorations eventually placed in the involved teeth in order to preserve the dentition. Enamel cannot regenerate; therefore the damage can be repaired only when this structure is restored.

Caries is treated as an infectious disease because it involves microorganisms. If it is not controlled, restorations will have only limited value because the teeth and restorations will develop additional lesions that may result in loss of the teeth. Therefore, curative treatment is started simultaneously with control measures. Patient cooperation will make it possible for the dentist to develop an oral environment that is conducive to dental cure. Control measures are explained in Chapter 18.

Following are some methods of control.[23]

Caries activity tests. These tests are used to obtain diagnostic data and to check on the effectiveness of the patient's home care therapy.

Dental health education. Methods are used to educate the patient on the value of teeth, the responsibility of maintaining dental health, and good oral hygiene measures.

Prophylactic procedures. Calcium deposits and stains are removed in cleaning the teeth. Hygienic measures for keeping the teeth clean and the tissues healthy should be demonstrated.

Systemic factors. If teeth are developing, the use of fluoride supplements is advisable in areas in which the communal water supply is not fluoridated. Information concerning selection of foods should also be given to point out the minerals and vitamins that are helpful in supporting tooth development.

Reinforcement of tooth surface. Topical fluorides should be applied for added protection of the teeth against acid solutions.

Diet methods. Analysis of the diet to determine the amount of fermentable carbohydrate consumed is helpful in acute cases. This service should include suggestions for restricting the intake of sugars and the recommendation of diets that satisfy nutritional requirements.

Mechanical methods. This step includes the treatment of chronic caries with proper selections of the tooth and filling material. In rampant cases, gross caries removal is performed to control the caries prior to the mechanical procedures.

Saliva problems. Medication for viscous saliva can be used in troublesome cases. An increase in the amount of saliva flow can be produced by dietary factors, mainly by the consumption of more citrus fruits. Medication for changing salivary flow and the use of astringent mouthwashes to aid food removal are usually inconvenient, however, and for this reason are not used for extended periods.

• • •

In studying control procedures it becomes apparent that several methods should be used for each patient. The treatment plan should not be initiated until success of the control methods is evident.

As will be explained in treatment planning, after satisfying the patient's chief complaint, the need for therapy and the treatment plan should be presented to the patient before restoration of the teeth. An understanding between the patient and the dentist is necessary, particularly in regard to the time and cost of the services. Briefly, the mechanical methods of treating clinical cases will be discussed.

Chronic caries. The number of teeth needing restorations is recorded on the chart. For economic reasons or because of patient disinterest it is sometimes necessary to restore the teeth only to stop the caries while hygiene is being improved. The patients are kept on the recall list until they decide to accept comprehensive treatment. The long-range diagnosis for the patient is always made in regard to periodontal improvements and prosthetic devices before some of the teeth are restored.

When a comprehensive treatment plan has been accepted and all the preliminary emergency work is finished, the dentist restores the teeth according to the most urgent needs. This is usually determined by the depth of the caries, by the existence of areas that are uncomfortable for pulpal or periodontal reasons, or by a need for improvement in esthetics. A regular time schedule is planned and followed until the treatment is completed. For protection of the dentist, financial arrangements should be made at the beginning of treatment to prevent a misunderstanding when the program is completed.

Acute caries (rampant). Acute caries is characterized by numerous, deeply involved lesions that result in "hourglass" configurations in the anterior teeth and near pulp exposure or abscess involvement in the molars. This type of caries commonly occurs in the 12- to 15-year age group, and because of the pressing nature of the condition the carious process is halted before placing any restorations.

A technique of gross caries removal (indirect pulp therapy) consists of excavating the superficial caries and sealing them with a sedative cement.[24] A small amount of caries is left in the excavation in order not to disturb the pulp tissue, and zinc oxide—eugenol cement is used to seal the tooth from the oral environment. The restorations become sedative treatments and are left in situ for 4 to 6 weeks to enable protective dentin to be formed. This procedure is also helpful in the mixed dentition. In children the number of pulpotomies and lost teeth are reduced when gross caries removal is employed; there are also benefits from using this treatment in adult patients. Gross caries removal quickly improves the oral environment and controls tooth pain during restorative care.

Only the gross lesions are excavated; usually one half or more of the thickness of the dentin has been damaged, making these areas easy to locate in the examination. If lesions are protected by enamel, they can be fractured with hand instruments or uncovered with burs. All four quadrants are excavated at the same time, and an anesthetic is seldom needed.

At the first appointment a practical program of hygiene is presented and a diet analysis is initiated. Removal of the caries and bacteria and correction of the diet reduces the caries potential. When a 6-week period has passed, the cement restorations are removed and the residual caries is excavated. The dentin wall is prophylactically capped or based and the tooth is restored. When the residual caries is removed, it can be decided whether the pulp is intact or whether endodontic or surgical procedures are necessary.

The lesions are restored with amalgam and tooth colored restorations except in unusual situations. These materials are more dependable in caries-prone patients or in patients who become negligent and lose interest in dental care. After a few years have passed and if the patient is still motivated, as determined by how well he follows the recall system and uses hygienic measures, a more permanent type of restoration can be placed.

DIAGNOSIS AND TREATMENT PLANNING

Patients come into the dental office for a purpose, and the first information obtained by the dentist should be the patient's chief complaint or the reason for making the appointment. Reasons for seeking dental care can be placed into three categories: (1) to have the dentition examined and restored, (2) to keep a maintenance appointment, or (3) to receive emergency treatment. Regardless of the reason, the procedures result in a treatment plan for the patient. The nature of the patient's complaint and the type of treatment needed must be established. Inaccuracies in setting up the correct type of appointment are common because the lay person usually does not know what the actual problem is; therefore, the emergencies should be cared for in short appointments.

Appointment objectives

Objectives of each type of appointment will be discussed.[22]

Diagnosis and restoration of the dentition. The complete oral examination and radiographic survey are used to study the oral cavity and the surrounding structures. Information concerning the patient's past medical history, dental problems, and use of drugs and medicine is collected. Study casts are made for the purpose of surveying or articulating the models to determine the shape of the teeth or the inclination and function of the existing dentition. The complete examination supplies the facts with which a diagnosis is made, which in turn is used to organize the ideal treatment plan for the patient.

Recall appointment. This appointment is used to scale and polish the teeth thoroughly, to make a screening examination of the oral cavity, and to add to the patient's record any changes detected in his medical or dental history. Preventive treatment by means of fluoride application is given at this time, and a postoperative evaluation of the restorative work is made. The new caries or periodontal problems can be observed in bitewing radiographs if they have been taken. The appointment schedule for the maintenance program is set up according to the individual's rate of calculus formation but usually necessitates an appointment at 6-month intervals.

Emergency appointment. This type of appointment is for patients who have pain in the teeth or the periodontium. Sometimes emergency care must be given for a fractured restoration. Patients are informed that the emergency appointment is being worked into the schedule and that radiographs and tests of the area of discomfort will be made. Medication and sedative cements are used for the relief of pain.

First appointment procedures

The treatment plans of all concerned patients should result in comprehensive care. This is an enduring cycle because dental care should continue throughout the lifetime of the patient. All new appointments are organized to fit into an efficient working pattern. In the first appointment the dentist should be certain that the chief complaint has been resolved or the patient will be dissatisfied. Although at the time only emergency care might be desired, the opportunity for examination and diagnosis should be available.

The information collected in the first visit is used for diagnosis of the patient's problems and formulation of a treatment plan. A plan is used in every case to serve as a guide for a logical, sequential, and thorough procedure for rehabilitation to produce optimum dental health. The sequence of treatment should be the most efficient possible in order to conserve the time and expense of both parties and to obviate unnecessary visits for the patient. Management of time, which is an important factor in all practices, must be accomplished in order to regulate the working day. This phase of the patient service is managed by the dental assistant after the schedule has been accepted by the patient.

Patients are reassured when the dentist carefully uses the accepted methods of detecting the emergency problem. The dentist should begin patient education at this time by telling the patient of the benefits of maintaining the natural dentition and the reasons for preserving the teeth. The type of practice and the possible plans for care should be explained in order to acquaint the individual with the possibilities of services. The dentist at this time will unknowingly convince the patient that his efforts are being directed toward the patient's welfare.

Patient interview. The medical history of the patient is one of the most overlooked and potentially hazardous factors in dental practice. The medical interview takes time, and since few patients are ill or poor risks, the dentist may gradually come to neglect this portion of the record. A complete questionnaire that includes information concerning common diseases and medications should be used to survey the patient's medical history. An individual interview is used to cover the possibilities of systemic problems.

Leading questions are asked between inquiries concerning the heart, blood pressure, respiratory diseases, kidney ailments, metabolic diseases, and sensitivities. In some cases a patient will overlook a condition that is under control but that could influence the treatment or type of drugs administered in the routine program. Important to the health of each patient is his history concerning local anesthetics and reactions to the various agents.

Printed questionnaires of varying lengths can be used by the dentist and hygienist. Forms are available that require only encirclement of relevant information and the signature of the patient to validate the information. This type of form is used mainly in the screening examination and it is very useful in becoming acquainted with the patient. The patient's name, telephone number, occupation, and address are obtained for the record. This information is given in the waiting room and read by the dentist prior to the interview. Additional inquiries can be made verbally and recorded at the bottom of the questionnaire.

If medical problems are discovered or if additional information concerning specific areas is needed, a physician should be consulted. If a medical risk is involved, nothing is done in the way of treatment unless clearance is given by the physician. The patient's safety is thus protected, and the dental treatment can be made subservient to the medical problem. Consultation with the physician protects the dentist by specifying the complicating factor. When juveniles are treated written consent should also be obtained from the parents.

Dental history. Following a cursory examination of the oral cavity the patient's dental history should be obtained. The time of the last visit to the dentist and the service rendered should be determined. The attitude of the patient toward dental care should be ascertained with the aim of finding out the knowledge he has of dental health. In some cases the actual purpose of the patient's visit is revealed at this time and the future course of analysis and treatment can be planned.

The quality of previous dental work should be observed and judged according to the effectiveness of function, periodontal protection, and successful esthetics. The feelings of the patient toward esthetics that could be included in treatment should be explored. The design of the restorations and the patient's appreciation of previous dental efforts should be determined before making any recommendations for treatment.

The survey of past dental experience should include inquiries about the patient's previous exposure to pain and his attitude toward long appointments. The patient's reaction to the injection technique and local anesthesia or any other unpleasant experiences should be discovered because the information supplied by these complaints or statements is helpful in evaluating the patient. The record usually contains a description of any unpleasant dental experiences or reveals the patient's appreciation of the services.

Diagnostic models. Casts can be made of the patient's mouth to study the dentition and to educate the patient. The models are not considered to be of diagnostic value until they are mounted on an articulator to duplicate the mandibular movement.[25] The models are made from an alginate impression and are poured in regular Hydrocal (Fig. 2-6). Whether models are needed is determined after the occlusal examination, and if so, they are included in the records for a complete examination.

At the time the models are made the patient will be interested in seeing the arrangement of his teeth. The bases should be neatly formed and all discrepancies removed that could cause confusion and unnecessary questions. The size and arrangement of the teeth and the estimated interdigitation are shown to the patient. Minor details such as the occlusal plane, the curve of Spee, and the arrangement and function of the anterior teeth can be pointed out. A desirable occlusion should be explained while simulating mastication with the models held in the dentist's hands or with demonstration models.

Tooth form and arrangement of the dentition can be observed in the

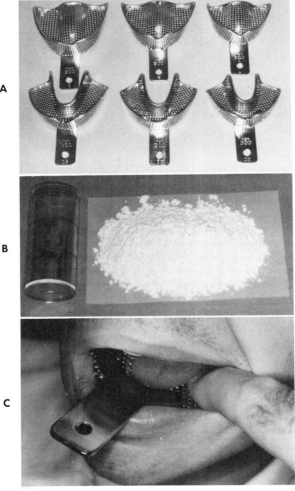

A

B

C

Continued.

Fig. 2-6. A, Stock alginate impression trays used for taking impression for diagnostic casts. **B,** Alginate powder and the water measure used to produce a consistent mix of impression material. **C,** The impression tray is placed in the mouth to see if the proper size has been selected and if there are tissue impingements.

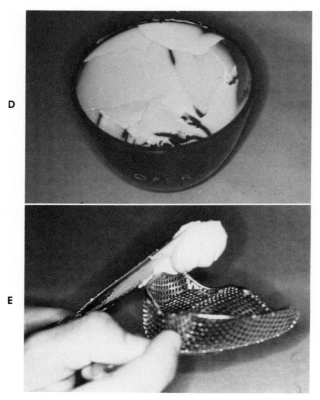

Fig. 2-6, cont'd. D, Alginate impression material. The material was mixed against the side of the bowl to prevent air entrapment. **E,** Loading the perforated impression tray with small increments of impression material. **F,** The seated impression tray following the gelation of the alginate material. **G,** Study casts. Observe the accurate duplication of the occlusal surfaces and the border trimmed to the mucobuccal fold.

edentulous spaces and the degree of tipping and rotation in the abutments. The models will be analyzed when they are mounted on the articulator, and the patient can observe his own masticatory apparatus at this time. The degree of tipping and the areas acceptable for clasping are analyzed on the surveyor.

Radiographs. For a complete examination a full radiographic survey should be made. This will include periapical films of all the teeth and bitewing films of all proximal surfaces between the distal surface of the cuspid and the terminal tooth. The radiographs are arranged in the sequence in which the teeth were examined, and the final analysis is made with the dry, mounted films at the time of the oral examination. The radiographs should be studied prior to the oral examination to detect any departure from the normal. The observations are recorded and placed in the chart until the mouth is examined. The carious lesions, osseous density and contour, location of the sinuses, pulp size, periodontal membrane thickness, and appearance of the bone surrounding the apex

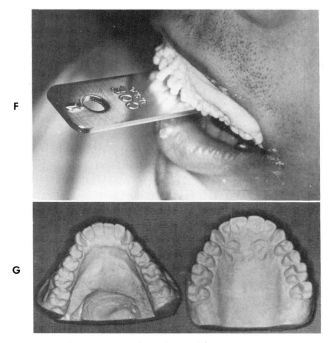

F

G

Fig. 2-6, cont'd. For legend see opposite page.

of the teeth should be observed. The radiographs are effective only when used in conjunction with the oral examination. The findings are charted and described for the case analysis.

A screening examination is made when the information for the record is collected. When the patient's medical and dental history is complete and the radiographs and study casts are made, the information is studied and another appointment is made for the oral examination and case presentation. Gross findings such as mobile teeth, soft tissue lesions, or abnormal tissue contour are examined at the first appointment. The teeth should be thoroughly cleaned of stain and calculus at the time the records are taken or during the appointment in which the case is presented. Clean teeth are desired for the examination. When performed adequately, the oral examination and case presentation require a long appointment in the office.

Examination of the oral cavity
Prophylactic care

As previously mentioned, the teeth must be thoroughly cleaned before the examination. If the periodontium has been neglected, it will be necessary to treat the condition as an emergency by grossly scaling the teeth on the first appointment, after the chief complaint has been satisfied.[19] The scaling procedure can be finished during the appointment at which the records are taken; this appointment should be scheduled a few days later to allow recovery from the initial calculus removal.

Regardless of the type of practice, prophylactic care of the teeth is integral to dental health and contributes as much to it as any other element. The thoroughness of the cleaning procedure before the oral examination, prior to the application of the rubber dam, and periodically for maintenance is as important as caries-control measures. Scaling and polishing the teeth is a simple procedure that, when done carefully, will be appreciated by the patient.

The use of small scalers that can be passed into the gingival embrasure without interference is indicated. The scaler must be passed between the cementum and free gingiva and must reach below the calculus to detach the deposit from the root surface. This procedure should be done without tearing the soft tissue attachment of the tooth and it is complicated by the dentist's inability to see the subgingival calculus. The scalers are limited in width and contain a sharp cutting edge for removing the calcium. The direction of the scaling edge is turned for convenience in scaling the posterior teeth. Scoring the cementum should be avoided because it may produce a future nidus for food entrapment.

Calculus deposits are more pronounced on the teeth that are near the openings of the salivary ducts. The lower incisors and upper molars usually have heavy deposits that require more attention and care. Although the exact mechanism is not known, the calcium phosphate from saliva is thought to become attached to a matrix on the tooth surface similar to the plaque. The rate of deposit varies widely, even in individuals with the same family background, and the consensus is that the deposit must be removed. If the calcium is left intact it becomes a local irritant and is the most common cause of periodontal disease.[19] Eventually the irritation causes deterioration of the bone and loss of tooth support. Calculus formation is retarded by good toothbrushing and other home care measures. Because the subgingival areas are inaccessible the use of periodic scaling is demanded.

Stain and calcium deposits in other areas of the tooth can be removed with special instruments. If left intact the rough edges on the enamel will irritate the tongue. The discoid instruments are helpful in the removal of these deposits, especially on the lingual surfaces of the incisors. They are placed in the concavities of the teeth and the cutting edge detaches the deposit. Repeated applications will be necessary because this type of calculus and stain is difficult to remove.

When the scaling has been completed, the teeth are polished with silica or pumice to remove the surface stain. The polishing material is mixed with water or glycerin and applied with a soft rubber cup. The abrasive is held in contact with the enamel surface and the cup is slowly revolved to remove the stain. The polishing, like the scaling, should be done systematically, always beginning and ending in the same areas. It is convenient to start with the upper buccal surfaces of the molars on the side of the operator. The mirror can be used to retract the cheek and the polishing can be observed directly. Complete polishing will result in smooth and clean enamel surfaces that are conducive to examination or treatment.

The interproximal spaces are cleaned to remove the abrasive, and before this is started the patient is instructed to rinse his mouth thoroughly. A strand of dental floss is wrapped around the index fingers in the same way as when examining for caries, and it is passed between all the teeth. The surfaces are polished gently and the floss is removed through the buccal or labial surface. If fluoride is to be applied at this time, it is recommended that unwaxed floss be used for maximum absorption of the solution on the proximal surface. When all the interproximal spaces are cleaned, the patient is instructed to rinse his mouth thoroughly again. If the scaling has been heavy and irritation is prevalent, it is advisable to have the patient rinse first with 3% hydrogen peroxide and then with water for aseptic purposes.

The teeth will be cleaned thoroughly if the system just described is used. Toothbrushing methods and use of dental floss should be reviewed to update the home care procedure, and the importance of a regular cleaning appointment should be emphasized. The method used for the recall system varies, but the appointment scheduling is regulated by the ancillary personnel.

Examination method

A detailed description of the method of conducting an oral examination can be obtained from a textbook on oral diagnosis.[22] The examination should be thorough and systematic so that no details or departures from the normal situation are overlooked. The use of preventive medical and dental treatment has improved the oral conditions of most patients that are examined in the office. With more emphasis on health and increased longevity, more routine examinations are being made. The tendency to overlook problems occurs because normal tissue is customary, but the dentist should be cautioned against overlooking pathologic conditions.

The routine bracket setup included in the dental unit is made available with all the records of the individual being examined. The soft tissue is observed first by using the mirror to reflect the tissue obscuring the vision. The index finger is used to palpate the tissues and oral landmarks such as the floor of the mouth, the buccal mucosa, the muscle attachments on the alveolar ridge, and the ducts of the salivary glands. If the tongue is asymmetric, it should be palpated; in addition the palate, tonsillar areas, and exostoses should be explored. Stains and inflammation are recorded, after which questions are asked in order to determine their etiology.

The gingival sulci and papillae are observed and, if necessary, the pocket depths around the periodontally involved teeth are measured. The mobility of the tooth is also tested at this time. The index fingers are used to support and push the weakened tooth in order to detect the movement in the jaw and to compare it with other teeth. At this time the occlusal relationship of the tooth is tested to see if it is related to the loss of alveolar bone.

The examination of the teeth for caries is done in the manner previously described. The radiographs should be illuminated with the view box so that they can be referred to for each tooth. The assistant can mark the tooth form in the record to show initial and recurrent lesions and defective restorations that need to be replaced. If this procedure is not followed, the radiograph mounting can be marked and the data can be assimilated when the treatment plan is written. It is important to dry each tooth and examine it thoroughly with the sharp explorer in order to detect caries and to study the groove formations and susceptibility to future caries.

Teeth that have atypical pulp symptoms and that show radiographic changes at the apex should be tested. A number of techniques can be used to determine vitality, which is necessary before planning the restorative care. The pulpally involved teeth must either be treated endodontically or removed because of the degenerated tissue causing systemic complications or abscess formation. The health of the pulp must be determined in all teeth that are to receive restorations or will be involved in the treatment plan.[26] It is usually necesssary to test only those teeth that have atypical symptoms.

A number of methods can be used to test pulp vitality, but the electric vitality test is considered to be the best way of making the evaluation. Electric pulp testers are included in many dental units and they can also be purchased as separate items. Direct current is utilized to prevent fluctuation of the electric stimulus, and the test takes only a few seconds. The electrode, which constitutes the tip of the instrument, is placed on that part of the labial or buccal surface where the middle and gingival thirds of the enamel join. The surface must be dry and the electrode must be placed on sound enamel, not on restorations. The current is increased until the pulp relays the stimulus and the numeric value of the stimulus is then recorded. This test is not painful and the patient should be relaxed in order to obtain a good evaluation.

The teeth adjacent to the one in question or the entire quadrant should be tested. The results are compared with those of other teeth in the same mouth; the readings have no value when compared with those of other patients. The type of pulp degeneration cannot be determined from the results of any test, including the ice or warm gutta-percha tests, but they do tell the dentist whether the tissue responds favorably and in the same way as other teeth in the quadrant. The other methods of testing vitality are used primarily to elicit painful responses that have been experienced, but they are not as rapid and standardized as the electric vitality test.

All the data that have been collected are recorded on the chart. A preliminary plan can be made at this time if the patient becomes curious about any of the findings. The condition of the soft tissue and caries will have been diagnosed sufficiently to know what teeth will be involved. In questionable teeth it is sometimes necessary to excavate the caries to determine whether the pulp is exposed; this can be done before the models are made. The exploration is helpful in determining pulp conditions if regular testing has been of no value.

Occlusal analysis

The type of occlusion and jaw relationship of the patient is important to the diagnosis. The analysis is made on an articulator that has been set to duplicate the mandibular movement. This type of analysis has been called a functional analysis, and it is used to determine the efficiency in the existing dentition.[22] The need for reshaping or restoring the teeth to improve function or the value of occlusal equilibration can also be determined.

The requirements for a desirable occlusion have been discussed for many years in the dental profession. Many concepts of the interdigitation of the teeth and the type of contacts that are made in the different positions of the jaw have developed. The type of occlusion that exists is important in the distribution of stress and the prevention of traumatic relationships. It is commonly agreed that occlusal contacts in the posterior teeth should occur only in centric occlusion to distribute the stresses evenly in the upper and lower teeth in a direction parallel to the long axis of the teeth.[27]

The study of occlusal relationships and jaw movements has been concentrated mainly in the areas of reconstruction and prosthodontics. Periodontics has contributed much to an understanding of occlusion due to the efforts of equilibrate teeth so as to prevent loss of the supporting tissues. The concept of balanced occlusion, or simultaneous contact of the teeth in eccentric movements, is used only in prosthetic replacements. The occurrence of balancing contacts causes horizontal forces on the tooth that result in wear facets on the enamel, breakdown of the periodontal membrane and alveolar bone, and occasionally temporomandibular joint disturbances. The horizontal contacts, when they are detected or clinically symptomatic, should be eliminated from the tooth or restoration. Intercuspation of the teeth in centric relation, with lack of contact in the posterior teeth in border movements, has been termed a natural or organic occlusion by Stuart and Stallard.

The determinants of occlusion, as described by gnathologists, are the two temporomandibular joints, the incisal guiding factors of the anterior teeth, the neuromuscular system that provides power, and the psychic factors used to coordinate the system.[28,29] These factors are used to determine the cusp and fossa locations in the teeth, the curve of Spee, and the occlusal plane for each patient. The determinants are used to diagnose mandibular movement, study occlusions, and design restorations.

All these factors are seen to influence the function of mastication and some of them can be measured and observed on the articulator. These factors cannot be changed in the patient, with the exception of some alteration of the incisal guidance. This means the anatomy of the restorations must fall within the functional range of jaw movements. However, the occlusal surfaces of the posterior teeth can be altered in reconstruction to harmonize with the determinants as they occur in the patient. Grinding the natural tooth structure when symptoms are not present is not necessary in all patients.[30]

In the study of occlusal relationships a number of terms are used that are helpful in recognizing problems.[31] The term "centric relation" is used to indicate the point of contact of the teeth when the condyles are in the rear-, mid-, and uppermost position of the glenoid fossae. This is an ideal jaw position for teeth, but it is considered a strained position in the joint, as are the eccentric positions. The mandible is in rest position when the arches are slightly open a distance of 3 to 5 mm. Ideally the teeth would have maximum interdigitation and desirable contacts when the condyles are in centric relation. Pure rotation occurs around the horizontal intercondylar axis, commonly called the hinge axis, which can be measured and relocated. Therefore the hinge axis mounting is used in reconstruction because it can be statically reproduced, and the movements and design of the restorations are started from an ideal position in centric relation.

The literature is abundant with methods for the diagnosis and correction of the premature contact. If uneven contours or poor relationships in the teeth cause early contact before interdigitation occurs, the condition is called a "prematurity." When the teeth are forced to close past the prematurity, the mandible slides forward to find an area of maximum occlusal contact, which is called a "mesial shift." This forward and lateral shift, caused by a number of premature contacts, is found in most patients. Differences in eruption, tooth size and position, rotation, and unplanned restorative care cause a gradual forward movement of the mandible throughout life. This is why two separate mandibular relationships can be found in most patients—the shifted bite, which is called centric occlusion, and maximum interdigitation in centric relation.

Many problems prevent the use of centric relation in the treatment plan. The difference between the two relationships can be 1 to 3 mm., and to get the mandible posterior for function would entail severe reshaping of most of the teeth that are in contact. This discrepancy supports the practice of making the restorations in the acquired centric occlusion.

The concept of normal occlusal arrangement of the teeth has developed through research and clinical evidence in much the same way as the theories of mandibular relationship. In cases of occlusal reconstruction the cusps and fossae are made to contact in centric relation, but in the routine clinical case the teeth must interdigitate to blend with the opposing teeth to avoid radical reshaping of the natural tooth structure.

For stability of the restoration in any jaw relationship the cusps should be located in fossae, but tooth position will sometimes require them to be placed on proximal marginal ridges.[27] The buccal cusps of the lower teeth should uniformly and evenly contact the fossae of the upper teeth and at the same time the lingual cusps of the upper teeth should contact the fossae of the lower teeth. The individual cusp-fossa contact should form a tripod by having three small contacts of the cusp in the fossa to eliminate shifting. In the working and idling position of the mandible the cusp tips should be adjusted so as to be able to escape through grooves in the opposing tooth. Chewing efficiency is determined by how close the cusp blades on the working side miss each other when returning to centric occlusion. The mastication of food is accomplished by the shearing action of the cusp blades.

Ideally the anterior teeth are the only ones that contact each other outside the chewing cycle.[27] The cuspids contact only in the extreme right and left eccentric positions. In the protrusive or end-to-end bite the lower anterior teeth will touch the lingual surface of the upper incisors. These descriptions refer to the ideal occlusion and are strived for in restorations.

In centric occlusion the lower anterior teeth will contact the upper lingual surfaces of the incisors. This relationship is measured by the horizontal and vertical overlap, which is responsible for developing the incisal guidance. This determinant of occlusion should be studied and worked out before restoration is begun because prematurities in anterior teeth in any jaw relationship contribute to rapid periodontal destruction and tooth loosening.

Occlusal analysis is made by observing the contacting surfaces to detect wear patterns. Some dentists have also advocated watching the patient chew different foods and then determining by direct questioning whether pain was experienced in the muscles of mastication or the temporomandibular joint area. The midline of the mouth can be observed to see how much deviation occurs from rest position, premature contact, and full closure.

The patient's head is tilted backward and centric relation is found by relaxing the patient and supporting the mandible during closure. The patient should be instructed to stop closure when the first contact is felt and should then be permitted to fully close; this procedure makes it possible to observe the amount of mandibular shift. The index finger can be placed on the alveolar ridge to determine which teeth are being grossly moved and in which areas the prematurities exist.

If the slide does not seem to be much of a problem or if teeth display pathologic signs caused by the prematurity, the damaging cause can be located during the examination. Thin articulating wax or paper is placed between the teeth, and the mandible is manipulated to contact once again in centric relation. The tooth or wax will be marked to determine which opposing teeth are in poor relationship and the problem is diagnosed. A small mounted stone can be used to correct the prematurities if they are obvious and are causing an acute problem. The complete analysis and reshaping is made on articulated models before the teeth are reduced in order to diagnose the undesirable contacts and to determine what could be gained by equilibration.

Selective grinding, a term used in occlusal equilibration, must be done

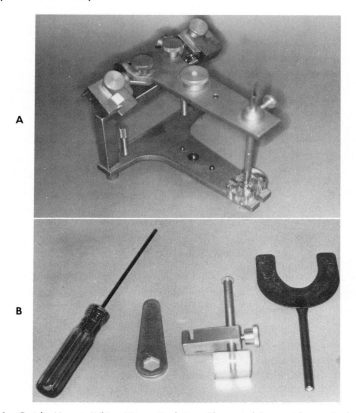

A

B

Fig. 2-7. A, Quick Mount Whip Mix articulator. The condylar guidance is located on the upper member of the articulator. **B,** Armamentarium for the articulator—adjustment and intercondylar wrenches, the nasion for the facebow, and the bite fork.

judiciously because the enamel cannot be replaced once it is removed. Care should be exercised not to unduly reduce the working cusps, i.e., the buccal surfaces of the lower teeth and the lingual surfaces of the upper teeth. The rule for equilibration in the acute area is that, when a tooth is high in centric occlusion, the fossa is deepened, and when a prematurity exists in lateral movement and centric relation, the cusp and the fossa are reduced.[25] Injudicious selective grinding is dangerous because the eccentric prematurities are hard to observe without models; and when a number of reductions are made, other uneven pressures develop, causing the diagnostician to become confused.

The complete occlusal analysis is accurately accomplished by fastening the study casts on an adjustable articulator (Fig. 2-7). The articulator should be adjustable and should closely duplicate the movements of the patient's mandible. The analysis includes mounting and shaping the models to remove the prematurities and to seat the mandible in a more posterior position on the articulator.

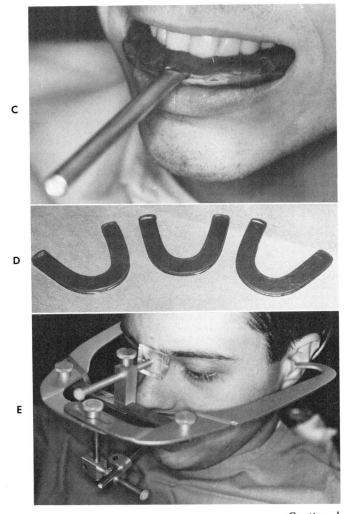

Continued.

Fig. 2-7, cont'd. C, Patient holding the bite fork by biting into two layers of wax. The bite fork is aligned in the midline. **D,** Wax bites used for the interocclusal records and for adjusting the guidance on the articulator. **E,** The facebow is retained by the bite fork and seated in the external auditory meatus. The nasion is used for the third reference point in mounting. The forward and middle screw on the facebow gives the intercondylar estimate of small, medium, or large.

A list of the adjustments made on the model serves as a guide for grinding the teeth if this becomes necessary.

The study casts that were previously made are used for the mounting. This procedure is recommended only for the patient who is going to receive numerous new restorations and replacements or for the patient with many prematurities and acute symptoms of periodontal disease. If the study casts have not been

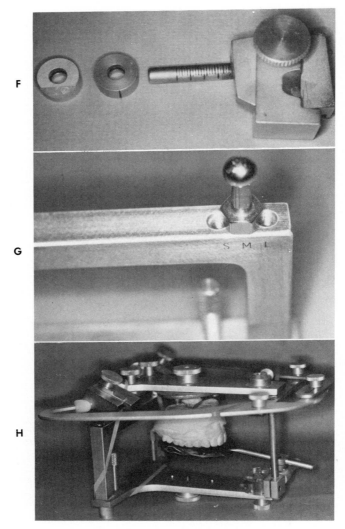

Fig. 2-7, cont'd. F, The guide plate and rings are used for the corresponding intercondylar distance. **G,** The articulator guidepost is adjusted to estimate the intercondylar distance. **H,** The facebow is attached to the articulator, with the upper model held in the bite-fork wax. The model is attached to the articulator at this time with quick-setting stone.

made, the alginate impressions are taken down to the mucobuccal fold. The models are trimmed to this border so that the teeth can be observed. Thick bases are not needed on casts for restorative purposes; casts are made only strong enough to support the model, and nodules that are interlocked with the mounting stone are placed on the bottom.

The casts are attached on the articulator mounting ring with the quick-setting stones. Numerous "bite stones" made of Hydrocal are available that harden

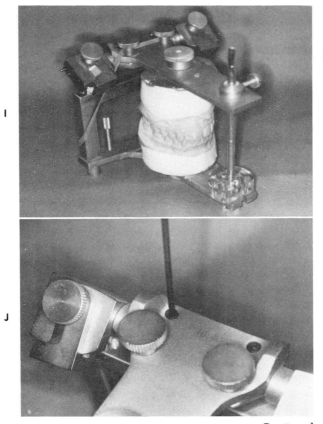

Continued.

Fig. 2-7, cont'd. I, Diagnostic casts mounted on the articulator. The centric wax bite is placed between the two models, and the lower model is attached to the lower member of the articulator. **J,** The wrench is used to loosen the condylar guide plate and the settings are made with the checkbite on the opposite side in place.

very quickly and have a minimum of setting expansion. These stones enable the mounting and adjustment of the articulator to be done quickly, making the analysis practical for the office routine.

Interocclusal wax records are taken to relate the casts to the articulator and to each other. A wax bite is taken in centric relation or occlusion and is used to position the lower cast. A right and left checkbite is taken to set the guiding mechanisms on the articulator. The Quick Mount articulator is used to present the technique for functional analysis. It is adjustable and can be used quickly to articulate the models.[32] Other products on the market are satisfactory, however, and will produce the same results.

A fully adjustable articulator is one that can be set to follow a pantograph, or curved Gothic arch tracing of the mandibular movement.[27] Following an

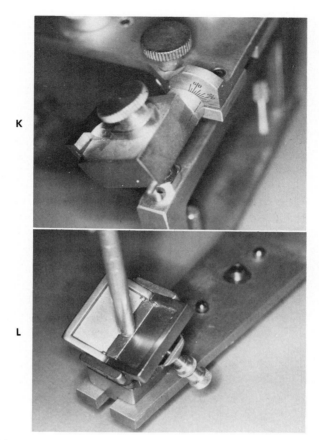

Fig. 2-7, cont'd. K, The measurement of the condylar guidance is recorded on the articulator. **L,** An adjustable guide plate that can be set to prevent wear on the contacting surfaces of the mounted models. **M,** A procedure similar to that just described being completed for the diagnostic casts on the Hanau articulator.

accurate location of the hinge axis, the tracing is made by numerous styluses that are directed by clutches cemented to the teeth. The fully adjustable articulator is used for occlusal reconstruction when all the teeth are restored with contours of an ideal occlusion in harmony with the temporomandibular joints. There are indications for this type of analysis and treatment, but in general it is too involved for the routine case. The sophisticated construction of the articulator is helpful in understanding the dynamics of occlusion.

The adjustable articulator, as used for the routine diagnosis and occlusal adjustment, is not as accurate as the fully adjustable articulator, but it places the models in the same order used in the treatment and in positions that can be compared to other cases. Three points of reference are used, two of which are the horizontal axis of the temporomandibular joint and the vertical measurement that uses certain anatomic landmarks for each articulator. The three reference

M

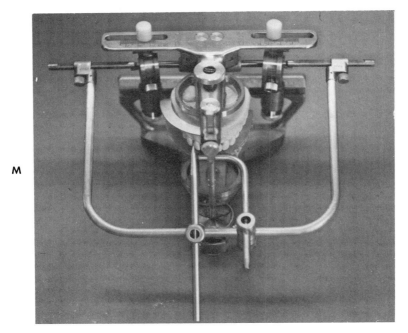

Fig. 2-7, cont'd. For legend see opposite page.

points make it possible to standardize the maxillary cast to the upper member of the articulator and to transfer the measurements of the patient to the articulator.

The anatomic landmarks commonly used in the vertical measurement are the nasion and infraorbital foramen. In gnathology a tattoo mark is placed at some standard measurement above the incisal edge of the cuspid. This point, located in the facebow standardized by the transfer, makes it possible to remount casts on the articulator for refining the restorative units. In remounting, the transfer and centric bite are used to place the casts back on the articulator, and the measurements that were recorded in analyzing the occlusion are adjusted. Recording the condylar guidance and "side shift" will eliminate the need of taking new checkbites to set the articulator.

The difference between the two types of articulators, adjustable and fully adjustable, is that the pantograph copies the Bennett movement of the mandible. In the Bennett movement the amount of sideward movement is timed. This measurement is critical but cannot be adjusted other than by trial and error in the mouth unless the fully adjustable articulator is used.

The adjustable articulator and the interocclusal wax checkbites are satisfactory for the functional analysis. Some adjustable articulators can be used in locating the hinge axis, but the only advantage of this procedure is in the diagnosis. The standardization and the fact that the actual occlusion can be

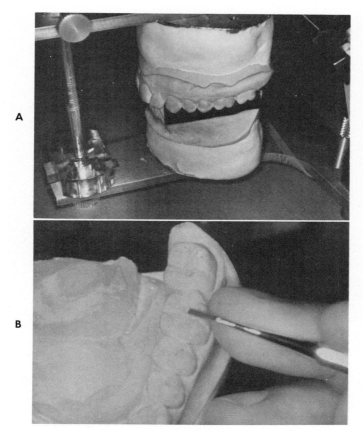

Fig. 2-8. A, Articulating paper between the diagnostic casts is used to mark the contacting areas on the models. **B,** Model adjustments are made with a sharp binangle chisel.

studied in no other way makes the use of the adjustable articulator preferable with full-arch models. Although the procedure described is used in diagnosis, it is similar to the use of the articulator in making castings.

Technique for mounting the cast. Two accurate models are obtained from alginate impressions. The casts are trimmed neatly and based for mounting purposes. To mount the upper model the facebow transfer is made. This is done by inserting the bite fork between the arches; the bite fork embedded in layers of wax is held forcefully by the patient. The facebow is attached to the bite fork and the arbitrary center of the condyle or the hinge axis mounting is made to contact the tissue over the joint while the vertical measurement is made on the soft facial tissue. The upper cast is mounted with quick-setting stone.

A centric occlusion (maximum acquired interdigitation) wax bite is taken for mounting the lower model. A centric relation record is made with the hinge axis mounting only for those patients requiring extensive occlusal adjustment. The lower model is mounted with the quick-setting stone by seating the cast in the bite on the inverted articulator. The eccentric wax records are taken on the right and left side by making the imprints in the wax with the cuspids end to end on the side being measured. A right and left lateral wax record is used for most articulators; however, some articulators require a protrusive bite to set the condylar inclination for use in edentulous patients.

The wax records are used to set the articulator. The individual checkbite, which is taken on the working or rotating side of the mandible, is inserted between the posts to set the opposite joint. The side that has been adjusted is the translating condyle, and the condylar guidance and side limit are set while the wax bite has the condyle suspended. The right checkbite is inserted between the models and the left joint is set as before. The setting is made by turning the upper and inside plates, representing the glenoid fossa, until they touch the ball, representing the condyle. The readings are made and recorded for the purpose of future remounting or building the cast.

The adjustable guide plate is set to preserve the models from abrasion or the plastic plate is contoured with quick-setting acrylic die. This will enable the anterior guidance to be made with the plate and guide pin of the articulator. The guide pin is used to move the models and study the relationship of the casts.

Adjustment of the casts. The models are marked with regular articulating paper and are shaped with a sharp binangle chisel (Fig. 2-8). This procedure removes the prematurities and permits movement of the lower model in a more posterior position. The desired occlusion is the "organic concept" advocated by Stuart, and the model analysis is made with this occlusal relationship as the goal. Following is a sequence outline by Stuart for diagnosis and adjustment of the occlusion on articulated models.

Occlusal adjustments*

Incisal relations are tested. If any bicuspids or molars contact, enough tooth structure is removed from the buccal cusps of the upper teeth and the lingual cusps of the lower teeth until no contact remains except on the edge-to-edge position of the anterior teeth. If a lower, tipped molar interferes, a groove is made in the distal surface of this lower molar for the upper cusp to pass through. This condition occurs when the lower, tipped molar is distal to the upper molars.

The cuspid relations in the lateral excursion are tested in the tip-to-tip contact. If any posterior cusps interfere or make simultaneous contact on the idling side, a groove is made in the upper teeth for the lower cusps to pass through. These grooves are sloped mesially from the markings on the upper teeth and distally from the markings on the lower teeth.

If there is interference or simultaneous contact between the bicuspids or

---

*This section was contributed by Charles E. Stuart of Ventura, Calif.

molars on the working side in the tip-to-tip relation, tooth structure is removed from the buccal cusps of the upper teeth and lingual cusps of the lower teeth.

After molar and bicuspid interferences have been eliminated on the idling and working sides in the tip-to-tip cuspid relation, the occlusion is tested nearer centric relation; that is, the occlusion is tested just a little inside the tip-to-tip cuspid relation. At this position the posterior cusp contacts are eliminated on the idling and working sides in the same way as in the cuspid tip-to-tip relation. Successive positions are taken nearer and nearer centric relation, eliminating the interferences at each position until the centric relation closure is reached. Repeat the procedure just described in the opposite lateral movement, beginning with the tip-to-tip cuspid relation and gradually working nearer and nearer centric relation. When testing in the lateral excursions, it is quite helpful to direct slight hand pressure toward the working side; pressure should be applied on the idling side to aid in securing the total side shift or Bennett movement.

The eccentric clearances on the posterior teeth should be so adequate that no carbon paper marks are obtainable and that the patient cannot feel contact. The centric relation is adjusted last by tipping the patient's head back and lightly closing the jaw in its posteriormost position. Carbon paper is placed between the teeth and the patient is instructed to close from the first contact to full inercuspation. The interferences are removed from the mesial slopes of the upper teeth and the distal slopes of the lower teeth. After these sloping contacts are removed, the fossae are deepened to give the centric-related intercuspation slightly more closure than was present in the former forward intercuspation. Finally, one should make certain that the patient's intercuspation has even pressure on both sides and that the bicuspids close simultaneously with the molars. Mesiodistal as well as bilateral equal closure is derived. The finished occlusion should have maximum intercuspation and the jaw rear-, and mid-, and uppermost intercuspation. Any other contact between the upper and lower teeth is relegated to the anterior teeth outside the chewing cycle.

After the biscuspids and molars are relieved of eccentric contacts, the centric-related intercuspation can be made because the eccentric relations have been considered. In waxing or in making any occlusal adjustment it is necessary to test the eccentric relations first to make sure that centric relation contacts are not destroyed in the eccentric excursions.

The adjusted models are shown to the patient, and the diagnosis and explanation of the reshaping that needs to be done is explained. Normally a patient should be treated by making only a few apparent improvements such as alteration of the plunger cusp or placement of working and idling grooves in teeth with heavy facets and symptoms of cusp splitting. The extensive occlusal adjustment can be made satisfactorily for many patients, but in others model adjustment will not be improved and therefore should not be performed clinically.

Tooth reduction is accomplished with small diamonds and then smoothed. The articulating paper is used in the mouth to produce the marks that appeared on the model, and the reduction is made by removing the marks from the teeth. The written guide that was recorded can be used to follow the same sequence as in reshaping the mounted casts.

Summary

The diagnosis is made after all the facts have been collected in the examination; it is an analysis of what needs to be done for the patient. The treatment plan is the schedule and sequence of the treatment that has been outlined. They are both arrived at by logical deduction and analysis of the patient's problems that have been determined from the results of the medical and dental history and the other parts of the examination.

The treatment plan is determined according to the urgency of each problem and the sequence of procedures that should be followed. The teeth should not be prepared for castings before the periodontal problem is corrected or a tooth should not be removed before the gingival lesion or lymph node involvement is diagnosed and treated. The outline to follow in making the plan is recommended by Kerr, Ash, and Millard.

Outline for treatment planning*

I. Systemic treatment
   A. Referral to a physician for systemic evaluation and treatment as indicated by history and clinical findings
   B. Appraisal of the influence of systemic treatment on the dental treatment plan
   C. Premedication with antibiotics or sedatives as indicated by the history
   D. Corrective therapy for oral infection

II. Preparatory treatment
   A. Oral surgery
   B. Endodontic therapy
   C. Caries control
   D. Periodontal therapy
   E. Orthodontic treatment
   F. Occlusal adjustment

III. Corrective treatment
   A. Operative dentistry
   B. Prosthetic dentistry

IV. Periodic recall examinations and maintenance treatment

This outline is presented to show the sequence in which operative dentistry should be performed. Obviously many conditions are discovered that require clearance or treatment by the physician. Any systemic disorder must be surveyed to relieve the dentist from the responsibility of problems that could occur during the treatment schedule because of pathologic conditions. The need to confer with a physician does not occur often and is usually not time-consuming, but assistance from a physician should be obtained in all cases in which it is needed.

---

*From Kerr, D. A., Ash, M. M., Jr., and Millard, H. D.: Oral diagnosis, ed. 3, St. Louis, 1970, The C. V. Mosby Co., p. 363.

In comprehensive planning there will be patients who need to be referred to a specialist. In cases involving difficult surgery and differential diagnosis of the dental structures and complicated periodontal problems the oral surgeon and the periodontist should be consulted frequently. Referral to a specialist should be explained to the patient, and all problems of a special nature must be corrected prior to restoration of the teeth. The soft tissues are treated, the teeth cleaned thoroughly, and caries-control measures effected before any tooth is prepared for a permanent restoration.

The caries and periodontal problems in the teeth are charted in the record. The bone height, missing teeth, and actual location of the carious lesions are drawn on the outline of the dentition. The serial method of numbering the teeth from 1 to 32 beginning with the maxillary right third molar is the system commonly used.

The caries location is marked on the chart in dark ink (Fig. 2-9). The treatment sequence for restoring the teeth is made according to the order of importance. Deep lesions that are acute and abutment teeth are restored first. If none of the lesions is obviously pressing, the anterior teeth can be restored first to improve the appearance of the patient. The treatment record will be used

DIAGNOSIS AND TREATMENT PLAN

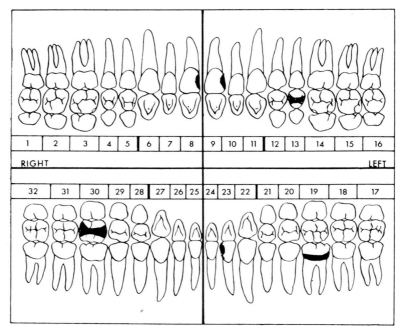

Fig. 2-9. Operative treatment chart. The carious lesions and probable restoration outlines are inked in on the chart. After the restoration they are marked as completed.

as a checklist after the patient is seated for the appointment. Changes will seldom need to be made prior to selecting the restorative task.

Presentation of the treatment plan should be done with an attitude of confidence and with a desire to do excellent work. The ideal method is presented first and, if social or economic problems make this service impossible, an optional conservative service should be offered. The advantages of ideal treatment and optimum health should be explained to the patient and demonstrated with models and diagrams if necessary. The patient's personal records, charts, radiographs, and diagnostic casts are presented to reveal the thoroughness of the examination, diagnosis, and construction of the treatment plan.

Some offices have special rooms for case presentation. They are pleasantly decorated and have instructional aids with which to inform the patient. The aids are not used as gimmicks to trick the patient into spending more money or accepting a useless service but are helpful in gaining acceptance of the ideal therapy. An open discussion of fees for the dental service should follow and the actual method of payment should be established. Plans are now available through business, insurance companies, and government agencies that help more people to obtain finances for optimum dental care. The business management aspect of the practice must supercede the service aspect unless credit measures and poor-risk patients do not concern the dentist.

The treatment plan is used to organize the work load and assure the patient that optimum care will be provided in the most efficient manner. The long-range benefits of dental health are explained and then provided for the patient by the recall examination and prophylaxis following the curative measures. Maintenance of the teeth costs much less per year than do other health or cosmetic services in the modern society.

The ancillary personnel controls the details of the appointment book. The treatment plan is used to set up the number of appointments and the spacing required between them. The assistant and the dentist should encourage long appointments because more care can be given per unit time. The patient is given a card, which emphasizes punctuality, containing the appointment schedule. Time units for each specific task should be allotted in the well-managed practice. Planning and punctuality on the part of the dentist also reap excellent results by making the day easier.

Treatment planning is also presented with other subjects in the book. The thoroughness of taking records, conducting the oral examination, making an accurate diagnosis, and planning treatment must be mastered before specific treatment is initiated.

REFERENCES

1. Blackwell, R. E.: Black's operative dentistry, ed. 9, Milwaukee, 1955, Medico-Dental Publishing Co., vol. 2.
2. Sumnicht, R. W.: Preventive dentistry and dental practice, Practical Dental Monographs, July, 1965, pp. 1-45.

3. Easlick, K.: Dental caries, mechanism and present control techniques—a workshop, St. Louis, 1948, The C. V. Mosby Co.
4. Selected dental findings in adults by age, race and sex, United States, 1960-1962, Publication No. 1000, Washington, D. C., 1962, U. S. Department of Health, Education, and Welfare.
5. Klein, H., Palmer, C. E., and Knutson, J. W.: Studies on dental caries. I. Dental status and dental needs of elementary school children, U. S. Public Health Rep. **53**:751, 1938.
6. American Dental Association, Bureau of Economic Research and Statistics: Survey of needs of dental care. VI. Summary and comparison with 1940 survey, J.A.D.A. **47**:572, 1953.
7. Hollinshead, B. S., director: The survey of dentistry; final report, Washington, D. C., 1961, American Council on Education.
8. Hennon, D. K., and Muhler, J. C.: Clinical use of fluorides, J. Indiana Dent. Assoc. **41**: 88, 1962.
9. Norquest, C., Dudding, N., and Muhler, J.: Questionnaire survey to Indiana dentists concerning preventive dentistry, J. Indiana Dent. Assoc. **42**:516, 1963.
10. Brudevold, F.: Fluorides in the prevention of dental caries, Dent. Clin. N. Am., July, 1962, pp. 397-409.
11. Miller, W. D.: New theories concerning decay of teeth, Dent. Cosmos **47**:1293, 1905.
12. Black, G. V.: Operative dentistry, ed. 3, Chicago, 1917, Medico-Dental Publishing Co., vol. 1.
13. McDonald, R. E.: Human saliva: a study of the rate of flow and viscosity and its relationship to dental caries, master's thesis, Indianapolis, Indiana University School of Dentistry.
14. Karshan, M.: Do calcium and phosphorus in saliva differ significantly in caries-free and active-caries groups? J. Dent. Res. **21**:83, 1942.
15. Afonsky, D.: Saliva and its relation to oral health; a survey of the literature, Tuscaloosa, 1961, University of Alabama Press.
16. Bibby, B. G.: Effect of sugar content on foodstuffs and their caries-producing potential, J.A.D.A. **51**:293, 1955.
17. Bunting, R. W.: Studies of the relation of Bacillus acidophilus to dental caries, J. Dent. Res. **8**:222, 1928.
18. Brauer, J. C.: Dentistry for children, ed. 5, New York, 1964, McGraw-Hill Book Co., Inc.
19. Goldman, H. M., and Cohen, W.: Periodontal therapy, ed. 5, St. Louis, 1973, The C. V. Mosby Co.
20. Bibby, B. G.: Do we tell the truth about preventing caries? J. Dent. Child. **33**:269, 1966.
21. Shafer, W. G., Hine, M. K., and Levy, B. M.: A textbook of oral pathology, ed. 2, Philadelphia, 1963, W. B. Saunders Co.
22. Kerr, D. A., Ash, M. M., Jr., and Millard, H. D.: Oral diagnosis, ed. 3, St. Louis, 1970, The C. V. Mosby Co.
23. Clinical preventive dentistry manual, Indianapolis, 1966, Indiana University School of Dentistry.
24. Massler, M.: Indirect pulp capping and vital pulpotomy for potential and actual pulp exposures, J. Tennessee Dent. Assoc. **35**:393, 1955.
25. Johnston, J. F., Phillips, R. W., and Dykema, R.: Modern practice in crown and bridge prosthodontics, ed. 2, Philadelphia, 1965, W. B. Saunders Co.
26. Gilmore, H. W.: Operative dentistry. In Goldman, H. M., Forrest, S. P., Byrd, D. L., and McDonald, R. E., editors: Current therapy in dentistry, St. Louis, 1964, The C. V. Mosby Co., chap. 12.
27. Stuart, C. E., and Stallard, H.: Principles involved in restoring occlusion to natural teeth, J. Prosth. Dent. **10**:304, 1960.
28. Stuart, C. E., and Stallard, H.: A syllabus on oral rehabiltiation and occlusion. II. Postgraduate education, San Francisco, 1965, School of Dentistry, University of California.
29. Pavone, B. W.: A syllabus on oral rehabilitation and occlusion. II. Postgraduate education, San Francisco, 1965, School of Dentistry, University of California.

30. Coolidge, E. D., and Hine, M. K.: Periodontia, ed. 2, Philadelphia, 1954, Lea & Febiger.
31. Ramfjord, S. P., and Ash, M. M.: Occlusion, ed. 1, Philadelphia, 1966, W. B. Saunders Co.
32. Instructional guide, Louisville, 1965, Whip Mix Corp.

chapter 3

Cavity preparation nomenclature, classification, and principles

NOMENCLATURE

The terminology of a science is known as the nomenclature. It is a system of terms specific to a particular science that must be understood before accurate communication can exist in discussion of the subject. The student, teacher, and research worker must know the terms in order to establish a mutual understanding when discussing the restoration of teeth. Since the terminology is used primarily in describing instrumentation and cavity preparation, it is necessary to master this phase of the subject in the beginning of the study.

Fortunately only a few terms need to be learned in operative dentistry. Many situations can be described by simply combining these terms, giving a simple but comprehensive classification of the field. Terms used in operative dentistry to discuss cavity preparation are borrowed from dental anatomy and serve to describe tooth surfaces and the walls involved in the prepared cavity form. The nomenclature of instruments is included in Chapter 4.

Cavity preparation is a surgical operation that removes caries and excises hard tissue to shape the form for the restoration. It is accomplished by extending and smoothing the cavity walls to produce a foundation to absorb the forces placed on the restoration. The design of the preparation includes margins located in caries-immune areas that keep the outline clean, and support is gained by boxlike mortise forms located within the preparation. Cavity preparations include intracoronal and extracoronal preparations and certain principles must be attained in both types. Cavity nomenclature as outlined by Black includes the names of cavities, groups of cavities, and internal parts of the cavity preparation. The internal parts of a cavity preparation are the walls and the lines and points where they are joined.

Cavity terminology

As discussed in the previous chapter, the term "cavity" is often used to refer to the lesion or condition of the tooth prior to operation. In discussing lesions the cavities are usually named for the surface on which they occur.[1,2] Lesions occurring on the mesial surface are called mesial lesions. The same method is used to name the occlusal, distal, and buccal cavities. Designation of the specific teeth is also included to further identify the location. An example would be a mesial lesion on the upper left first bicuspid or a distal lesion on the lower second molar. Individual tooth numbers can also be used; this system is the most practical way in which to inform a colleague about a mesial cavity on the No. 19 tooth, for example, or an occlusal lesion on the No. 30 tooth.

Following are examples of lesions named for the surface and tooth on which they occur. Cavities occurring on the buccal surfaces of bicuspids and molars are called buccal cavities; lesions occurring on the lingual surfaces of the same teeth are referred to as lingual cavities. Cavities occurring on the lingual surfaces of incisors are referred to as incisor lingual cavities; cavities occurring on the labial surface of incisors and cuspids are called labial or facial cavities. Lesions occurring on the proximal surfaces of the teeth are sometimes referred to as proximal cavities. Proximal cavities can be further divided into incisor proximal cavities or bicuspid and molar proximal cavities and sometimes include the designation of a surface, that is, a mesial or distal incisor proximal cavity. Surface designations are derived from the anatomic surface on which the lesion is located.

A simple cavity is one involving a single surface. This type of cavity is usually noted for being less extensive, having a smaller carious involvement, and requiring a less difficult restoration. A complex cavity is one involving two or more surfaces. This type of cavity includes two or more surface lesions caused by the spread of caries, and the restoration outline requires extension because it is located on the boundary of a caries-susceptible surface.

The types of lesions listed have specific ways in which they are restored because of similar patterns of caries development. Dental literature uses special terms to describe research findings about the natural dentition and new techniques of restoring it.

Cavities and cavity preparations are broadly divided into pit and fissure and smooth surface types. The incidence, etiology, and surgical procedures are common within each respective group. Pit and fissure cavities result from poorly coalesced areas on the tooth surfaces called defects. The areas are produced by poor and inadequate union of the calcification lobes. Poorly coalesced enamel is found on the occlusal surfaces of bicuspids and molars, the lingual surfaces of the maxillary incisors, the lingual grooves of the maxillary molars, and the buccal grooves of the mandibular molars. The caries usually begins in a pit, which is an undesirable union of three calcification lobes. As it develops, the lesion undermines the enamel, necessitating its removal as well as that of the poorly formed grooves in contact with the edge of the weakened enamel. Pit and fissure caries occurs most commonly on the occlusal surface of the molars and bicuspids. The degree of coalescence is similar in all dentitions but varies among individuals.

Smooth surface cavities are attributed to neglect because they occur on surfaces that have sound enamel which is usually free of defects (Fig. 3-1). This type of lesion is found on the axial surfaces of the teeth in areas that are habitually uncleaned. The same result occurs in the clean mouth, however, when tooth position prevents sound hygienic practices. Smooth surface lesions are activated by the apposition of bacteria and food with the teeth. Apposition is measured by the contact time of the food with the enamel and by the degree of fermentation and acid production, factors that influence the progress of caries. The lesion develops on the hidden interproximal surface and usually spreads laterally until an area is reached that is regularly cleaned in the process of mastication. As in the development of pit caries, after the smooth surface lesion has reached this point, further damage to the tooth is caused by undermining of the enamel through dentin destruction. This factor has caused the smooth surface lesion to be called a surface phenomenon in contrast to the way in which the pit lesion develops.

The pit and fissure type of lesion has characteristics opposite those of the smooth surface lesion. The pit caries begins on a surface that is habitually clean and is attributed to food and bacterial impaction in the small defects. The grooves hold material in the niduses because they cannot be cleaned during normal mastication. The entrapped food breaks down, forms acid, and decalcifies the surrounding area. The lesion characteristically progresses by undermining the enamel and producing a brittle tooth covering. The size of the caries is determined by the type of food and bacteria that continues to be trapped in the defect. The pit and fissure cavity usually occurs on a clean tooth surface, undermines the enamel, and penetrates the dentin.

Pit and fissure caries communicates with pits of other surfaces by way of the dentin. It is common to find involvement of the lingual grooves of upper molars and the buccal grooves of lower molars with the occlusal cavity. By joining the two surfaces the cavity preparation results in only one outline. Extensive lesions of this nature may also undermine the smooth surface, and the problem is not always solved by replacing the wall with a restoration.

The cavities located in the gingival portion of the buccal and lingual surfaces are of the smooth surface type. These are caused by neglect and by faulty cleaning of the tooth below the height of contour, and they are repaired by specific methods of isolation and instrumentation. The collected food rests in contact with the enamel at the border of the gingival tissue. Débridement of this material is accomplished by adequate toothbrushing and gingival massage during the brushing procedure.

Extensive involvement of caries, or the complex cavity, results in lesions

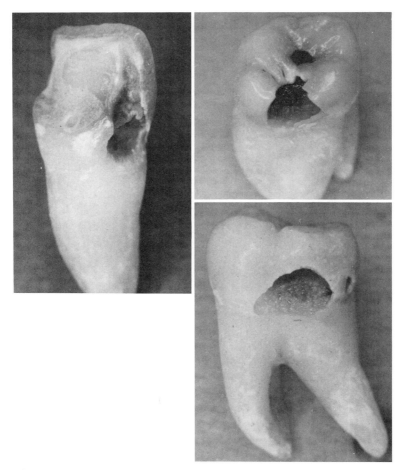

Fig. 3-1. Three examples of caries caused by neglect that commonly result in loss of the tooth from pulp degeneration.

that include both pit and fissure and smooth surface areas. The tooth is prepared so as to include all the involved areas plus susceptible surfaces that contact the edge of the lesion. Rules for extension and management of the enamel occasionally result in the restoration of numerous contiguous surfaces of the tooth.

The characteristics of each type of lesion have been discussed in connection with dental caries, but a few facts relevant to the subject of nomenclature should be mentioned. Pit and fissure lesions occur soon after the eruption of teeth. The proximal surfaces are protected at this time and their involvement occurs later in the clinical life of the tooth. Groove defects in bicuspids, molars, and incisors should be closely watched and treated in the young patient. Knowledge of the eruption date and pattern of caries development has led to the categorization of cavities according to age groups and lesion types.

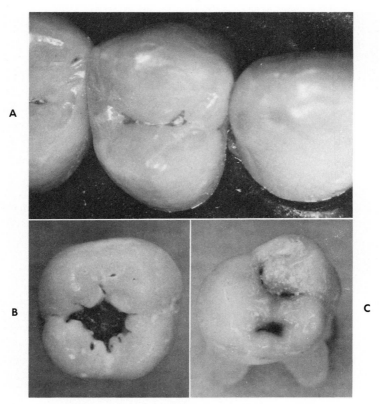

Fig. 3-2. A, A solid pre-carious occlusal groove that, if restored, would involve a conservative outline form. **B,** Extensive Class I lesion requiring a large diamond-shaped outline form. **C,** Occlusal caries that can be restored with two separate outline forms to preserve the oblique ridge. **D,** Class II caries on a maxillary molar. **E,** Class III caries on a central incisor that displays undermined enamel. **F,** Class IV caries involving loss of the incisal angle of the tooth. **G,** Numerous Class V lesions that demonstrate the variety of extension needed in restorations.

Black's classification

Certain types of cavities classified by Black into groups that require special consideration and instrumentation (Fig. 3-2) are as follows:

Class   I   Cavities occurring in the pit and fissure defects in the occlusal surfaces of the bicuspids and molars, the lingual surfaces of the upper incisors, and the buccal and lingual grooves that are found occasionally on the occlusal surfaces of molars

Class   II   Cavities in the proximal surfaces of bicuspids and molars

Class III   Cavities in the proximal surfaces of the incisors and cuspids that *do not* require removal and restoration of the incisal angle

Class IV   Cavities in the proximal surfaces of incisors and cuspids that require removal and restoration of the incisal angle

Class   V   Cavities in the gingival one third of teeth (not in pits) and below the

Fig. 3-2, cont'd. For legend see opposite page.

height of contour on the labial, buccal, and lingual surfaces of the teeth

Class VI   Cavities in the incisal edges and smooth surfaces of teeth above the height of contour (not included by Black).

It should be noted that Classes II to V are all smooth surface lesions. Each class has an instrumentation that is similar for the specific tooth being restored and problems peculiar to the restorative material being used. The hand-cutting and rotary instruments reduce the tooth in a special way and are assisted by certain rubber dam clamps, retracting devices, and separating devices for each cavity classification.

Nomenclature for cavity preparation

Each component of the cavity preparation is named so that it can be discussed and described in detail. This includes not only the walls of the preparation but also the areas where they are joined. The boxlike mortise form is used in all classes involving intracoronal preparations. Again, a similar anatomic nomenclature that corresponds to anatomic surfaces has been developed for all internal parts of the cavity preparation.

Walls of the cavity preparation. In general the surrounding walls of the preparation take the name of the surface toward which they are derived.

An occlusal Class I preparation has four surrounding walls (Fig. 3-3):

Distal wall	Buccal wall
Mesial wall	Lingual wall

A proximal Class III preparation has the following surrounding walls:

Labial wall	Gingival wall
Lingual wall	Incisal wall (only occasionally)

Cavity preparations have floors or bases that have also been given specific

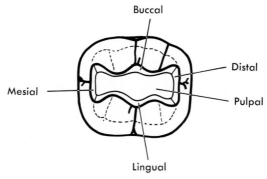

Fig. 3-3. The walls of an occlusal cavity preparation in a molar tooth.

names. The wall of the prepared cavity that covers the pulp and serves as the floor of the preparation is in a plane at right angles to the long axis of the tooth and is called the pulpal wall. Black states that, when the pulp is removed and the cavity extension includes the floor of the chamber, this foundation is called the subpulpal wall. In addition to the four surrounding walls for the Class I occlusal preparation the pulpal wall must be included to complete the box form.

The cavity wall directed toward the axial surfaces of the tooth is called the axial wall. It covers and approximates the pulp tissue. The axial wall is added to the Class III cavity preparation to complete the box form. In a similar manner the Class V cavity preparation has an axial wall that completes the box form for the gingival preparation.

The next cavity size is the complex cavity in which two or more surfaces are included in the preparation. Because two surfaces are involved, one of the surrounding walls will be missing. These walls are named by including the involved surfaces such as a mesio-occlusal cavity preparation or a mesio-occlusal-distal cavity preparation. Most of the time the proximal and occlusal cavities are joined to produce a nonconfined cavity preparation.

The mesio-occlusal Class II preparation on a molar or bicuspid has the following surrounding walls:

Distal wall	Pulpal wall
Lingual wall	Axial wall
Buccal wall	Gingival wall

Black's system of cavity wall nomenclature can be used for all types of preparations. It is impossible to cut an angulation on the inside of the preparation that cannot be named and then located by another observer.

Angles of the cavity preparation. As previously mentioned, the cavity preparation has a box form. All walls and angles of the box are named in each type of preparation because their location must be described.

The rules for designating angles in the Black system are as follows:

1. All line angles are formed by the junction of two walls along a line and are named by combining the names of the walls that join to form the angle. Therefore line angles are named for two anatomic surfaces.

2. All point angles are formed by the junction of three walls making a corner. Since they are named according to the walls of the anatomic surfaces involved, they are composed of three terms.

3. All angles of the cavity preparations are named according to the *specific* walls that are joined to form the angle. The same method of nomenclature is used for both line and point angles, with no particular order being used in selecting individual walls.

Following are examples of the nomenclature of angles according to the rules just mentioned.

A simple occlusal prepared cavity has the following sets of line (1 and 2) and point (3) angles:

1. Mesial-buccal angle
    Mesial-lingual angle
    Distal-buccal angle
    Distal-occlusal angle
2. Buccal-lingual angle
    Lingual-pulpal angle

    Mesial-pulpal angle
    Distal-pulpal angle
3. Mesial-buccal-pulpal angle
    Distal-buccal-pulpal angle
    Mesial-lingual-pulpal angle
    Distal-lingual-pulpal angle

A buccal or lingual prepared cavity has the following line (1 and 2) and point (3) angles:

1. Mesial-gingival angle
    Distal-gingival angle
    Mesial-occlusal angle
    Distal-occlusal angle
2. Axial-gingival angle
    Axial-mesial angle

    Axial-occlusal angle
    Axial-distal angle
3. Axial-mesial-gingival angle
    Axial-mesial-occlusal angle
    Axial-distal-occlusal angle
    Axial-distal-gingival angle

A simple proximal cavity will have a nomenclature similar to that just given. In most cases the occlusal area is excised to produce a complex preparation that involves a missing wall. In this situation the proximal line (1 and 2) and point (3) angles are named in the following way:

1. Buccal-gingival angle
    Lingual-gingival angle
2. Buccal-axial angle
    Lingual-axial angle
    Axial-gingival angle

3. Axial-labial-gingival angle
    Axial-lingual-gingival angle

Because of the joining of the labial and lingual plates near the incisal edge in Class III cavities, it becomes difficult to find the incisal line angle. Usually an undercut retention form is all that is present to designate the angle as an incisal point angle.

An angle formed by the axial and pulpal walls is called an axial-pulpal line angle. These angles are found in complex cavity preparations and are noted for their ability to accumulate stresses. The location and formation of this line angle receive much attention when the cavity preparation is designed.

An understanding of the internal angle nomenclature is necessary before con sidering the cavity design. Since this system of nomenclature is workable and nearly infallible, it is unnecessary to memorize all the possibilities.

Prepared cavity wall. The prepared wall of the mortise form can be divided into parts that describe different areas. Junctions in the wall that regulate the depth of cutting have been given specific names.

Cavosurface margin. The cavosurface margin is the area formed by the cavity wall and an external tooth surface. This junction can be located in enamel or cementum. The discussion here involves the cavosurface relationships of enamel to the marginal edge of the restorative material (Fig. 3-4). When located in enamel, it is called the cavosurface margin. It is either beveled or refined to a

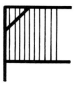

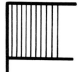

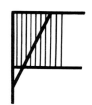

Fig. 3-4. Drawing to illustrate the cavosurface relationships necessary for restorative materials.

right-angle structure, and the terms "beveled" or "plane" cavosurface margin are used to describe whichever condition is present. The cavosurface margin surrounds the entire outline of the cavity preparation. An attempt is made to locate the margin in a clean area, and it is then refined for the purpose of supporting the restorative materials.

Enamel wall. The enamel wall is the portion of the prepared cavity wall that is enamel. It is located between the cavosurface margin and the dentinoenamel junction. The enamel is brittle, and it is prepared in a direction that is related to the histologic structure in that it is somewhat parallel with the rods. Rules are followed during the finishing of the enamel wall to remove detectable brittle or unsupported enamel.

Dentinoenamel junction. The dentinoenamel junction is the line formed by the joining of the enamel and dentin. It is used to judge the depth of the internal cavity. The intracoronal thickness of restorations is greater than the width of the enamel covering when this demarcation is passed in the cavity wall.

Dentin wall. The dentin wall is usually an extension of the enamel wall and is on the same plane. The dentin portion of the wall is resilient and contains the retention forms that are placed in the tooth for auxiliary support. Ideally, preparations end 0.2 mm. past the dentinoenamel junction, and this portion of the cavity wall, together with the axial and pulpal walls, is made up of dentin tissue.

Other helpful terms used to locate cavity or preparation areas are the various planes and surface divisions of the tooth. A dental anatomy text should be consulted if assistance is needed.

PROPERTIES OF TOOTH STRUCTURE

The tooth is composed of several kinds of tissue and therefore it is classified as an organ. The ectodermal enamel and the mesodermal dentin are formed by apposition of the cells of the embryologic layers. The enamel forms a protective shell for the crown of the tooth. The interior and major parts of the tooth are composed of dentin, which is associated with the vital functioning pulp tissue.[3]

Enamel

Enamel is the hardest known biologic substance and serves as a protective shell for the crown of the tooth.[4] Enamel has no regenerative power so that when it is penetrated by caries or fractured it must be mechanically repaired. The extreme hardness of enamel causes it to be brittle, and it is therefore prone to fracture when not supported by dentin. The hardness and structure of the enamel, which will be discussed in detail later, are complications that must be dealt with in cavity preparation.

Hydroxyapatite accounts for 95% of the weight of enamel, and organic matter and water account for the remaining 5%. The individual structural unit of enamel is known as the rod, or prism, which in cross section has a keyhole shape and is about 5μ in diameter. The prisms extend from the dentin to the external surface of the tooth and their paths take various directions. In certain areas, near the outer half of the enamel, the rods are nearly parallel, whereas closer to the dentin they are intertwined.

Each rod is surrounded by a band of organic matter known as the rod sheath. It is organic in composition and susceptible to dissolution by acid. Caries attacks this portion of the enamel to penetrate the surface by decalcification and thus reach the dentin. In addition to the rod sheath it is reported that a very fine submicroscopic organic network extends throughout the enamel.

The enamel crystals are reported to be hexagonal in shape and ribbonlike. The individual crystals are 50 to 100 Å in diameter and are estimated to be at least 1,500 Å in length. The long axes of the crystals are reportedly parallel to the direction of the rod, and there is evidence of considerable intercrystalline space. One of the problems in developing adhesion to the enamel is found in the watery organic component occupying this intercrystalline space, which complicates bond formation. It is concluded that this organic material is keratinlike in composition, which is responsible for the small degree of permeability observed in enamel.

The surface of enamel is very porous, and when viewed with an electron microscope, its appearance is like that of the surface of the moon. The voids in the enamel make it impossible to clean the tooth perfectly, and they could contribute to the initiation of caries. This also produces problems in cleaning the tooth following the cavity preparation and in creating a surface that is conducive to the bonding of the restorative material. On the other hand, the voids could also be helpful in making areas available for the interchange of ions that serve a protective purpose.

Fluoride solutions interact to change the properties of the enamel surface. Not only does solubility decrease but hardness increases in the enamel surface, regardless of its inert qualities.[5] After this occurs, methods of increasing the protective property of enamel are available and are useful in improving the physical characteristics of enamel. However, these methods are mainly useful when the tooth is forming and calcifying.

Although the enamel surface is considered to be protective, it is vulnerable to many factors present in the oral cavity. The restorative procedures are directed toward conserving the natural enamel in order to support the tooth in function and to maintain esthetics. Tooth-colored materials that are available do not exhibit the "lifelike" esthetic qualities observed in the intact enamel surface.

Through years of use the thickness of the enamel surface is gradually reduced. Attrition is caused by the abrasive action of foods and cleaning compounds and the natural rubbing of the teeth on the occlusal and proximal surfaces during mastication. The thinner enamel and the increased thickness of the dentin are considered to be physiologic phenomena that account for the slight darkening or yellowing that occurs in the teeth of aging persons. Enamel is essential in that it continues to function and provides protective contours to preserve supporting tissues. The esthetic appearance of the natural tooth is made possible by the enamel layer.

Histologic structure of enamel in relation to cavity preparation

The brittleness of enamel makes it difficult to produce a smooth cavity wall. The rough texture of the cavity wall must be refined in order to remove the unsupported enamel. The enamel remaining around the lesion is usually whiter in color and will fracture or crumble when force is applied. This enamel is removed by fracturing it with hand-cutting or rotary instruments and then it is replaced with a restoration.

As previously discussed, enamel rods are crystalline structures that are surrounded by a cementing substance. Penetration occurs through the interface between rod core and sheath (the rod sheath is acid resistant). Lack of matrix support causes the rods to be displaced from the surface and, as a result, the caries penetrates the underlying dentin. The cementing substance makes a natural area for enamel cleavage because it is weak. It has always been supposed that fracture of the enamel occurs in this area and that the separation is parallel to the enamel rod.

The rule requiring only full-length supported enamel on the cavosurface

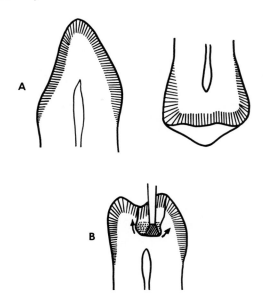

Fig. 3-5. **A,** Schematic representation of the inclination of the enamel rods that influences cavity preparation. **B,** Undermining the enamel with the inverted cone bur to complement the efficiency of tooth reduction with regular-speed burs.

margin has caused beginning students to study the inclination or direction of the enamel rods as they radiate from the dentin (Fig. 3-5). The cutting of enamel with regular-speed burs is accomplished by undermining and fracturing the enamel, while the hand instruments are used to cleave the tissue in a direction parallel to the rods. The need for sound enamel in the cavity wall has produced different wall angulations that are named for the way in which they follow the directions of cleavage lines in forming the cavity preparation.

Generally the enamel rods are not straight and exactly parallel to each other. Rather they are gnarled around the dentin surface like a pine knot bur and straighten out as they approach the external surface. The direction of the rods can be observed by etching longitudinal sections with dilute hydrochloric acid. Generally the individual rods are perpendicular to the external surface, and it is this portion of the enamel wall that guides the formation of the preparation because the rods are somewhat parallel in this area. The cavity wall angulations are determined by the direction of the surface rods.

Areas of abrupt rod turning. There are several areas in tooth reduction that require special consideration regarding the angulation of rods. Convex tooth curvatures cause abrupt turns in the direction of the rods in these areas of the tooth. Naturally this condition must be accounted for in providing a cavity wall that is supported by dentin.

Areas having abrupt rod turning include the incisal edges and the buccal cusp tips of teeth. In these areas rods turn rapidly because of the junction of two surfaces. The gingival one third of the tooth also has a great degree of curvature because of the cervical bulge areas that serve as protective contours of gingival tissue. Primary occlusal grooves in posterior teeth exhibit a rapid change in angulation. In this case the degree of curvature is favorable to the support of the tooth and the restoration. The degree of angulation can dictate the extension and occlusal width of the outline because in these areas the cavity walls are usually made parallel to each other and perpendicular to the pulpal wall. Lateral primary groove extremities are to be noted also because they take an abrupt turn to the outside of the tooth. This dictates the use of a flared wall; therefore the fissure bur is turned to accomplish the task. The occlusal marginal ridges must be considered in the simple occlusal cavity preparation. The wall next to the marginal ridge is the terminal portion of the dovetail that is extended to include the fossa area. As in the groove extremities, this wall is flared to prevent weak enamel from remaining on the margin. The lingual marginal ridge of incisors and cuspids is another area in which the rods turn rapidly. The problem involved in making the lingual wall of anterior proximal preparations is obvious. In this area the wall is angled to produce full-length enamel rods and to provide the convenience form for inserting the restorative material. As in most of the areas considered here, this wall is one in which the insertion of the restoration complements the design of the cavity preparation.

The cavosurface margin, which was discussed in the section on the enamel wall, is designed to remove loose surface rods. This procedure is performed in order to secure smooth enamel on the surface. The smoothing is accomplished regardless of the beveling used for gold restoratives and of the right-angle joint used with restorative materials weaker than enamel. The marginal finishing is proportional to the breakdown on the cavosurface area, where fracture of the entire wall is a problem involving improper flaring.

The rule for the enamel wall is that the surface rods must be supported by sound dentin or by other enamel rods. In no area, with the exception of the labial wall of anterior teeth, may enamel be left without dentin support. The fact that dentin tissue is vital and resilient generated the original theory that its function was to cushion the enamel.

Although the inclination of enamel can be studied in a number of ways, it is most helpful for the student to make hemisections of different types of teeth. The sections should be flattened and then etched with dilute hydrochloric acid to dissolve the cementing substance. Powdered graphite is rubbed onto the etched surface and the specimen can be observed under a high-power microscope. After the surface inclinations are observed in various specimens, the chisel can be used to fracture the different areas and observe the directions of cleavage.

The advent of quality carbon steel hand instruments has made the opinion that enamel can be fractured only parallel to the rods obsolete. A freshly sharpened chisel can be used with only moderate force to cut enamel in any plane.

It is thought that surface rods are gradually crushed and the enamel smoothed only by repeated applications of the cutting edge.

The description of the hard and brittle properties of enamel and the inclination of enamel rods makes the reason why the histology of the tooth must be learned self-explanatory. The fragility of calcified tissue makes the use of sharp hand instruments and slow-turning burs with light handpiece loads necessary for cavity refinement.

Dentin

Dentin is considered to be vital tissue and it serves mainly to protect the functioning pulp tissue. It accounts for most of the weight of the tooth, and it is covered by enamel in the crown and cementum in the root. Dentin tissue is an efficient thermal and chemical barrier and, when exposed, it is permeable. Normal wear or trauma to the tooth causes the dentin to respond by depositing additional tissue adjacent to the pulp. This response is a built-in protective mechanism furnished by the dentin that gradually fills in the pulp chamber to accommodate for external influences on the tooth.

Dentin contains about 70% mineral matter, 20% organic matter, and 10% water. The mineral matter is hydroxyapatite, such as that found in enamel, but the crystals in dentin are estimated to be only one tenth the size of those in enamel. Less is known about the structure of dentin than about that of enamel, but it is thought that crystal distribution is governed by the collagen matrix. The precise orientation of dentin crystals is reported to differ from that observed in enamel. The organic matrix of dentin is composed of collagen, and the dentinal tubules are more curved and irregular than those in enamel.

The histologic appearance of dentin shows a system of S-shaped tubules between the pulp and enamel. These calcified tubules surround the process or terminal fiber of the odontoblast cell, which is responsible for dentin formation. The odontoblast is characterized by having one end in contact with vital pulp and the other end touching calcified tissue. The actual mechanism of dentin formation is not known. The wall of the tubule is a highly calcified band of matrix about 1μ in width called the peritubular dentin. The process of the dentin cells is also reported to be 1μ in diameter. The system of tubules in dentin causes the tissue to be permeable.

The different types of dentin are classified according to their appearance or structure. Primary dentin is formed first and is more regular than the other types. When the tooth begins to function, the odontoblasts form secondary dentin that acts as a chemical barrier. There is evidence that the dentin is penetrated by isotopes from around the edges of restorations, which indicates that certain dyes and stains could damage the superficial portion of dentinal tissue. The dentin, however, is considered an effective barrier that is helpful in neutralizing and blocking the chemical constituents of restorative materials.

After tooth eruption the primary dentin becomes sealed and inert and can show radiographic changes. If it changes, the tissue becomes calcified or vacuolated and is called sclerotic or translucent dentin.

Secondary dentin continues to be formed throughout the life of the tooth because it is stimulated by attritional factors. The main deposits of secondary dentin are on the occlusal surface of the tooth and inside the proximal contact areas. Its formation is accelerated when caries attacks the tooth and microorganisms invade the tubules. The protective action of secondary dentin is confined to the wall in the area where the tubules are penetrated.

Cavity preparation causes the third type of dentin, reparative dentin, to be formed. The cutting action of the bur is associated with pressure and temperature that cause the formation of "osteoidlike" material below the wall of the preparation. This material is called traumatic dentin. Its formation has been attributed to osteoblastic type cells, and its structure resembles the calcific bridges that result from capping procedures. Traumatic dentin also serves to protect pulp tissue in time of need and at the site of injury.[6]

Thermal insulation is another advantage derived from having a layer of dentin under the restoration. The tissue is a poor thermal conductor, having a value of 2.29×10^{-3}, which is comparable to the thermal conductivity of glass, concrete, and zinc phosphate cement.[7] The dentin tissue prevents temperature transfer from the bur during cavity preparation and its thermal transfer is much lower than the value of metallic restorative materials. Thermal conductivity is often a problem for 2 to 4 weeks following the insertion of a deep restoration. After this time the response decreases because more dentin has formed next to the pulp to provide additional insulation.

The severity of the pulp response to heat has been studied. Temperatures up to 600° F. on dentin surfaces did not prevent recovery of the pulp tissue from injury.[8] The elevation of temperature during cavity preparation is not believed to reach this figure, but the protection against damaging temperatures is revealed by the data.

Research has demonstrated that the thickness of the remaining dentin (RD) is directly related to the success of the restoration. It has been stated that if 2 mm. of dentin are preserved between the wall of the cavity preparation and the pulp the trauma will be resolved regardless of the way in which the tooth is restored.[9] The preservation of dentin is therefore a major goal in cavity design and in the selection of restorative material because it preserves the vitality of the pulp.

Many different surface configurations and chemical compositions of tooth structure have been presented to point out the considerations that are necessary in surgical procedures. Cavity preparation will produce many relationships with the histologic structures of enamel and dentin. The chemical nature and cleansing difficulties of these structures are considered deterrents in the development of a truly adhesive restorative material. The material presented points out the necessity of reliance on mechanical factors when restoring the individual tooth.

PRINCIPLES OF CAVITY PREPARATION

The cavity preparation is the foundation of the restoration, and the thoroughness of the preparation naturally determines the success of the operative procedure. Rotary and hand-cutting instruments are employed to prepare the tooth to receive and support the restoration. In each preparation a biologic outline must be developed to prevent recurrent caries at the edge of the restoration; certain depths and angulations in the cavity walls are needed to support and retain the restorative material after it is placed in the tooth. To develop an orderly procedure and satisfy the requirements of different cavity designs, specific principles must be followed for each restoration.

For half a century cavity preparation was a "slipshod" procedure. When instrumentation was improved, issues concerning extension, contour, outlines, and separation were raised. The publications by Black were the first in which the methods of tooth reduction were refined and categorized. He is responsible for the rules of extension and for the boxlike mortise forms that are designed for all teeth. Black listed instrumentation sequences for each type of preparation, and these principles have served as guides in operative dentistry for three quarters of a century. Although the techniques have been refined and outlines have been modified, Black's principles are still used in each preparation and therefore must be mastered prior to patient treatment.

The principles of cavity preparation are listed and defined as follows[1]:

1. Outline form—the shape and border of the restoration that is curved on the tooth surface
2. Resistance form—the thickness and form given to the restoration and tooth to prevent fracture of either structure
3. Retention form—properties placed in the tooth structure to prevent dislodgement of the restoration
4. Convenience form—methods used to prepare the cavity to gain access for inserting and finishing the restorative material
5. Removal of caries—procedure of removing decayed and decalcified enamel and dentin; if necessary, followed by placement of intermediary bases
6. Finish of the enamel wall—process of smoothing, angling, and beveling the walls of the cavity preparation
7. Toilet of the cavity preparation—the cleaning of the preparation following instrumentation, including the removal of tooth particles and any other sediment remaining in the preparation as well as the application of liners and medicaments to enhance restorative properties or to protect the pulp

An attempt should be made to complete each step in the order it is listed, although it will sometimes be necessary to remove caries following the outline form to determine the depth and extent of the lesion. Modern instrumentation accomplishes a number of these principles in a short time.

The principles of cavity preparation are discussed on a biomechanical basis.[10] They are either concerned with the biologic processes of tissue or with the mechanical factors that complement the physical properties of the restorative material. The biologic principles include the outline form and the removal of caries. These two procedures are concerned with locating the margin in immune areas, controlling the bacteriology of caries, and protecting the vital pulp. The hard and soft tissues are preserved in order to promote the relationship of the tooth and peripheral circulation. When this fails, vitality in the tissues is terminated and the tooth is usually lost.

Mechanical procedures protect the restoration and support the tooth. In the management of tooth structure the utilization of engineering principles with exacting instrumentation satisfies the principles of retention, resistance form, and finish of the enamel wall. Definitely shaped cutting instruments are used to place the forms in tooth structure. The cavity depth and the cutting method used should not interfere with the biologic processes previously discussed. Mechanical factors are not as important when considering the health of the tooth as the biologic factors, but they are vital in protecting the restoration.

A conservative approach is followed in reducing the tooth.[11,12] Reduction is concerned mostly with the mechanical factors of cavity depth and wall angulation. These factors must be in keeping with the outline form and are varied according to the physical properties of the restorative material. Enamel has no regenerative power and conservative measures are used for this reason. The rule that "the tooth is prepared minimally to satisfy the requirements of the restorative material" should be followed.

It is often possible to estimate the size of the finished preparation. To do this the variables of size, shape, and location of the tooth and the caries involvement are observed. Pulp size is also a variable, and the need for bases on axial-pulpal walls is considered. Tooth morphology and the extent of the caries can be determined by radiographs and clinical examination. Cavity preparation is not started until the extent of the reduction is estimated.

Outline form

The outline form is the shape of the marginal area of the preparation, and it is determined by many factors. The outline encompasses the carious lesion and the caries-susceptible areas on the surface being restored. The margins are located on smooth tooth structures that are either cleaned naturally during mastication or that can be reached by hygienic devices. To include these areas the outline form results in a gentle, sweeping curve on the tooth surface. It appears to be harmonious and is designed for esthetics as well as for the prevention of recurrent caries. Since the restorative materials do not have antibacterial properties, cleaning the margin is an excellent way of preventing plaque from forming in the cavosurface area.

Factors influencing the outline form

The cavosurface relationship is part of the outline form. A clean enamel margin is made to protect the tooth, but the relationship is dictated by the physical properties of the restorative material. The cavosurface is beveled when materials that are stronger than the tooth are used. If weaker materials are used, the cavosurface is refined to a 90-degree angle. Gold restoratives are the only preparations that require beveling the cavosurface margin. Enamel on the marginal outline is supported by subjacent enamel and by dentin. Finding the supported wall influences the width of the outline form.

Another group of factors that helps determine the outline form are the rules governing "extension for prevention" or "cutting for immunity." These factors dictate where the final cavity outline will be located. The preparation is extended through caries-susceptible areas that contact the edge of the carious lesion. Because of extension the outline form occupies a greater surface area than does the caries.

Since extension for prevention means cutting the cavity to include the susceptible areas within the outline, these areas must be understood in order to determine the outline form. Tooth areas that are caries-susceptible include the poorly coalesced primary and secondary grooves on the occlusal surfaces of the posterior teeth as well as the buccal and lingual extension of these grooves and the pits in the lingual surfaces of the upper incisor teeth. In addition the proximal surfaces of all teeth just below the contact area and in an area just inside the line angle of the tooth are caries-susceptible, as are the buccal and lingual surfaces below the height of contour and the surface along the border of the gingival tissue.

Caries-immune areas are found on smooth surfaces about the height of contour. These areas include the cusp planes, buccal and lingual surfaces, incisal edges, and cusp tips, all of which are constantly cleaned by mastication. These areas are included in the outline only when the "self-cleansing" enamel has been undermined by caries.

The importance of adequate extension was pointed out in a study of recurrent caries; the survey included over 5,000 restored surfaces in the teeth of naval recruits. Laswell found that secondary caries occurs more frequently in some areas than initial lesions.[13] The data suggested that the margins of restorations, a majority of which were amalgam, are more prone to caries than are susceptible enamel surfaces, making the recurrence incidence higher than that attributed to this area of liability. Areas observed to have a high incidence of secondary lesions were the buccal surfaces of the upper molars and the lingual surfaces of the lower molars. Secondary caries was often located in inadequately extended occlusal grooves. These statistics point out the dangers in inadequately extending the cavity preparation (Fig. 3-6). Regardless of the classification or tooth, there are immune boundaries that need to be reached in the outline form.

The mechanism of caries and the differences in the shape of pit and fissure and smooth surface types of lesions were discussed previously. The greater amount of undermined enamel associated with the pit and fissure lesion accounts for the difference in shape. The criteria to follow in making the outline form include (1) the surface involvement of the enamel (usually a decalcification), (2) the lateral spread of caries at the dentinoenamel junction (degree of undermining), and (3) the areas involved in extension for prevention (placing the margin in immune areas). The first two criteria are regulated by the lesion, while the last, cavity extension, is regulated by the anatomy of the involved surface.

Pit and fissure outlines are extended through uncoalesced grooves and are placed on cusp planes and marginal ridges. The margin is located just outside the stain line to assure oral cleaning. Some secondary grooves usually need to be excised, causing the occlusal outline to rest on the cusp planes in depressions

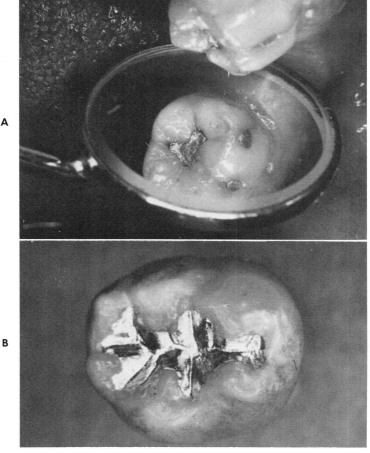

A

B

Continued.

Fig. 3-6. A, Failure of amalgam restoration because of improper "extension for prevention." **B,** Desirable occlusal outline form that obliterates the caries-susceptible areas of the surface. **C,** Desirable occlusal outline form. **D,** Occlusal amalgam restorations on molars, with lingual extensions for pre-carious grooves.

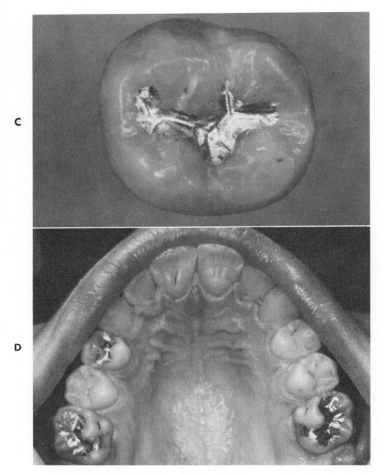

Fig. 3-6, cont'd. For legend see p. 83.

where the grooves end. A butterfly design ending in a dovetail is characteristic of the occlusal preparation. The design of the outline in this case is dictated by the caries and by the anatomic configuration of the occlusal surface.

The proximal surfaces of posterior teeth require extension to more definite areas. Proximal caries is more confined and results in a standardized proximal outline. The buccal and lingual walls are located outside the embrasure but neatly inside the line angles of the tooth. The gingival wall usually terminates below the crest of the gingival tissue. Loss or disease of the gingival tissue necessitates placing the wall near the cementoenamel junction rather than unduly extending the tooth in a cervical direction.

In order to preserve self-cleansing the buccal and lingual proximal margins must be out of contact with the adjacent tooth (Fig. 3-7). This means that the design of the posterior proximal outline is dictated by the caries, the surface

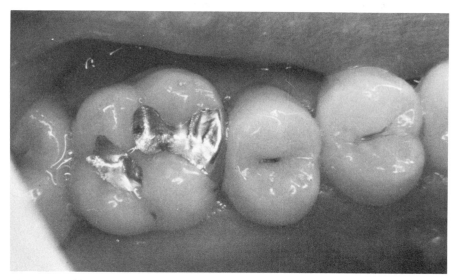

Fig. 3-7. Desirable proximal outline form in which the margins, being out of contact with the adjacent tooth, can be cleaned yet will be somewhat protected from stress.

contour, and the location of the adjacent tooth. The actual size and form of the contact area, the embrasures, and the location of the gingival tissue are observed in order to determine the proximal outline. Extension is also needed to insert the matrix band and to polish and carve the restoration. The proximal outline is a definite structure that is aligned with the occlusal margin to decrease the exposed surface area and to join the two surfaces of the restoration.

Prophylactic odontotomy is included in a discussion of the outline form.[14] In 1933 the Hyatt research group in New York advocated that the defective occlusal surfaces of posterior teeth be restored or polished, depending on the configuration of the groove. The purpose of this procedure is to remove the nidus for caries and to restore the tooth conservatively before lesions have a chance to develop. The procedure is still used by some, but since most precarious areas are not conducive to polishing, they are usually restored instead. The concept is preventive in nature in that the tooth is restored before caries develops.

The polishing technique of prophylactic odontotomy cannot be used often. It is accomplished by cutting and polishing the tooth structure to remove poorly coalesced grooves. A small round bur is placed in the pit or groove and the enamel is opened until the bottom of the fissure can be examined. If enamel is on the floor of the groove, a larger size round bur is pushed through the groove, gradually opening the area to a point at which it can be artificially cleaned. Groove polishing is not permitted often because of the contour of most occlusal surfaces (the cusp planes are too steep) and because exposed dentin is usually present in the bottom of the opened groove, presenting another disadvantage.

The use of prophylactic odontotomy has declined. Other preventive measures, mainly the use of topical fluoride and sealants, are proving to be beneficial. These other preventive measures protect pre-carious areas from decalcification, and if the enamel is broken, the fluoride limits the size of the lesion, encouraging an ideal outline form. This type of preventive care avoids needless restorations.

The anterior proximal outline follows the same general rules as the posterior proximal outline. The walls must be located out of contact with the adjacent tooth, but they must also conform to esthetic requirements. Labial and lingual walls are located outside the embrasure and inside line angles, with the labial wall being more limited. Anterior teeth are easier to clean and most insertion procedures are begun from the lingual wall to make it possible to preserve the labial enamel. The gingival wall is again located below the tissue or close to the cementoenamel line in cases in which an acceptable condition does not exist.

The Class III preparation is triangular in shape, and efforts are made to preserve the contact point and incisal edge. Extension in this location varies with the shape of the tooth, and it does not always result in taking the margin out of contact with the adjacent tooth. This is possible only in ovoid teeth where more proximal curvature exists. On square or tapering teeth only the upper half of the contact is removed to prevent fracture of the incisal edge. This embrasure does not present a problem in cleaning and the wall should be removed only far enough to satisfy the requirements of esthetics and convenience.

The gingival restoration also requires a certain amount of extension. The lesion is located along the gingival tissue, dictating that all margins of the typical outline, with the exception of the occlusal margin, be placed below the tissue. When the typical Class V outline is not used, the lesion should be restored as a pit lesion and made as small as possible.

The typical Class V outline is extended to the height of contour in an occlusal direction. The excursive action of food will clean the margin in this location. Mesial and distal margins are extended past the line angles and end below the gingival papillae. The cervical wall is located below the healthy tissue where it can be protected from the accumulation of food. If the proper cervical bulge is placed in the restoration, food particles will be shunted over the soft tissue, minimizing the accumulation of food material.

There are other factors that influence the shape and size of the outline form. The patient variables of age, caries liability, and saliva properties and the type of restorative material that is used are factors to be considered in extension for prevention. The need for adequate cleansing of the restoration and the type of outline that is suitable from an esthetic standpoint must be taken into account in selecting some restorative materials. Following are the secondary factors regulating cavity extension:

1. When a conservative approach is followed in treatment, the cavity is prepared in such a way as to save all immune and functioning tooth structures.[15] The histologic structure of the enamel rods is followed to flare the walls in groove extremities and dovetails and to make the outline parallel with the marginal ridges.[16] When possible the buccal and lingual extensions are restored as pits and not as steps. The oblique and marginal ridges are left intact when they are well coalesced to maintain the integrity of the tooth. Fine and delicate instruments are used to place the final margin in order to avoid unnecessary cutting and overextension of the tooth. This concept of conservative care is used when the oral cavity is relatively caries-free or in conjunction with a thorough preventive program.

2. Enamel etchings are included in the outline form. When an occlusal lesion is restored and the proximal surface is decalcified, the outline is made into a complex preparation. Chances of breakdown and enamel penetration are apt to occur later, and the outline is made conservatively by including the incipient lesion.

3. Different types of restorative materials are used with different extensions. Direct gold and amalgam restorations are treated conservatively because of esthetic problems and limited marginal strength. The cast inlay is more extended in order to promote better marginal cleaning and to facilitate the polishing of the metal. The tooth-colored materials are placed in limited extensions because of the short clinical life associated with silicate cement and resins. The outline is limited when materials having anticariogenic properties are used.

4. Access is produced by extending the outline form or by flaring the enamel wall. To gain access the margin can be extended to enable the instrumentation for the internal wall design and the insertion of the material to be accomplished. Extension for access is done in those areas not visible to the observer.

5. Tooth size and arch position influence the design to be used. Rotated teeth have unusual outlines because they must be restored out of contact with the adjacent tooth. Steep cusp inclines require extra extension, but typical gingival contours and tissue relationships allow a typical outline to be used.

6. Esthetic requirements also dictate the use of special outlines. Cohesive, gold castings and amalgam restorations can be refined only to avoid an unnecessary display of metal. Rapid separation is occasionally used to limit the outline form, and when this is not possible, tooth-colored materials are used.

7. Tooth cleansing influences the extension of the outline form. Poor patient motivation and salivary and dietary problems influence the type of cleaning the tooth receives. More extension is required when these factors cannot be controlled.

The outline form is the border between the restoration and the tooth. Problems in smoothing the enamel and placing a precise restoration have resulted in locating the margin in protected areas. The outline form is critical and the preparation is not started until the design is estimated.

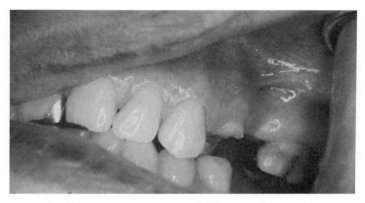

Fig. 3-8. Failure of the resistance form in the bicuspid as noted by the loss of the restoration and a part of the tooth.

Resistance form

The resistance form should prevent fracture of the restoration or of the tooth (Fig. 3-8). This is accomplished by placing the mortise form in the tooth and applying some engineering principles. The thickness of the restoration and the design of the cavity walls are intended to divert or absorb stresses. Failure of resistance form is noted by a fractured restoration that remains locked in the preparation or by the loss of a large portion of the tooth such as the cusp or buccal surface.

Factors influencing the resistance form

There are several factors that influence the resistance form. For instance, internal cavity walls are prepared in such a way that they join at perpendicular and parallel directions to the line of force, and definite full-length walls are produced in order to complement resistance. Cavity depth is adequately placed in order to develop an occlusal-cervical thickness of the restorative material. Internal line angles of the mortise form are definite and rounded. Physical properties of the restorative material also influence resistance. Metal restorations are suitable only for stresses in posterior teeth or in other places where there is a direct application of force. Finally, the type of leverage placed on the restoration is related to resistance. The surface area in Class II and Class IV restorations is increased to reduce the leverage and resultant torque.[17]

These properties are closely related to retentive qualities and sometimes overlap in discussion. The use of conservative measures in the width, not the depth, of the mortise form maintains the resistance form of the treated tooth most satisfactorily. The depth, not the width, of the axial and pulpal walls complements resistance.

Force normally occurs in a direction parallel to the long axis of posterior teeth, and the internal walls are made perpendicular and parallel to this direc-

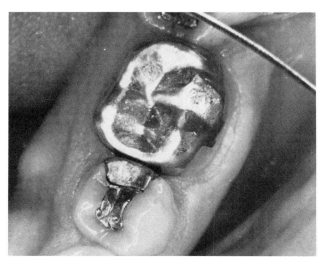

Fig. 3-9. Failure of the resistance form because lack of proper cavity depth resulted in isthmus fracture.

tion. Pulpal and cervical walls are made flat and perpendicular to the axial wall. These and the other surrounding cavity walls constitute the footing for the absorption of stress. The surrounding walls are made parallel to the line of force or to the axial walls. Exceptions are made in cases in which the walls are flared, but this is necessary to protect tooth structure. This architecture will resist the occlusal force of mastication that is developed in the centric contacts and prevent breakage of the tooth when the shear forces are applied during function.

The proper thickness of restorative materials is assured when the axial and pulpal walls are placed 0.2 mm. within the dentinoenamel junction. The tooth is prepared to this depth or based out to the measurement for protection of the pulp. This cavity depth is accepted as adequate if normal occlusal forces are placed on the tooth and maximum strength properties are present in the restoration. Resistance form is best provided by cavity depth, not width, because extra-buccal and lingual extension weakens the cusps (Fig. 3-9).

Angulation of the walls of the mortise form affects resistance. A "dish-shaped" cavity is not conducive to good support and results in dislodgment. The angulation factor is associated closely with frictional wall retention. Inlay preparations that are purposely tapered for withdrawal and insertion must not be overdone. The highly tapered inlay presents a problem because it is continually being dislodged since it has poor resistance form and little retention form.

Line angles prevent rotation of the restoration out of the prepared cavity. Demarcation of the walls is produced in order to make the internal dimensions exact, and line angle placement is helpful in establishing uniform depth of pulpal and axial walls.

The type of material that is used influences the resistance form of the restoration and the internal design. If the tensile and compressive strengths are high, the material can be used in a preparation with less boxing. The gold inlay is limited in depth for conservative purposes because it is retained with auxiliaries, posts, and surface coverage. Silver amalgam is brittle and requires a boxed form to create thickness both in the body and in the margin of the restoration.

Class III restorations are noted for being difficult to retain. Because of the small bulk of tooth structure in incisors, the resistance form is difficult to make. The forces on maxillary incisors are placed on the lingual surface and to counteract this the labial wall is preserved. The gingival and lingual walls are shaped at right angles to the axial wall, but not much stability is gained from this procedure. Mechanical undercuts keep the restoration seated better than angulation of the cavity walls.

The resistance form completes most of the cavity excavation. The remaining principles of cavity preparation are satisfied by refining the mortise form.

Retention form

The purpose of the retention form is to prevent dislodgment of the restoration. Prevention of dislodgment of the restoration is equally important to the resistance form and is accomplished by some type of mechanical interlocking between the cavity wall and the restorative material.

Types of retention forms

The retention form includes (1) frictional wall retention, (2) mechanical undercuts, and (3) accessory forms of grooves, postholes and dovetails, and pins.

Frictional wall retention is caused by the interlocking of the filling material. Within reason, the rougher the cavity wall, the better the retention of the restoration. Surface apposition or interlocking is related to particle size and technique, and it is the greatest factor complementing retention form. Angulation of the cavity wall provides greater resistance, but parallel walls and intimate interlocking are the ideal properties for retaining the restoration. The cavity wall is not purposely roughened or grossly undercut to satisfy the principles of cavity preparation; regular instrumentation creates the rough wall.

Mechanical undercuts are placed in the corners and extremities of the preparation. In some cases they serve as point angles or convenience points for beginning the direct gold restoration. They are placed in the dentin and should not be overdone because of the undermining that would be produced in the enamel. The undercuts are not useful if the procedure that is used does not fill the forms with the restorative material.

When other methods are not available for retention, as in the extensive lesion, grooves and postholes can be used. These are primarily used and discussed with inlay restorations. As the length of the groove and the posthole is increased, the casting becomes more retentive. A number of these auxiliaries can be used in con-

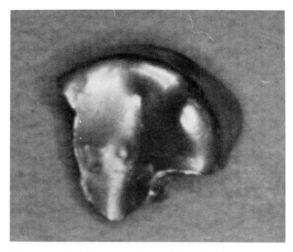

Fig. 3-10. Failure of the retention form as observed by displacement of the intact restoration from the tooth.

junction with dovetails or retentive boxes when the retention is increased. The abutment tooth is modified to produce more than usual retention in order to prevent dislodgment of the restorative material during surface reduction for full-coverage restorations.

The Class II and Class IV restorations have been discussed in connection with leverage produced on the restorations. Three types of levers are possible, and they produce different mechanical advantages. In the Class II and Class IV restorations the dovetail and posthole are placed as far away from the cervical wall as possible to resist the forces of the Class I and Class II levers.[17] This is accomplished by added extension and is very helpful in retaining the restoration. The levers cause torque to develop, which dislodges the casting (Fig. 3-10).

Retention form has been improved by the use of pins. There are several types of pins and procedures that are used for extra retention of the amalgam restoration. The use of parallel pins with the gold casting has been popularized, as well as the use of pin retention with plastic restorations in anterior teeth. These pins are useful in a large restoration, but they are only auxiliary methods and should not cause the other principles to be sacrificed.

Convenience form

Gaining access to prepare the tooth and insert the restoration is essential. Many methods can be used that are helpful, and no preparation is advocated that has walls that cannot be reached. This means that at one time or another all the parts of the preparation must be observed to determine whether the principles of cavity preparation have been established. Such observation is a requirement for the construction of the internal form and for the insertion of the prepared material.

Methods of obtaining the convenience form

Following is a list of methods for obtaining the convenience form.

1. *Extending the cavity preparation.* The tooth can be prepared to allow access to caries and dentin. This is done by varying the angulation of the wall or by removing sound enamel.
2. *Selection of instruments.* The use of smaller or specially designed instruments enables the cavity to be prepared when surfaces are difficult to reach. The contra-angle handpiece is an example of this type of instrument.
3. *Mechanical methods.* The application of slow and rapid separation and gingival retraction can provide convenience in making the cavity preparation.

Many of the preparations for cohesive gold restorations utilize a number of factors in producing convenience. The walls of the preparation are flared to allow entry of the hand instruments for shaping the dentin. The teeth are sometimes separated to prevent an excessive display of gold on the labial surfaces. The design of special gold condensers, namely the Ferrier and Woodbury series, provides excellent access to the preparations for building the gold restoration. Jeffery's concept of "lingual approach" utilizes a special preparation and instrumentation for developing an esthetic gold foil restoration.

Lesions on the buccal and lingual surfaces of second molars usually have limited access. If the lesion cannot be reached when the patient opens his mouth, sound tissue must occasionally be sacrificed in order to operate on the tooth. Cusp removal or overextension of the carious surface is occasionally required to reach the bottom of the carious lesion. The extra reduction is not desirable because of the liability of the surface to secondary caries. However, when the tooth cannot be retained in any other way, this method must be used. The ramus of the mandible prevents proper use of the handpiece in this situation.

Miniature contra-angle handpieces and short burs can be placed in areas where there is reduced operating room. These instruments are available for both air turbines and regular-speed power sources and are useful in the second molar regions. Pedodontists use these handpieces routinely and the same convenience is provided in adult patients who have difficulty in opening the mouth wide enough.

Hand-cutting instruments are made in various sizes. Measurements vary from one manufacturer to the other, but generally the smaller the instrument the more delicately it is used. The preparations requiring convenience form are usually critical in outline and indicate that the small-dimension hand-cutting instruments be employed. Duplicates of small chisels, monangles, hatchets, and angle formers should be obtained because there is seldom need of large hand-cutting instruments. The carbon steel alloy has resulted in a long life for instruments, even when they are sharpened as indicated.

Convenience form is necessary for the operative procedure because without access the proper dimensions and refinement cannot be placed.

Removal of caries

The permanent restoration should not be placed until all the caries has been removed from the lesion. Carious material is infectious tissue that is soft or spongy, making it unsuitable for the foundation of the restoration, and it is removed to produce a solid dentin wall. The excavation is often stained by chromatogenic bacteria, but this area is not removed because it is solid dentin. It is claimed by some investigators to be the sterile portion of the lesion.

Complete caries removal is necessary to determine the proximity of the pulp and the need for basing. Deep cavities are prophylactically lined with calcium hydroxide, but if an exposure is found, some type of endodontic therapy is usually planned. Pulp capping promotes healing of the pulp in the undetected exposure and stimulates the deposit of secondary dentin. The prognosis would be poor if these conditions were not made possible by complete excavation.

Other problems could occur if active caries was left under the restoration. Studies have demonstrated that caries development stops when the lesion is sealed but that the organisms remain viable.[18] Any time the bacteria receive nutrients the caries activity is stimulated, and this could happen in the clinical situation. The restoration covering microorganisms could fracture, causing fluids to penetrate the residual caries. This condition would be impossible to detect and caries development would be accelerated (more so than in the normal lesion) within a short period of time. This possibility is another reason why the tooth is thoroughly excavated and cleaned prior to the insertion of any restorative material.

In the previous chapter techniques were described for sealing caries in the tooth for a 4- to 6-week period. Gross caries removal or indirect pulp therapy is used in the patient with acute caries, and these procedures should not be confused with the principle of caries removal.[19] Gross removal is used to rehabilitate the patient at the onset of treatment by removing the caries, adjusting the diet, improving the toothbrushing techniques, and altering the bacterial flora in the mouth. When gross removal is performed, the teeth with temporary restorations and residual caries are completely excavated after secondary dentin is formed. Then permanent types of restorations are placed over the excavated dentin, following the rules just advocated.

Removal of caries eliminates irritants to tooth structure. The fact that carious tissue is soft and diseased makes it incompatible with the restoration.

Finish of the enamel wall

Finishing the enamel wall is the most delicate phase of cavity refinement. The walls are smoothed to a certain extent regardless of the type of material being used. The final angulation of the wall is done during the planing and finishing stage.

Special attention is now given to the cavosurface margin. It is either refined to a right angle or beveled to complement the physical properties of the selected restoration. This procedure is also performed to protect the tooth and requires minimal instrumentation. It is impossible to produce a perfectly smoothed wall, but methods can be employed to remove gross discrepancies. The combined use of regular-speed rotary and sharp hand-cutting instruments is the method of choice for finishing the cavity wall.

The adaptation of certain materials has been improved by a roughened cavity wall. More interlocking probably occurs with the use of amalgam as a result of the increase in the surface area of the wall. This improved adaptation to a rough surface dictates that the bottom portion of the wall be designed for this purpose. This procedure is routine for the amalgam restoration. The rim of enamel, however, is smoothed in all preparations to produce the best possible cavosurface margin. The smoothed and definite cavity wall enhances all the principles of cavity preparation.[20]

Toilet of the cavity

Cleaning the finished preparation is the last principle to be accomplished. Black strongly advocated that no tooth should be restored that was not cleaned and dried for inspection. Cleaning out the debris such as tooth chips, blood, saliva, and mucin in the cavity enhances the adaptation of the restoration to the cavity wall. Lack of cavity cleaning is considered a deterrent to the development of material that bonds to the tooth. Contamination is lessened by using the rubber dam to isolate the tooth.

Many types of cleaning agents and medicaments have been used for cleaning the cavity. Nothing should be used as a cavity wash that is irritating because of the potential damage to the pulp and gingival tissue. The cleaning agent of common choice is 3% hydrogen peroxide applied directly from the unit spray. The peroxide solution is effective in removing contamination inside the prepared cavity. This solution is also used during the cavity preparation to improve the surgical field.

Warm applications of air are used to complete the cleaning procedure. The tooth is thoroughly dried and examined with a sharp explorer. The tip of the explorer is placed in the retentions to clean out the sediment, and the air is again applied until the degree of cleanliness is acceptable. The final inspection is made with magnification and if corrections are needed they should be minimal.

• • •

Cavity preparation is a surgical procedure governed by certain principles. These principles include biomechanical factors that are universally accepted by the profession. The application of sound principles is characteristic of all health professions and will always be required in cavity preparation unless dental caries and restorative materials are both drastically changed.

INSTRUMENTATION USED TO ACCOMPLISH THE PRINCIPLES

The various instrumentations used to achieve the principles of cavity preparation are as follows:

1. Outline form—The Black method, using a No. ½ round bur entry and No. 34 inverted cone bur extension in regular-speed rotary instruments operating at 6,000 rpm, is accepted. For ultraspeed rotary instruments of 250,000 rpm the small fissure burs (Nos. 556, 557, 699, and 700) are used.

2. Resistance form—Regular-speed fissure burs (Nos. 557 and 701) are used. Some of the mortise form is made with hand-cutting chisels and enamel hatchets.

3. Retention form—Undercuts are placed with a No. 33½ inverted cone bur and postholes with a No. 700 inverted cone bur and Spirec burs, all of which are operated within regular-speed range.

4. Convenience form—Small delicate hand instruments and small fissure burs are accepted. The straight handpiece bur is employed for convenience because the longer and thinner shank of the bur is helpful in anterior preparations.

5. Removal of caries—The initial large amounts of carious material are removed with a spoon excavator. Residual caries is removed with the large round burs (Nos. 4 to 6) revolving at the lowest speed possible.

6. Finish of the enamel wall—The plane fissure burs operating at the lowest regular speed are used for smoothing. The margin is refined with sharp chisels following the use of the bur.

7. Toilet of the cavity—Pledgets of cotton saturated with 3% hydrogen peroxide are acceptable for cleaning the finished preparation.

Favorite instruments and procedures can be used by the experienced operator. During the evaluation of instrumentation that is accepted for these tasks, the steps listed are closely followed and the instruments are used at regular speeds.

REFERENCES

1. Black, G. V.: Operative dentistry, ed. 3, Chicago, 1917, Medico-Dental Publishing Co., vol. 2.
2. McGeehee, W. H., True, H. A., and Inskipp, E. F.: A textbook of operative dentistry, ed. 4, New York, 1956, McGraw-Hill Book Co., Inc.
3. Bhaskar, S. N.: Synopsis of oral histology, ed. 3, St. Louis, 1969, The C. V. Mosby Co.
4. Adhesive restorative materials, requirements and test methods, Publication No. 1433, Washington, D. C., 1969, U. S. Public Health Service.
5. Phillips, R. W., and Swartz, M. L.: Additional studies on the effect of fluorides on the hardness of enamel, J.A.D.A. **40**:513, 1950.
6. Sicher, H., and Bhaskar, S. N.: Orban's oral histology and embryology, ed. 7, St. Louis, 1972, The C. V. Mosby Co.
7. Lisonti, V. F., and Zander, H. A.: Thermal conductivity of dentin, J. Dent. Res. **29**:493, 1950.
8. Zach, L., and Cohen, G.: Thermogenesis in operative techniques, J. Prosth. Dent. **12**:977, 1962.
9. Stanley, H. R.: Changing concepts of the dental pulp based on recent investigations, J. Dist. Columbia Dent. Soc. **37**:6, 1962.
10. Ingraham, R.: The application of sound biomechanical principles in the design of inlay, amalgam and gold foil restorations, J.A.D.A. **40**:402, 1950.
11. Ryge, G., Foley, D. E., and Fairhurst, C. W.: Micro-indentation hardness, J. Dent. Res. **40**:1116, 1961.

12. Craig, R. G., Gehring, P. E., and Peyton, F. A.: Relation of structure to the microhardness of human dentin, J. Dent. Res. **38**:642, 1959.
13. Laswell, H. L.: A prevalence study of secondary caries occurring in a young adult male population, M.S.D. thesis, Indianapolis, 1966, Indiana University School of Dentistry,
14. Hyatt Study Club of New York: Prophylactic odontotomy, New York, 1933, The Macmillan Co.
15. Hollenback, G. M.: A plea for a more conservative approach in certain dental procedures, J. Alabama Dent. Assoc. **46**:16, 1962.
16. Mahler, D. B., and Terkla, L. G.: Relationship of cavity design to restorative materials, Den. Clin. N. Am., Mar. 1965, pp. 149-157.
17. Randolph, K. V.: Principles of mechanical retention of restorations, W. Virginia Dent. J. **38**:2, 1964.
18. Besic, F. C.: Fate of bacteria sealed in dental cavities, J. Dent. Res. **22**:349, 1943.
19. Massler, M.: Indirect pulp capping and vital pulpotomy for potential and actual pulp exposures, J. Tennessee Dent. Assoc. **35**:393, 1955.
20. Charbeneau, G. T., Peyton, F. A., and Anthony, D. H.: Profile characteristics of cut tooth surfaces developed by rotating instruments, J. Dent. Res. **3**:957, 1957.

chapter 4

Instrumentation

Tooth reduction is complicated by factors not often associated with other surgical procedures. The arrangement of the teeth and surrounding structures causes problems of convenience and lighting. The area of the tooth being restored must be in full vision, and access to the limits of the preparation must be accomplished with the selected instruments. Since the tooth is the hardest biologic substance, the instruments must be sufficiently hard to fracture, mill, or grind the enamel and dentin. The exacting surgical procedures are accomplished by using an efficiently designed set of rotary and hand-cutting instruments.

The methods and philosophy of tooth reduction have changed significantly in the last decade. The first foot-operated and electric engines for rotary cutting used large burs to excise the tooth, which resulted in rough cavity walls, vibration, and pulp stimulation. The hand instruments commonly used at this time had large cutting edges that assisted rotary cutting by grossly fracturing the unsupported enamel. The preparations were not as refined as present ones because the methods used occasionally resulted in what is now considered "overextended preparations." Hand instrumentation was used to reduce the amount of rotary cutting rather than to refine the preparation.

Through the years an evaluation of high-speed rotary cutting has led to the development of a system for preparations that enables ideal dimensions to be accomplished with less effort and trauma. The ultraspeed method, in which the air turbine is commonly used, produces an ideal cavity form, and it has gained wide acceptance by the profession. Regular-speed rotary and hand instruments are still necessary, but only for refinement. Cutting instruments commonly used for refinement have been reduced in size for greater precision. The present-day system of cavity preparation with its improvements in design and cutting efficiency makes possible longer lasting restorations, a much needed improvement since people today retain their natural dentition longer.

Standardization of design and specific usage of instruments are helpful for both rotary and hand-cutting instruments. The instruments are classified by a system of nomenclature and dimension, used in an orderly sequence, and stored in regular places in the cabinet for ready use. The degree of proficiency and the quality of the work depend on maintenance of the instruments. The conscientious dental surgeon will use an adequate number of instruments and keep them clean and sharpened at all times. Only hand instruments with sharp cutting edges should be used.

The design, classification, and application of the hand and rotary instruments will be discussed to assist the student in mastering instrumentation.

HAND-CUTTING INSTRUMENTS
Manufacturing process

Hand instruments are used to assist in cavity preparation and to insert or finish the restorative material. They contain a handle (or shaft), a shank, and a cutting edge or working point (also called a nib). Initially many types and shapes of instruments were used, which made the teaching of cavity preparation difficult. The present identification system was established by Black and is the only one used for hand instruments. The purpose was to establish a system of nomenclature and to standardize the manufacture of hand-cutting instruments.

The metal used for hand-cutting instruments must be hard but not too brittle for cutting the tooth. The ideal metals to use are alloys of carbon steel. The alloy used by most manufacturers contains iron and 0.5% to 1.5% carbon. This carbon steel alloy is characterized by its sharpness, but it has the disadvantage of being susceptible to corrosion in metallic salt solutions. Also, careful handling is necessary because if these instruments are dropped they will probably fracture. These disadvantages are tolerated because of the outstandingly sharp cutting edge produced by the alloy.

Early practitioners made their own dental instruments, and early dental schools used construction techniques as beginning exercises. The problems of availability and the expense involved made individual fabrication impracticable, and the responsibility of producing acceptable instruments is now vested in the manufacturer.

In the manufacturing process, blank steel is bent to the degree of angulation needed in the shank and blade. The edges are then milled to produce the proposed edge and structural design. The formed piece is heated to 1,500° to 1,600° F. and then quenched to harden the working edge. Not more than 5 mm. of the tip is heated for hardening purposes since beyond this area an edge cannot be reestablished by sharpening. Cutting edges are usually tempered to produce additional hardness and to remove some of the brittle qualities. To accomplish this the tip is reheated at a lower temperature than before and quenched in solutions of oil, acid, or mercury. Hard steel is highly capable of being tempered, and additional treatment supplements the qualities of the alloy. The temperature ranges and colors characteristic of each series of instruments are listed in Table 4-1.

After the cutting edges are tempered the shanks of the instruments containing

Table 4-1. Temperatures used for tempering some hand instruments*

Temperature	Color	Use
423° to 450° F. (217° to 232° C.)	Light yellow	Enamel chisels, burnishers
469.4° F. (243° C.)	Medium yellow	Excavators, scalers
496.4° F. (258° C.)	Brown-yellow	Condensers
510.8° F. (266° C.)	Brown-purple	Saws, shanks of instruments
534.2° to 570.2° F.		
(279° to 299° C.)	Blue	Spring temper

*From McGeehee, W. H., True, H. A., and Inskipp, E. F.: A textbook of operative dentistry, ed. 4, New York, 1956, McGraw-Hill Book Co., Inc.

the hardened cutting edge are swaged into handles and pressure-welded. The same metal is not used for the handle as for the cutting edge because of the prohibitive cost and danger of breakage. The handles and a portion of the shank are then chrome-plated to prevent unsightly tarnish and corrosion. The tip of the blade and working surface of the nib are the only areas prone to discoloration and corrosion in sterilizing solutions. This corrosion is caused by an attack on the grain boundaries of the carbon steel by the metals in the sterilizing solution. This problem has been partially solved by coating the susceptible surfaces of the blade. The micro-thin coating layer is passive to ions and maintains the same appearance throughout the life of the instrument. Other commercial products employ the same coating procedure to protect the cutting edge; this surface layer has been inaccurately called stainless steel. The coating has been found to augment the sharpness of the cutting edge.

Hand-cutting instruments are useless unless sharpness is maintained. Therefore they have to be routinely sharpened after use, which causes a gradual reduction in the length of the blade. The dentist must observe the length of the blade and be prepared to replace the instruments regularly. If he does not do so, after a time the cutting set will be ineffective in producing cavity detail, and the quality of the work will decline.

Stainless steel alloys are also used to make hand-cutting instruments. A common stainless steel dental alloy contains 15% to 25% chromium, 1% carbon, and the remainder iron. The chromium in the alloy reduces the corroding tendency by depositing a small invisible oxide layer on the surface of the metal. The problem with the stainless steel alloys is that the cutting edge cannot be resharpened to the original quality. The problem of sharpness has resulted in stainless steel alloys being used primarily for working points in condensers and instruments for inserting cement rather than in cutting instruments. Although the unit cost of the instrument is increased by the additional alloying, this expense is offset because the instruments last longer. Tarno steel, a popular alloy in dental instruments, is used in procedures in which the metal contacts cement or other medicinal products capable of corroding carbon steel.

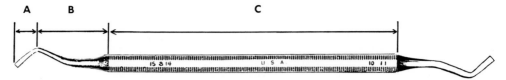

Fig. 4-1. Numbering system placed on handles of dental instruments. The left numbers indicate formula numbers, the right manufacturers' identification. **A,** Blade; **B,** shank; **C,** handle.

Another alloy often used in instruments is stellite. It consists of 65% to 90% cobalt and 10% to 35% chromium, with trace amounts of tungsten, molybdenum, and iron. High resistance to acids and hardness are its chief characteristics. This alloy is also used in instruments for mixing and inserting cements.

Parts of the hand instrument

Handle (shaft). The component parts of the hand instrument have different shapes. The handle can be formed for developing pressures and for better grasping. The diameter of the handle is about the same as a pencil. Hand instruments can have either double- or single-ended cutting edges. The purpose of the handle is to hold the instrument and to direct the cutting of tooth structure. Both the number series and manufacturer's name appear on the handle (Fig. 4-1). These are small and difficult to read and are not routinely used for identification. Constant use and comparison with other instruments enables the individual to select the correct instrument by observing its cutting edge or working point.

Cone-socket handles are used with working points that require much sharpening and that wear rapidly. The cone-socket handle holds a screw type of blade or nib, which can be replaced when worn rather than discarding the instrument. The cone-socket handles are larger and are held in the palm of the working hand in order to apply more pressure on the cutting edge. These handles can be obtained in ebony or stainless steel and are selected according to the type of sterilization used (Fig. 4-2).

Shank. The shank connects the handle with the working point and is gradually tapered from the shaft down to the blade or nib. This part of the hand instrument produces the access for the cutting edge because it is angled to offer many approaches. The shaft may be straight or have one, two, or three angles; the instruments are accordingly called straight, monangle, binangle, triple angle, or back-action instruments.

The angle is regulated by having the working point within 3 mm. of the center of the handle. If the working point is not aligned, torque develops and results in a poorly balanced instrument for regulating the working pressures. When this rule is not followed, the instrument is used only for inserting the filling rather than for cutting tooth structure.

Blade or nib. The blade or nib is the working point of the hand instrument.

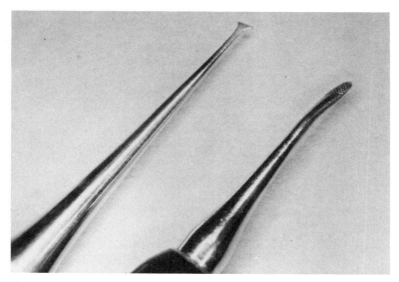

Fig. 4-2. Screw-tip No. 228 gold foil instrument in an ebony handle and universal No. 13 gold foil foot condenser.

The blade is a cutting edge that is used for cleaving and smoothing enamel and dentin. The nib contains a face or working surface and is used to insert, condense, and finish the restorative materials.

The cutting edge is formed by a 45-degree angle on the blade to produce a maximum thickness on the cutting edge that contributes to sharpness, and the angle is maintained by sharpening. Some instruments are bibeveled and are useful in placing undercuts in preparations. The blade of the bibeveled instrument is much smaller than the regular cutting edge, and this instrument is not used as frequently as the regular sets of cutting instruments.

The nibs are usually found on condensers and are used to impact and adapt the materials in the cavity form. The working faces of the nib are either plain or serrated, depending upon the materials being used. The serrations serve to increase the surface area of the face of the nib to provide more complete condensation and a greater degree of density in the restoration. The serrations also help to adapt the material to the tooth surface prior to the application of force.

Black's instrument formula

Several numbers are stamped on the instrument handle. The numbers classify each instrument by designating the measurements that produce the design of the shaft and cutting edge. The numbers selected by Black are used in sequences of three and are the component measurements listed to the left of the manufacturer's name. The first number is the width of the blade in tenths of millimeters, the second number is the length of the blade in millimeters, and the third number is the angulation of the blade with the handle in centigrade degrees. These numbers are commonly referred to during the surgical procedure by using the first number, the angulation of the shaft, and/or the type of excavator. A No. 10 binangle chisel is an example of a chairside request that is made of the assistant.

Kit number

The kit number appears on the handle at the end opposite the measurement numbers. Most instruments belong to a kit designed for broad and specific usage, and the series of instruments can be used for regular preparations or for specific techniques. For coding purposes the instruments are assigned a kit number. Next to this number is placed an R or an L, depending on whether the instrument has a right or left cutting application. Instruments should be placed in the cabinet and instrument tray according to their kit numbers. The Ferrier, Woodbury, and Loma Linda powdered gold series are examples of the kit numbering system.

Manufacturing number

For the purpose of die records a manufacturing number appears on the handle between the trade name and kit number. It is placed there for commercial use and should not be confused with the numbers for instrument recognition.

The student need not memorize the numbers on the instruments but he should be familiar with the three numbers selected by Black for the measurements, particularly with the first of the series because it will be referred to most often. The size and angulation of the blade must be understood. The tasks associated with the instrument angulation will be self-explanatory.

When Black developed this classification of instruments, he also designed a kit of 102 instruments to be used for cutting tooth structure. Every possible size and angulation of cutting instrument was made by Black, and these kits are still available from some manufacturers. At Northwestern University it was soon realized that Black's kit was an overproduction, and it was reduced to 48 hand instruments. The trend in operating is to use the smallest number of instruments that have the largest number of applications. By grasping an instrument differently or changing the force and angulation of the handle, other uses and conveniences are obtained for making the cavity preparation. Only repeated applications of the instruments in preparing teeth will enable their endless possibilities to be discovered.

Dental schools have instrument lists determined by the faculty that are set as minimum requirements for a program in restorative dentistry. Not only is the cost of education controlled in this way but a broader usage of each instrument must then be discovered by the student since only the basic instruments are used. The student develops favorite sequences and selections and, following graduation, he may purchase an additional number of instruments with different designs that serve his individual practice more adequately. A particular manu-

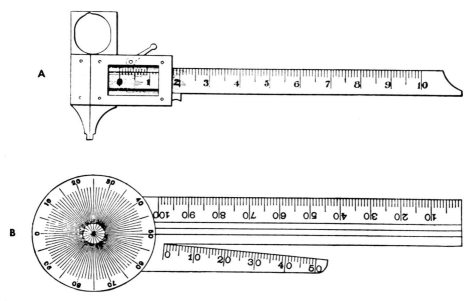

Fig. 4-3. A, Dental instrument gauge. **B,** Boley gauge. (From Black, G. V.: Operative dentistry, ed. 3, Milwaukee, 1917, Medico-Dental Publishing Co., vol. 2.)

facturer's products may be appealing because of variations in weight, balance, and metallic constituents. The value of Black's measurement system is acclaimed by the fact that it provides both the purchaser and manufacturer with a guide and classification of the hand instruments used in the dental profession.

Measuring devices

The dental instrument gauge is used to measure the individual parts of an instrument (Fig. 4-3). Long ago there was much variation in the size of instruments made by each company, and dentists preferred measuring the dimensions before accepting a purchase. Improvements in metallurgy, die casting, and gross production have alleviated the problem, and many gauges are no longer in use.

The instrument gauge has a millimeter scale to measure the length of the blade and a groove calibrated in tenths of millimeters to measure the width of the blade. A 100-degree centigrade circle measures the angulation of the blade to the handle. The long axis of the handle is placed on the central line of the rule and the blade angulation is observed on the circle. The shank angulation is expressed in centigrades; the 100-degree centigrade circle should not be confused with the 360-degree astronomic circle. The term "centigrade" has been used in operative dentistry since the classification was devised. The manufacturers like this system of measurement because it eliminates the need for placing three-digit numbers on the instrument handle. Use of this particular measurement spread to other areas of the field, and early dimensions in cavity

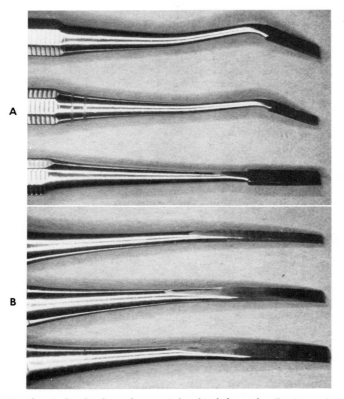

Fig. 4-4. A, Two binangle chisels and a straight chisel from the Ferrier series. **B,** Three sizes of Wedelstaedt chisels. (**A** courtesy Suter Co.)

preparation and lines of force were expressed in centigrades. Today these angulations are expressed in astronomic degrees, and the use of the centigrade system is limited to hand-cutting instruments.

The Boley gauge is helpful in measuring small thicknesses or widths of objects. The vernier scale measures in tenths of millimeters at the same time that the regular millimeter dimension is being recorded. Every dental office should have a Boley gauge because it can measure other items such as the thickness of the rubber dam, the proximal contact size, and the dimensions of prosthetic teeth.

Types of cutting instruments

The terminology for cutting instruments, all of which are called excavators, is derived from the angulation of the cutting edge. Common descriptions of each type can also be given that correspond to other working tools. Excavators are used to cleave unsupported enamel, to form dentin walls into exact forms, and to remove carious tooth substance. The categories and primary applications of the excavators will be described.

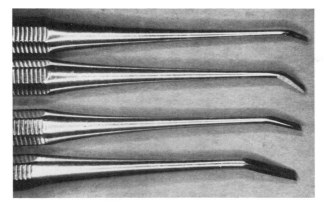

Fig. 4-5. Four types of monangle cutting instruments.

Chisels (Fig. 4-4). The blade and cutting edge of chisels are in line with the center of the handle. Chisels are used to cleave the labial surfaces of incisors, the buccal surfaces of the posterior teeth, and the lingual walls of the proximal preparation in maxillary teeth. The small straight chisel is helpful in gaining access to caries in anterior proximal preparations.

The Wedelstaedt chisels are some of the most adaptable cutting instruments available. They come in three widths and are curved for use on both the labial and lingual surfaces in both dental arches. The cutting edges are placed in such a way that they have mesial and distal application, which further increases their usefulness. The chisels are used for both cleaving and refining the tooth structure. Thorough application of the Wedelstaedt chisels will eliminate the need for many other instruments.

Monangle chisels (Fig. 4-5). These chisels have one angle in the shaft. They can be used like the straight chisel or with a pull motion. They are also called hoes. A monangle chisel is primarily used to smooth the walls of the preparation.

Binangle chisels. Binangle chisels have two bends in the shank to produce additional access. They are helpful when working on the buccal walls of the maxillary Class II preparation. The bends aid in cleaving the lingual wall of the anterior proximal preparation. A binangle chisel can be placed in more areas than the straight or monangle chisel.

Hatchets (Fig. 4-6). The cutting edge of the hatchet is perpendicular to the long axis of the handle. Hatchets are used for cleaving enamel in a vertical direction and are helpful when working on the occlusal surfaces of posterior teeth and the walls in proximal posterior preparations. They are regularly used to smooth the gingival wall and place resistance factors in the proximal portion of the Class II preparation. "Off-angled" hatchets are used to produce better force applications on the posterior teeth. The blade and cutting edge of the off-angled hatchets are rotated. All hatchets are made with right and left cutting blades.

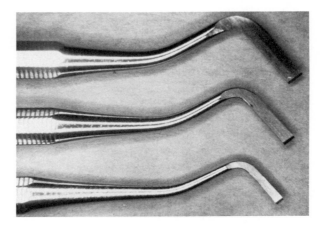

Fig. 4-6. Three sizes of enamel hatchets.

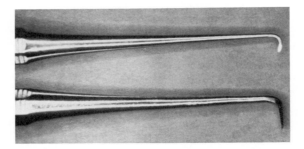

Fig. 4-7. Bibeveled hatchet and monangle cutting instrument.

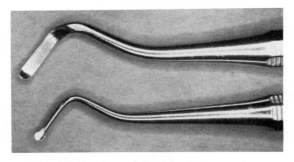

Fig. 4-8. Regular and discoid spoon excavators.

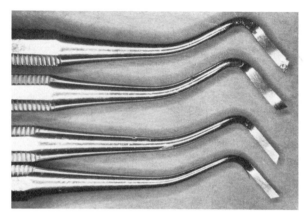

Fig. 4-9. Two sizes of margin trimmers.

Bibeveled hatchets (Fig. 4-7). These small hatchets have two bevels on the cutting edge. They are used with a chopping motion and confined to the dentin tissue. The instrument is used primarily for cutting out the incisal retention form in Class III preparations.

Spoons (Fig. 4-8). These instruments are used to remove large amounts of residual caries in the upper portion of the lesion. The shanks are curved and the end is sharp and rounded to facilitate scooping the softened tooth structure. The end of the spoon resembles the blade of a round bur, which is also used for caries excavation. The spoons come in two types, regular and discoid, and personal preference dictates which type will be used. The spoon excavators also come in pairs to provide right and left cutting applications. Large carious lesions can be quickly removed after the decayed area is made accessible. The spoon is inserted toward sound dentin and lifted to rotate most of the diseased tooth tissue out of the damaged area.

Margin trimmers (Fig. 4-9). Margin trimmers are used to smooth and bevel cavosurface margins. The margin trimmer shaft is curved and angled to produce right and left applications for both mesial and distal surfaces. A complete group of margin trimmers includes four instruments that are used to bevel cervical walls and to produce sharp retentive areas in the internal line and point angles in some cavity forms.

Angle formers (Fig. 4-10). These instruments are shaped like binangle chisels and have their cutting edges pointed at right and left angles. The pointed cutting edges are used with a push or pull motion in order to place mechanical undercuts in the dentin. These retentive forms are convenience points that are used in the gingival corners of Class III preparations to start condensation of direct gold fillings.

Discoids (Fig. 4-11). Discoids are rounded monangle excavators that are no longer used as such. Discoids are spoon shaped and are commonly used as

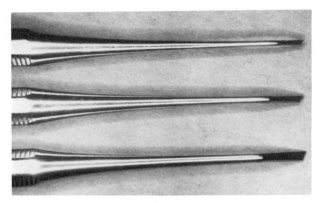

Fig. 4-10. Three examples of angle formers.

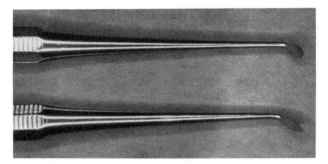

Fig. 4-11. Discoid and cleoid carving instruments.

carving instruments for metallic restorations. The disk-shaped head of the instrument accounts for its name.

Cleoids. These instruments are small claw-shaped monangle excavators and are similar to discoids. The cleoid is also used for carving but is used very little for excavation. Because of its pointed end it is used to form the occlusal fossae in metallic restorations and to carve the lingual contour of anterior gold restorations.

Reverse bevel instruments. Most excavating instruments can be obtained with two different bevels—regular and reversed—and usually come as double-ended instruments. The bevels are also referred to as mesial and distal cutting edges and are helpful in producing additional access. The binangle chisel and the Merchant angle formers are examples of instruments having two different bevels. Some instruments feature side bevels. Side bevels extend down the side of the blade and join with the cutting edge at the tip. The side cutters are useful in breaking through interproximal spaces to establish a self-cleansing dimension for the cavity preparation. Although they are not used often, situations do occur that are best handled with side-cutting instruments.

• • •

Through the years several kits of hand instruments have been designed. The most widely used kit was developed by Woodbury. Refinements made in some of the Black instruments resulted in the production of new designs. Angle formers were designed by Woodbury and were influential in gaining wide acceptance of his kit in dental schools and private practice. The main advantages of the Woodbury kit are that the designs are more delicate and precise and that the instruments conform to Black's system of cavity preparation. Manufacturers became more interested in producing instruments with better balance and uniform measurements with the advent of the kits.

Not long after this refinement in hand instruments occurred, Ferrier designed a series that was the last major improvement made in this area. The thickness of the blades in all cutting instruments was standardized, producing a design that provides access and qualities of exactness. A group of condensers and finishing instruments was also developed for use in the Ferrier preparations and in the placement of esthetic gold foil restorations. The quality of the Ferrier kit of instruments is exceptional. The uniform thickness of the blades provides better balance and control.

Ferrier's teachings inspired Alexander Jeffery to develop the "lingual approach" gold foil procedures. These gold foil operations are performed entirely from the lingual surface in the maxillary anterior teeth, and the technique requires a specially designed set of instruments. Cutting instruments and condensers are included in the set to develop the invisible gold foil restoration. The procedure, if done properly, requires knowledge of all the instruments in the Jeffery kit and skill in using them. The kit is another example of outstanding originality.

A number of single instruments have been designed for specific uses in operative dentistry (Fig. 4-12). The Jones knife, the Smith BBS instrument, and the Spratley burnisher are just a few of those that could be mentioned. Some are not even catalogued, but they may be observed during postgraduate work and study club activity. These instruments are useful in many cases and, if appropriate, they should be included in the routine individual tooth restoration.

Instruments should be arranged in the drawers so that those most commonly used are located in the most convenient areas. Chisels and hatchets should be placed next to mirrors and explorers because they are needed in most tooth operations. It is helpful to label the drawers so that assistants can return sterilized instruments to their proper place. This arrangement aids in rapid recognition and location of instruments. The chairside assistant must learn the dentist's routine in order to anticipate the need and use of instruments.

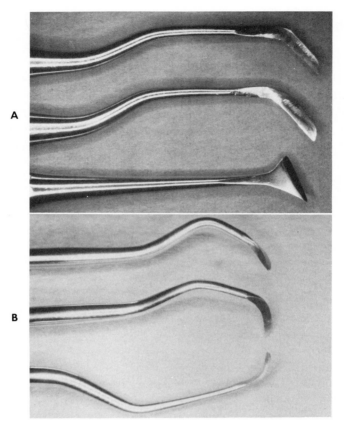

Fig. 4-12. A, Gold finishing knives. **B,** Periodontal scalers that must be sharpened with a cylindric mounted stone.

Sharpening

As stated previously, the hand instruments must be sharpened regularly to be effective in cutting tooth structure. It is necessary to sharpen an instrument after it has been used a few times in order to keep the entire selection of instruments in the cabinet in acceptable working condition. Some cavity preparations require sharpening during the procedure, making it necessary to keep the sharpening device available at all times. The dentist should sharpen the instruments because the assistant does not know what degree of beveling is to be maintained on the cutting edge.

The method of choice for sharpening hand instruments is the Arkansas oilstone (Fig. 4-13). The stone is wetted with regular engine oil to lubricate the metal and the slab. The metal edge is cut slowly, preventing rapid abrasion and loss of the instrument. This method teaches one to recognize the angulation and exactness of the individual cutting edge. The excavating hand instruments can

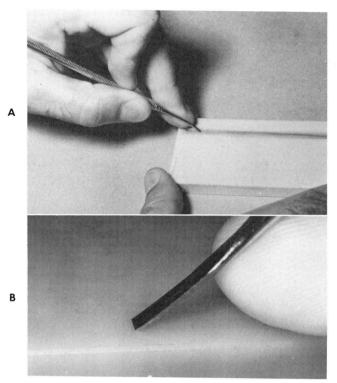

Fig. 4-13. A, Sharpening a hand instrument on the Arkansas stone. **B,** Setting the bevel on the Arkansas stone before sharpening.

all be sharpened with the Arkansas stone. To set the bevel the instrument is grasped by placing the cutting edge firmly on the slab. The wrist is locked to maintain the angulation of the bevel, and the arm is moved to activate the instrument back and forth on the slab. The third and fourth fingers are used as guides and should be rested upon the slab to prevent uneven sharpening or rounding of corners. The instrument can be held so that arm movement is either parallel to or at right angles with the slab. Both arm positions should be tried to select the more comfortable one. The degree of sharpening is validated by a black deposit of metal on the stone. After sharpening, the instruments are wiped with an alcohol sponge to remove the oil. They are then placed in the sterilizing media and returned to the cabinet, ready for use. Recognition of an acceptable cutting edge and mastery of the sharpening procedure will soon become part of the office routine. The use of sharp cutting instruments prevents many of the worries and problems involved in finishing preparations and restorations.

Mechanical sharpeners useful in the office have been designed (Fig. 4-14). Emory or carborundum wheels that are abrasive enough to reduce the cutting edge are mounted on small electric engines. Keying plates are mounted over

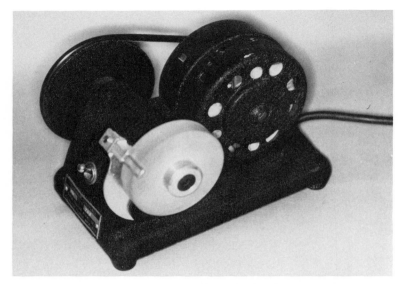

Fig. 4-14. Mechanical sharpening device for hand-cutting instruments.

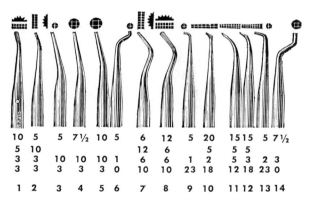

10	5		5	7½	10	5		6	12		5	20		15	15	5	7½
5	10							12	6			5		5	5		
3	3		10	10	10	1		6	6		1	2		5	3	2	3
3	3		3	3	3	0		10	10		23	18		12	18	23	0
1	2		3	4	5	6		7	8		9	10		11	12	13	14

Fig. 4-15. Black's universal gold condenser points. (Courtesy Cleveland Dental Manufacturing Co.)

the wheel to hold the instruments. Caution must be used in regulating pressure on the metal. The sharpeners are convenient, but loupes and light pressure should be used to prevent overcutting the blades with the mechanical sharpener.

Working points

Hand instruments also have working points and are classified as condensers, knives, files, and burnishers. They are used to insert and finish restoration materials. Thorough descriptions of the common working points will be presented

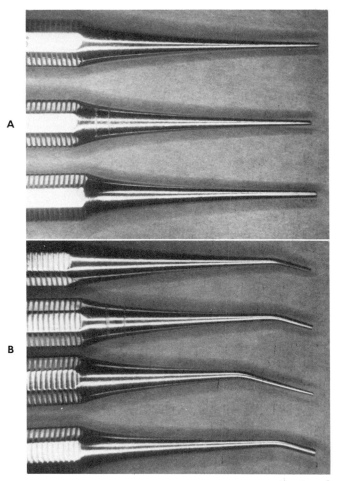

Continued.

Fig. 4-16. Ferrier condensers. **A,** Three small, round gold foil condensers. **B,** Round monangle condensers. **C,** Bayonet condensers. **D,** Right-angle condenser and foot condenser. **E,** Two condensers that are used to place the noncohesive cylinders of gold.

in the chapters on restorative procedures. Since they are classified as hand instruments, they are briefly presented in this chapter.

The long hand condensers are used with the hand mallet to impact gold foil (Fig. 4-15). The handles are drawn out and tapered longer than other instruments and they have a flat end. The end is malleted to produce a hard surface on the gold. Many shapes of nibs are available that can be used in different portions of the restoration with varying amounts of force. The nibs all have serrated faces (Fig. 4-16), which prevents slippage on the gold pellet and seats the condenser in the metal when forces are applied. Certain condensers are used for hand pressure with powdered gold or for the insertion of amalgam. The

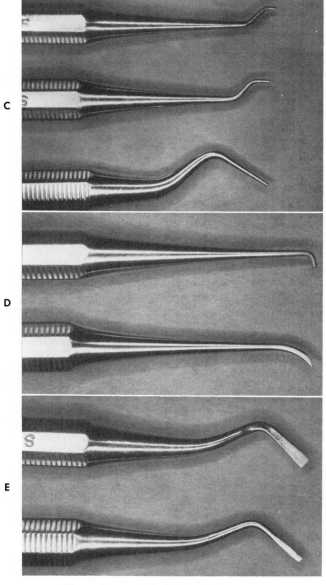

Fig. 4-16, cont'd. For legend see p. 113.

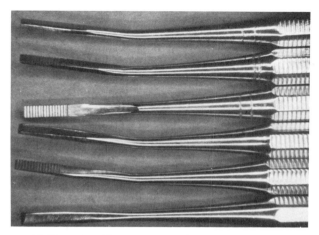

Fig. 4-17. Ferrier gold files. The files are manipulated in a push and pull direction. The angulation of the head produces access to the restoration.

serrations are not quite as prominent in these types, and in large-diameter nibs that are used for pressuring material they are located farther apart. The serrations are kept free of filling material to enable thorough condensation. The numbering system on the handles of the condensers will either have one digit near the nib or be imprinted with both a number and the name of the designer. The numbers used on cutting instruments are not present on condensers.

Many types of files are manufactured for adapting gold materials to tooth structure (Fig. 4-17). Soft gold will elongate, and success in some procedures depends on pulling the metal closer to the cavosurface margin. Files are numbered in sequence like the condensers and are to be used with a push or pull hand force. Selection of files is based on the different angulations and sizes of the file nib.

Burnishers are used to polish and finish other metallic materials. They can be used to draw mercury into the overpacked layer of amalgam or to harden the surface of the direct gold restoration prior to filing. The smaller the surface contact the greater the pressure that can be applied to burnish the gold. In operative dentistry the burnisher has application in those cases in which pressure is useful and can be applied with a blunt instrument.

Contouring restorations is facilitated by the use of finishing knives. Proximal contours and embrasure forms are carved with amalgam and gold knives. For the amalgam restoration the blades are placed at right and left angles, and for the proximal gold restoration they are straight and much smaller. They carry only one number and require sharpening following each finishing procedure. Excessive and rapid wear of the blade occurs because the metal is thin. For this reason the knives are often used with a screw type of handle to keep replacement cost minimal.

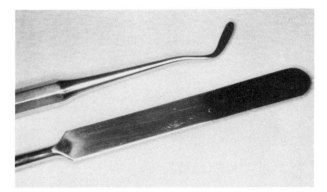

Fig. 4-18. Cement instrument and spatula that are used for mixing and placing various types of cement.

A number of special instruments in this category have been designed. New types of materials and cavity preparations will always necessitate changes and new designs in the manufacture of instruments (Fig. 4-18).

Instrument grasping and operating hand positions

Successful instrumentation requires satisfactory body posture and correct hand grasps and positions (Fig. 4-19). The patient associates firm and delicate cutting using sharp instruments with excellent treatment. The instruments must be held and stabilized properly to promote confidence. Basically two grasps are used, and they can be varied with the task or the location of the tooth and cavity preparation.

Pen grasp. The pen grasp is the most commonly used grasp and is accomplished by positioning the hand as for writing. The instrument is held between the thumb and first two fingers, with the handle centered in the cushions of both fingers. The middle finger rests on the shaft and work surface to stabilize the cutting edge. This grasp is used for the delicate cutting and finishing techniques discussed in conjunction with the principles of cavity preparation. Although the pen grasp is not considered powerful, heavy pressures can be developed with practice. This grasp is used when direct vision is possible, and it is considered to offer the best control because the thumb and two fingers provide a tripod for the instrument. The pen grasp should be used whenever possible because of the accuracy that is attained with it.

Palm and thumb grasp. In the palm and thumb grasp the instrument handle rests in the palm and the cutting edge is directed by the four fingers and thumb. In some cases the thumb rests on another tooth surface, usually the tooth adjacent to the one being prepared, to support the movements. This grasp is used more often with the upper teeth, primarily the occlusal and buccal surfaces of posterior teeth and the lingual surface of anterior teeth, because it is

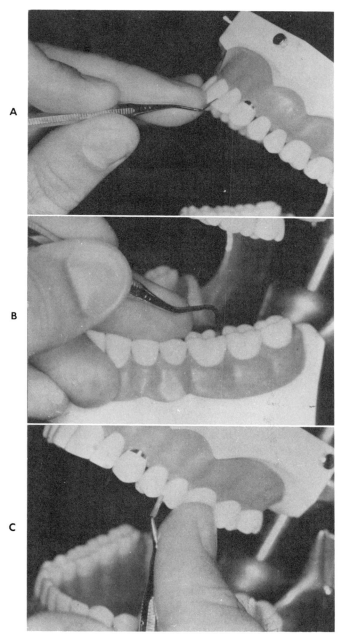

Fig. 4-19. A, Pen grasp of the chisel to cleave enamel on anterior teeth. **B,** Pen grasp of the enamel hatchet on posterior teeth. **C,** Palm grasp of cutting instruments for leverage.

uncomfortable to use the pen grasp in these areas unless the patient is reclined.

The palm and thumb grasp is used when more force is needed than can otherwise be produced. Stability is not as easy to attain as with the pen grasp, but when the instrument and rests are properly placed, the grasp is helpful in grossly fracturing tooth structure.

The inverted pen grasp and palm-thrust grasp are occasionally used, but they are only slight variations of the two just described.

Rests. The fingers that are not used to grasp the instrument support and stabilize the working hand. These fingers provide the rests necessary to keep the instrument confined to the preparation, to prevent injury of the tissue. Rests should always be on firm tissue—the teeth. It is ideal to rest on teeth adjacent to the one being operated on. Free-hand operating may be necessary for minute details that cannot be produced with stability, but it is very undesirable. The two small fingers provide rests for the pen grasp, and the thumb provides a rest for the palm grasp. The rest is established before any cutting is done on the tooth. When possible the rests are on teeth adjacent to and in the same arch as the tooth being prepared.

Guards. The free hand of the operator is used to stabilize the surgical field or the patient's head, which also helps prevent instrument slippage during tooth reduction. The thumb and forefinger of the free hand, which is usually the left hand, are placed opposite the working point to resist forces and prevent the teeth in the arch from moving. Problems of instability are found to occur more often in mandibular teeth since the mandible is the free-moving portion of the head. The lower border of the mandible is occasionally used for support, but if access permits, adjacent teeth should be used. It is helpful to keep the guard close to the tooth being restored, because this provides more balance for the operator. When restoring the inaccessible molar regions, it is necessary to use the protective guard on the opposite side of the patient's head.

The use of rests and guards is essential for good instrumentation and for the protection of the patient.

Instrument sterilization

The hand instruments are contaminated after each patient application. Driclave or cold sterilizing solutions are used to eliminate microorganisms from the metal. Fomites that are present on instruments may inoculate the soft tissue if it is punctured during cavity preparation.

The instruments are prepared before they are placed in the sterilizing medium. When the patient is dismissed, the bracket cover is removed and the collection of instruments is taken to the sink. The instruments are held by the middle of the handle and the working points are scrubbed thoroughly with soap and water. The instruments are rotated in the hand until all debris is removed from the metal surfaces. They are then placed under a forceful stream of water until the soap is removed. At this time they are placed in the solution in the tray or in bags for driclaving.

Sterilization has harmful effects on hand instruments, particularly if the technique is neglectfully performed. The metal can become corroded, rendering the instrument dull and ineffective, but this can be held to a minimum if it is thoroughly scrubbed. As previously mentioned, carbon steel is highly susceptible to corrosion, but this problem is tolerated because it produces the best cutting edge.

Some equipment in the operatory is not cleaned in the way just described because, if it were, it would be permanently damaged. The devices having moving parts or threads are given special attention because corrosion would render these instruments useless. If necessary the individual pieces should be scrubbed with soap and water and quickly dried with the air syringe on the unit. The article is then thoroughly wiped with a small sponge saturated with the cleaning solution, isopropyl alcohol. Items that are cleaned in this way are the separators, rubber dam punch, and forceps. Before they are placed back into the cabinet a drop of engine oil is occasionally spread on the adjustable parts.

Following the rules of instrument sterilization preserves the life of the equipment. Instruments should not be left too long in solutions and should be dried thoroughly before being replaced in the drawer. The driclaving method cannot be altered; damage to the metal is tolerated because driclaving is effective against a greater number of organisms. Cleanliness and sterilization of the operatory and of all equipment are required for an aseptic area for treatment. Constant care of carbon steel alloys is necessary because of the corrosion caused by the sterilizing medium.

ROTARY INSTRUMENTS

Rotary cutting instruments are used for the bulk of tooth reduction. They are the instruments most frequently discussed by the patient and are thought to be the most unpleasant equipment in the office. Patient reactions to an appointment are influenced by the type and length of rotary cutting that is used to restore the teeth. This area of practice has been improved more than any other as a result of the development of ultraspeed cutting power sources and handpieces. Ultraspeeds are used for gross reduction and regular speeds are employed for smoothing the preparation. The two systems make possible a tooth preparation that is more ideal and less traumatic to the patient. The combination of rotary methods has made it possible to increase the workload and quality of the practice.

Rotary cutting is used mainly for gross reduction of the tooth. The initial opening, extension, squaring, and flaring of the preparation are done with the bur held and turned by the handpiece. The cavity margin, outline, and mortise forms are produced with differently shaped burs, and most of the refinement and smoothing is accomplished with hand instruments for the individual restoration. The ideal preparation for a single tooth employs a combination of rotary and hand instruments. Rotary reduction is made possible by means of a power source that turns the bur. The handpiece holds the bur on the tooth while the cutting is being done. The type of cutting and the trauma and patient reaction that are produced vary widely according to the technique and instrumentation employed.

Rotary reduction has been improved in regard to both power sources and cutting points. The first major improvement occurred in 1932 when the electric engine replaced the foot engine. The first electric engine was adjusted to reduce the noise and heat, which were considered the primary problems. A variable rheostat was wired into the circuit to provide different speed ranges. The regular-speed electric engines are basically the same today, with speeds from 2,000 to 6,000 rpm.

Shortly after World War II the profession became interested in reducing tooth structure at accelerated speeds. Modifications that are still being used were made on the engine to increase the revolutions per minute and the amount of tooth structure reduced per unit time. Problems naturally occurred, but the interest in increasing cutting efficiency is still mounting in research and practice. The resistance was shunted and the belt and handpiece pulleys were changed to enable the bur to cut at speeds between 20,000 and 50,000 rpm. The problems of this increased speed were obvious, and new supportive systems were rapidly developed. Additional increase in speed prevented use of the conventional pulley and handpieces because wear and vibration caused frequent breakdowns. The first departure from the adjusted engine was an electronic vibrating instrument, which was a completely new concept in tooth preparation. Although the resulting research was useful, the vibration instrument did not produce as exact a cavity form as the rotary devices. A slurry of aluminum hydroxide flooded the field, blocking vision. Neither this instrument nor the airbrasive unit was used for long, because exacting dimensions could not be produced in the cavity form with them. Although the vibratory motion resulted in the design of scaling and condensing devices that are quite useful in practice, the concept is not used for cavity preparation.

A few years later the turbine system was developed as a power source. The water turbine appeared first and rotary speeds up to 60,000 rpm were developed. Copious amounts of water are used as a coolant, and the entire system is driven by a water pump. Special cutting points, both burs and diamonds, were produced that are helpful in crown and bridge procedures. They are longer than the conventional burs and are advantageous in smoothing the full-coverage preparation. Introduction of air systems and the need for an additional cabinet in the operatory has limited the acceptance of the water turbine.

The development that caused a diametric change in rotary cutting and instrumentation was the air turbine. It increased the operating speed range to 250,000 rpm which, because it is above the vibratory perception of the patient, resulted in acceptance by the public. The sharp increase in speed resulted in a voluminous amount of research on the biologic response to and technique for using the air turbine. The efficiency of the air turbine has enabled the dentist to restore and save a greater number of badly damaged teeth and to construct more fixed prosthodontic units. The dentition is thus being cared for more effectively. The system will inevitably contribute to a reduction in removable appliances.

The air turbine is now used to accomplish gross tooth reduction in short periods of time. The regular-speed and other high-speed rotary instruments are used for smoothing and finishing procedures that are dependent on the design of the preparation. The air turbine has been universally accepted, as witnessed by the purchases of graduating students. Modern practice utilizes all three major speed ranges to produce various types of preparations. This chapter will explain how each system is employed.

Operating speed ranges

Regular speed (2,000 to 6,000 rpm) is accomplished with sleeve and cog-driven handpieces; medium speed (10,000 to 60,000 rpm) is accomplished with ball-bearing, low-speed, air-driven and mounted electric handpieces; and ultra-speed (250,000 rpm) is accomplished with the air turbine and some belt-driven handpieces.

Regular speed. This speed range is conventional for the dental unit and is used for prophylaxis and polishing of restorations in addition to tooth reduction. This speed range was used for designing burs and resulted in the Black instru-

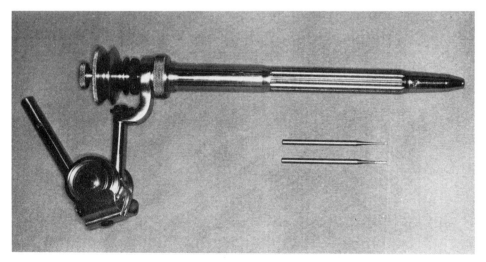

Fig. 4-20. Straight doriot handpiece used in the regular-speed range.

mentation that is common for all types of preparations. It is the first speed range used by the student to master the benefits derived from the histologic structure of the enamel walls. Angulation of the enamel rods in the different locations of the teeth is learned with the regular-speed range.

The conventional handpieces are used with the unit engine for the regular-speed range (Fig. 4-20). In the straight-sleeve handpiece a long straight steel bur is used for cutting. The bur is held in the handpiece by two spindles and a collet chuck. The assembly is covered by a sleeve and the mechanism is turned by the drive pulley on the base of the handpiece. The action of the handpiece results in metal turning against metal, and wear and eccentricity are soon produced. The brass parts of the instrument are sometimes protectively coated to prevent wear and heat production in the moving parts.

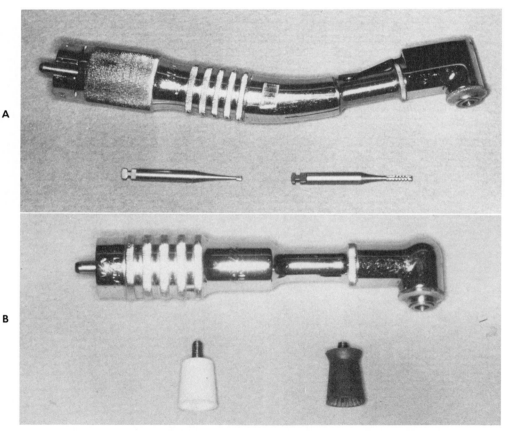

Fig. 4-21. A, Contra-angle handpiece in which latch burs are used. **B,** Polishing angle handpiece. The white cup is used for tooth prophylaxis and the dark cup is used for polishing metallic restorations.

The regular contra-angle handpiece is used for cavity preparations except those in the anterior teeth (Fig. 4-21). The contra-angle has two angles that project from the straight handpiece, which places the bur nearly vertical to the long axis of the straight handpiece. The tip of the bur is located within 3 mm. of the central axis of the straight handpiece in order to reduce torque. The contra-angle has two sets of gears, the drive and the pinion, that are used to turn the bur. The bur tube is connected to the pinion gears in the handpiece head.

The regular-speed handpieces are used with the Black instrumentation or for smoothing the walls of the preparation following reduction with the air turbine. The low speeds produce the smoothest cavity wall, and during refinement a better regulated extension demands that regular-speed cutting be used for finishing all cavity forms. The regular speeds employ a pulley system to deliver energy from the power source to the bur, and as a result considerable vibration from the pulleys and engine belt is transferred to the tooth. This causes bone-conducted vibration and noises that are unpleasant to the patient. Use of the regular speeds is held to a minimum for this reason.

In anterior teeth not much extension is required for the ideal preparation. In addition to the danger of overcutting, this fact dictates the use of only regular speeds for anterior preparations. It is helpful to use only the straight handpiece unless a lingual insertion of the restorative material is planned. Access to the lesion is gained by breaking down the enamel covering with hand instruments. The bur is placed in the dentin and the cavity is quickly prepared by using the undermining technique to remove the enamel. Smoothing and angulation are accomplished at the same time by changing burs to eliminate the use of accelerated speeds.

Medium speed. As described in Chapter 6, additional accelerated speeds are produced with the regular electric engine. Wiring adjustments and handpiece attachments cause speeds to be increased up to 50,000 rpm. This speed requires that a ball-bearing pulley and handpiece system be used, because in this range wear and vibration are pronounced.

The ball-bearing handpiece is more expensive because of its improved design and the type of material used. Two ball bearings suspend the spindle and bur chuck in the straight handpiece. They are sealed and should not be serviced by the dentist. Tungsten carbide burs and diamond points are used with these handpieces and this speed range because of the temperature produced with the instrumentation. The ball-bearing contra-angle is used with this straight handpiece. One or two sets of ball bearings in the contra-angle produces smoother cutting and less vibration than the regular type. The drive gear usually contains the bearing, and the pinion gear is speed-coated for working in the medium-speed range.

The medium-speed range is used for surface reduction and smoothing. Burs cut effectively but are more suitably used with air turbines. Diamond instruments are used more frequently in the medium-speed range when cooled with copious amounts of water. The diamonds are advocated for the gross wall reduction, angulation, and smoothing that is necessary for full-coverage preparations. Vibration is lessened by the increase in speed, which results in less unfavorable patient reaction. The cutting, however, is more traumatic and the water used to lubricate the diamond is also needed to minimize temperature.

Ultraspeed. Some belt-driven equipment is capable of producing ultraspeeds but it is not commonly used. The air turbine, commonly called the airotor, is the instrument used by the majority of practitioners. The air turbine is driven by an air compressor and operates above vibratory perception to eliminate many of the unpleasant factors involved in tooth preparation. This speed range produces rapid cutting that does not respect the histology of the tooth, so the outline form is limited only by the judgment of the operator. The air column is directed against a turbine located in the head of the handpiece. The bur is suspended in the center of the turbine, which runs on a bearing that works only when light loads are placed on the handpiece. The turbines are lubricated with an oil mist that contaminates the preparation and the operatory. This oil mixes with pulverized tooth structure and is troublesome in cleaning the tooth. Some turbines are packed with grease and work effectively with less debris.

The cutting efficiency that is possible with the air turbine causes it to be used for gross tooth reduction. Although it is considered a "blocking out" tool, the air turbine has a great deal of accuracy when compared with other methods that have been used for accelerated tooth reduction. Overextension of the cavity causes pulp damage with any speed range, and this must be regulated when using the air turbine with operating loads of less than 6 ounces. The gross outline form of the axial or pulpal wall for any intracoronal preparation should be taken no farther than 0.2 mm. below the dentinoenamel junction.

The ease of cutting reduces the number of burs needed to produce the outline. Temperature is regulated with small-diameter burs, and the greatest efficiency is produced with a cylindric type of bur. The design of the bur is proportional to the amount of tooth structure that has to be removed. Diamonds are not found to be as effective with this speed range. One good feature of the air turbine is that burs need not be changed too often. Small fissure burs are featured when there is no danger of abrading an adjacent tooth, and small inverted cone burs are used when a proximal lesion is opened adjacent to a sound surface.

Cutting points

Two different methods are used in the mechanics of tooth reduction. The burs are milling devices and function by chip removal of the tooth (Fig. 4-22). Other cutting points such as diamonds, stones, and abrasives cut by grinding the tooth surface. The effectiveness of burs and diamonds varies with the design of the point, the operating load, the coolant, and the speed range employed.

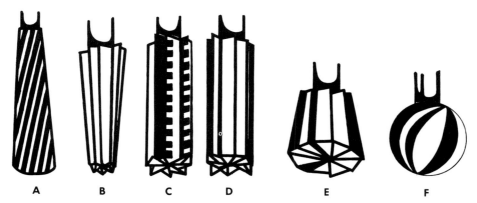

Fig. 4-22. Variation of bur design. **A,** Pear-shaped fissure bur; **B,** tapered fissure bur; **C,** straight cross-cut fissure bur; **D,** straight fissure bur; **E,** inverted cone; **F,** round bur.

Burs

Two kinds of burs are available that differ in hardness and composition. The regular bur is a carbon steel product made by cutting a blank piece of metal. The blades are milled by machines, and the bur is hardened and tempered for use. The steel bur is considerably harder than tooth structure, but it does not last long when pressed against enamel while revolving. The hardness of the tooth and the increased temperature in cutting cause the metal to fracture and discolor, producing an ineffective bur. The steel burs turn black or dark blue with excessive cutting temperatures, which indicates that they are permanently damaged. The steel burs are used in tooth reduction to undermine and fracture the enamel. They are also effective for cutting dentin. They are employed with light pressure for smoothing and placing retention forms in cavity walls. The steel burs are used only with regular-speed instruments, last only a short time, and can be purchased at a reasonable price.

For accelerated cutting the tungsten carbide burs are used. They are also made of carbon steel alloys and are much harder and more effective in milling teeth. The burs are made by powder metallurgy in which the metal constituents are mixed and a packed mold is sintered at high temperatures for fusion. The mold specimen is milled to produce the head of the bur, which is later welded to a regular steel blank that furnishes the shank (Fig. 4-23). A mixture of 5% to 10% cobalt and the remainder of tungsten carbide accounts for the additional hardness of the bur. The carbide burs are used both for accelerated speeds and for producing the outline at regular speeds. The burs are sufficiently hard to fracture or cleave the enamel in order to produce the outline form in opening and extending the carious lesion. Tungsten carbide burs are useful at medium speeds for undermining enamel and at ultraspeeds for gross reduction of any part of the extra- or intracoronal preparation.

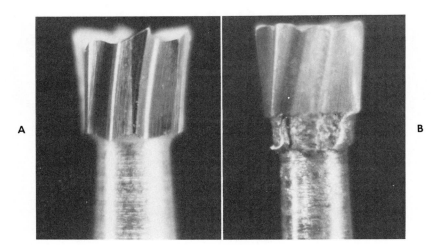

Fig. 4-23. A, Carbide bur made from a single blank of steel. **B,** Carbide bur head that has been welded to a regular steel shaft. (Courtesy Kerr Manufacturing Co.)

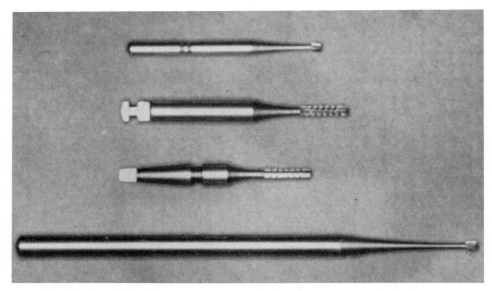

Fig. 4-24. Four types of burs commonly employed. From top to bottom: the friction-grip bur for air turbines, the latch bur for contra-angle handpieces, the tapered bur for contra-angle handpieces, and the straight bur for doriot handpieces.

Bur parts. The parts of a bur have a nomenclature similar to that of hand instruments.

Shank. The shank is secured to the handpiece for the purpose of driving the bur. The length and shape of the shank vary with the chucking mechanism. The regular doriot handpiece requires a long straight handpiece bur and the contra-angle handpiece requires different types of short burs. The latch and tapered short burs are used for regular- and medium-speed instruments and the friction-grip bur is used for the ultraspeed air turbine and all the other type handpieces (Fig. 4-24).

The straight handpiece and bur should be used whenever a choice can be made. They have fewer moving parts and the straight bur can be maneuvered to produce more access. The bur shank is thinner and greater accuracy is obtained with the more centrically running straight handpiece.

The contra-angle handpieces for all speed ranges have been studied for eccentricity. The collet chuck mechanisms are more accurate than the plastic bur tubes for the air turbines. At regular speeds the latch-type contra-angle handpiece exhibits more wear than the tapered-type handpiece. Naturally more vibration and eccentricity are associated with the latch-type handpiece, but it is commonly used because of the simplicity in changing the bur. The latch-type handpiece can be rebuilt to avoid the inaccuracy caused by wear of the bur tube. The actual rotary force is caused by the pinion gear in the contra-angle turning the drive flange on the end of the latch bur.

Shaft. The shaft connects the head of the bur with the shank. As discussed previously, the straight bur has a longer shaft, which is helpful in providing more access. The shaft of contra-angle burs is shorter to permit them to be used in the posterior teeth.

Head. This part of the bur does the cutting by means of small blades located on the metal. The shape and design of the blades on the head classify the bur as to how it is used in the preparation. Other factors such as the diameter of the head and the number of cutting blades also influence the efficiency of tooth removal. An increase in speed is responsible for the cutting action.

Because of differences in the design and cutting efficiency, burs have specific tasks for each particular speed range. They are classified in relation to the regular-speed range and are requested by specific numbers. The two basic groups of burs are the extending and excavating burs, and they are made with blades that cut when rotated to the right (clockwise). Left cutting burs are obtained only by special order and are useful in certain applications. For cavity refinement the bur should be pulled in the direction of the wall.

Inverted cone burs (Nos. 33½ to 37). Small to large sizes are available in inverted cone burs (Fig. 4-25). They have truncated shapes, the widest portion being at the tip of the bur. Inverted cone burs are used primarily for extension and retention. The No. 34 bur is the popular size for extension and the No. 33½ bur is commonly used for retentive undercuts. The other sizes can be used for

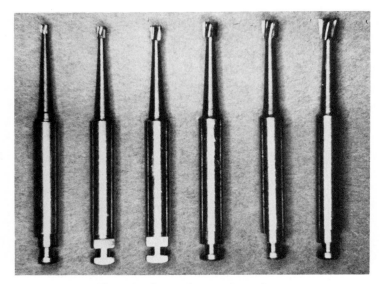

Fig. 4-25. Series of inverted cone burs.

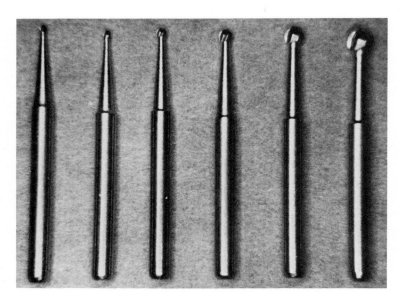

Fig. 4-26. Series of round burs.

extremely large lesions, but they produce more vibration in cutting and make a wider outline.

The inverted cone bur is used to undermine and fracture the enamel in extension for prevention. The bur is inserted into the deepest pit just inside the dentin and then pushed under the enamel. The revolving bur is then pulled upward through the occlusal surface to cleave the enamel in the direction of the rods. This is the common procedure used with regular-speed instruments when the uncoalesced grooves abutting the caries are excised to produce the self-cleansing outline. For a guide the No. 34 bur is pushed through the groove, with the bur being evenly divided to produce an accurate initial opening.

The small No. 33½ bur is ideally shaped to produce pyramidal retention forms in the dentin. It is pushed laterally in the dentin to produce an undercut under the enamel. The bur is inserted to locate the convenience points in the gingival corners of the Class III gold foil preparation. In some cases undercuts are placed with the bur in the ends of the occlusal grooves and in the proximal walls of the Class II preparation. They produce a mechanical locking that assists in starting condensation and in building the gold shelf in the proximal direct gold restoration.

Round burs (Nos. ¼ to 8). These burs are circular shaped and are indicated for the excavation of caries (Fig. 4-26). The blade of the bur is curved and resembles the spoon excavator, which is also used for removing decay. The bur is placed into carious dentin and revolved slowly while light force is applied from the side of the crater. The caries is rapidly scooped out with spoon excavators and the round bur is inserted to clean the dentin surface, which is used as the footing for the restoration and therefore must be aseptic and solid. The Nos. 2 to 4 round burs are the sizes commonly employed for caries removal.

The round burs have other applications. Class III lesions are penetrated with the No. ½ bur to undermine the enamel so that the plate can be fractured for access of the extension bur. The No. ½ bur is also used to initiate retention forms in the Class III preparations in much the same way as the small inverted cone burs.

The No. 4 round bur is used to contour the surfaces of metal restorations during the polishing procedure. The same bur is helpful in shaping tooth-colored restorations.

Regular plane fissure burs (Nos. 56 to 59). These burs are used to square and flare the walls of the cavity preparation to the dimension dictated by the histology of enamel and the type of restorative material. The fissure burs have end- and side-cutting blades that can be used to plane two walls simultaneously in order to form sharp line angles. This series of burs produces the mortise form in depth and angulation, in addition to smoothing the cavosurface margin. Lighter operating loads are applied to the margin than to the cavity walls.

There are several variations in the design of fissure burs. Some fissure bur blades are made with crosscuts, which are small indentations that increase the

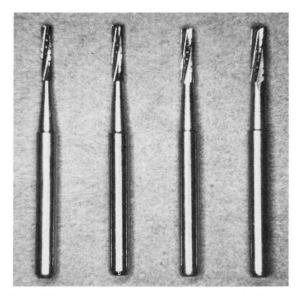

Fig. 4-27. Regular fissure burs with crosscuts in the blades.

surface area (Fig. 4-27). These burs are also called "enamel shavers" and are numbered from 557 to 559. The crosscuts produce a rough enamel wall, which is helpful in improving the interlocking of the amalgam restoration. The No. 557 crosscut fissure bur is commonly used for this design, and the blades supposedly increase cutting ability at regular speed because of the larger surface contact.

Other variations in design include the direction of the blade on the head of the bur. The spiral design is used to encourage a larger chip removal and is popular with some manufacturers. The difference in efficiency of the two blade directions has not been studied but should be considered because of the increased use of straight-bladed fissure burs with the air turbine handpiece.

Tapered fissure burs (Nos. 699 to 701). These burs are of cylindric design but are tapered a few degrees in order to place wall inclinations for the cast gold inlay (Fig. 4-28). The taper in the wall facilitates withdrawal of the wax pattern and insertion of the inlay. After the outline form is made the No. 701 tapered fissure bur is used to taper all the surrounding walls of the cavity preparation.

The Nos. 699 and 700 burs are selected to produce undercut grooves for the retention of the proximal amalgam restoration. The same bur produces tapered grooves that guide the inlay to the seated position. The same type of crosscuts and spiral blades are available in the tapered fissure burs as in the regular plane fissure burs.

Finishing burs. Plane-bladed burs with round and cylindric heads are used for finishing and polishing metallic restorations. The blades are shorter and closer

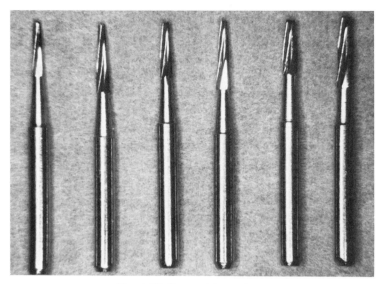

Fig. 4-28. Tapered fissure burs.

together than those in other burs in order to produce a burnishing effect on metal. Finishing burs are pulled from metal to tooth structure when the margin of the restoration is being corrected. They cannot be employed to close a poor marginal relationship, but they are helpful in refining the marginal metal for inlays that are made to rest over the cavosurface margin.

Bur design. The manner in which the blades are arranged and the shape of the bur head influence the amount of cutting that can be done per unit of time (Fig. 4-29). The face of the bur blade, which is the surface in front of the cutting edge, is angled differently in various burs. The so-called attack angles are measured in relation to the radial line of the blade. The positive rake angle, in which the face of the blade is located behind the radial line, is the most effective cutter. It reduces a larger portion of the tooth surface and is the characteristic design for most tungsten carbide burs. A negative rake angle, in which the face of the blade is located in front of the radial line, is used for regular steel burs. Regular steel burs require this angle because it is less conducive to fracture. Because of the negative angulation of the blade a smaller amount of tooth structure is removed.

Accelerated speed burs are designed to last longer and are more effective in chip removal than other types of burs. For this reason a land is placed on the blade to increase the thickness of the cutting edge. This technique is common in industrial milling and has been used on most of the new burs designed for air turbines.

The chip space, or flute, located between the bur teeth has been increased by

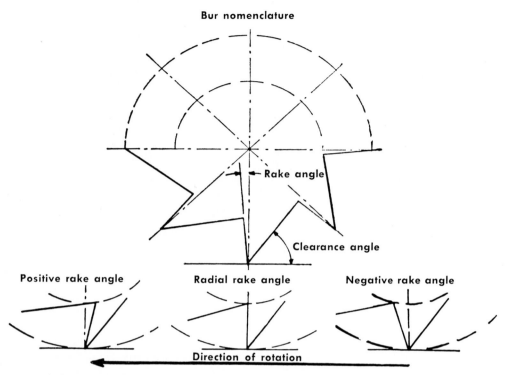

Fig. 4-29. Diagram showing the design of dental burs. (From Henry, E. E., and Peyton, F. A.: J. Dent. Res. **33:**281, 1954.)

placing only six or eight blades on the bur. The increased size of this space creates a larger clearance angle (angle between the back of the blade and the tooth surface) and provides room for removal of the fractured piece of tooth. These two features are helpful when operating at high speeds because less interference occurs when the blade is placed on the enamel surface.

The improvements just mentioned have also been placed in the inverted cone and fissure burs. The individual design varies with manufacturers, and effectiveness is determined by the amount of reduction, the temperature produced, and the life of the bur. Evaluation of these factors is made by the way the handpiece feels while the bur is cutting and by the number of successive cuts possible before the bur turns dark and fractures on the edge.

Biologic factors. A number of biologic factors in the design of burs favor efficient tooth reduction. Variations in design and technique are all secondary to the biologic response associated with the preparation. No reduction procedure should cause a response in the pulp greater than the pathologic condition itself. The cavity preparation should be a stimulation rather than an irritation and should cause no irreversible inflammation or degeneration in pulp tissue.

In an ideal cavity preparation the response is confined to the cut dentin tubules and there is no deep tissue involvement. The histologic picture shows increased circulation in the superficial layers and activity in the odontoblastic layers. Proliferation is observed by the formation of fibroblasts, which is thought to be the precursor of protective dentin. This histologic picture is associated with good postoperative results and should be strived for in all techniques. Protective dentin is a physiologic structure that protects the pulp from the thermal changes and ion diffusion indicative of some new restorative materials.

Pulp response to cutting procedures has been studied by a number of investigators. Their results have confirmed that the ultraspeed instrument is the least traumatic of all rotary instruments. A number of criteria are used to study pulp response and trauma, which must be controlled regardless of the speed range used. Within each speed range the operating load, revolutions per minute of the cutting point, diameter of the bur, temperature rise on the tooth surface, and type of coolant influence pulp response.

In Table 4-2 the factors associated with each speed range are categorized according to research findings. The information is helpful in understanding the accepted methods of rotary cutting. Proficiency and lack of trauma prevail only with careful application of the techniques advocated for each speed range.

The most controversy concerns the amount of trauma prevented by use of air turbine coolants. Both water and air coolants are available with the air turbine handpiece, and the advantages and disadvantages of each have been studied by tissue sections, high-speed photography, and subjective patient symptoms. The data are somewhat conflicting and are therefore confusing to the practicing dentist. Accurate comparisons of research findings cannot be made because different criteria were used to study the biologic response. Using water as a coolant presents a problem because it blocks the vision in the operating field. This is exasperating when copious amounts of water (100 to 200 ml. per minute) are used, and the method requires vacuum elimination to keep the surgical field cleared. It has been reported that, if 2 mm. of sound dentin are present between the bur and pulp tissue, there will be no irreversible pulp response no matter what rotary method is used. There are reports that burn lesions and abscesses of the pulp occur when large cylindric diamonds and excessive pressure are used with air turbines. Conversely, other studies demonstrate that limited pulp response occurs with the turbines when small-diameter burs are used with normal 4-ounce operating loads and air coolants alone. It is apparent that the beginning student and "heavy-handed" operator should use water as a coolant prophylactically. This is necessary because of the overextension that invariably results with the initial use of the air turbine handpiece. If the rules for using ultraspeeds are abused, the pulp tissue cannot tolerate the additional cutting.

The 2-mm. safety dimension for the pulp is composed of dentin. The protection it affords is thought to result from the insulating qualities of the dentin layer. The thermal conductivity of dentin has been determined at 2.29×10^{-3},

Table 4-2. Classification of rotary cutting

	Main use	Common burs	Cutting mechanism	Handpiece load	Temperature production and coolant
Regular speed, 2,000 to 6,000 rpm (standard engine)	Excavation or refinement	Inverted cone for opening; fissure bur for refining	Undermining and fracturing	1 to 4 pounds, intermittent	Mild; air
High speed, 20,000 to 50,000 rpm (adjusted engine)	Surface reduction or smoothing	Diamonds, mainly tapered	Grinding (surface apposition)	½ to 2 pounds, steady or regular	Severe; water (50 to 100 ml.)
Ultraspeed, 150,000 to 250,000 rpm (airotors)	Gross cutting	Fissure burs, Nos. 57 to 556 and 699 to 700 (Nos. 34 to 33 only for proximal surfaces)	Milling (chip removal)	4 to 6 ounces, intermittent	Negative or severe; air and water used separately or as spray (5 to 40 ml./ minute)

which is comparable to the values of concrete, glass, and zinc phosphate cement. The dentin minimizes temperature transfer to pulp tissue and is particularly helpful when large metallic restorations are used. The dentin also protects the pulp by blocking the diffusion of solutions and ions from the restoration; although the dentin tissue is permeable, it is considered to be an effective chemical barrier.

The protection afforded by dentin has been studied by subjecting the surface of cavity preparations to elevated temperatures. In one study the pulps were viewed histologically and were found to recover after temperatures of 600° F. were applied to the tooth surface. When the dentin layer is estimated to be thin, an intermediary base is used to furnish insulation to the pulp. The greater the thickness of the dentin remaining in the tooth restoration, the more successful the service will be from the aspect of pulp protection.

The variable of pressure, or operating load on the handpiece, is thought to be the most traumatic aspect of rotary tooth reduction. An increase in pressure will elevate the surface temperature, and if the protective dentin thickness is not present, an irreversible response can occur. Temperature is elevated by an increase in the revolutions per minute and the diameter of the bur, but the pulp response is regulated by the pressure on the cutting point. All speed ranges, regardless of the bur or preparation being used, necessitate a water or air coolant during the operation.

The water coolants are used when the recommended pressure is damaging. The medium-speed range is critical in this regard, requiring a heavy stream of water to cool the bur and tooth surface. A spray-bottle attachment is used to

Recommended bur diameter	Maintenance	Hazards	Use in preparation	Patient comfort and acceptance
1 to 1.2 mm.	Daily care and supervision; minimal cost; oil lubricant	Moderate temperature rise; torque on bur	+	Negative—vibration
0.8 to 1 mm.	Weekly care and supervision; grease lubricant; maximum adjustments; belt wear	Severe temperature; torque on diamond	++	Moderate—vibration reduced
0.75 to 0.8 mm.	Minimal care; daily supervision; oil lubricant; air and wire cleaning of air lines	Oil mist; bacterial and fomite contamination; hearing damage	+++	Maximum—complaints of dust, noise, and odor

produce 50 to 150 ml. of water per minute; it is required when diamonds are used. Water-evacuating units are then necessary to keep the surgical field clear because regular unit aspiration with the saliva ejector is not adequate. Air turbine handpieces have coolant tubes that are directed onto the bur tip and tooth surface. The water coolants are directed from the bur by the "air swirl" at the cutting site. The inexperienced operator should use the water coolant with the burs for additional protection; when diamonds are placed in the air turbine, the water is needed to clean the cutting point.

The air and water coolants only assist the operation; of primary importance is the regulation of the pressure on the bur.

Abrasives

Abrasive cutting points are employed to abrade tooth surfaces. The procedure is slower than burs and is associated with elevated temperatures. Abrasives are used with a coolant and primarily for surface reduction. Different types of abrasives are placed on the shank or wheel and the edges of the exposed abrasive particle cause the reduction. The nature of the cutting mechanism causes abrasives to be confined primarily to surface smoothing and beveling. Abrasives are used for numerous types of work surfaces. The classification of these cutting instruments follows.

Diamonds. The most popular rotating abrasives are thought to be the diamonds. Diamond particles are used for hardness, and they are fused to steel blanks that are shaped as cylinders, wheels, and tapering points. They are more

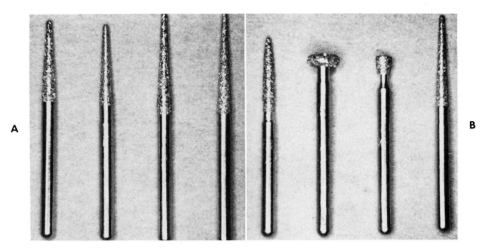

Fig. 4-30. A, Different shapes of diamond abrasives. **B,** Abrasive points.

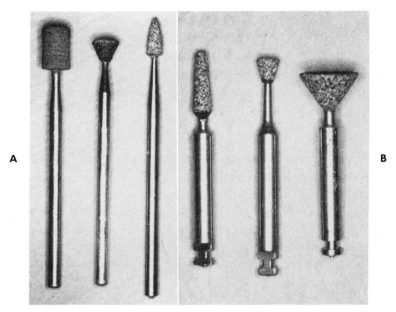

Fig. 4-31. A, Ruby sharpening stone and two mounted carborundum stones for the doriot handpiece. **B,** Mounted carborundum stones for the contra-angle handpiece.

effective with the medium-speed range if a generous coolant of 50 to 100 ml. of water per minute is utilized. The water is required to clean the tooth particles from between the diamond particles since the tooth surface cannot be reduced if the diamond particles are clogged. Commercial diamonds are sorted by mesh sizes that leave a corresponding roughness on the cavity wall. In some cases the imprint is not acceptable for the finished preparation. The diamond produces a better wall when numerous mesh sizes are used, and the smaller the particle size the smoother the imparted imprint.

Flame-shaped and tapered diamonds are selected to place gingival bevels and to smooth the cappings and wall flares of the preparation (Fig. 4-30). The tip must be pointed and small enough to reach the corners of the outline. The acceptance of the air turbine and the results obtained with burs have reduced the use of diamonds. The abrasive action of the diamond is dangerous in intra-coronal preparations because of the problem of temperature control.

Mounted stones. Small finishing and polishing carborundum stones are mounted on long or short handpiece shanks. They are useful in smoothing tooth structure and in polishing metallic surfaces at regular speeds. The stones are manufactured in different sizes and have many applications for refining inlay preparations and preparing gold castings for cementation (Fig. 4-31). The carborundum particles are molded under pressure and fused with a silica binder to produce the stone. They cannot be used with accelerated speed because the binder and the particles break down. The mounted stones are capable of smoothing tooth structure similar to the plane fissure bur. They are kept centric by a truing stone; an uneven edge would result in fracture of the stone. Mounted stones are also helpful in smoothing tooth structure that has been adjusted or the edges of teeth that have been fractured.

Unmounted stones. Abrasive wheels and points made of corundum and carborundum are used for polishing. The abrasiveness of the wheels is related to the hardness and size of the particle. The hardest particles are used for polishing chromium cobalt castings, and steel and the softer types are used for polishing gold castings and appliances. The unmounted stones are not as accurate as the mounted stones because they are attached to mandrels. The cost of the unmounted stones is low since only the material is purchased and the sizes can be obtained for long or short mandrels. The stones are not applied often to tooth structure.

Rubber wheels. Many types of rubber wheels can be obtained for polishing (Fig. 4-32). Burlew rubber wheels are popular because they are soft and bend into the contours of the restoration. The Burlew disk is used for polishing and also in laboratory exercises. Temperature is controlled with an air coolant when the rubber wheels are used on the teeth. The rubber abrasive is an intermediate step in the polishing of metal. Other rubber wheels can be used that are more abrasive and therefore more effective in smoothing harder metals such as stainless steel.

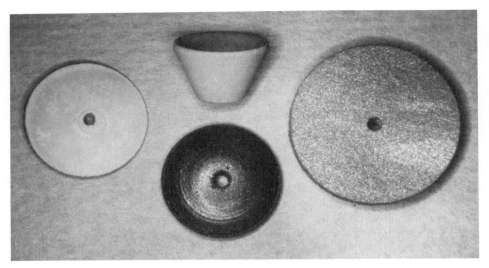

Fig. 4-32. Rubber abrasive wheels for polishing metal.

Sandpaper disks. Different grits of sandpaper are glued to paper with shellac to produce various degrees of abrasiveness (Fig. 4-33). The most popular disks are garnet and cuttlefish. The particle size of these two abrasives is graded, and the disks are used in an order of descending abrasiveness. This procedure gradually smooths the surface and imprints the wall similar to diamond instruments. The disks are attached to a screw mandrel in the handpiece. If they are used in the oral cavity, the disks are coated with cocoa butter to prevent the shellac binder from getting wet. Although loss of the particles is retarded, the disk will last only a short time in saliva. Not only is this problem alleviated by the dry rubber dam field, but the gingival tissue is also protected from the disk by the sheet of latex.

The common disks come in diameters of ⅜, ½, ⅝, and ¾ inch. The smaller disks are applied more often because they reach more areas when polishing. The grits are marked from No. 0 to No. 000, which is a rough to smooth gradation for both the garnet and the cuttlefish disks. Intraoral finishing is useful in casting work, but intraoral polishing must be done cautiously and confined to the restoration. If care is not taken, the disk will damage the enamel and cementum around the metal and become a nidus for staining and bacteria.

Crocus disks. These are paper disks charged with iron oxide. The crocus disks are used to smooth the margins of castings after the sandpaper abrasives have been used. The disks come in different sizes and are used on the margin lightly, only to polish the gold. Other abrasives are not necessary after use of crocus disks and they are not placed in the oral cavity. Regular screw mandrel mounting holds the disk while it is being turned.

Many other types of abrasives are available that can be used for smoothing

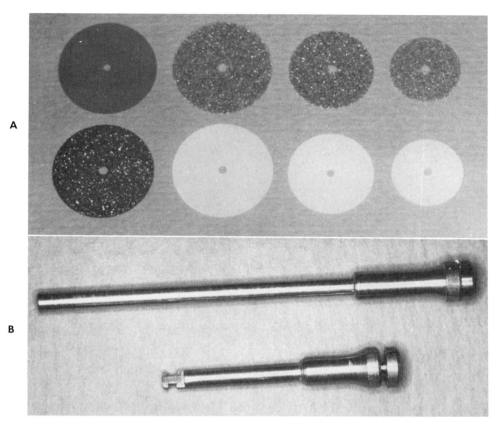

Fig. 4-33. A, Top row: a crocus disk and garnet sandpaper disks. Bottom row: a separating corundum disk and cuttlefish sandpaper disks. **B,** Polishing mandrels used with straight and contra-angle handpieces.

and polishing (Fig. 4-34). These materials include wax compounds or powders that are held on the surface by soft brushes or rubber cups.

Polishing compounds

Polishing the restoration is the last phase of the operative procedure. The metal surface of the restoration is first burnished and smoothed and then polished, creating an amorphous surface layer that is more passive to the attack of corroding ions. The luster of the restoration is attained by polishing, and the metal will feel as smooth as the tooth to the patient. Polishing materials include silica, pumice, and metallic oxides that are applied with a soft rubber cup or brush wheel. The compounds can be used dry or wet, depending on the location of the tooth in the mouth, the type of surgical field, and the sensitivity of the tooth to temperature change. Although vision is better with dry polishing, the surface apposition of the abrasive is not as effective. Polishing the restoration is necessary both for comfort and for the acceptance of the restoration by the soft tissue.

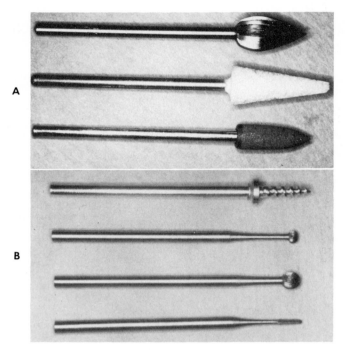

Fig. 4-34. A, The top two abrasives are acrylic finishing points and the other abrasive is a rubber polishing point. **B,** Screw-thread mandrel and three gold finishing burs.

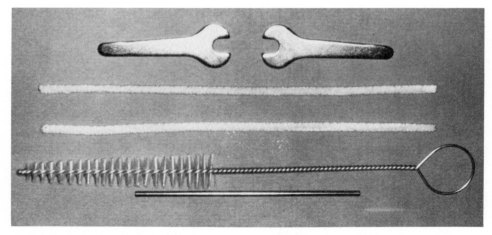

Fig. 4-35. Straight handpiece cleaning kit that includes wrenches, pipe cleaners, brush, and plunger.

The luster on the surfaces should be produced quickly and inspected for the finished restoration.

Handpiece maintenance

Regular care must be given to the handpieces in the office or wear and breakdown will be costly. The unit having accessories is certain to break down on occasion and problems with the power sources are corrected by the dealer. The timing and methods of lubricating the handpieces are provided by the manufacturer at the time of purchase. The requirements should be studied and presented to the office personnel who care for the equipment. The usual procedures in caring for equipment are as follows:

The regular-speed handpieces (doriot type) are opened and wiped with alcohol to remove the old oil and debris from the spindle casting (Fig. 4-35). The components of the handpiece are then coated with engine oil and put back together. The contra-angle handpiece is opened and rotated in cleaning and lubricating solutions. The handpieces are taken from the container and placed in a soiled towel before being driven at high speed in order to throw out excess oil before being used on the patient. This cleaning and lubrication should be done after each appointment in which the handpiece is used.

Medium-speed, ball-bearing handpieces are opened, wiped with alcohol, and lubricated with grease only once a week. If necessary the cleaning can be done more often, but the lubrication of the bearings must not be excessive. The higher operating speed requires the use of heavier lubricants that will adhere to the bearings, and the grease should be placed in the holes marked and diagrammed for the handpiece. Further breakdown of the handpiece will necessitate factory repair.

In ultraspeed air turbines the bearing in the head of the handpiece is lubricated with an oil mist through the air-drive tube. The oil coats the bearings at a rate of 15 to 30 drops per minute while they are functioning. The oil comes from a reservoir in the control box, and care should be taken to keep the solution above the fill line in the container. The oil level should be checked daily, and oil should be added when the level is too low. Running the handpiece without oil will cause the bearings to overheat and fracture. The oil drop rate can be checked by observing the glass on the top of the control box. If bearing lubrication is discovered to be inadequate, the dealer should be contacted. Some air turbines have the advantage of having a grease-packed bearing. Maintenance is accomplished by forcing the grease into the head of the handpiece at the end of each day. This type of lubrication minimizes the problems of air contamination in the operatory, causing less soilage on the surgical field.

Sterilization

Problems occur in keeping the burs and handpieces aseptic. There are many moving parts that need constant lubrication and that would be corroded if subjected to sterilizing procedures. Methods are used only to alleviate the problem of contamination, and the handpiece is considered to be a major problem in sterile hospital surgery.

The burs are cleaned with a wire brush and wiped thoroughly with alcohol. The scrubbed bur is placed in the sterilizing solution or driclave container with the hand instruments. If a sterilizing solution is used, the burs should be dried before being replaced in the storage block or cabinet trays. The most important phase of bur sterilization is the scrubbing, which removes debris from the small cervices in the bur.

Only the sleeve of the doriot handpiece is driclaved. The sleeve is removed and cleaned before being placed in the driclave container with the other instruments. The sleeve is often scrubbed thoroughly and wiped with alcohol, but this procedure is considered less effective than driclaving.

The instruments available for reducing tooth structure are classified as hand cutting and rotary instruments. The effectiveness and variables associated with different designs must be understood before the teeth can be adequately restored.

ADDITIONAL READINGS

Blackwell, R. E.: Black's operative dentistry, ed. 9, Milwaukee, 1955, Medico-Dental Publishing Co., vol. 2.

Bouschor, C. F., and Mathews, J. L.: The use of the air turbine with air spray as coolant, Texas Dent. J. **79**:8, 1961.

Gilmore, H. W.: A method of teaching ultraspeed instrumentation to undergraduate students, J. Dent. Educ. **27**:318, 1964.

Henry, E. E.: The influence of design factors on the performance of the inverted cone bur, J. Dent. Res. **35**:704, 1956.

Henry, E. E., and Peyton, F. A.: The relationship between design and cutting efficiency of dental burs, J. Dent. Res. **33**:281, 1954.

Lammie, G. A.: A comparison of the cutting efficiency and heat production of tungsten carbide and steel burs, Brit. Dent. J. **90**:251, 1951.

Lammie, G. A.: A study of some different tungsten carbide burs, Dent. Rec. **72**:285, 1952.

McGeehee, W. H., True, H. A., and Inskipp, E. F.: A textbook of operative dentistry, ed. 4, New York, 1956, McGraw-Hill Book Co., Inc.

Morrison, A. H., and Grinnell, H. W.: The theoretical and functional evaluation of higher speed rotary instrumentation, J. Prosth. Dent. **8**:297, 1958.

Osborne, J., Anderson, J. N., and Lammie, G. A.: Tungsten carbide and its application to the dental bur, Brit. Dent. J. **90**:229, 1951.

Peyton, F. A.: Modern methods of shaping cavities in teeth, Fort. Rev. Chicago Dent. Soc. **34**:11, 1957.

Schuchard, A.: Action of water coolants with ultra-high rotating speeds, J. Prosth. Dent. **12**:559, 1962.

Schuchard, A.: Pulpal response at 160,000 r.p.m. using air coolant, J. Calif. Dent. Assoc. **38**:26, 1962.

Skinner, E. W., and Phillips, R. W.: The science of dental materials, Philadelphia, 1960, W. B. Saunders Co.

Stanley, H. R.: Traumatic capacity of high speed and ultrasonic dental instrumentation, J.A.D.A. **63**:749, 1961.

Stanley, H. R., and Swerdlow, H.: Reaction of the human pulp to cavity preparation: results produced by eight different operative grinding techniques, J.A.D.A. **58**:49, 1959.

chapter 5

Selection of restorative materials, bases, and liners

There are numerous materials that can be used to restore teeth. The materials are classified as permanent or temporary, metallic or nonmetallic. The physical properties of the materials differ according to their particular chemical compositions and manipulative techniques. The differences inherent with dental caries, motivation of the patient, economic factors, and diagnostic acumen of dentists have contributed to many concepts on selecting the filling material.

Dentists vary in regard to the use of materials. Criteria for selection are available and have been regularly revised to include new materials. The reports have included research on the physical properties of materials, the stress distribution in the natural dentition, and the factors of oral biology that influence the dental restoration. There are many approaches to the restoration of teeth in ideal patient treatment. The conservation of natural tooth structure and in turn the preservation of a normally functioning pulp are necessary in any restoration. When restoring the tooth, the problems need to be fully evaluated. When conditions in the oral cavity do not permit an acceptable approach, the oral environment must be improved with hygiene.

In some cases restorative materials are used for more than one purpose. In the following list the materials are classified according to their use in clinical practice (Fig. 5-1).

1. Permanent restorations. Materials for permanent restorations must satisfy the objectives of the restoration for periods of 20 to 30 years. When manipulated properly, the cohesive gold fillings, gold inlays, and silver amalgam restorations meet the requirements of this category. An ideal restoration would be one that lasted as long as the tooth.

2. Temporary restorations. These materials last for shorter periods when compared to the life of the tooth. The temporary restoration should seal the tooth or maintain its position until a permanent service can be offered. The temporary materials need to be replaced often. This includes the silicate cement and resin

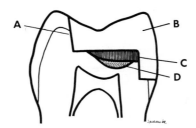

Fig. 5-1. A, Cavity liners. **B,** Permanent restoration. **C,** Intermediate base. **D,** Pulp capping.

restorations and the zinc phosphate and zinc oxide–eugenol cements. Copper cements and gutta-percha were formerly used as temporary restorations but have since been discarded because of toxicity problems.

3. Intermediary bases. Certain compounds are placed between the restoration and tooth structure to protect the vital pulp. These are called intermediary bases. The base should block the chemical irritants from the surface of the restoration and provide the pulp with some insulation from temperature changes. The base material should not be irritating since it is close to the pulp tissue and is used to replace the dentin under the restoration. The intermediary bases are used under metallic restorations in areas of stress and are commonly made of zinc phosphate, polycarboxylate, and reinforced zinc oxide–eugenol cements. They are used as an aid to established resistance form.

4. Liners. These materials are placed on the cavity walls either to sedate the pulp and seal the dentinal tubules or to improve the adaptation of the restorative material to tooth structure. Cavity varnish and calcium hydroxide are best suited for lining the cavity. They are an adjunct to the method of restoration and are routinely indicated for some services.

Black outlined the attributes that an ideal filling material should possess.[1] These qualities were placed in categories of primary and secondary importance and are still used to evaluate the efficiency of new materials or the development of new techniques.

PRIMARY FACTORS

The properties of restorative materials that are of primary importance are as follows:

1. Indestructibility in the fluids of the mouth (Fig. 5-2). The restoration should not dissolve in the oral cavity. This property is described as the solubility of a material, and it is measured by the actual weight loss after the restoration is placed in different environments or solutions.

2. Adaptability to the walls of cavities (Figs. 5-3 and 5-4). Adaptability refers to the degree of mechanical interlocking and sealing between the material and the wall of the cavity preparation. This property is studied by observing

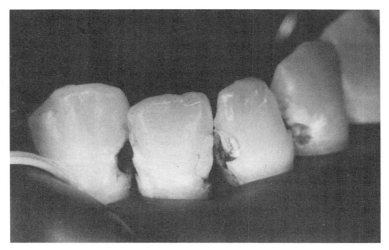

Fig. 5-2. Several examples of the clinical solubility of silicate cement.

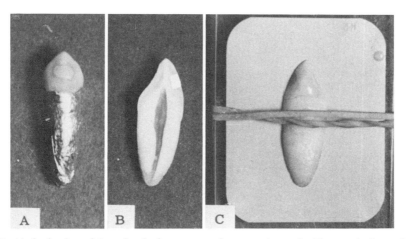

Fig. 5-3. Method of studying the leakage around restorations. **A,** The tooth is sealed and placed in radioactive calcium chloride. **B,** The tooth is sectioned. **C,** The tooth and restoration are placed on the x-ray plate. Leakage is assessed by the black line; the reduction of the plate is caused by the radioactive calcium that surrounds the restoration. (Courtesy Marjorie Swartz.)

the amount of penetration of radioisotopes, dyes, and bacteria into the space between the restoration and the tooth structure.

3. _Freedom from shrinkage or expansion following placement in the cavity form._ This linear dimensional stability or change is measured in microns. The change results from the setting reaction or from the thermal expansion and contraction of the material.

4. _Resistance to attrition._ This property is measured by the resistance of the

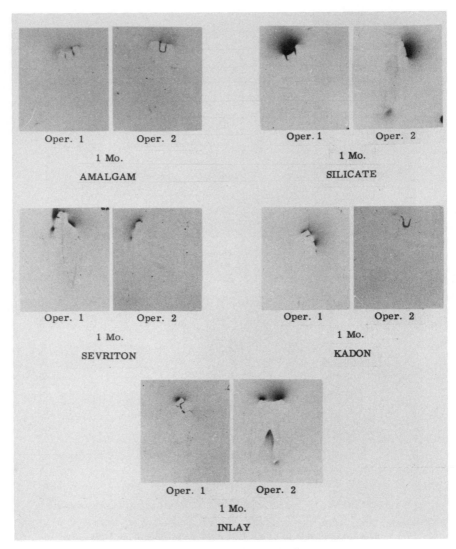

Fig. 5-4. Leakage associated with certain materials and the differences that exist between clinicians. (Courtesy Marjorie Swartz.)

material to certain abrasives and is compared with profile characteristics of the surface to determine the amount of material lost or surface change.

5. Sustaining power against the force of mastication. This property is measured by the compressive and tensile strengths of the material. The strengths are important because a combination of these forces occurs in mastication. Compressive strength has been studied more than the other properties. A universally accepted shear test has not yet been designed.

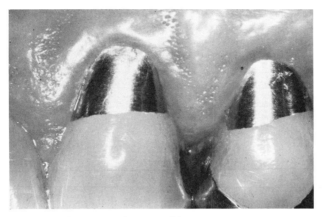

Fig. 5-5. Surface integrity of 5-year cohesive gold restorations. Note the lack of tarnish and corrosion and observe the excellent gingival response.

SECONDARY FACTORS

Properties of restorative materials that are of secondary importance are as follows:

1. Color or appearance. Satisfactory esthetics is occasionally difficult to achieve with metallic restorations. When the cavity margin is visible, esthetics is augmented by using a neat outline form in the preparation or by selecting a tooth-colored restorative material. In some cases esthetic considerations are of primary importance.

2. Low thermal conductivity. Thermal conductivity must be controlled in order to prevent painful pulp responses. Thermal conductivity is measured in calories per second; it is influenced by the type of base material as well as by the thickness of the insulating base.

3. Convenience of manipulation. This property refers to ease in handling specific instruments, and for this purpose devices have been designed to condense or pack the material into the cavity preparation. Although this factor should not greatly influence the selection of the material, measures should be taken to reduce the strain of the operation whenever possible.

4. Resistance to tarnish and corrosion (Fig. 5-5). This property prevents surface or chemical contamination, and it is measured by direct observation of the restoration after storage in different solutions. A noble metal such as pure gold is one that does not readily tarnish or corrode in the oral fluids. Tarnish and corrosion are encouraged when dissimilar metals contact in the mouth.

The dentist should know the attributes of restorative materials and the accepted standards for each. The actual purchase of specific materials should be governed by experience gained while working with acceptable products, and all the materials should be approved by the Bureau of Standards of the American Dental Association. Materials that have no specification should be selected on the basis of reliable research or upon recommendation of a dental school in the area.

SELECTION OF RESTORATIVE MATERIALS

In addition to the attributes of ideal restorative materials, Black also listed a number of factors that influence their selection.[1] They are included with some modifications in the following discussion.

Physical properties

The occlusal surfaces of the posterior teeth and the incisal edges of the anterior teeth are areas that receive stress in masticatory function. Restoration of these areas requires a material of high strength to withstand the forces and resist fracture. Only the metallic restorations and the full-coverage acrylic and porcelain crowns adequately satisfy this requirement. The gold alloy casting is best suited for stressful areas, and it can be used to form the shapes and contacts in the teeth that are necessary for individual and group function in the dentition. Although the gold casting is difficult to fabricate accurately and the cement that is used for luting is vulnerable, the properties of the gold alloy are acceptable for rebuilding tooth structure.

The compressive strength is not only related to the physical properties but also to the thickness of the restoration that is placed in the tooth. The more bulk in depth, the less likely a gross fracture will occur. This rule concerning bulk is followed in placing the amalgam restoration. The resistance of silver amalgam to compressive forces is adequate when the bulk requirement is satisfied, but the problem of fracture at the edge of the restoration still exists.[2] The marginal breakdown is attributed to the low tensile and shear strengths and is one disadvantage of the amalgam restoration.

The tensile and shear strengths maintain the marginal integrity of the restoration (Fig. 5-6). The cohesive golds are known for excellent marginal quality, which is enhanced by the ductility of the metal.[3] It is thought that elongation of the margin occurs during finishing, and the increased tensile forces of the instrumentation require that the restoration be placed in more intimate contact with the tooth. The gold casting also has this advantage, but it cannot be perfected to the same degree in the cavity preparation because of its greater hardness and the presence of the cement liner.

Although other physical properties are important, strength appears to be discussed and considered more often than the others. The tooth-colored compounds—silicate cement and acrylic resins—are not sufficiently strong to resist the functional forces and should be used only in areas where there is no direct application of stress. Such areas include the proximal surfaces of the anterior teeth where the angle is not involved and the labial or buccal surfaces of the teeth.

Adaptability to the cavity wall is the most important property of restorative

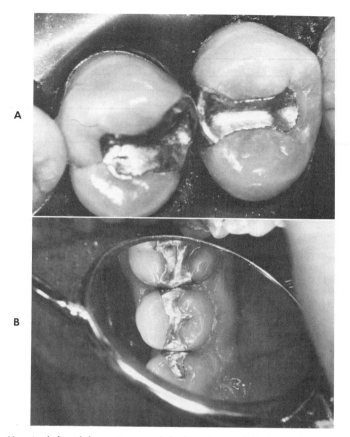

Fig. 5-6. A, Marginal breakdown in a polished and unpolished amalgam restoration. Both restorations are 7 years old. **B,** Typical result of marginal integrity in a polished, conservative amalgam restoration after 5 years.

materials.[4] To achieve a perfect restorative material an acceptable chemical and physical bond to tooth structure would have to be developed. A hermetic seal of the cavity form could then be produced by the restoration to prevent additional involvement of caries and pulp irritation. Other properties of strength, color, and manipulative ease could then be added to complete the perfect material.

The amount of leakage around different types of restorations has been assessed both in vitro and under clinical conditions. Leagage is found to occur around all the restorative materials now being utilized.[5,6] Extracted and clinical teeth have been restored; subjected to media containing radioisotopes, dyes, and bacteria; and later sectioned in order to measure the ingress of oral fluids. The degree of adaptation is assessed by the amount of leakage between the restoration and tooth.

The metallic restorations, particularly amalgam and the direct golds, seal the cavity preparation more effectively, and leakage around these materials decreases with time. Among the many factors that influence adaptation are the surface characteristics of the tooth structure, the particle size or type of material being used, and the insertion technique. From the standpoint of adaptation the statement that "the amalgam restoration is better than it looks" is true. This is attributed to a gradual oxide formation on the wall of the restoration that acts as a mechanical plug. The cohesive golds are also found to be acceptable when tested by isotopes, but the leakage varies widely with the method of condensation and the type of gold that is used.

The leakage around the restoration must be controlled in all teeth on which operative procedures are used. The saliva guarantees moisture in the space between the restoration and tooth, and the environment that is created is produced by bacteria and acid formed from ingested food. If the oral solution is capable of decalcifying tooth structure, the damage will continue regardless of the hygienic measures employed by the patient. The ability of the material or technique to seal the preparation should be determined prior to clinical usage.

Size of the carious lesion

The surface decalcification and depth of the caries are observed before selecting the material. In posterior teeth the greater the involvement, the more likely that a gold casting should be used for strength. In anterior teeth the involvement of numerous surfaces dictates the full-coverage restoration. When this cannot be done, methods of retaining and supporting other materials can be used, but they do not serve as adequately. Incipient lesions in anterior teeth can be restored with a number of materials, and the selection is governed by consideration of the other factors.

Caries susceptibility

When new caries develops and control methods are being instituted, a less permanent restorative material should be used. The amalgam restoration, with its sealing ability, and the silicate cement, with its ability to reduce the solubility of enamel, are inserted to protect the tooth in caries-susceptible patients. The acid environment, together with the caries, dissolves the cement that holds the inlay in position, and use of the gold casting is therefore contraindicated.[7] If the lesion is exceptionally large, the tooth can be held in position by the pin-retained amalgam restoration and continue to function.

When caries persists, the diagnostic aids for bacteriologic activity and salivary and dietary problems should be used. Rather than merely restoring each new lesion the main contributing factors should be determined and controlled. When control measures are used by the dentist and the patient, caries susceptibility can be diminished.

Condition of the pulp tissue

If a healthy functioning pulp is not apparent or if the electric vitality tests do not indicate normal tissue, a permanent restoration should not be inserted.[8] The treatment plan should be formulated after the tooth has been excavated or extracted if endodontic therapy is not feasible. The tooth in question should be sealed with a reinforced mix of zinc oxide–eugenol to prevent pain until the diagnosis or treatment has been made.[9]

The restoration must protect the pulp at all times. If an endodontic opening is made, subsequent degeneration results in loss of the tooth or damage to the restoration. Precautions are taken by using controlled instrumentation, preserving the dentin, and selecting proper bases and liners. The condition of the pulp is studied by excavation, examination, and electric vitality testing. The tissue must be normal before the treatment plan can be made.

In providing a healthy pulp, biologic considerations must be observed by using a material that does not contain toxic qualities.[10] The pulp and periodontal tissues would be damaged if irritants leaked from the restoration, and the tissue abutting the restoration would become necrotic or irritated. Moreover, absorption into the bloodstream could alter the physiology. The cements have been studied because of the acid present on the surface, but damage resulting from use of the cements is prevented by using liners properly.[11] Liners have been advocated for some of the new resin compounds because of their toxicity.

Application of the rubber dam

The type of surgical field that is used influences the choice of the material because of the deleterious effects of moisture on the setting reactions and adaptation of some materials. If the rubber dam cannot be placed to produce an ideal surgical environment, an involved and expensive restorative service should not be selected. The design of rubber dam clamps and the greater thickness of latex rubber have simplified the application of the rubber dam. Problems in stabilizing the clamp to retain the dam occur in partially erupted or grossly fractured teeth, but the new designs are useful in these conditions. If a restoration is needed, the cements can be used to limit the caries until more eruption occurs or until the gingival tissue can be altered to receive the rubber dam clamp. The cement can be removed after a few months and a permanent restoration can be placed in the properly isolated tooth.

Ability of the operator

The skill of the individual dentist has much to do with the selection of a material or technique. If he is not absolutely proficient, as the new graduate sometimes is not, the tendency is to refer the case to a more qualified individual or to use an alternate procedure. Operative skills are developed by continual practice, and more involved procedures can be performed as diagnostic acumen improves. No tooth operation should be attempted unless the operator has the necessary confidence and knowledge.

Esthetics

The appearance of the teeth influences the type of treatment recommended for the patient. Personal desires and the actual display or prominence of the teeth influence the selection of the material. As discussed previously, the white tooth-colored materials have undesirable properties and need replacement within a few years, indicating that they should not be used unless the outline includes a visible tooth surface. The permanent, metallic type of restoration is difficult to hide in the extensive outline form having a labial or buccal exposure.

Other problems are confronted in improving esthetics. Radical methods of creating a desirable appearance include the full-coverage veneered castings or porcelain jacket crowns. The pulp size and the expense involved in this service limit its use. The display of metal and discoloration involved in silver amalgam restorations have caused many dentists to use only gold in the bicuspids. Patient variables often eliminate a selection of this nature, but if an obvious interest in esthetics is discovered during the examination, the use of gold should be presented. When the patient is not satisfied with the appearance of his teeth, he is usually unhappy about the care received.

Economic factors

The time and expense involved with the service are commonly used as the basis for establishing fees. Many procedures that are indicated cannot be performed because of inadequate financing on the part of the patient. To preserve the natural dentition an alternate service that is not as costly is provided. Although some degree of function or esthetics is sacrificed, the loss is far less severe than loss of the vital teeth.

Payment plans can be established with the aid of the dentist, professional societies, or a financial agency. The schedule of payments is agreed upon at the time the treatment plan is presented. There are many payment plans and dental care programs available so that the ideal treatment plan is within reach of most people. Fee schedules are formulated by the dental society or the local organization of dentists. The cost of services is usually in accord with the economic status of the community. The additional cost of a specialist's services or of an unusual case is regulated only by the dentist providing the care. Unreasonable fee schedules are ethical problems and are as detrimental to the profession as inadequate fees.

The least expensive treatment program employs preventive concepts and conservative restoration of the teeth. These objectives are accomplished when the ideal treatment plan is fulfilled and usually result in only a few costly restorations. In considering the initial cost the patient should be reminded that replacements and new lesions will practically be eliminated and that subsequent costs will primarily involve maintenance. This cost per year is much lower than most health care and cosmetic services. This type of conservative dental plan is a creditable program and it helps to alleviate the problem of fees.

Patient motivation

The attitude of the patient toward dental care and the importance he places on health influences the selection of materials. In the modern society most families are interested in their dental health. The public relations methods used by medical and dental societies educate, to a limited degree, most of the population as to the importance of saving the teeth. Motivation increases in parents when caries in their children's teeth is controlled or when a restoration functions well for a number of years. The dentist sincerely involved in educating his patients suddenly has more work than time will permit. However, some patients have undesirable attitudes toward dental treatment, and they should be selected for comprehensive planning. Health care measures for these people should include a thorough maintenance program and instructional aids that will help to improve their attitudes. Until motivation and appreciation are established, time should not be wasted in planning comprehensive treatment for the unwilling patient.

Office procedures should include distribution of information about the accepted methods of restorative dentistry. Literature can be furnished and sent home with patients or presented in the course of treatment during the appointment. Patients who consistently appear for the recall examination indicate improved attitudes. Regardless of the type of appointment, diagnosis of the problem and the means necessary to restore optimum function are presented. When this procedure is followed, the dentist cannot be criticized for neglecting to inform the patient of his dental condition, and this mutual understanding helps to improve patient attitudes.

• • •

Black listed a number of other factors that are sometimes helpful in determining which restorative material should be used.[1] Variables such as age of the patient, position and alignment of the tooth, avoiding use of dissimilar metals, and other factors are recognized as helpful. The accuracy with which the selection is made and the treatment given differs widely with variables in teeth, patients, and caries. Individual skill will always be important, and postoperative examinations will reveal the efficacy of the service. The individual practice should not be confined to the use of one or two materials but should offer the patient a full selection of services. Close scrutiny of the case will indicate which materials would be most suitable for the individual.

THE DENTAL PULP

The dental pulp is a highly vascular and innervated piece of connective tissue that occupies the tooth chamber.[12] It is responsible for the vitality of the tooth because it is directly connected to the systemic circulation. The pulp is a sensitive organ because it reacts to external stimuli, and it is also formative because it is responsible for the production of protective dentin. The deposition of protective dentin gradually reduces the size of the chamber and pulp tissue during the clinical life of the tooth, but this process does not interfere with the health of the tissue. Once degeneration begins, the pulp becomes inflamed and then necrotic, resulting in liquefaction and abscess in the periapical bone. Unless endodontic procedures are executed, the infection results in loss of the tooth.

The pulp tissue is divided into a superficial and a deep zone.[13] The superficial tissue contains the odontoblasts and the cell-free and cell-rich zones. A majority of pulp reactions involve only the superficial layers and commonly result in recovery. The deep tissue contains fibroblasts, ground substance, and blood vessels. The severe responses observed in these take the pulp longer to resolve, and sometimes they are conducive to degeneration. The more severe the stimulus the greater the amount of secondary dentin that is deposited under the area of the tooth receiving the injury.

The pulp vessels do not contain much smooth muscle, but the tissue does have a self-regulating blood mechanism. This is helpful in carrying away local irritants or solutions and in regulating the temperature produced in the tissue during cavity preparation. The pulp has resolved temperatures of 600° F., indicating that the tissue is resistant to injury and that the circulatory mechanism is effective.[14] Few restorative procedures cause such an elevation in the surface dentin temperature, which indicates that thermogenesis is not a problem in cavity preparation unless the tissue comes in contact with the bur.

The reaction of the pulp to cavity preparation and to filling materials has been extensively studied. A meaningful early paper on the subject was written by Van Huysen and Gurley.[15] It was demonstrated in several teeth that the deeper the cavity preparation, the greater the response produced in the pulp. For many years standardized cavity preparations were used to study the irritating qualities of materials. All these studies verified that a direct relationship exists between cavity depth and inflammation. The results of these studies could be summarized by saying materials cause responses that are not severe enough to prevent full recovery of the surface tissue unless the pulp is exposed. This consensus would indicate that cavity preparations or actual pulp exposures masked the true chemical and physical responses of the restorations in the early studies.[16]

New data to substantiate this opinion were collected with the aid of the operating microscope. A technique was developed for producing a pulp exposure without causing an inflammatory response (Fig. 5-7).[17,18] The technique was used to study the toxic properties of restorations that produced only a minimal inflammatory response when the pulp had not been penetrated. Without direct exposure or undue pressure and fracture of the dentin floor the pulp recovered after having developed only a few inflammatory cells and formed traumatic dentin that resembled osteoid tissue.

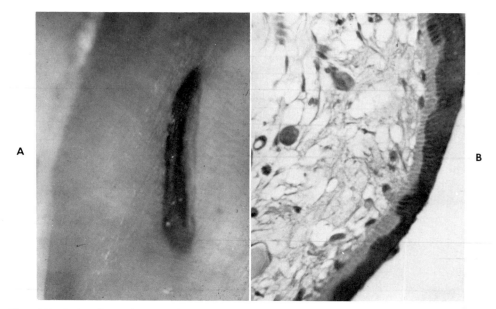

Fig. 5-7. A, Nonhemorrhagic pulp exposure with a drop of pulp fluid in the bottom of the wound. **B,** Lack of inflammation associated with the mechanical nonhemorrhagic pulp exposure. The pulp appears to be a normal histologic structure. (**A** courtesy Dr. Grant Van Huysen.)

An interesting sidelight of the procedure was the detection of pulp fluid that flowed through the bloodless mechanical exposures. The fluid had previously been reported by Haldi and analyzed as being chemically the same as blood serum.[19] The pulp fluid was collected by extending the deep preparation until the red outline of the pulp appeared. The remaining thin dentin wall was flexed until it became thin enough to fracture. Within a few minutes a clear, nonhemorrhagic solution, "dental pulp fluid," appeared in the floor of the cavity. It has been suggested that the fluid mechanism would be helpful in the small clinical exposure because of the outward pressure to prevent the medicaments from contacting the tissue. It appears that the pulp will resolve adverse responses unless an exposure is present and that the normal tissue has a specific defense mechanism.

The atraumatic exposure procedure was also used to study the mechanism of dentin formation. A protein dye was placed in the bloodstream of dogs at timed intervals following cavity preparation.[18] A capping material was also mixed to include a dye, and the reparative dentin was histologically sectioned to detect where its precursor was formed for the actual calcification. The reparative dentin revealed that the injected protein, which was detoxified and placed in circulation by the liver, was responsible for forming the dentin. This would discourage the direct application of special drugs and formulas on the pulp tissue and dictate instead the use of a neutral and nonirritating compound to allow the systemic mechanism to seal off the tissue with secondary dentin.

These data suggest that toothache following restoration results from a minute undetected pulp exposure in the bottom of the cavity. This type of exposure is nonhemorrhagic; it is often caused by the recessional lines of the pulp, and the pain is found to occur at extended periods following the placement of the restoration. Therefore all deep cavity preparations should be prophylactically lined with calcium hydroxide in case an undetected exposure exists.[20] This liner is used because the compounds have a neutral pH and are painted on the dentin by a flow technique. This causes only a superficial necrosis of the pulp tissue and does not initiate degeneration by displacing the tissue in the chamber.

The recuperative power and protective mechanism of the pulp was further demonstrated by Mitchell.[21] Silicate cement was previously blamed for many pulp deaths. In monkeys the histologic results were not as expected in cavities that were exposed to saliva or restored with silicate cement. The pulp tissues recovered if 600μ of sound dentin remained between the cavity floor and the tissue. The cut surfaces exposed to saliva recovered with the deposition of dentin. The acid on the surface was damaging, but only in near or actual pulp exposures.

The use of medicaments and drugs to assist in healing the pulp tissue is not indicated. Most cleaning solutions cause more irritation than they prevent. Experiments with the corticosteroids have revealed a reduction in inflammation following cavity preparation, but the significance of this in relation to repair has not been explained.[22] The reduction in the number of leukocytes might not be desirable if the pulp tissue has been injured. Solutions of this nature are not really helpful except to prevent toothache or to postpone endodontic therapy. Chemical treatment of the dentin is not recommended. A better understanding of the mechanism for medicaments is necessary because of the outward pressure of the dental pulp fluid. How can the applied solutions reach the tissue?

The studies that have been conducted concerning pulp reactions to both instrumentation and filling materials indicate that the future is promising for restorative dentistry. Any procedure that is done properly does not produce an untoward pulp reaction. The damage is caused by a carious or mechanical exposure and superficially by tearing or displacing the tissue in the chamber or by bacterial contamination of the surface.

More teeth are being saved by restoration because of better instrumentation and pulp protection. The regulatory and repair mechanisms of the blood are also helpful in maintaining vitality when the tissue has not been exposed.

BASES AND LINERS

Bases and liners support the restoration and protect the pulp tissue while the deep lesion is being restored.[23] Some liners improve physical properties. The properties of an ideal base or liner are as follows:

1. The base or liner should improve the marginal seal and cavity wall adaptation.
2. The thermal conductivity of the restoration (metallic) should be reduced by the base.

3. The base or liner should prevent chemical exchange between the restoration and the tooth.
4. The process of galvanic action should be reduced by the sedative base or liner.
5. When placed on the tooth structure, the base or liner should not irritate the pulp or interfere with the setting reaction of the restoration.
6. The material should be easy to apply and should not contaminate areas of the tooth outside the cavity preparation.

Not all materials possess these qualities, but these are the criteria for selection. Because of the presence of moisture in the tooth and the dissimilar metals used in restorations, nothing can stop a true galvanic response. However, galvanic pain can be relieved by removing the restoration. It has been suggested that pulp exposure could be responsible for this response, and most galvanic problems do occur in the deep restoration.

Materials available

Calcium hydroxide. Calcium hydroxide can be used as a base or a liner and, as mentioned previously, it is the material of choice for prophylactic pulp capping (Fig. 5-8). The compounds are alkaline in composition and have a high degree of flow. Controversy has existed for years over which material is best suited for pulp tissue, and calcium hydroxide is commonly agreed upon. Its opponent, zinc oxide–eugenol, is best suited as a base for relief of toothache because the eugenol is a rubefacient that acts to sedate the diseased pulp.

Pulp capping is not advocated for all exposures in permanent teeth. Calcium hydroxide is used for routine protection and only rarely in cases in which traumatic factors produce mechanical exposure. The mechanical opening must be done in a dry cavity, which is provided by the rubber dam, to minimize the bacterial contamination of the tissue. Pulp capping will be effective in limited cases, but when painful symptoms are involved in a deep restoration, it is believed that unsuccessful capping is responsible for the degenerative symptoms.

Procedures of pulpectomy, pulpotomy, and capping are indicated in deciduous teeth because of the shorter period of tooth retention coupled with a smaller and dynamic pulp tissue.[24] A successful technique is the formocresol pulpotomy in which the remaining pulp tissue is fixed before the restoration is placed. Bacterial contamination and inadequate removal of diseased tissue are deleterious aspects of the capping procedure. Pulp capping is employed as a temporary measure or to postpone extraction.

Cases have been reported in which partial pulpectomy has been successful in fractured anterior teeth. This procedure is accomplished by opening and removing the coronal portion of the exposed pulp immediately following injury and placing calcium hydroxide over the remaining stump. Within a few weeks a calcium bridge is formed directly below the material that seals off the remaining vital tissue.

Restoration of the treated incisor is accomplished by removing the temporary

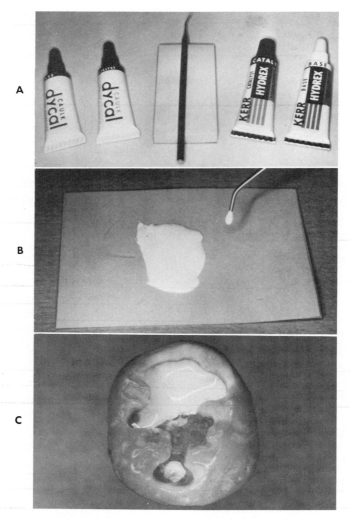

Fig. 5-8. A, Commercial preparations of calcium hydroxide. **B,** The mix and carrying instrument coated with calcium hydroxide. **C,** Calcium hydroxide placed in the excavation of the prepared form for prophylactic pulp capping.

coronal restoration and cementing an orthodontic tube to act as a core.[25] The placement of a jacket crown restoration or one of the sulfinic acid resin materials over the core completes the treatment. Needless to say, diagnosis and timing are extremely important in the partial pulpectomy. In pedodontics the procedure has been useful in incisors with incompletely formed roots that preclude endodontic therapy. Advantages gained by retaining the fractured tooth include esthetics and space maintenance.

Manipulation of the commercial preparations of calcium hydroxide is easy.

Table 5-1. Compressive strength of base material after 30 minutes*

Material	Compressive strength (psi)
Zinc oxide–eugenol	
Cavitec	400
Pulprotex	700
Caulk Z-O-E	800
Temrex	4,200
Calcium hydroxide	
Dycal	500
Hydrex	900
Zinc phosphate	12,000 to 15,000

*From Phillips, R. W.: Dent. Clin. N. Am., Mar., 1965, p. 159.

Small tubes of catalyst and base are usually used, and the contents are proportioned on the mixing slab in equal amounts. The paste is made by mixing the contents thoroughly with a specially designed instrument. The paste is then painted on the solid dentin wall that forms the floor of the carious lesion. The compounds are detectable on radiographs, are water soluble, and exhibit very low strengths. Only a thin layer of the calcium hydroxide is placed over the tooth structure because thick applications crumble.

The strength of calcium hydroxide has been measured at different intervals and compared to the strength of other base materials (Table 5-1).[26] A strength of 400 pounds per square inch is maximum and has been used to support the condensation of amalgam in simple cavities. In the extensive lesion or complex cavity the base should be veneered with a strong cement to prevent fracture during condensation of the restoration. A piece of broken base would act as an inclusion in the amalgam, and although it might not be troublesome, it is hardly a procedure that can be recommended.

When calcium hydroxide liners are applied under large inlays, particularly in a quadrant series, a strong and well-adapted base of zinc phosphate cement should be used to cover the capping (Fig. 5-9). A well-sealed temporary restoration is then placed over this because of the solubility of calcium hydroxide in water. If the calcium hydroxide dissolves, gross leakage results and the bases are dislodged when the impression is removed. Special care must be exercised in the basing to place the compounds on dry tooth structure to ensure the adaptation and hardness of the base. The dry dentin surface is the only satisfactory medium on which the calcium hydroxide can be placed. The mix will flow freely and cover the deepest portion of the wall. When moisture is present, the set of the paste is accelerated, making good coverage of the excavated wall difficult.

To repeat, calcium hydroxide is used mainly as a liner for the deep cavity. It is used in teeth that do not have degenerative symptoms in order to protect

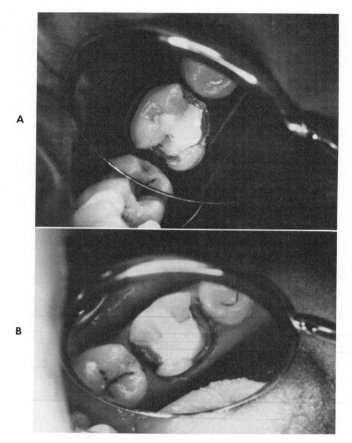

Fig. 5-9. A, Extensive inlay preparation lined with calcium hydroxide. **B,** Preparation veneered with zinc phosphate cement for strength.

an undetected exposure. The amalgam, gold inlay, and silicate restorations should be protected, and if the lesion is extensive in the posterior teeth, it is advisable to veneer the capping with a thin layer of cement. In anterior teeth or the shallow cavity the axial or pulpal wall of the base is located 0.2 mm. inside the dentinoenamel junction. In this case there will not be space for the cement veneer.

The preparations make calcium ions available on the surface of the liner. The calcium ions are free to contact the pulp tissue on one side and are available to neutralize free acid on the other. Their primary purpose is to promote health in the pulp tissue or at least to permit the recuperative powers of the tissue to act.

When a calcium hydroxide liner contacts the pulp tissue, a calcific bridge is formed that seals off the vital tissue.[27] Microscopically, the superficial layer of the pulp degenerates and the tissue withdraws 50 to 150μ from the capping agent.

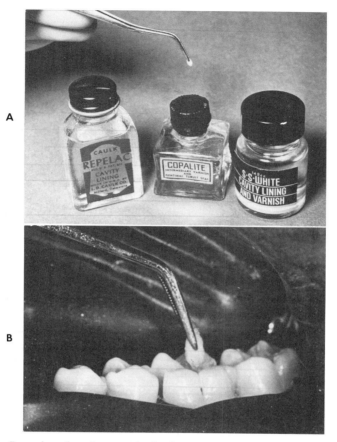

Fig. 5-10. A, Examples of cavity varnish. **B,** Cavity varnish being applied with cotton to the internal parts of the cavity preparation.

Within 4 to 6 weeks the bridge can be radiographed, and the film is used to evaluate the success of the capping. The new dentin is similar to osteoid layer tissue, and it spans the opened area. In some cases there are imperfections in the calcific bridge that resemble stalactites, which are undesirable but which cannot be avoided. The formation of the osteoid bridge, the reaction of the surface of the pulp tissue, the pressure exerted during capping, and bacterial contamination are factors that are difficult to control and that lead to discrepancies in capping procedures.

In the anterior resin preparation in which a base is needed, calcium hydroxide should be used. Cavity varnish will dissolve in the liquid monomer of the resin, contaminating the restoration and the cavity form. A protective cement base could be irritating in this situation, and the problem has been partially solved by use of the new compounds for pulp capping.

Cavity varnish. These liners have recently gained in popularity and are being widely used in restorative dentistry (Fig. 5-10). Cavity varnish is an organic copal or resin gum suspended in solutions of ether or chloroform. These solutions are solvent and dehydrate rapidly after the varnish is placed on the tooth, leaving a thin organic residue on the cavity wall. The thickness of the layer varies from 5 to 25μ, depending on the type of solvent and the number of applications.[28]

The dentist can enhance the result of the restoration within seconds by using varnish because the liner acts not only as an inert plug between the tooth and the restoration but also as a semipermeable membrane. Briefly, by using cavity varnish as a liner, the sealing ability of amalgam is improved, the cement acids are partially blocked, and other ions that are advantageous are harnessed from the restorative materials, particularly amalgam. As previously explained, cavity varnish is not used with restorative resins because the gum dissolves in the monomer.

The varnish is applied with small pieces of cotton that are held with the cotton pliers or curved explorer. The small pledgets can be made in advance or when needed from the bracket dispenser, and the cotton is placed in the solution only once to avoid contamination of the bottle of varnish. The cotton is wetted, and the cavity walls are wiped thoroughly and allowed to dry. The varnish should be applied twice; this is accomplished by wetting another pledget of cotton and following the procedure just described. Coating the inside walls is of primary concern, but if the solution spills over the cavosurface margin, no severe problem will develop to hamper the placement of the restoration. Some clinicians prefer to apply the varnish with small wire loops to minimize the excess.

Solvents are placed in the varnish kits and are used to remove the liner from the external tooth surface. However, rather than forfeit the benefits of having a layer of varnish on the upper portion of the enamel wall, the solvent is seldom used and the sticky debris is tolerated. Special attention is given to the amalgam carving because a greater amount of overhanging metal is encouraged with varnish excess. With the amalgam carving, polishing must be done sooner to prevent fracture or else the overhang must be controlled by using extremely sharp carving instruments.

Another problem in using varnish is to prevent the development of too thick a solution in the bottle. The bottle should be kept over one-half full at all times. Although evaporation occurs rapidly when the cap is removed, the solution level can be controlled by adding more solvent. When thick varnish is applied, the liner does not dry quickly enough and the film is too thick for practical purposes.

The application of cavity varnish is not difficult, its benefits are numerous, and its acceptance by the practicing dentist is increasing. Cavity varnish has specific applications. It is used to line the cavity preparation for amalgam in order to improve the marginal seal. The inert layer of varnish acts as a mechanical plug and, together with the formed oxides, measurably decreases leakage.

This technique causes a reduction in the postoperative sensitivity and inflammation of the restored tooth when compared to methods using no liner. The varnish also helps in the amalgam restoration to retard ion migration into the dentin. This results in noticeably less tooth discoloration, particularly in the bicuspids.

In the direct gold restorations the varnish layer is helpful in minimizing the postoperative symptoms. This is attributed to a reduction in the leakage and not to thermal insulation since it is too thin for this purpose.

Prior to the application of zinc phosphate cement the varnish is applied to partially block the acid. This is advantageous in basing procedures and in seating castings. The "sting" will be eliminated from cementation when the cavity walls are lined with varnish because of the confinement of the free acid.

Cavity varnish is used sparingly in the shallow silicate preparation. This type of preparation does not provide space for the calcium hydroxide, and the varnish is confined to the axial wall dentin. Coverage of the enamel with varnish would block the transfer of fluoride from the silicate restoration, which is usually the main reason for selecting the material.

Zinc phosphate cement. Intermediary bases are used to reduce thermal conductivity in metallic restorations and to block out undercuts in the cavity wall when the tooth is being restored with a casting.[29] The thickness of the base is not responsible for controlling temperature change, but somehow the layer of cement improves postoperative comfort by minimizing thermal transfer from the restoration to the pulp.

The base material that is used most often is zinc phosphate cement (Fig. 5-11). A zinc phosphate powder and phosphoric acid are mixed to form a crystalline mass that is strong enough to be brittle and to support the restoration. The actual strength needed in an intermediary base is not known, but the hard surface is helpful in shaping the desired mortise form inside the cavity. The free acid associated with the surface of the cement is a pulp irritant, and methods employing cavity varnish are used to seal the dentinal tubuli.

The solubility of zinc phosphate cement is difficult to control.[7] Dilute organic acids are harmful on the cement because of the dissolution they cause in the media. Lactic and citric acids are associated with significant weight loss in the cement, and these acids are commonly found in the oral cavity as a result of the diet or carious process. The dissolution of the cement occurs around gold castings or under restorations that have fractured and been penetrated by the saliva.

Two types of mixes are made with zinc phosphate cement. The creamy mix is used for luting castings, and the thick mix is used for basing procedures because of the ease with which it is molded and adapted. The same general procedure is employed for making the thick mix; that is, as much powder as possible is placed in the mass, and spatulation is continued until molding properties are apparent.

The base is placed in the cavity with the Tarno cement instrument. The condenser end is used to tamp the mix against the cavity walls, and the blade

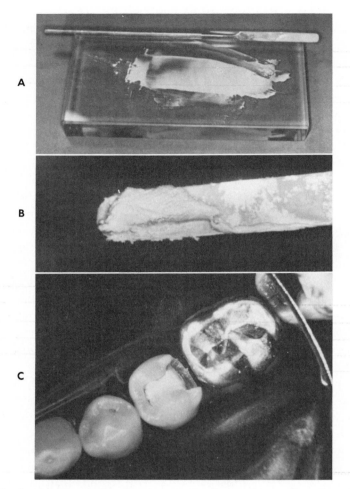

A

B

C

Fig. 5-11. A, A thick mix of zinc phosphate cement for an intermediary base. **B,** Consistency of zinc phosphate cement needed for basing procedures. **C,** Zinc phosphate cement base in the second bicuspid.

is used to form and angulate the surface. An alcohol solution is placed in the dappen dish into which the instrument is dipped. This will prevent the cement from sticking to the Tarno instrument and facilitate the shaping of the intermediary base. Cement bases that are used to reduce thermal transfer are merely placed over the dentin and the surfaces are rounded to provide bulk in the amalgam restoration. The thickness is not as important in reducing thermal transfer as the axial-pulpal surface coverage. The base must not cover an enamel wall or contact the cavosurface margin; therefore, it is necessary to shape the cement with a fissure bur or sharp explorer.

The basing procedure for inlays is done with more care. The cement is placed against the tooth and formed to create a desirable shape for the lost dentin. The bases are squared and smoothed and finally located 0.5 mm. inside the dentinoenamel junction. The tapered fissure burs are used to angulate the base so as to eliminate undercuts in the surrounding walls and to produce an inclination that will encourage withdrawal of the wax pattern.

The cement for the bases should be manipulated by the assistant to reduce the time of the operation. The mixing can be initiated while the toilet of the cavity is being made; the cement is then placed into the transfer area by the assistant and adapted to the tooth by the dentist. A thick mix and well-adapted base will be stronger and therefore less susceptible to the dissolution that could occur from exposure to saliva.

Zinc oxide–eugenol cement. This material is used to a limited degree for intermediary bases. The mix has a bland and sedative action, and in deep cavities the cement is helpful for relieving toothaches. Problems associated with zinc oxide cement include its difficult manipulation and solubility. Commercial preparations have been produced with improved manipulative qualities and strengths. The zinc oxide bases are used mainly in deciduous teeth, but there is no distinct contraindication for their use in the permanent dentition. The deep excavated lesion should not be lined with eugenol because the pulp tissue does not form as good a calcific bridge when an exposure is present.

A thick mix of zinc oxide–eugenol is desirable but difficult to make. Strength is required for spatulation in order to incorporate the powder into the mix. A regular mix can be developed to a thick consistency or the cement can be reinforced with cotton fibers for strength (Fig. 5-12). Although the molding and shaping of zinc oxide–eugenol is similar to that for zinc phosphate cement, this material is not advocated for inlays because of its tendency to fracture. The cement can be used for temporary restorations, in inlay restorations, or for treatment fillings in teeth awaiting extraction or endodontic therapy. Polycarboxylate cements have similar properties but at this time are used primarily for cementation of restorations.

TEMPORARY RESTORATIONS

Temporizing is a procedure used to protect a vital tooth for short periods of time. Temporary restorations can be sedative in nature for the inflamed or freshly stimulated pulp, or they can be rigid to stabilize the arch position of the tooth and to provide function. Aside from alleviating the pain of toothaches, the temporary restoration maintains the teeth for a period of 1 to 2 weeks while they are being prepared for castings. Zinc oxide–eugenol cement and acrylic materials are commonly selected because of the protection and stability they afford the pulpal and periodontal tissues. Obviously, to be effective, the temporary restoration must be comfortable to the patient.

Objectives

The objectives of temporary restorations are as follows:
1. The teeth must be stabilized to prevent drift or movement because of the

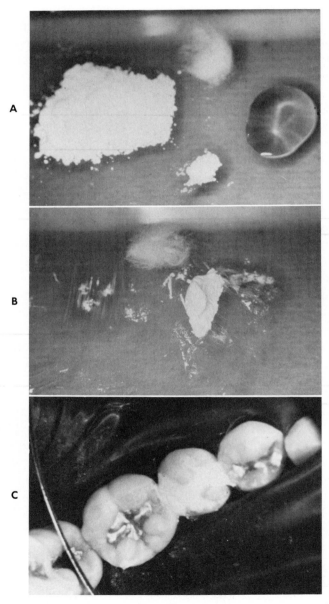

Fig. 5-12. A, Items necessary for a reinforced mix of zinc oxide—eugenol include the powder, liquid, acetate crystals, and cotton fibers. **B,** Mix is completed before the cotton fibers are added. **C,** Reinforced mix placed in the second bicuspid serves as a temporary restoration.

damage that would otherwise occur in the supporting structures and the changes that would be necessary in the casting.

2. The soft tissue must be protected while the temporary restorations are in place. Rough edges and poor contour will cause gingival irritation and hypertrophy.

3. Since the pulps of the teeth should not be disturbed, a sedative dressing or a cementing medium should be used as the temporary restoration. Apposition of the reduced dentin with the sedative cement works as an obtundent and prevents additional pulp injury after the teeth are prepared.

4. The temporary restorations should be comfortable to the patient. Contact with rough surfaces and sharp margins will irritate the tongue and mucosa.

5. The temporary material should seal the preparation in order to prevent discomfort in the interim period. With some compounds this problem has encouraged the use of cements.

Types

Many types of temporary restorations can be used. The materials are selected according to the number of teeth needing protection, the type and location of the cavity preparation, and the demand for esthetics.

Zinc oxide–eugenol cement. A regular mix of zinc oxide–eugenol cement is used for small and protected areas, whereas the extended preparation requires the cement to be reinforced with cotton. A stiff mix is made on the slab, and zinc acetate crystals are added to accelerate setting. The small cotton strands are forced into the mix after the proper consistency has developed. The recommended pack has a doughy consistency and can be picked up and tamped into the excavated tooth. The surface is smoothed with a moistened cotton roll, and the contour and occlusal relationship are tested and adjusted with a large round bur. The cotton strands are cut off the absorbent bracket supply with sharp scissors. Enough strands are added so that they appear on all surfaces of the mix. The size of the pack corresponds to that of the tooth, and the consistency of the mix is regulated by the drops of eugenol that are added.

When multiple preparations are being protected, regular and reinforced mixes are inserted to stabilize the quadrant. The regular mix is inserted into the interproximal spaces and covers the tissue to the level of the pulpal walls of the cavity preparations. The reinforced mix is placed across the occlusal surfaces of the teeth, being carefully shaped with the index fingers and tamped with moistened cotton. A noninterfering occlusal relationship is made with the round bur. The pack serves to lock the teeth in position, while at the same time the adaptation and contour provide the tissues with protection. Zinc oxide–eugenol cement is often used with inlays and is criticized only because of its rough surface. When bell-shaped teeth are being restored with intracoronal preparations, it is the most suitable material that can be used for the temporary restoration.

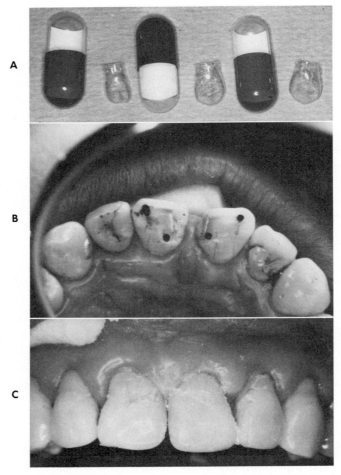

Fig. 5-13. A, Examples of celluloid crown forms. **B,** Postholes blocked with nylon fibers in the inlay preparations. **C,** Crown forms filled with resin to serve as temporary restorations.

Gutta-percha. Gutta-percha is a rubberlike compound placed in the tooth by warming the stick in a flame and packing and holding the mass in the tooth under pressure. Some dentists use the material because of the rigidity that can be gained with adjacent teeth to regulate drifting of the teeth. The problem with gutta-percha is that it seals the cavity wall inadequately. The leaky temporary restoration then becomes loose, and the movement of the material forces saliva in and out of the dentinal tubules. If a gutta-percha pack is selected, it should be removed after cooling and then cemented with zinc oxide–eugenol.

Caution must be exercised when placing gutta-percha because the material or the warmed instruments can severely burn the soft tissue. Patients also complain about the roughness of the gutta-percha surface, which can be partially

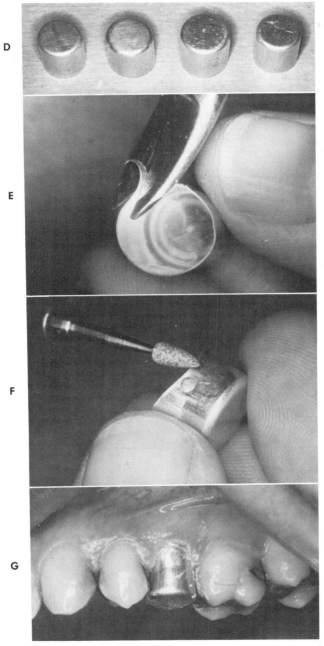

Continued.

Fig. 5-13, cont'd. D, Aluminum crown forms used for temporary-coverage restorations. **E,** Festooning of the aluminum crown with curved scissors. **F,** Smoothing the border of the crown form with the mounted stone. **G,** Aluminum crown form restoration.

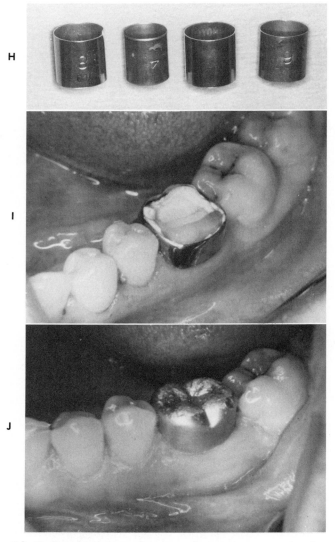

Fig. 5-13, cont'd. H, Seamless copper bands used as temporary restorations or matrices for amalgam and cement. **I,** Copper band holding cement restoration during endodontic therapy. **J,** Anatomic aluminum crown temporary restoration.

corrected by smoothing with warm burnishers. When gutta-percha alone is used as a stopping material, its best application is for plugging endodontic openings, which are usually small and simple to smooth. The seal, which is undesirable, can be made only by holding the warm material in the tooth under pressure.

Crown forms. Plastic, tin, and aluminum crown forms are used for temporary restorations (Fig. 5-13). The plastic varieties are used in anterior teeth and are filled with quick-curing acrylic resin for esthetic purposes. The metal crown forms are used for the posterior teeth and are retained with zinc oxide–eugenol cement. The crown forms that have anatomic shapes are the most effective because of the function and protection they afford the tissues. The techniques for trimming and placing all types of crown forms are similar.

The plastic or metal crown form is trimmed with the curved scissors and results in a festooned margin that has the same contour as the gingival tissue or periodontal attachment. The crown is selected according to the diameter, and the metal is made to contact all around the cervical line of the tooth in the gingival space. When this procedure, which allows full seating of the crown form to rest on the occlusal surface of the preparation, is accomplished, the cut edges are smoothed with a mounted stone and rubber wheel to prevent irritation of the gingival tissue covering.

A regular mix of zinc oxide–eugenol cement is made with the zinc acetate accelerator and is used to coat the inside of the crown. The preparation is dried and the temporary restoration is seated with pressure. All the excess cement is cleaned from the gingival crevice with an explorer, and the temporary crown and teeth are wiped with a moistened sponge or sprayed with 3% hydrogen peroxide.

The plastic temporary crown form is filled in a similar manner with the sulfinic acid catalyst resin. The crown is seated and allowed to polymerize in the preparation. If the preparation is extensive, the plastic is removed and then seated with the palliative zinc oxide–eugenol cement. The polymerized plastic is also cleaned from the gingival crevice with an explorer.

The temporary shell crown is used most often on the full-coverage or three-surface casting preparation that has been capped. The crowns cannot cover the occlusal surface unless the area has been reduced, which means that cement alone is used for many intracoronal temporary restorations.

Acrylic temporary restorations. The quick-setting acrylic resins are used for temporary restorations and best fulfill the objectives listed (Fig. 5-14). Although this procedure requires more time, it can be used for inlays, crowns, and bridges to produce an accurately fitting and functional temporary replacement. The cured resin restoration is seated with zinc oxide–eugenol cement, but the liner is thinner because the restoration fits more accurately.

A wax impression is taken of the teeth before they are prepared. The acrylic resin is mixed and placed in the wax impression, and once again the impression is seated firmly and held under pressure for the 5- to 8-minute curing period. The temporary restorations are recovered by taking the impression off the teeth and pulling the plastic out of the mold. These acrylic materials do not allow time for trial packing, which causes some excess plastic to surround the prepared teeth.

The acrylic temporary restoration is cut with burs and rubber wheels to pro-

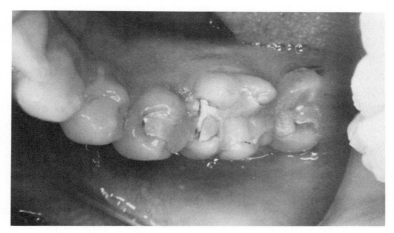

Fig. 5-14. Acrylic temporary restorations seated with cement.

vide definite edges, reasonable surface contours, and desirable occlusal relationships. The inside of the full-coverage or extensive inlay preparation is relieved to provide room for the cement. The preparations can be lined with a base if difficulty of withdrawal is anticipated. Bridge spaces are filled by waxing a pontic on a cast and copying the model with a rubber impression. The disadvantage of acrylic temporary restorations is the time required for the procedure. However, the accuracy, appearance, and function achieved in the technique strongly indicate its use.

Temporizing procedures are necessary to protect the teeth while the castings are being made or a planned procedure is awaited. Careful selection and manipulation of materials will lead to patient comfort and to a healthy periodontium when the temporary restorations are removed.

The selection of restorative materials presents no great problem because certain factors can be used to determine which material is most appropriate in regard to the size of the preparation and the type of patient. The factors that are influential in the selection of materials have been discussed, and it has been shown that the physical properties of materials limit their applications more than do the other factors.

REFERENCES
1. Blackwell, R. E.: Black's operative dentistry, ed. 9, Milwaukee, 1955, Medico-Dental Publishing Co., vol. 2.
2. Nadal, R.: A clinical investigation on the strength requirements of amalgam and the influence of residual mercury upon this type of restoration, M.S.D. thesis, Indianapolis, 1959, Indiana University School of Dentistry.
3. Welk, D. A.: Physical properties of 24 karat gold restorative materials, J.A.D.A. 9:26, 1966.
4. Phillips, R. W., and Ryge, G.: Adhesive restorative dental materials, Spencer, Ind., 1961, Owen Litho Service.

5. Going, R. E., and Massler, M.: Influence of cavity liners under amalgam restorations on penetration by radioactive isotopes, J. Prosth. Dent. 2:298, 1961.
6. Swartz, M. L., and Phillips, R. W.: Influence of manipulative variables on the marginal adaptation of certain restorative materials, J. Prosth. Dent. 12:172, 1962.
7. Norman, R. D., Swartz, M. L., and Phillips, R. W.: Studies on the solubility of certain dental materials, J. Dent. Res. 36:977, 1957.
8. Gilmore, H. W.: Methods of pulp protection for gold foil procedures, J. Am. Acad. Gold Foil Operators 9:16, 1966.
9. Massler, M.: Indirect pulp capping and vital pulpotomy for potential and actual pulp exposures, J. Tennessee Dent. Assoc. 35:393, 1955.
10. Shapiro, M.: The scientific bases of dentistry, Philadelphia, 1966, W. B. Saunders Co.
11. Swartz, M. L., and Phillips, R. W.: Permeability of cavity liners to certain agents, J. Dent. Res. 39:1232, 1960.
12. Healey, H. J.: Endodontics, St. Louis, 1960, The C. V. Mosby Co.
13. Swerdlow, H., and Stanley, H. R.: Reaction of the human pulp to cavity preparation: results produced by eight different operative grinding techniques, J.A.D.A. 58:49, 1959.
14. Zach, L., and Cohen, G.: Thermogenesis in operative techniques, J. Prosth. Dent. 12:977, 1962.
15. Gurley, W. B., and Van Huysen, G.: Histologic changes in teeth due to plastic filling materials, J.A.D.A. 24:1806, 1937.
16. Gilmore, H. W.: Pulpal considerations for operative dentistry, J. Prosth. Dent. 14:752, 1964.
17. Marzouk, M. A.: Effect of deep cavity preparation on the tooth pulp using the operating microscope as well as serial histologic sections, M.S.D. thesis, Indianapolis, 1963, Indiana University School of Dentistry.
18. Hassan, E. H., Van Huysen, G. V., and Gilmore, H. W.: Deep cavity preparation and the pulp, J. Prosth. Dent. 16:751, 1966.
19. Haldi, J., Wynn, W., and Culpepper, W. D.: Dental pulp fluid. I. Relationship between dental pulp fluid and blood plasma in protein, glucose and inorganic element content, Arch. Oral Biol. 3:201, 1961.
20. Mohammed, Y. R., Van Huysen, G., and Boyd, D. A.: Filling base materials and the unexposed and exposed tooth pulp, J. Prosth. Dent. 11:503, 1961.
21. Mitchell, D. F., Buonocore, M. G., and Schafer, S.: Pulp reaction to silicate cement and other materials: relation to cavity depth, J. Dent. Res. 41:591, 1962.
22. Mosteller, J. H.: Use of prednisolone in the elimination of postoperative thermal sensitivity, J. Prosth. Dent. 12:1176, 1962.
23. Mosteller, J. H.: An evaluation of cavity liners and intermediate base materials, Dent. Clin. N. Am., Nov., 1958, pp. 585-592.
24. Starkey, P. E.: Management of deep caries and pulpally involved teeth in children. In Goldman, H. M., Forrest, S. P., Byrd, D. L., and McDonald, R. E., editors: Current therapy in dentistry, vol. III, St. Louis, 1964, The C. V. Mosby Co.
25. Castaldi, C. R.: The management of some common pedodontic problems, J. Canad. Dent. Assoc. 28:80, 1962.
26. Phillips, R. W.: Cavity varnishes and bases, Dent. Clin. N. Am., Mar., 1965, pp. 159-168.
27. Glass, R. L., and Zander, H. A.: Pulp healing, J. Dent. Res. 28:97, 1949.
28. Eames, W. B., and Hollenback, G. M.: Cavity liner thicknesses and retentive characteristics, J.A.D.A. 72:69, 1966.
29. Voth, E. D.: A study of the thermal diffusion through amalgam and various liners, M.S.D. thesis, Indianapolis, 1959, Indiana University School of Dentistry.

chapter 6

Dental operatory, working positions, and instrument arrangement

The dental operatory is analogous to the operating room in a hospital, and it is here that the dentist spends most of his time. The operatory contains the materials and equipment used by the dentist and the assistant for treating the patient. The room should be organized and attractive to the dental team and the patients.

Although the operatory is only part of the office, much thought must be given to its location and to the design of equipment. The type of practice, general or specific, and the operating method are considered first by the dentist. Geographic location, economic strata, and treatment specialization all influence the type of practice and the nature of the work. A practice that includes primarily operative cases requires only a few instruments and pieces of equipment. Quality of the care and adherence to principles are axiomatic in all practices.

The location of the dental operatory is determined by the traffic pattern. The operatory should be arranged to prevent congestion and to ensure privacy. Requirements for plumbing and other utility lines will naturally dictate the location of the operatories in most dental offices.

The operatory should be well lighted and decorated in a pleasing color. It should be possible to clean the room quickly and efficiently because the working area must always be clean and organized. The equipment, instruments, and supplies are kept in cabinets to prevent contamination. Light green, blue, or brown wall colors, louvered lights, and attractive views or murals provide a pleasing atmosphere in which to treat the patient.

The room is kept at an optimum working temperature of 68° to 70° F., which requires an adequate ventilating system. Proper temperature and humidity take much of the strain out of the working day and prevent many untoward patient reactions. The ventilating system should be filtered and should remove unpleasant odors from outside sources and materials. The clean operatory reflects an efficient operation.

The selection of specific types of equipment depends upon personal evaluation. Many new designs and concepts have been developed within the last few years. Some of the unit designs differ enough to considerably change the procedures used in a practice. Operatory equipment should be carefully evaluated before purchase because of the expense. Whenever possible the dentist contemplating a change should use all the desirable types of equipment to determine whether the design fits his particular dental practice. Changes in the equipment should be made for improvement, not for the sake of being different.

The construction and modification of buildings or existing spaces make it possible to have any type of office that the dentist prefers. It is helpful to work closely with the architect and the dental dealer because of their experience and training. Auxiliary personnel can help by informing the dentist of their personal preferences; their knowledge of the dentist's habits and working patterns will also be valuable. The success of the project often depends upon combined efforts and planning. Pride in the dental office usually reflects the standards of patient treatment. Achievement of this objective in dentistry requires personal contact and the dental operatory must therefore be kept surgically clean at all times.

COMPONENTS OF THE OPERATORY

The dental unit is usually the central piece of equipment in the operatory. Whether the unit is of the standard design or the bracket type, it contains most of the items necessary for restoring the teeth. The location of the chair and the position of the operating team are determined by the accessibility of the dental unit. Unit designs differ in the placement of the components.

The standard dental unit is an upright, enclosed cabinet connected to the floor. It has air, gas, electric, and waste lines (Fig. 6-1). The unit contains a dental engine that has a capacity of 4,500 to 50,000 rpm, which is the power source for cutting instruments. The four basic lines activate the components of the unit. The air and water outlets attach to syringes used in the oral cavity during the operating procedure, the electric current powers the light and engine, and the waste line is connected to the saliva ejector and the cuspidor. The deluxe unit has more accessory items than the standard unit, is more expensive, and requires more maintenance. The added accessories are helpful in restorative dentistry. The main difference between the two units is an electric input with a low-voltage panel that transforms a current of 6 to 8 volts from the regular line. The panel is wired to a heated air syringe, cautery, mouth lamp, and occasionally a spray attachment. If restorative treatment is performed frequently, a deluxe unit should be employed.

A small electric engine mounted on top of the unit drives the rotary cutting instruments (Fig. 6-2). The speed range of the engine varies for the degree of

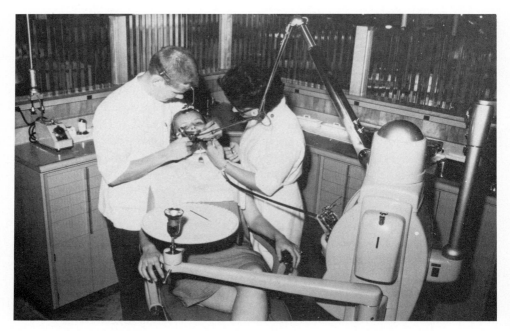

Fig. 6-1. Standard dental unit and proper operating position for the dentist and the assistant.

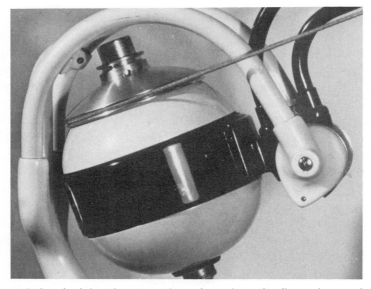

Fig. 6-2. Standard dental engine with accelerated-speed pulley and engine belt.

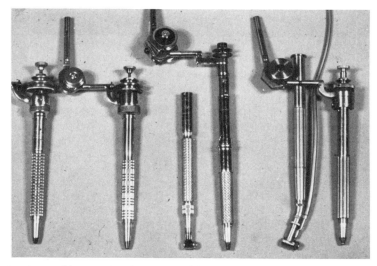

Fig. 6-3. Ball-bearing handpieces capable of working in the high-speed range.

refinement necessary in the cavity preparation. The engine works off a magnetic field that is developed in the armature. The electric line current is distributed to the armature by carbon brushes. The speed in the engine is controlled by a rheostat that is located on the floor and that is foot operated. Four resistances in the rheostat control the four general speed ranges available with the engine. Other methods of controlling the speed of the rotary instruments will be discussed later in this chapter. Deluxe units contain a two-way switch, called the high-low switch, that removes an additional resistance and permits the engine to run faster. The speed is elevated to 25,000 to 50,000 rpm and the resistance is placed in the current line between the engine and the rheostat. The electric engines are capable of 1/20 horsepower and are used for some tooth reduction, most of the cavity refinement, and prophylactic procedures.

The power is transferred from the engine to the cutting instrument by a belt and pulley system. The bur, suspended in the handpiece, is driven by the engine belt (Fig. 6-3). Noises and vibrations conducted by the system are the undesirable aspects of tooth reduction. Waxed engine belts and ball-bearing pulleys help to reduce these undesirable factors. The engine belt produces much torque on the bur, which is advantageous in perfecting the cavity preparation.

Drive pulleys are fastened to the armature of the engine and to the spindle of the handpiece. Two pulleys are located at each bend of the engine arm. The tension on the engine belt is regulated by an adjustable screw that slides the arm in and out in order to determine the amount of tension that will reduce strain on the engine and vibration in the pulleys.

The air line on the unit comes directly from a compressor capable of developing between 45 to 60 pounds per square inch. The air is regulated by a syringe that is used to dry the teeth for inspection and to remove deposits collected in tooth reduction. The deluxe unit syringes have a heated filament in the nozzle or tip to warm the air as it is directed on the tooth. The air syringes are also used to control the temperature on the tooth surface while it is being reduced.

The air compressor is used to propel the air turbine handpiece. This power source is capable of driving the bur at 250,000 rpm or higher. The air is directed to the turbine through a tube connected to the handpiece. The same air supply used to drive the turbine in which the bur is held is also employed to cool the tooth surface.

The air for the handpiece is regulated by a two-position switch that opens and closes the air valve. Some manufacturers are now producing variable-speed air turbines with switches to control the amount of opening in the air valve, making it possible to adjust the velocity of cutting in the ultraspeed range. The greater the current, the more the valve is opened.

The air turbine handpiece is connected to a control box on or inside the master unit. The power is regulated in the control box by two solenoids, one each for the water and air coolant lines, with a separate valve and filter. The water for the coolant in the handpiece comes directly from the unit line and has only this pressure to force the solution out of the tube and onto the bur. The water line is capable of delivering 30 to 50 ml. per minute on the turning bur and the tooth. The valves and filters regulate the amount and cleanliness of the coolants.

Some air turbines have an oil mist lubricant that is delivered to the turbine and to the handpiece. Other turbines are grease-packed or have a floating type of bearing that requires no special attention. The oil reservoir in the control box must be kept above the fill line at all times. The lubricant is dripped into the line at 30 drops per minute and is exploded down the air line tube to spray the bearings in the turbine. The turbine bearings will burn out rapidly if the rate of the drops is not maintained. The air turbine system requires little maintenance, but several functioning parts should be examined daily.

The water syringe is located near the air syringe because both are used frequently during the appointment. The water syringe is regulated by a thumb lever that opens and closes the valve to the unit water line. The water is directed onto the tooth to reduce the surface temperature or to wash out the debris following restoration procedures or prophylaxis. The water line will become calcined and thus interfere with the flow of water. When this occurs, the tip should be opened and cleaned with a small wire or bur to remove the calcium deposits.

The spray syringe is a variation of the air and water syringes. The regular water syringe is connected to the air line that travels through a reservoir. The spray syringe can be filled with mouthwash or hydrogen peroxide for washing out areas that are diseased or hemorrhaging, to produce a more aseptic area following treatment.

Recently all three component syringes have been made into a single unit called a three-in-one syringe or multiple syringe. The syringe aids the assistant by minimizing the number of instrument movements. The material needed during the appointment is selected by a switch on the syringe.

A bracket table is attached to the unit to hold the instruments used during the operation. The brackets are either round or rectangular and are adjustable to different heights. This enables the instruments to be placed at any desirable position for both the dentist and the assistant, whether the team works in a standing or a sitting position. The bracket table is usually in front of and below the direct vision of the patient in order to make the instruments readily accessible to the dentist. The brackets have been eliminated in some offices.

Some units have pulp testers that are helpful for diagnostic purposes. The testers are electric and have direct current converters that assure a constant input to the electrodes that deliver the current to the tooth. This eliminates the problem of alternating line currents, which interject error into the testing, especially when the pulp tester is used at different times during the day. The direct current is delivered through small electrodes placed on the tooth surface. The response is recorded by the calibrations that appear on the handle of the pulp tester when the stimulus in the tooth is detected. The pulp testers are used to detect teeth that are degenerating rather than to determine the type of pathology that exists in the tooth.

Near the unit is the water heater, which is used for the syringe and for the coolants for the handpieces. Isothermal water at body temperature is maintained in a reservoir that is heated by a filament activated from the regular line current. Pulp trauma and painful responses are supposedly reduced when warm water is used. Heated water is also helpful in cleaning areas around sensitive root surfaces.

An important part of the unit is the light used to illuminate the oral cavity. The light is powered by the regular line current and is supported by an arm or pedestal attached to the unit. It is recommended that the light produce 1,500 foot-candles of illumination and be in a 4:1 ratio with the overhead lighting. This arrangement produces optimum lighting of the oral cavity and minimizes the amount of visual accommodation needed when changing from two intensities during the operation. Proper illumination by the unit light during the dental procedure is one of the most important requirements in the operatory. The lights should be covered by a shield to prevent dust contamination inside the casing.

A basic component of the dental unit is the saliva ejector utilizing a sterile disposable tip. The suction apparatus works by the Venturi principle from the water line. The suction is pulled through a tube that is connected to the ejector tip placed in the sublingual space. The force pulls out excessive saliva that accumulates during the operative procedure. The ejector tubes are protected by

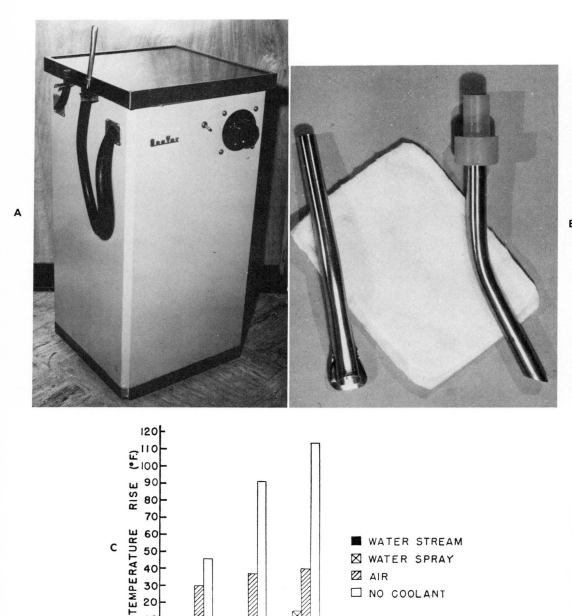

Fig. 6-4. A, Oral evacuation unit that is used by a chairside assistant. **B,** Evacuator tips. **C,** Evidence of the usefulness of the water coolant in the high-speed range. (From Peyton, F. A.: J.A.D.A. **56:**664, 1958.)

screens because they are narrow and are easily blocked. The screens should be cleaned regularly with the air syringe and water stream to reduce noise in the office and to eliminate waste more efficiently. Impression compounds and filing materials will rapidly block the ejector screen. The ejector is painful and its position must be carefully observed during restoration because it may injure the mucosa.

If this method of oral evacuation is not adequate, the high-velocity suction apparatus can be used (Fig. 6-4). Occasionally this vacuum is developed in a separate unit by a fan that utilizes an intake and exhaust line. The resultant vacuum is taken through a filter and the waste is dropped in a reservoir. The suction hose has many working tips that can be employed by the assistant to remove extra saliva, waste, or water used in accelerated cutting. The washed-field technique employs this type of evacuator to remove the 250 to 400 ml. of water per minute from the working area. In the office setting a central vacuum system is most commonly used.

Some units contain a cautery, which has limited application but is useful in some restorative procedures where tissue removal is necessary. The cautery is a wire that is heated from the low-voltage panel. The working tips consist of many different shaped wires to permit access to the tissue. When the wire is near the tissue, the current is regulated by a rheostat in the holding piece. Hypertrophied tissue can be removed with this attachment at the time the impressions are taken because use of the cautery does not induce bleeding. Commercial electrosurgery units are used for the same purpose.

Work-efficiency operatories are the result of time and motion studies and are being used to reduce stress in the operatory (Fig. 6-5). Newly designed equipment has changed the appearance of the dental office and in some cases has eliminated the need for the unit. Manufacturers have introduced attachments that are mounted on the back or side of the dental chair. Compactly designed kits attached to the pedestal of the chair base can be positioned over the patient when needed. The key to work simplification is efficient utilization of the dental assistant, which has been termed "four-handed dentistry."

Another purpose of work-efficiency operatories is to hide the dental unit from the patient's view. Again, the type of practice and office is determined by the design of the equipment and the allocated space in the operatory. Most operating rooms measure 10 by 12 feet, but the type, age, and construction of the building affect the dimensions. This new approach in equipment design usually requires a sitting position and four hands to perform the work. The use of this procedure depends on the arrangement of the cabinets behind the chair; thus it is desirable to have larger rooms when this system is selected.

If the regular dental unit is not employed, the chair becomes the focal point of space allocation in the operatory. There are basically two types of chairs—the conventional upright chair and the contoured chair—although some chairs combine both principles. The chairs should be motor-driven to adjust the vertical

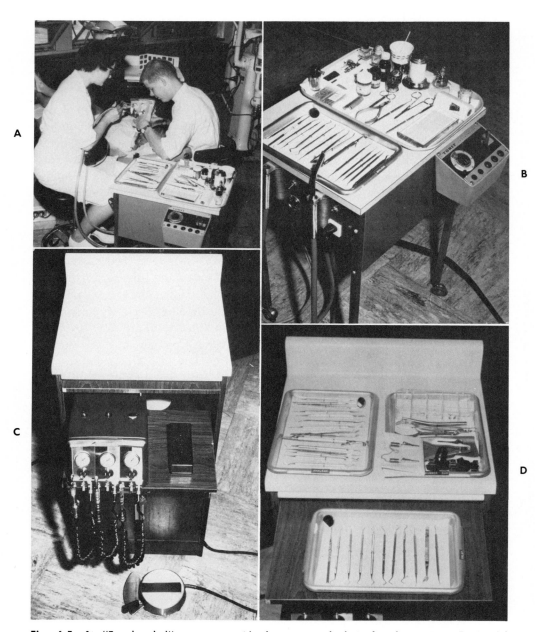

Fig. 6-5. A, "Four-handed" operatory with the contoured chair for the patient. **B,** Dental assistant's unit with all the accessories, instruments, and supplies. **C,** Dentist's cabinet with the handpieces, burs, and rheostat. **D,** Preset trays used for different operations and for application of the rubber dam. **E,** Transfer area where operational movements are accomplished. (From Kilpatrick, H. C.: Work simplification in dental practice, Philadelphia, 1964, W. B. Saunders Co.)

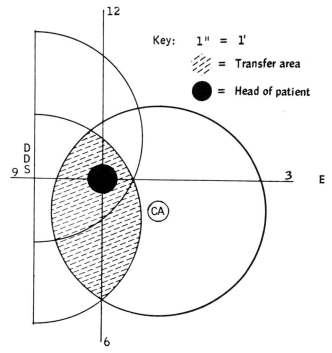

Fig. 6-5, cont'd. For legend see opposite page.

height, and some models include a horizontal motor adjustment for the back of the chair. The selection of one particular chair for a specific unit is not necessary; they can be interchanged to fit a space or adapted to the treatment routines of the office (Fig. 6-6). The regular upright chair stabilizes the patient in the working position and requires less space than the contoured chair. The contoured or "lounge-type" chair is the more modern design. It is supposedly more comfortable for the patient during a long appointment because it supports the entire body. Contoured chairs are used more often in the work-efficiency operatory because this system requires that the patient be in a supine position. The location of the patient's head during the operation makes the sitting position ideal for the dentist because the working field can be sufficiently lowered.

The design of the storage cabinets differs according to the type of equipment system. The cabinet should be large enough to conceal all the medicament bottles and loose equipment that must be readily accessible for patient treatment. Adequate storage space calls for a compact cabinet and an organized system to quickly move the material in and out of the drawers. It is helpful to have rollers installed on the upright cabinets containing drawers because this allows for the relocation of equipment in the room and for versatility of use. A movable cabinet with a work space on top for materials is helpful to the dental

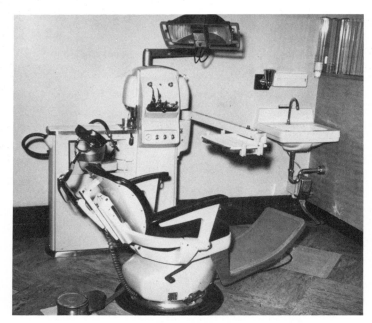

Fig. 6-6. A unit that can be used in the standard operatory or in a work-efficiency operatory.

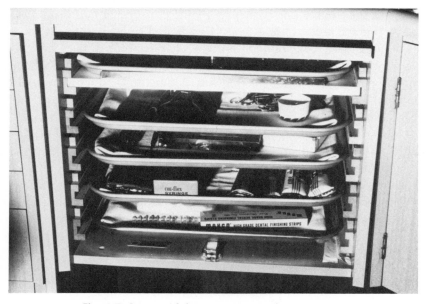

Fig. 6-7. Storage of the preset trays in the operatory.

assistant. The hand instruments are stored in the top drawers. Storage space for the other items is determined by the frequency with which they are used. For example, drape napkins are used for all patients so they should not be placed in the bottom drawer, since this necessitates excessive bending for the assistant.

Built-in or modular cabinets are designed for many of the new offices. The "modulars" are placed around the work-efficiency equipment and have a dual setup for the assistant and the dentist. Twin sinks and large working surfaces are usually included. The dental assistant has the greatest portion of the working area because she does most of the mixing of materials.

Basic to the modular cabinets is the color-coding system and preloaded trays essential for each operative procedure (Fig. 6-7). The trays are organized by groups of instruments and devices required for a specific technique. Small plastic bands of different colors are slipped over the shaft of the instrument. The colors designate on which tray and in which area each instrument is located. Individual colors and preloaded trays are used for amalgam, tooth-colored, direct gold, and cast restorations. The system adds to the operatory organization and increases the time available for the intraoral phases of treatment.

Following each appointment the instruments are sterilized, replaced on the tray, and put back in the designated position. The assistant prepares the trays in advance or at various times during the working day in order to be ready for each appointment. The color and location of plastic bands on the instruments makes rapid identification possible and improves the timing of instrument transfer.

A trend has developed for working in a sitting position, requiring a stool for both the dentist and his assistant. The stools are located close to the unit base or have built-in rollers to allow for movement in the transfer area. Adjustable stools with contoured seats and back supports have been designed for added comfort and serve to increase the use of stools. The position of the operator must be comfortable and must allow him to function as efficiently as he would in the standing position. The working area must also be visible and accessible. The dentist should change sitting positions regularly during the day to prevent circulatory problems from developing in his legs. The acceptable sitting position requires tilting the chair backward, but this is a minor problem that has been alleviated by the contoured chairs.

Some dentists prefer to design their own office and to construct their own equipment. The actual design and construction of the equipment is supervised or done by the dentist in the custom-made office, but the procedure is slower and more expensive than the more common practice of consultation and regular installation. Because of the lack of training and the need to conserve the time and effort of others, the average dentist should be discouraged from developing a personal system unless architectural design and crafting is a hobby. Equipment repair is still best handled by the dental dealer.

For a century the design of the dental operatory was not changed appreciably.

Recently, however, the impact of the time and motion studies and the findings of efficiency engineers began to influence the profession. At first the dental unit was modernized in appearance but not much change was made in the attachments. The traditional office procedure involved the use of the common unit and the upright chair, which required the standing operating position and varying degrees of participation by the dental assistant. The work load continued to increase over the years, and productivity was limited by this arrangement despite the extra value offered by the assistant.

The work-efficiency operatory is different in that the dental assistant assumes a role comparable in importance to that of the dentist. The system has been termed "four-handed dentistry," and it cannot be used to advantage unless there are two workers who understand the tasks. If not used properly the system is limited and the equipment must be used in a conventional manner. Research on time and motion has been conducted to study the many facets of the dental operation. The role of physiology and the design of the equipment have been studied in an attempt to discover where stress occurs during the operation. The caloric expenditures and the effect on blood pressure, respiration, and galvanic skin response in tissue have been determined, but the actual causes of stress remain unknown. The psychologic aspects of the practice are considered to be influential in producing stress, and thus the worrying is as much a factor as the working. The unknown factors of stress have encouraged authorities to advocate the use of equipment and systems that are less troublesome to the dentist. As long as the quality of dental care is not adversely affected, no limits are placed on the dentist in the adoption of improved concepts. The design of the equipment in the operatory can be chosen to suit the dentist. Combining trial and error with common knowledge is necessary to organize the individual office.

THE DENTAL ASSISTANT

Much information has been published on the advantages of employing a dental assistant. The daily work load can be increased from 25% to 75%, depending on how the services of the dental assistant are used and the type of production for which the office is designed. The dental assistant helps the dentist by managing patients, providing chairside assistance, handling business matters, and performing housekeeping duties. The assistant's principal purpose is to alleviate problems in the office and to assist the dentist in providing more and efficient dental care. The assistant must keep the practice running smoothly so that the dentist can devote himself to his work in the operatory.

Chairside assistance is the most important duty of the assistant. Books concerning practice management should be consulted to learn the business aspects of the practice.

The duties of the assistant in the operatory are similar to those of a nurse in the hospital operating room. The assistant prepares the sets of instruments and passes and receives instruments as the dentist requires them during preparation and restoration of the tooth. A knowledge of the instruments and the sequence in which they are used is mandatory. The effective assistant can place the desired instruments in the dentist's hand before he requests them.

The assistant must prepare the operatory prior to seating each patient. The unit and the cabinets must be checked for debris from the last appointment, and all surfaces in the area that were used should be wiped with a moistened towel or napkin. The accessories on the unit are sponged with alcohol to remove contaminating material from the tips and handles of the syringes. If necessary a small wire brush should be used to clean out cracks and crevices before the metal is wiped thoroughly with alcohol. The cuspidor, engine hood, bracket arm, and other dust collectors are cleaned and checked before each patient is seated in order to keep the operatory and unit surgically clean.

The dental assistant then escorts the next patient into the operatory and sees that he is comfortably seated in the chair. The conversation should be friendly and cordial to alleviate any anxiety of the patient before beginning the appointment. The napkin or drape is placed on the patient and a clean cup is inserted in the mount and then filled to demonstrate that the container is fresh. The patient's prosthetic appliances are placed in a fresh cup of water and, if necessary, his glasses are removed. The patient is now ready for the dentist to begin treatment. A final chair adjustment for comfort and position is made by the dentist when he first enters the room.

The patient's records are placed on the top of the work surface within reach of the dentist, and the routine setup is placed on the bracket table. The chart containing the previous work record and treatment plan should be in full view of the dentist. The most recent radiographs are placed at the top of the record to re-confirm tooth selection, formulate plans for the cavity preparation, and assist in making the choice of an anesthetic. The procedure for the appointment is then explained by the dentist to help the patient understand the maneuvers during the session and to alert the assistant to prepare the anesthetic syringe and instruments needed for the restoration.

The bracket table setup is routine for each operative appointment and it is placed in its customary place, based on equipment design, after the patient is seated (Fig. 6-8). The mirror and explorer armamentarium is needed for the cursory tooth examination after the treatment plan is consulted. Other instruments such as hand-cutting instruments, scalers, and condensers are placed on the work surface or bracket when the actual tooth selection is made. The instruments in the setup as well as those needed for the rubber dam application are usually kept on the work surface in the order in which they are used. When working alone, the dentist places the hand instruments on the bracket table. The items necessary for a basic bracket setup are as follows:

1. Mouth mirrors are needed for the illumination and examination of the teeth and the deflection of the soft tissue.
2. Explorers are used to examine the tooth surfaces and to detect caries in-

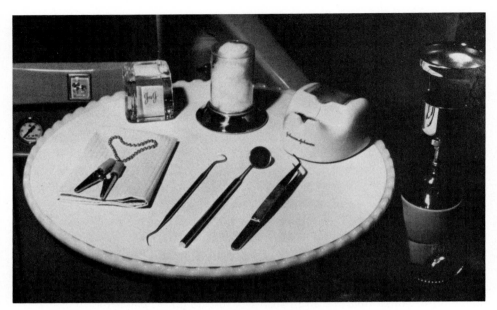

Fig. 6-8. Standard bracket table setup.

volvements or defects that are usually located in pits and fissures and in
hypoplastic areas.

3. Cotton pliers are utilized to pick up cotton to dry the tooth surfaces or to
carry medicaments and topical anesthetics to the tissues. They are also
used to remove loose restorations or foreign bodies that have been inad-
vertently dropped in the mouth during treatment.

4. Dental floss is employed to examine the proximal surfaces of the teeth to
detect caries and to examine the size and relationship of the contacting
surfaces. Food debris is removed and rough edges on the teeth are detected with dental floss. These procedures are the first steps taken in placing
the rubber dam or in cleaning the teeth that will be isolated in the surgical
field.

5. Cotton is placed in a dispenser located toward the back of the bracket.
Its use has been previously described in conjunction with the cotton pliers.

6. The waste receiver is a small receptacle to hold all the soiled items used in
placing the restoration. It is changed after each appointment. Pieces of
cotton, floss, and applicators are a few of the items that become soiled
and that must be discarded or concealed from the patient.

A clean bracket cover is placed on the tray prior to seating the patient. The
basic items previously listed are then spaced neatly on the clean cover. This
armamentarium is basic and is used for all operative or prophylactic appointments. While waiting for the anesthesia to take effect, the dental assistant places
the instruments required for the specific procedure and the rubber dam arma-

mentarium on the work surface. The rubber dam equipment should be arranged from left to right, beginning with the punch, the dam, the forceps, the clamps, and the napkin. It will then be easy for the dentist or the assistant to locate the items in the sequence needed.

The sterile, sharpened hand-cutting instruments are placed in order and within reach of the dentist or the assistant, depending on the system selected for the operation. If preloaded trays are used, the entire tray is placed on the work surface. If the dentist works alone, hand instruments are usually placed in one corner of the bracket. Space is left between each item to permit an easy pickup and return following the application to the tooth. Color coding is advantageous with both methods because it enables the assistant to properly locate each instrument in its designated place for storage or during use.

The small burs have always created a problem in the operatory. Although air turbine handpieces require fewer bur designs and sizes, it is still inconvenient for the assistant to remove or replace burs in the storage block or to keep them in proper position on the bracket table. The full-time chair assistant changes all the burs. This requires three hands and precise movements; while the dentist holds the handpiece, the assistant inserts the bur with one hand and secures it in the tube with the other. Knowledge and anticipation on the part of the assistant is necessary to accomplish this task effectively and efficiently. The burs are kept in one block. It is unwise to place them on the preloaded trays because they are small and easy to lose. After each appointment they are scrubbed with the wire brush, either wiped with sterilizing solution or driclaved, and then replaced in the bur block.

The surgical pass is employed to transfer the instruments from the work surface to the dentist's operating hand. The assistant passes the instrument with the left hand and receives it with the right hand. A firm quick pass places the middle of the shaft in the palm of the operator's hand, enabling him to apply the instrument to the surgical field, using the palm or pen grasp, to begin the tooth reduction. The assistant retrieves the soiled instrument with the thumb and first two fingers, being careful not to lacerate the soft tissue, while at the same time passing another instrument to the operator. A routine pattern will develop for each procedure. The anticipation of the assistant must be keen in order to stay ahead of the dentist at all times. It is impossible to read the mind of the operator, but repeated operations will reveal distinct patterns and personal desires that are followed most of the time.

The assistant operates the air syringe throughout most of the time required for cavity preparation. This keeps the preparation clear and improves vision, removes the grindings from the mirror, and reduces the temperature in the tooth caused by the rotary cutting instruments. The air should be directed toward the tooth during reduction but away from the patient and the operator. The time required for making the cavity preparation is significantly reduced when the air syringe is effectively used by the assistant.

Greater efficiency is achieved during the operation when the assistant prepares and mixes the restorative materials. The necessary supplies are kept within reach so that the well-trained assistant can quickly prepare the materials for insertion when requested to do so by the operator. Correct timing is important to avoid unnecessary delay during manipulation. The assistant must not only understand the manipulation and timing but must also master the technique needed for developing dental materials in respect to their physical properties.

The assistant should begin straightening the operatory while the dentist inspects the restoration after removal of the rubber dam and checks for proper occlusion and the condition of the soft tissues. When everything is satisfactory, the assistant removes the napkin and cleans the patient's face of debris if necessary. The dentist completes the records at this time and enters the treatment and cost of the service on the record. The assistant takes the record and escorts the patient from the operatory to settle financial matters and schedule the next appointment or place the individual's name on the recall list. The assistant can do much at this time to maintain rapport with the patient. In many cases the attitude of the patient will be influenced by the manner in which he is treated by the office personnel.

The assistant performs an important role in most dental practices because her efforts serve to increase efficiency and reduce problems in the dental office. Each practitioner has definite working habits and patterns that must be learned by the assistant if she is to become an asset to the practice. The kindness she shows and the responsibility she assumes in handling patients are of great value to the dental practice.

INSTRUMENT ARRANGEMENT

Regardless of the office design, a work surface must be available for the armamentarium and the instruments required in each operative appointment. The equipment is placed nearest to the person handling the items; this can be either the assistant or the dentist, depending on the operatory design. Combinations of equipment can be used, but most work-efficiency operatories require the services of a full-time dental assistant. Regardless of the type of setup, the instruments are placed in the order in which they are used and in the same location for each appointment. They are replaced in the same position when discarded, making it possible to recover or reuse the item if necessary. Standardization of the procedure is primary to a well-functioning office and to proper placement of the instruments.

Basic instruments on the working surface (arranged from left to right)

The order in which the instruments are arranged is as follows (Fig. 6-9):
1. The universal scaler, prophylaxis angle with rubber cup, and dappen dish with silica are used for scaling and polishing the teeth before the application of the rubber dam. The stain and calculus are removed from the teeth that are to be isolated immediately after the anesthetic is administered.

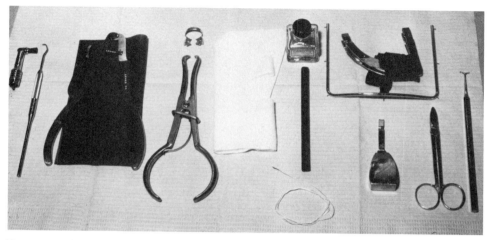

Fig. 6-9. Cabinet top setup for operative treatment, which is arranged prior to seating the patient.

2. The rubber dam armamentarium includes the dental floss, punch, rubber dam, clamp forceps, clamps, napkin, and retainer. The items are arranged from left to right. The saliva ejector is included in case the patient requires it, but the work should be attempted without the ejector because of the danger of injuring the floor of the mouth.

3. The anesthetic equipment includes a topical anesthetic, cotton swab, syringe, and carpule. These should be located in one area. The dentist applies the topical anesthetic to the covering tissues while the assistant removes the needle cover and holds the syringe out of sight of the patient. When the anatomic landmarks are located, the dentist injects the anesthetic. The syringe is returned to the assistant in such a way that the patient does not see it.

4. Patient records are placed on top of the instrument cabinets in large offices. The treatment plan and work record are kept readily accessible, and the radiographs are placed at the top of the record for possible reference during cavity preparation.

The organization of the operatory is reflected in the treatment of the patient. The hand instruments are arranged in the outlined sequence and used with exacting movements to obtain the optimum benefit of each design.

THE DENTAL CHAIR

The location of the dental chair is fundamental to the arrangement of the operatory. The chair must be near the unit so that the patient's head will be within reach of the working attachments. The location of the working field dictates the positions of the dentist and his assistant. When there is no unit, the

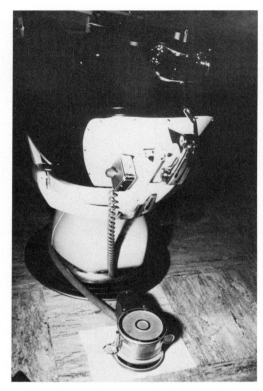

Fig. 6-10. Proper position of the rheostat with the pedal at right angles to the chair axis.

components are placed on the brackets, and thus the location of the chair becomes the primary factor in planning the operatory (Fig. 6-10).

Most patients and dentists have accepted the contoured chair, which fixes the patient in a relaxing curved position and allows him to be more comfortable during the appointment. This type of chair requires more room because the patient is placed in a supine position. Regardless of chair position, the same rest curve is maintained to equalize pressure on the body. The patient's head must be in a position that allows the operator and the assistant to have easy access to the surgical field.

The conventional upright dental chair is still widely used because it has certain advantages. The chair is more stable for securing the patient but is not as comfortable as the contoured chair. The headrest and upright position prevent drift during the operation because the head is held firmly in the occipital region.

The positioning of the patient's head is the most important factor for the dental team. Regardless of the type of chair or the position of the operator, the selected teeth must be at an ideal working distance. The patient's head must be level with the lower half of the dentist's upper arm. When the patient's mouth is open, the operating field is even with the operator's elbow, which permits a restful working position. The assistant should assume the same position and, if shorter than the dentist, should stand on a box in order to equal the dentist's height.

The patient's mouth must be fully illuminated at all times. When treating mandibular teeth, the lower occlusal plane should be parallel to the floor when the mouth is open. When operating in the upper arch, the maxillary teeth should form a 45-degree angle with the floor to permit illumination and either a direct or indirect view of the structures. This head position allows for good posture when the dentist is working in a standing position.

If the patient is seated in a conventional dental chair, the chair back is reclined to place the majority of the patient's weight or center of gravity at the bottom of the spine. The headrest is adjusted to support his head in the occipital region. If the patient slides forward and assumes a poor posture, the entire chair is reclined in order to properly locate the oral cavity. The chair arms are moved in or out to support the forearms. When these procedures are followed, the patient is more comfortable because his body receives proper support.

Contoured chairs require few adjustments. When the patient is seated, the headrest is adjusted to the position just described. Usually only the position of the headrest and the height of the chair require adjustment. The same working position is maintained by the dentist in relation to the patient, regardless of the body position of the two individuals. The sitting position requires the chair to be lowered and tilted backward. The operator usually works with his thighs under the chair back to attain the previously described relationships.

While the patient should be made as comfortable as possible during the appointment, the working position of the dentist dictates the positioning of the patient because the operator's comfort is of prime importance. The trend in practice is to employ contour chairs for comfort and efficiency.

WORKING POSITIONS AND POSTURE

The best way for the dentist to assure production over a period of years is to use good posture. A visual range of 10 to 14 inches from the surgical field should be maintained without bending the neck unduly in any direction. This distance will vary with the vision, the type of optical correction, and the use of magnifying loupes. Whenever possible the head should be held vertical to prevent muscular strains and skeletal changes in the cervical area.

The back of the operator should be straight and the shoulders erect. However, this position is not possible when working in the maxillary arch because the operator's arm must encircle the patient's head in order to retain the mirror for vision. The forearms are held parallel to the floor and the elbows are kept close to the side. When this position 10 to 14 inches from the surgical field is maintained, the ideal standing position is achieved. During the operation, the dentist should place his feet 10 to 12 inches apart and direct them slightly outward for good balance and weight distribution. The weight can be shifted by using the balls of the feet. This spacing is also maintained when sitting because balance becomes more difficult when working in the sitting position. The dentist shifts his weight to the heel when activating the rheostat for the engine. When the engine is used for an extended period, the weight can be shifted back to the ball of the foot. Balance is maintained and leg fatigue is avoided when proper foot positioning is practiced.

The position of the torso remains unchanged in the sitting position. The same general rules of preventing leg fatigue also apply to this position. Alternate standing and sitting positions should be used throughout the day because lack of muscular movement causes a stasis of blood in the legs. Circulation problems will soon develop if the position is not alternated or an exercise program to stimulate circulation is not initiated.

The dental assistant is advised to assume the same general posture. Extra duties allow the assistant to leave the chair or change her position more frequently than the dentist. The manipulation of dental materials, the passing of instruments, and other chairside duties should all take place within 26 inches of the patient's head. The assistant should return to the unit with a professional and restful posture. Good posture preserves the operating team for the entire work day and prevents the development of bad habits and postural defects.

The working posture is considered to be an occupational hazard. Exercise, both in and away from the office, prevents changes in the musculature and skeleton caused by the unnatural working positions necessary in the operatory. A regular program of exercise that exerts antagonistic forces on the structures that are strained while working will do much to preserve the posture of the dentist. Many physical fitness programs can be followed that improve circulation, stretch connective tissue to aid in preventing joint problems, and increase respiratory capacity. Exercise also helps to regulate the body weight, thus preventing the fatigue and strain associated with an overweight condition.

As already discussed, the dentist may assume four chairside positions in relation to the patient. A dentist who works with his right hand will station himself on the right side and in front of or behind the patient. The left-handed dentist will work on the left side of the chair in the forward or backward position. Thus the working hand determines the body position.

Any of the four basic positions may be used, but the choice is left to the individual operator. The preferred working position must provide the best possible vision and permit an ideal operating posture. The forward position is commonly used for treating the anterior teeth and the mandibular posterior teeth. The backward position is commonly employed when using the mirror to view the maxillary teeth. The same position is also used for some preparations on the maxillary anterior teeth. During an extensive procedure the dentist should move to the opposite side of the chair to be on the same side as the tooth that requires treatment. This switch in positions is usually restful and the regular operating muscles are allowed to relax. Operating in an unfamiliar position is difficult so this system is not used extensively, but it is a restful method of working on the opposite side of the arch where limited access and vision present a problem.

•   •   •

There are many office designs and types of equipment. The system should conform to the type of practice and enhance the dentist's performance. Stress is a natural occurrence in dental practices because of the extensive work load and the exacting procedures. Therefore, the selection of operatory equipment should minimize stress on the dental team and be pleasing to the patient.

ADDITIONAL READINGS

Blackwell, R. B.: Black's operative dentistry, ed. 9, Milwaukee, 1955, Medico-Dental Publishing Co., vol. 2.

Kilpatrick, H. C.: Work simplification in dental practice, ed. 2, Philadelphia, 1969, W. B. Saunders Co.

McGeehee, W. H., True, H. A., and Inskipp, E. F.: A textbook of operative dentistry, New York, 1956, McGraw-Hill Book Co., Inc.

chapter 7

The operating field

The oral cavity is an extremely difficult area in which to work. Vision and access are impaired by the cheeks and tongue. Restorative care must be accomplished without damaging these or other soft tissue structures, which sometimes makes traction and indirect vision necessary in the working area. Indirect vision is provided by the mirror and traction by special instruments designed to retract the tissue for short periods of time. The nature and content of saliva also complicate operating conditions. This seromucous exudate is necessary for mastication and digestion of food. The flow of saliva is usually activated during the dental appointment. By one method or another the saliva must be prevented from contacting the teeth because its presence in the operating area results in a less favorable restorative service. Once saliva dries, a mucinous deposit remains on the wall of the tooth and the cavity preparation, creating an undesirable foundation or lining for restorations.

To restore the teeth properly an ideal working field must be established. In medical operations a surgical field is one that has been cleaned of bacteria and other types of contaminants. The field is isolated and washed prior to the operation to provide a relatively sterile environment for the operation. The teeth should be clean, relatively free of bacteria, and thoroughly dry before beginning tooth reduction. If these ideal conditions are established and maintained, cavity preparation becomes a surgical procedure. It must be realized that teeth are vital structures important to the general health of the patient. Asepsis is as important in dentistry as in any other health profession, and the establishment of an ideal field for restorative procedures is the first step toward acceptable treatment.

RUBBER DAM

The best possible operating field in restorative dentistry is achieved with the rubber dam. The dam is made of latex rubber that is punched and placed around the teeth in order to isolate them from the oral environment. The use of the dam makes it possible to keep the teeth dry for the duration of the appointment, except for the moisture inherent in tooth structure. The patient appre-

ciates the rubber dam because the rubber partially retracts the perioral musculature and aids in keeping the jaws separated. The improvement in the surgical
environment has led to an immediate improvement in the quality of dental care.

The rubber dam was introduced to the profession by Robert Barnum in New
York City in 1864, and with this innovation it became possible to produce a contoured restoration. Prior to this the term "filling" was literally true because
restorative techniques consisted of wedging metals between the walls of the
crudely prepared tooth. The dam enabled the cohesive properties of gold foil to
be utilized for the contoured restoration. The inventor deserves much credit for
the development of the rubber dam because no other material or technique provides a more suitable operating environment.

The popularity of the rubber dam was quickly established in the early clinics.
The advantages of using the rubber dam were self-evident, and a large percentage of practitioners began using the technique. The rubber dam was useful in
the early research on amalgam and cavity preparation and it was widely advocated by the pioneer dentists.

The value of the isolation technique has survived the test of time in clinical
dentistry. The discovery of the workability of the rubber dam has led to the refinement of the technique. With the use of increased speed ranges the problem
of maintaining the tooth and bur at acceptable or atraumatic temperatures was
presented. Study of the problem led to the "washed-field technique" in which
large amounts of water were placed in the preparation during tooth reduction.
This technique naturally discouraged the use of the rubber dam for a short time.
Refinement of the coolant systems, proper utilization of the dental assistant, and
development of new evacuator systems resulted in the revival of rubber dam
isolation. It has been proved that when the rubber dam is used in conjunction
with these combined factors even greater efficiency and quality are achieved.
The dental assistant is a valuable adjunct and shares with the dentist the responsibility of applying the dam. Moreover, the high-velocity evacuators make
it possible to use any volume of water coolant during the preparation because
the evacuator easily removes 400 ml. per minute, which is maximum delivery at
the cutting site.

Study clubs throughout the country have done much to promote the use of
the rubber dam. The clubs that demonstrate clinical procedures, regardless of
whether or not they are concerned with the use of gold foil, require that an ideal
field be maintained for demonstration purposes. Each club usually requires an
established outline to be followed in applying the rubber dam, and the rules
usually include a pledge to use the technique whenever possible. The influence
of the clubs, through motivation toward good dentistry and the transfer of
knowledge, has led to a gradual increase in the use of the rubber dam for
practical purposes. The value of study clubs is evident from this observation, and
all dentists should participate in this type of activity as a part of their continuing
education.

Advantages

In general the rubber dam should be used in all places where a posterior tooth can be clamped. It is used primarily to improve vision and to establish a dry field. Ideally the restorative service should be accomplished without injury to any of the tissues. The rubber dam provides the best environment in which to accomplish these objectives. J. M. Prime has elaborated on the indications for use of the rubber dam. Only its salient advantages will be discussed here.

Cavity preparation

More precise tooth reduction is possible with the improved access and vision afforded by the rubber dam. The dark contrasting rubber field allows better vision of the tooth being restored, and the dryness obtained increases the accuracy of the internal architecture of the preparation. Smooth, full-length walls are readily prepared and an easy evaluation can be made of the wall angulation and line-angle sharpness. The amount of retention required in the preparation can also be determined since the complete extension can be observed.

When the teeth are isolated in groups or quadrants, the production of the outline form is simplified. The anatomic curves and shapes and the location of the adjacent teeth become more apparent. The gentle sweeping curve of the outline form can be made to blend with the gross anatomic features of the tooth. When the teeth are dry, the extent and coalescence of the occlusal grooves can be observed. The coalescence and involvement of the buccal and lingual grooves can also be evaluated at this time. In some cases the degree of enamel undermining is observed, which helps to preestimate the amount of tooth structure that must be removed in the initial cutting of the outline form.

A critical and final phase of cavity preparation is the cavosurface relationship of the reduced enamel surface. The cavosurface enamel is meticulously refined to meet the demands of the physical properties of the restorative material. For metals that are stronger than enamel the tooth structure is beveled to receive the restoration. A right-angle joint is required with all materials weaker than enamel; this procedure is probably more critical because of the difficulty in cleaving enamel. Marginal accuracies greatly influence the life of the restoration, and the improved vision provided by the rubber dam helps to accomplish accurate refinement. Better margins are routinely observed postoperatively when the rubber dam is utilized.

Properties of restorative materials

Because efficient isolation eliminates moisture, the physical properties of the restorative materials are enhanced. Ideally a restorative material would produce a chemical-mechanical bond to tooth structure and prevent leakage down the walls of the cavity preparation. Since no material provides a perfect bond to tooth structure, the operator must do everything possible to assist the mechanical interlocking of the material. Such interlocking is aided by a clean cavity wall and by a thorough toilet of the cavity prior to restoration. The presence of moisture and tooth grindings inside the preparation will reduce the chances of good adaptation of the restorative material. If bases and liners are used in the wet cavity, it is impossible to achieve the performance that is normally expected of the specific material being used. In such cases the physical properties of the liners are reduced and do not act to the advantage of the restoration.

The setting reactions of materials are allowed to proceed at a normal rate in the dry cavity preparation. The presence of moisture in freshly mixed materials will interfere with the dimensional change or chemical reaction of the materials after they are placed in the tooth. This in turn might affect the marginal adaptation, hardness, or accuracy after setting.

The amalgam restoration is very susceptible to moisture because, when contaminated, a severe delayed expansion of the material occurs. This expansion has been measured at 500μ and is accompanied by blister formation on the surface of the metal. Amalgam is allowed a maximum expansion of only 25μ according to the specifications of the American Dental Association. Amalgam expansion usually occurs in cervical restorations where the rubber dam cannot be applied. The surface becomes quite rough and acts as a gingival irritant, necessitating another restoration in the same area. When this situation occurs, a nonzinc alloy should be used and extension in the cavity preparation should be limited. The nonzinc alloy is not susceptible to the delayed expansion caused by moisture and will therefore serve more adequately for the restoration.

Plastic materials are quite susceptible to moisture. Another complication with plastic occurs when hemorrhage of the gingival tissues is stimulated during tooth reduction. If ignored, the hemorrhage will soon stop but will result in a black stain inside the preparation. If the tooth is restored in this condition, the enamel-colored materials will soon be darkened and the tooth will have a shadowed appearance. This "capillary creep" around plastics is even a problem when the rubber dam is used, although to a lesser degree. When this occurs, a gingival string may be placed in the epithelial sulcus to produce displacement. These strings are placed after the dam has been inverted with the blunt instrument. Some gingival strings contain hemostatic agents and work very well in this situation. At no time should the tooth be restored when there is blood in the cavity preparation.

The silicate restoration is also sensitive to moisture. The saliva can interfere with the gel structure of the silicate and cause a weakened restoration. This means that the silicate restoration will be more susceptible to stains and dissolution during its clinical life. Although the silicate should not be polished during the insertion appointment, a better restoration is produced if it is allowed to set in a dry cavity preparation.

The direct resin restoration is more susceptible to contamination than are the other materials. The catalysts will not effect complete polymerization when the sulfinic acid compounds are contaminated with moisture. As a safeguard the dentist should carefully observe the restoration for soft margins so that any defective restorations can be removed immediately. Caution should always be used in evaluating the resin restoration because of the damage that contamination causes. A standard rule to follow is to use resin materials only when the rubber dam is in place and the cavity preparation is absolutely dry.

To make use of the luting properties of zinc phosphate cement this material must also be placed on a dry surface. Moisture is very deleterious to an effective mechanical bond of cement with the cavity preparation. Wet surfaces make it almost impossible to place intermediary bases and liners because the material will not stay in place while the mortise is being formed. Cavity depth and the soundness of dentin cannot be accurately judged when moisture obscures direct vision.

The cast gold inlay and crown are also vulnerable because they are held in place with zinc phosphate cement. Prior to seating a casting the rubber dam should be applied and the cavity preparation thoroughly dried. The castings are seated with a creamy mix of cement and retained in place by force in order to combat the hydraulic pressure under the casting. Upon completion of the setting reaction the cement will be difficult to remove from the dry enamel surface. The quality of this type of cementation will produce bias when compared to other procedures for placing castings and will require rubber dam to be used.

Application of drugs and medicaments

There are many advantages of having the teeth dry when drugs and solutions are applied during the appointment. It makes it possible to prepare the teeth for maximum absorption of the solution and prevents the drugs from contacting the tissues. This will assure the greatest benefit to the tooth and at the same time protect the soft tissue from the irritating effects of the solutions. When the teeth are being worked on in quadrants, it is advantageous to apply a fluoride solution to the cavity form and to the eroded areas in order to harden the tooth surfaces and reduce the solubility of the damaged area. In some cases the rubber dam can be used when applying fluoride pastes to pre-carious areas in the enamel and cementum. Prior to the application of different types of medicaments and after the rubber dam is applied it is helpful to remove the stain and calculus from the teeth being treated. The fact that the teeth are dry simplifies the task of removing the contaminants and produces a greater surface area on which the applied solutions can react.

Drugs are applied most often in endodontic procedures. For root canal therapy special clamps have been designed and procedures indicated for single tooth isolation, especially in the treatment of anterior teeth. In these teeth it is usually necessary to make only a lingual opening in the crown in order to perform the operation. The canal is enlarged and all medicaments are inserted through the lingual opening to render the root canal chamber aseptic. The clamps used for single tooth isolation are of the hatch design and possess a double bow.

When these clamps are used, it is very important that stability of the clamps be maintained in order to prevent the gingival tissue from being torn where the jaw of the clamp approximates the root surface. Any twisting or turning of the clamp on the epithelial attachment can lacerate the tissue involved. It is quite helpful to stabilize the teeth with compound in order to prevent movement of the clamp during the manipulative procedures of root canal therapy. The drugs used in endodontic therapy are usually concentrated and are capable of producing irritating effects in the gingival tissues. These solutions must be carried in and out to the back of the tooth through the lingual opening in the crown. At times the solutions are placed on cotton pledgets, and in some cases absorbent points are employed to carry the solution throughout the entire length of the canal. If careful application of the drugs is not exercised, it is possible to cause irritation of the soft tissues even with the rubber dam.

When the root canal appointment has been completed, the rubber dam offers additional advantages. It is necessary to produce a cement seal in the lingual opening of the tooth. If this seal is broken or not adequately established, it will allow saliva and bacteria to flow into the root canal chamber being treated, which will produce bacterial contamination. The rubber dam helps produce dryness in the root canal opening, making it possible to accomplish a more efficient cement seal and to minimize the risk of contamination between appointments. Because of the emphasis on sterile conditions in root canal therapy, it would be impossible to enjoy any type of success in this field without the application of the rubber dam.

Efficiency

As previously discussed, the rubber dam enables the dentist to accomplish more work per unit of time. Because the rubber dam provides a true isolation and surgical field, efficiency is greatly increased as a result of the improved vision that results from the dark contrasting background of the rubber dam and from the dry teeth. The rubber dam makes it possible to more accurately prejudge and estimate the amount of cutting and outline form needed because the anatomic details of each individual tooth can be observed. As previously discussed, the length and type of groove coalescence can be observed especially with the aid of operating loupes, and when the stains that remain are readily visible, they are included in the pre-carious areas. Efficiency is somewhat improved by all of these factors because a more thorough understanding of what is needed to satisfactorily prepare the tooth is achieved.

The dry tooth also makes it possible to thoroughly observe the caries excavation. Sometimes, when the tooth structure is dried, it will clearly reveal the presence of caries because of the moist leathery texture of the lesion. Also, when the caries is removed, the solidity of the remaining dentin can be tested and fully observed. This procedure simplifies the cavity wall refinement, which can take place either before or after the placement of a sedative treatment or intermediary base. Preparation time is reduced and much better work is produced by encouraging more refinement.

The rubber dam is quite useful in quadrant procedures in restorative dentistry. The restorations are placed in quadrants and one rubber dam application is used for the restoration of two or more teeth in one appointment. This technique makes it necessary to anesthetize the section of the mouth being worked on and to increase the duration of the dental appointment. With the proper type of isolation, it is possible to prepare and restore many teeth in one appointment. The use of the dental assistant enables the dentist to complete more work during the day, and the rubber dam certainly contributes to an improvement in working conditions. It is helpful to explain the rubber dam application, the type and number of restorations, and the advantages of this procedure. It is important that there be a definite understanding between the dentist and the patient regarding fee assessment for the work schedule using the rubber dam.

Silence on the part of the patient makes for greater efficiency in dental procedures. When the rubber dam is applied, it is possible for the dentist to be in sole command. The patient does not use the cuspidor and has only to become comfortable in the dental chair and submit to the wisdom of the operator. The dentist can use the time during which the rubber dam is applied for patient education. Although the needs of the patient have been previously discussed, they can be reemphasized and evaluated while the dental appointment is in progress. Home care and periodic recall appointments can be stressed, and when these procedures are utilized, it is possible to motivate a patient to preserve his natural dentition. Also, if additional carious lesions or edentulous spaces are present, this can be indicated, and the patient will become receptive to the restorative treatment that is needed. The case needs can be emphasized at this time, and an understanding will certainly develop between the parties involved. It is important for the patient to understand the amount and type of work that is received, and the alert dentist will use the time when the rubber dam is applied for this purpose.

Examination and diagnosis

In some cases radiographs and routine examinations are not sufficient to determine whether or not caries is present in a tooth. When teeth are rotated or overlapped, an adequate radiograph cannot always be obtained. Usually the teeth are superimposed labiolingually and blockage of the embrasure is caused by an abundance of tooth structure. Sometimes dental floss can be passed between the teeth and, if a tear occurs in the string, a lesion is suspected. When these procedures are inadequate, the rubber dam should be applied, the teeth separated, and the enamel surface observed directly. In most cases it will be necessary to separate the teeth slightly in order to see between the proximal surfaces. This procedure is quite useful in detecting incipient caries and in determining whether the tooth needs a restoration. There are decided advantages in restoring lesions in the incipient stage, and this is especially true in anterior teeth where multiple restorations might result in subsequent fracture, with loss of the angle of the tooth. Prevention is exercised by using the rubber dam for examination purposes and limiting the restoration in this case to the Class III classification.

Another diagnostic method that is quite useful in neglected teeth is gross caries removal. In this situation caries control is of primary concern to the operator, and organizing or analyzing the final types of restorations that can be placed in the involved teeth is of secondary concern. In some deep lesions it is not radiographically possible to determine whether an exposure is present because the caries and pulp are superimposed on the film. In some cases teeth that possess gross or open carious lesions have no symptoms and there is no other way to determine the prognosis of the tooth than by excavation of the carious material. In neglected teeth or cases of acute caries these types of lesions occur in multiples, which makes it necessary to excavate many teeth prior to the placement of restorations.

When multiple excavation is necessary, the rubber dam can be applied and the caries removed a quadrant at a time. Because of the nature of caries it is not necessary to use an anesthetic for superficial removal. In this procedure only the gross caries is removed, and when sensitivity is apparent, the excavation is stopped and sedative zinc oxide–eugenol cement treatment fillings are placed in the concavities. At a later date the treatment filling is removed, and it is then possible to excavate the tooth completely and to examine the dry dentinal floor. If no exposure or undue symptoms are present, the restoration is attempted at this time because the field has already been established. The teeth are lined with calcium hydroxide and restored with amalgam as described in the discussion on caries control. Teeth that are sensitive and that appear questionable after the excavation has been completed should be sealed with sedative fillings for longer periods. Teeth that need to be extracted can be removed at this time to allow the healing process to be completed before restoring the excavated teeth. The rubber dam greatly simplifies the treatment of acute caries.

Gingival retraction

A good sealing rubber dam causes a large amount of gingival retraction, better termed compression, in the interproximal spaces. This is especially true of the heavier weight rubber dams. It is possible to routinely compress 1 mm. or more of the dental papilla. As can be imagined, this is used to advantage when placing any interproximal type of restoration. With the tooth structure visible, it is possible to observe the entire length of the cut and depth of the gingival wall in the cavity preparation. After the gingival wall is prepared, the retraction helps make the loose and friable enamel rods in the cervical area visible.

The Class II amalgam restoration is somewhat simplified because the gingival wall is visible. A wood wedge is placed interproximally over the retracted dam and is abutted to prevent the bur from tearing the rubber material around the teeth. The cavity preparation can be estimated by placing the gingival wall down to the wedge as long as the wall does not contact the adjacent tooth, because this margin will be located below the healthy gingival tissue. This type of gingival retraction is utilized in adapting and wedging the matrix band for the amalgam restoration. It should be noted that the wedge will hold more adequately if it is wet, and it should be placed in sterilizing solution before it is inserted between the metal band and the adjacent tooth. If this procedure fails to provide adequate stability, a compound block can be placed in the embrasure to provide more backing for the matrix band. Once the band is removed the gingival retraction allows the condensed amalgam to be observed. At this time the cervical margin can be carved with the instruments and smoothed with dental floss. Since it is impossible to polish this area of the restoration, as smooth a condition as possible should be established at this time. The better the junction of the cervical wall and the tooth structure, the less irritation will occur in the gingival tissue that contacts the restoration. For health of the supporting tissue it is absolutely necessary that a good relationship be established during this phase of the Class II amalgam restoration, and accomplishing this objective is simplified by retraction by the rubber dam.

It is possible to utilize the tissue compression afforded by the rubber dam with the indirect inlay and crown and bridge impression procedure. When any elastic impression material is used, the gingival tissue must be displaced from the wall of the cavosurface margin. This procedure can be accomplished by either chemical or mechanical methods or by a combination of the two. The rubber dam is quite useful in that the tissue requires no medicaments, which in some cases alter the health of the gingiva following restoration of the tooth. The heavier weight rubber dam provides interproximal compression of the mechanically displaced gingiva. The same type of procedure is used as with the amalgam restoration, and certainly many impressions can be taken adequately when the tissue is completely reflected from the cavity preparation.

ARMAMENTARIUM (Fig. 7-1)
Rubber dam material

Several types of rubber dam are available. The rubber comes in different colors, sizes, and weights. The use of a dark rubber dam is universally accepted because of the color contrast in the operative field. Although practically no one uses the white rubber dams, it should be mentioned that they are still manufactured. The thicker or heavier gauged rubber dams provide more contrast because they are darker, and there is a tendency to use this type of material.

In the early days dentists were cautioned to wash the rubber dam before applying it to the patient's mouth. This was done to remove the powder employed in the packaging process because the material contained trace amounts of arsenic. Some dentists believed that if enough rubber dam applications were used the arsenic absorption could possibly harm the patient. The powder is now

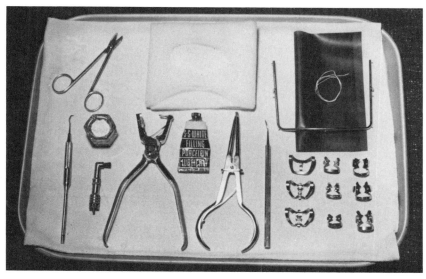

Fig. 7-1. Rubber dam armamentarium arranged according to the order in which the equipment is used during the application.

removed in order to provide a darker rubber dam surface for more contrast. If it is washed, the dam should be dried before it is applied.

The commercial products are available in rolls and in 5 × 5 and 6 × 6 inch squares (Fig. 7-2). Many dentists still purchase the material in rolls so that they can cut different sizes as different cases are presented. The 5-inch squares are used for children and the 6-inch squares are used for adults. Some operators advocate that a 5 × 6 inch rubber dam be used in adults for anterior teeth and that a 6 × 6 inch dam be used for the posterior teeth. The extra inch for the posterior teeth is necessary to cover the lip adequately and to isolate the teeth from the oral cavity. There are many variations in rubber dam application and certainly a type of material is available to suit the individual dentist's preference. The operator should use a technique that works well for him, and the use of rubber dam in rolls is advantageous because it does not limit the size of the application that the dentist must use.

The weight of rubber dams—their gauge or thickness—ranges from light to extra heavy. The measurements vary, of course, for each thickness, and there is diverse opinion as to the optimum dimension. The disadvantage of using a lightweight rubber dam is that it is easily torn during the operation. The tears can result from faulty or rough margins on restorations or dental caries or from contact with the rotating instruments. There seems to be a significant trend toward using the thicker gauged rubber dams.

Most people feel that a heavyweight dam should be used for operative procedures. In some cases it is possible to use a lightweight rubber dam for endo-

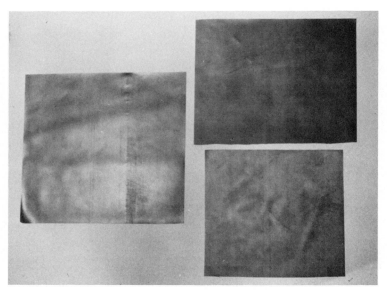

Fig. 7-2. Three common sizes of dark, heavyweight rubber dams. The dimensions are 6 × 6, 5 × 6, and 5 × 5 inches.

dontic procedures, but this technique affords no great advantage in single tooth applications. The heavyweight dams are helpful in operative procedures because they do not tear or cut readily when applied to the teeth. In addition this weight of rubber can be punched in precise holes because of its thickness, and it seems to afford more stability when being held in the retainer. The heavyweight rubber dam certainly has an advantage in that clamps are not always needed to retain the material when working anterior to the molar teeth. The rubber is thick and resilient enough to resist dislodgment from the teeth once it has been passed below the embrasures of the bicuspid teeth. When the teeth are dried, it is nearly impossible to dislodge the inverted rubber dam during the appointment. The special heavyweight rubber dam is used for Class V or gingival restorations. This weight causes an unusual amount of tissue compression. When this thickness is used in conjunction with the Schultz or the No. 212 gingival clamps or with other types of retractors, the epithelial tissue is literally pushed away from the cervical area of the tooth without harming the attachment. It should be realized that the special heavyweight dam provides a great amount of retraction and vision. Once the rubber dam technique has been employed, its advantages will be observed, and an improvement in restorative procedures will result from the additional access and cleanliness it provides.

The universal approach and the one common to most operators in adult restorative dentistry is to use a 6 × 6 inch dark, heavyweight rubber dam. Only a short time is needed to master the use and application of this material. Until this technique is mastered, a highly refined operative service cannot be provided because of the physiologic factors of the oral cavity.

Lubricants

The application of the rubber dam is simplified by the use of lubricants. Lubricants are placed on the tissue side of the rubber to facilitate passing the material between the contacts of the teeth. The advantages of lubrication are readily seen in cases in which tight contacts or many defective and rough tooth surfaces exist in the isolated quadrant. The lubricant should be placed only over the punched holes since these are the only areas of the rubber that pass between the teeth. The compounds that are used should not provide continuous lubrication and should be soluble in saliva so that they can be more easily removed from the exposed teeth. This is very important because a dry tooth surface serves to quickly invert the rubber dam and to produce the seal that is necessary for the operation.

Many solutions and ointments have been advocated for use as lubricants. The most popular of these seem to be surgical soap, shaving cream, and castor oil flavored with syrup of orange. All of these compounds are readily removed from the enamel surfaces after the dam has been passed through the contacts, and they effectively assist the application. Water-soluble oils that have excellent lubricating abilities are available from the druggist.

The importance of using lubricants cannot be overemphasized. The selection of Vaseline and cocoa butter as lubricants is not encouraged since they may leave a contaminant film on the tooth surfaces. In most offices it is convenient to use surgical soap for lubrication; this soap is contained in a dispenser and is used for washing the hands. The surgical soap should be applied immediately prior to the application of the dam in order to combat dehydration of the media, since the soap is ineffective once it has dried on the rubber.

Punches

In order to surround the tooth with the rubber dam a hole must first be punched in the latex. The hole should be a precise and even circle so that tears and rips in the dam will be minimized during the application technique (Fig. 7-3). One hole is punched in the rubber for each tooth, and locating the proper site is not difficult when the rules are followed. The hole to be punched should correspond to the center of each tooth being isolated. This makes it possible to surround the tooth with enough rubber to compress the soft tissue and to obviate tissue strangulation or leakage around the cervical areas that results from an inadequate amount of rubber. The ideal rubber dam punch has five or six holes in the punch plate (Fig. 7-4). Teeth vary in size and the correct diameter for each tooth is selected from the punch plate. The holes are punched accurately in regard to size and arch alignment so that no discrepancies occur when the rubber is applied. The holes in the plate are graduated from small to

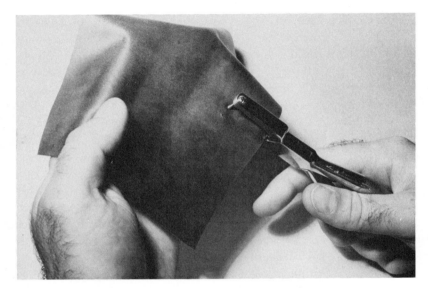

Fig. 7-3. Sharply punched hole in the rubber dam.

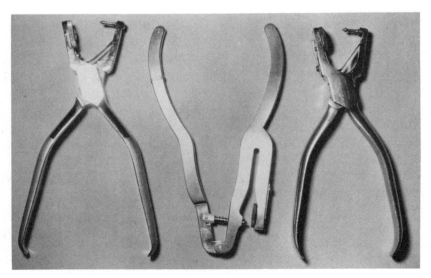

Fig. 7-4. Different types of rubber dam punches.

large and are used for the lower incisors up to the large molars. The cervical diameter of the teeth being isolated dictates the size of the hole selected.

The rubber dam punch is a simple apparatus that must be kept in excellent condition at all times. The dam is punched by a small pointed cone that projects into the holes on the punch plate and is activated by a spring in the handle. The spring is necessary to keep the sphere disengaged in the punch plate when it is not being used. The metal parts will be damaged if the punch is operated without rubber in the plate. When the punch is used without a thickness of rubber, the edges of the holes on the plate will be flattened and the angulation of the sphere will be changed, causing inaccurate punching and scalloped edges in the holes.

The efficiency and thoroughness of the punching are most important. If the rubber dam punch is not operating properly, a new punch plate should be purchased. It is sometimes possible to reshape and sharpen punch plates, the areas causing most discrepancies, and thus improve the usefulness of the punch. The surface of the plates can be sharpened on an Arkansas stone to improve the sharpness of the metal edges. A small amount of oil is placed on the stone and the plate is moved back and forth with light pressure in order to smooth the metal. An even, regular pressure should be exerted in order to develop a level cutting edge around the holes on the plate.

Since the rubber dam punch is used for all applications of the surgical field, it should naturally be aseptically maintained. The punches are cleaned by merely wiping all the parts with a sponge soaked in alcohol. The rubber dam punches are permanently ruined if they are placed in sterilizing solutions. The corrosive products of the solutions clog the inside of the punch plate and the other movable parts, making a sharp punch impossible. Only dry heat sterilization or alcohol sponges should be used to clean the punch.

Because of the number of times the punch is cleaned, it will be mandatory to periodically lubricate the moving parts. A small amount of engine oil (two or three drops) should be placed around the spring, in the handle joint and in the turning joint of the punch plate. If an excess of oil is used, it can be wiped off with an alcohol sponge. Usually sterilization of the punch is not too great a problem since the dentist has scrubbed his hands thoroughly immediately before punching the rubber dam; therefore, the rubber dam punch is usually cleaned with the alcohol sponges and then stored in the drawer near the syringes to simplify the manipulation of these instruments during the appointment. The syringe and the punch are both needed at approximately the same time and they can be removed from the instrument drawer simultaneously in order to eliminate unnecessary movement for the dentist or assistant.

Retainer

A retaining device is needed when applying the rubber dam in order to grasp and stabilize it around the patient's face to prevent blocking the field of

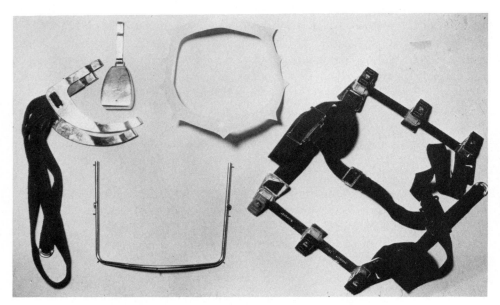

Fig. 7-5. Examples of the strap and frame retainers.

operation (Fig. 7-5). Tension is created between the retainer, which is an extra-oral device, and the clamp that secures the rubber to the teeth and retracts the cheeks and the tongue away from the working area.

Retainers are necessary to provide stability and to hold the rubber dam out of the field of vision. Special care should be taken to prevent any of the tissues from being damaged because of the length of time during which the retainer is in contact with the tissues. The retainer should be easy to apply and should not disturb the cosmetic appearance of the patient. The retainer of choice provides a great deal of access and retraction of the tissues to improve the vision. Retainers are sometimes selected solely on this basis because of the problem of access in some dental operations. The most stable type of retainers are the strap apparatuses that provide two or three clamps for the rubber on each side of the face. These provide the best surgical field, but they take a few seconds longer to apply and disturb the patient's hair arrangement. These considerations are of minor importance, however, and should not discourage the use of the strap retainers. For all long appointments or quadrant type of operations the strap retainers should be used because they afford greater retraction around the teeth.

Although use of the strap retainers has been challenged, there is no significant difference in the time it takes to apply these devices. At first the use of these retainers seems more difficult because of the critical amount and positioning of rubber that is necessary for the attachment at the sides of the face. However, proper location of the punched holes allows the application of the strap retainer

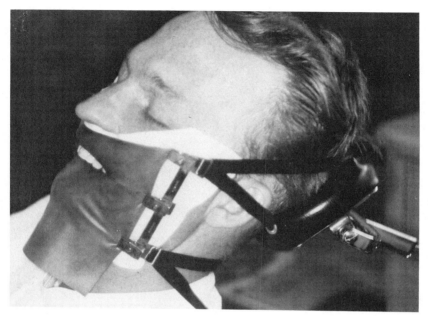

Fig. 7-6. Application of the Woodbury-True retainer.

to be completed in a short time. Because this type of retainer has obvious advantages, the dentist should describe the technique to the patient in order to encourage its acceptance during the lengthy appointment. When this technique becomes routine, hardly any other type of retainer will be used.

The two most common types of strap retainers are the Woodbury-True and the Wizzard retainers. The Woodbury-True apparatus includes two straps with metal attachments containing three clamps for each side of the face (Fig. 7-6). The two straps are connected in the back of the head to keep the pieces in a proper relationship during the appointment. The Woodbury-True retainer is the most stable type available. The Wizzard retaining apparatus is also a strap retainer; it has two metal clamps for each side of the face. A weight is needed for the lower half of the latex to hold this portion of the dam down, producing retraction in the field of operation (Fig. 7-7). Any type of weight can be used as long as it is heavy enough to retract the part of the rubber dam that projects below the mandibular teeth. The lower half of the dam is not as critical as the upper half because it cannot block the line of vision.

The frame type of retainers are used in some offices. These are usually circular or U-shaped frames that retain the rubber dam by means of projections located on the outside of the frame. They are used for quick or simple applications and have excellent adaptation in pedodontics. However, access and stability are sacrificed in this quick procedure, and any work of an extensive nature is best performed with other types of retainers. The frame retainer is more

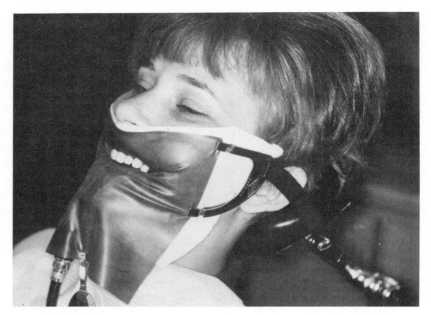

Fig. 7-7. Application of the Wizzard retainer with a rubber dam weight.

practical the farther anterior the tooth is located. Usually only one or two teeth are isolated, and if these are anterior or bicuspid teeth, the frame sometimes serves a useful purpose for young patients. The popular types of frame design are the Young and Nygard retainers. Both of these frames are suitable for the fast procedure, but in general neither makes a neat-appearing application. To reduce the chance of leakage, not as many teeth are isolated with these retainers because the frame is sometimes moved during the operation. Some of the problems associated with use of the frame retainer include catching sleeves or bumping the edge of the frame when reaching for instruments, and these mishaps sometimes move the rubber away from the teeth and break the seal against saliva. The main advantage in using the frame retainers is that they allow a rapid and simple application that is useful in minor procedures such as a simple occlusal restoration, amalgam polishing, and gross caries removal. If stability and access are desired in the operating field and if the appointment is expected to be longer than usual, strap retainers are used to provide the necessary stability and access.

Rubber dam napkins

To enhance the rubber dam application an absorbent napkin should be used to protect the tissue underlying the rubber dam. A napkin, several of which have been designed for specific use, occupies the space immediately under the rubber and acts as a liner. The napkin catches the saliva that spills over the lips and at the same time keeps the rubber off the facial tissues. The rubber dam napkin encourages a neater application of the dam and makes the patient more comfortable during the operation. These napkins are helpful in working with patients who have allergies or in preventing the irritation and cracked facial tissue that result from prolonged contact with moisture. The rubber dam application is begun by placing zinc oxide ointment in the corners of the mouth and, with use of the napkin, most of the tissue reactions from this will be prevented. The napkin is also helpful when the dam is removed. The soft, absorbent material can be used to remove any debris from the face and the corners of the mouth that may have collected during the dental operation. The rubber dam napkin is usually the last part of the armamentarium to be removed, and it is convenient to use the napkin to clean the patient's face and mouth before his departure.

Many types of rubber dam napkins are available. Napkins can be custommade by the assistant out of bird's-eye or diaper cloth. Patterns are available for different types of napkins that can be cut and fitted to conform to certain types of retainers. A flannel cloth napkin can also be obtained commercially. In some cities civic clubs and organizations have projects for producing the flannel napkins, which are cut from patterns with regular scissors. The material for the napkin should be clean, soft, and readily absorbent. Any material that fulfills these requirements, regardless of its color, will serve the purpose and will make the patient more comfortable. Like other commercial products, a disposable napkin is popular.

Forceps

Important for the patient's comfort during the rubber dam application is the method used to seat the clamp on the tooth (Fig. 7-8). The forceps will naturally influence the way in which the clamp is seated and removed from the tooth before and after the operative treatment. The clamp placement requires good judgment in order to prevent injury to the soft tissue, which is accomplished only with adequately contoured and fitted rubber dam forceps. The clamps should be seated firmly so that they will not move or rock on the forceps beaks. If this procedure is followed, the dam will be retained in the quadrant and damage to the cementum and periodontium will be minimized. A universal type of forceps should be used so that all types of clamps that are used in operative procedures can be utilized. The curved, narrow offset beaks can be employed with most of the clamps.

The forceps are designed to be comfortable in the operator's hand. In seating the clamp on the tooth, the forceps should not be bunglesome or unstable. Some situations demand that the clamps be held under tension, making it necessary for the handle to accurately fit the operator's curved palm. The terminal teeth in the arch produce these situations because the surrounding tissue must be deflected while the clamp is seated. The forceps are accurately grasped because the clamp is opened under tension for a longer time when being seated.

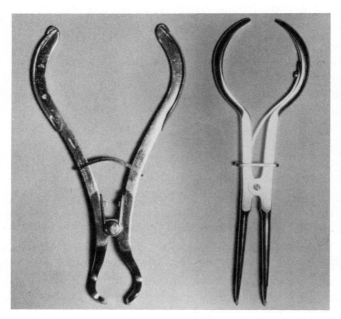

Fig. 7-8. Rubber dam forceps.

Many types of forceps are available since most manufacturers have made different designs to enhance the workability of the forceps. Ideally, forceps should have a narrow beak and should be offset to enable them to grasp the perforation in the wing of the clamp and to facilitate separation following tooth placement. If the offset or prominences on the beaks are too large and interfere with the clamp, they should be disked to reduce the size. Once the clamp is released the forceps should be drawn freely from the holes in the metal and should not move the clamp on the tooth. It is necessary to have a right-angle bend or curvature in the beaks of the forceps so that the jaws of the clamp can be cleared on withdrawal. The bend is extremely helpful with the double-bowed gingival clamps because of the conflict that results when the forceps interferes with the mesial half of the clamp. The forceps designed to place the No. 212 gingival clamp is advocated for use in operative cases.

The handle lock on the forceps is a safety device. The lock will hold the forceps open and retain clamps on the bracket while they are under tension. The handle spring is needed to help regulate the pressure in opening the clamp.

Maintenance of the rubber dam forceps is similar to that of the punch in that alcohol sponges are used for cleaning both of them. The forceps can also be driclaved, but they must not be placed in any type of sterilizing solution. If the joint is not freely movable and will not secure and release the clamps, a few drops of oil should be placed in the joint. It is absolutely necessary to have a free-moving forceps at all times because improper release of the clamp is traumatic for the patient.

Clamps

The rubber dam is usually secured to the teeth by means of a clamp. The clamp is placed upon the most distal tooth in the selected field in order to secure and anchor the dam and to facilitate the application of the rubber around the teeth. Seating of the rubber dam clamp should be a painless procedure, and the dam should be firmly secured in order to prevent any movement during the operation. Movement causes the trauma that was previously discussed. In some cases in which the anterior teeth are being restored and the heavier weights of rubber have been selected, it is possible to apply the rubber dam without the use of a clamp. When a clamp is not needed, it should not be used. All dentists, however, should master clamp selection, adaptation, and placement because most situations require the use of the clamp.

A description of the clamps is necessary to understand how they should be selected. All clamps have beveled jaws that contact the tooth and a bow that connects the jaws. Since the clamp is placed upon the teeth with the forceps, it contains holes or small depressions that facilitate its placement and stabilization. To a limited degree the clamps are designed for specific purposes and accordingly differ in shape. The clamps retain the rubber dam or retract the gingival tissue. The metal of the clamp is plated or made of stainless steel, and the most acceptable metal is one having an anodized surface that is impervious to the surface stain caused by the corrosive products. The clamps have some spring and are manufactured with precision to provide standardization of shape and positive retention on the tooth. The stainless steel products last longer.

The clamps can be purchased with or without wings. The wings are placed adjacent to and behind the jaw of the clamp, and they also come in different sizes. It is the function of the wings to provide extra retraction of the rubber on the buccolingual surfaces of the teeth. A special technique is needed for placing the clamp with wings because of the difficulties encountered in passing the rubber over the enlarged structure. If a favorite clamp does not come wingless it is simple to remove the wings by grinding, thus facilitating the rubber dam application. The clamps with wings are placed in the rubber dam before they are seated on the tooth. After the clamp is attached, the rubber dam is edged off of the wing in order to control seepage. This procedure is thought to be disadvantageous because the jaws of the clamp cannot be guided properly when it is seated on the tooth.

Clamp selection is critical to the rubber dam application. The clamps are selected mainly according to the size and type of jaws they have. There are two distinct theories on the type of clamp jaw that is most useful. Some dentists use the four-pronged type of clamp that rests firmly on the teeth in the line-angle areas. The other basic type is the jaw that has the same buccolingual

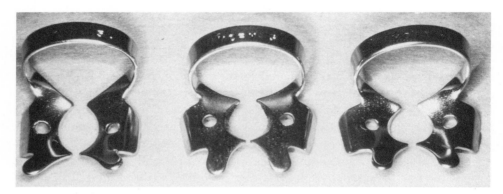

Fig. 7-9. Rubber dam clamps contoured to conform to the buccolingual tooth curvature.

contour as the tooth being secured (Fig. 7-9). Regardless of the type of jaw that is used, the requirement of stability must be fulfilled in order to keep the dam from moving and to negate the possibility of tissue damage. The four-pronged jaw clamp appears to be the most satisfactory and the most universally used. These clamps (No. W8A and No. 14A) can be reshaped and adapted to almost any type of tooth and easily secured below the height of contour. This type of clamp provides more retention on the tooth and extra stability, in addition to producing more tissue retraction. With the angulation of the prongs, it is possible to use matrix bands and impression procedures on the teeth that serve to hold the clamps. The prongs are directed toward the tissue and provide room for metal matrices and other types of materials necessary in the proximal restoration. These clamps must be specially ground. A disadvantage in using the contoured design is that many more clamps are needed. Teeth differ measurably as to size and curvature, and many clamps are needed in order to fit every situation. The operators who use the rubber dam routinely employ the four-pronged clamp because it requires fewer clamps and allows the operator to spend little time in selecting the clamp. Moreover, the stability and tissue retraction it affords instill more confidence in the rubber dam technique.

Selective grinding of the rubber dam clamps is necessary to produce a universal set for the operatory. The small carborundum stones are used to reshape most of the clamps that are purchased. The size and angulation of the apertures in the jaws can be adjusted to fit different types and sizes of teeth and also to accommodate the rotated or displaced tooth in the dental arch. During the grinding of the clamps it is necessary to remove sharp points and imperfections on the jaw. All clamps should be slightly beveled but should have no roughened areas that abrade the tooth surface. It is unusual if the rubber dam clamp does not have to be adjusted or smoothed with the mounted stone. It is easy for the dentist to select the proper clamp for the operation because he has made the adjustments himself and knows in what ways the designs and modifications will work to his advantage. Some operators feel that part of the temper should be taken out of the clamps in order to reduce tension, but this is conjectural. It is not difficult to determine which clamp will be overretained. Usage of the clamp for long periods of time will reduce the spring in the bow. When the temper is taken out of the clamp, the surface is damaged and will allow contamination and corrosion to occur. Unless bending the metal is indicated it will probably be unnecessary to alter the temper of the metal. The dentist should rely on careful grinding and readjustment of the clamp jaws to provide the ideal situation for retaining the dam.

The clamps that are most commonly modified are the Ivory No. W8A and the S. S. White No. 212 Ferrier clamps. These clamps have broad application and are shaped to fit the majority of operative cases. Before modifying a large number of clamps each operator should first master the technique of reshaping. This will develop judgment concerning the need for clamp adjustment and provide the necessary knowledge for clamp modification to increase the workability of the armamentarium. It will also increase the use of the rubber dam in operative procedures.

Ivory No. W8A clamp

The Ivory No. W8A clamp is used to develop three universal molar clamps. The new clamp should be evaluated to determine the dimension and direction of all four projections in the jaws. The top of the metal jaw surfaces are reduced by one half to create more room for the proximal matrix and impression procedures.

Small mounted stones are used to open the aperture in the center of the clamp (Fig. 7-10). The mesial and distal projections are opened 3, 4, and 5 mm. to facilitate the clamping of small, medium, and large teeth. The numbers, inscribed in the center of the bow with the round bur, correspond to the inside distance and the clamps are referred to by this number in the office. The reduced edges are smoothed with Burlew rubber wheels or with sandpaper to prevent the dam from being torn or the teeth from being abraded. The only molar, upper or lower, that cannot be secured with one of these clamps is the extremely large molar. A No. 14A clamp is used to secure this tooth. When the No. W8A clamps are adequately shaped, there will seldom be a need to use any other clamp in the office.

No. 212 rubber dam clamp

This clamp was designed by Ferrier specifically for isolation of the Class V gold foil restoration. The clamp retracts as well as retains the rubber dam. The No. 212 clamp is seated after the rubber dam has been applied. It has two bows that are secured to the isolated teeth to ensure stability. The jaws of the clamp remain in place during the operation and the compound locks are used as finger rests, which is beneficial to both the patient and the operator.

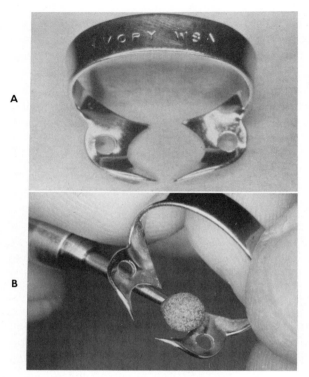

A

B

Fig. 7-10. A, Ivory No. W8A clamp as it appears when purchased and prior to any modification. **B,** Inside reduction and top surface thinning of the No. W8A clamp. **C,** Rubber abrasive disk being used to smooth the reduced metal. **D,** Measurement of the front opening of the clamp. **E,** Clamp modifications for 3, 4, and 5 mm. openings for different sizes of molar teeth.

The No. 212 clamp was designed to be used with as many types of lesions as possible. Many operative dentists find it necessary to modify the clamp by reshaping the metal. This is advocated because of the errors in manufacturing and the many clinical variations encountered. Factors such as tooth size, rotation or angulation, and cervical location of the lesion require a number of modifications in the original clamp design. Occasionally a clamp will need to be adjusted or reduced for an individual tooth to fulfill the purpose for which it was designed.

The labial bow of the No. 212 clamp is opened to create access for placing the restoration. Many hatch-type and endodontic clamps have constrictions in the labial bows that prevent the operator from reaching the tooth or the restoration. Care should be taken not to mistakenly select the wrong clamp. The No. 212 clamp is also utilized in the gingival amalgam restoration. The clamp can be used for other types of tissue retraction in the same way as the Schultz clamps are selected for the gingival amalgam restoration.

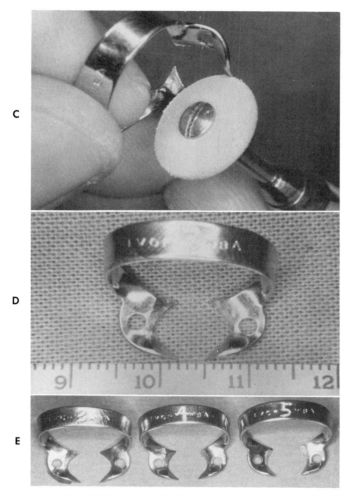

Fig. 7-10, cont'd. For legend see opposite page.

The clamp is made of stainless steel and is spring tempered for permanency. The metal is not influenced by cold sterilizing solutions, and it is receptive to adhesion of the compound. The spring in the bows and the constriction of the jaws limit movement after the clamp is seated. Any movement causes abrasion of the cementum and leakage in the surgical field. Both factors are eliminated when the clamp is stabilized by the use of compound under each bow.

Clamp selection is important for each individual patient. The location of the lesion and the shape of the tooth determine the choice of the various types of No. 212 clamps. The clamp selected must have the same curvature as the buccal surface of the cementum on which it is placed. The other criterion is the width of the labial jaw of the clamp; it should be the same width as the

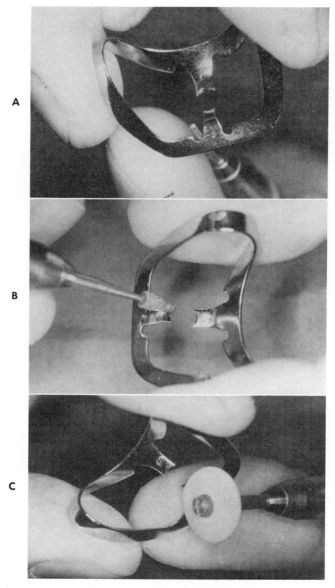

Fig. 7-11. A, Deepening the four grooves on the clamp with a No. 558 bur. **B,** Reducing and shaping the stainless steel clamp with a mounted stone. **C,** Smoothing the altered metal with a rubber abrasive wheel.

tooth. Proper clamp selection and placement will ensure excellent isolation and stabilization. The jaw of the clamp does not abrade the cementum. When cavity reduction is begun, the jaw serves as a guide for the initial cutting. The gingival wall of the preparation should be made parallel to the labial jaw of the clamp and be located 1 mm. above the metal. The critical relationship and guideline provided by the labial jaw of the No. 212 clamp make it necessary to seat the clamp in proper alignment. The clamp is placed squarely on the tooth, with the labial jaw usually parallel to the occlusal plane of the posterior teeth. Therefore, the clamp is helpful in judging the outline form and extension needed in the cavity walls.

As previously mentioned, because of variations in tooth size, lesion location, and arch relationship, the No. 212 clamp must be modified (Fig. 7-11). There are five basic modifications that fulfill the requirements of the majority of clinical situations. With these modified clamps in the armamentarium it will seldom be necessary to make further adjustments for individual needs. The clamp adjustments are made with fissure burs, carborundum or acrylic stones, and rubber abrasive wheels. The following are the modifications made in the No. 212 clamps after they are received from the manufacturer.

1. The four grooves adjacent to the clamp jaws should all be deepened 1 mm. with a No. 558 bur. This modification facilitates carrying the clamp on and off the tooth with the forceps. The depressions should only be accentuated, with caution taken not to notch the areas. With the forceps (preferably the University of Washington design or one with a similar curvature) the depressions in the clamp are engaged so that they will not slip and damage the cementum, restoration, or gingival tissue.

The No. 558 bur is then used to smooth the metal jaws and remove uneven or barbed areas that could abrade the tooth structure. The bur is used with light pressure to smooth and uniformly set the bevel of the labial and lingual jaws where they touch the tooth. These two modifications are made for all No. 212 clamps regardless of the additional modifications. One clamp with this design should always be available because it is used for most cuspid and bicuspid teeth. This clamp will be the one that is used most often. Four other modifications are made to develop a set of five No. 212 clamps for each operatory.

2. One clamp is modified for narrow teeth. The width of the labial jaw is reduced with the stones. It is ideal to reduce nearly half the width of the original dimension of the labial jaw of the clamp. This clamp is used for lower incisors and narrow cuspids and bicuspids. The extensive cervical constriction of these teeth make this adjustment necessary.

3. Another clamp is adjusted for lesions located far cervically on the tooth. This usually occurs with extensive lesions on large teeth, commonly cuspids. The adjustment is made on the lingual jaw of the clamp to enable the clamp to reach below this type of lesion. The angulation of the labial jaw is never changed because access to the cavity would be blocked. Ferrier designed the No. 212

clamp to provide access and to change the angulation of the labial jaw would destroy the principal purpose of the clamp.

Before bending the lingual jaw the temper must be removed from the clamp. To do this the lingual jaw is held directly in the bunsen flame and heated until the metal develops a cherry red color. The clamp is removed from the flame and stabilized with two contouring pliers. The pliers on the lingual jaw is used to turn the metal upward or toward the occlusal surface. Different angulations can be produced that will permit the labial jaw to be placed more cervically on the tooth.

The spring must be placed back in the clamp before it can be used. To do so, the clamp is reheated until it becomes a bright red color once again and then rapidly quenched in water. Some operators place the clamps in inlay ovens for 45 minutes and then remove them and quench them in cold water. The spring is then placed back into the clamp and it can be used on the tooth in this condition. Any carbon or residue on the clamp can be removed with pickling acid and then washed.

4. Two of the clamps are shaped for use on rotated teeth. The insides of the jaws are removed with small cylinder stones to adapt to mesially and distally rotated teeth. These are called right and left clamps and they are used for many of the eroded areas that need to be restored. Erosions occur in prominent teeth and in many cases this is a result of the rotation caused by crowding in the arch. After the insides of the jaws are removed for angulation the bevel is then reestablished with the No. 558 bur.

After the clamps have all been reshaped it is desirable to go over the areas with rubber abrasive wheels. This will remove the projections and smooth the surface of the metal. The tarnishing tendency of roughened metal is reduced by using the rubber abrasive on the modified clamps (Fig. 7-12).

One of the modified clamps will appear to be more ideal when all the factors are considered. The No. 212 clamp is selected after making the following observations.

1. The width of the tooth 1 mm. below the border of the gingiva is noted.
2. The amount of rotation of the tooth is observed in addition to the location of the most prominent area of the root surface.
3. The location of the gingival lesion is noted. The gingival depth, extension, and tooth size might dictate the use of a special clamp.
4. The height of the gingival tissue on the tooth and its corresponding health and sulcus width should be observed. These factors will determine the outline form of the restoration and the most suitable clamp in the set that has been prepared.

Schultz clamps

The Schultz clamps are useful for gingival restorations. The S1, S2, and S3 clamps are used for the specific purposes of preparing and cementing full-

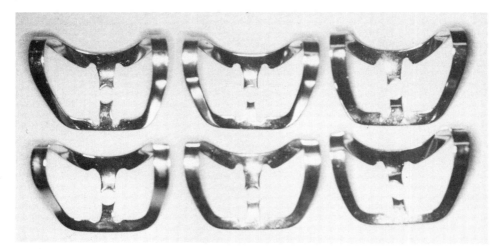

Fig. 7-12. Compare the five shaped No. 212 clamps with the unmodified clamp in the bottom left corner. The technique for shaping is described in the text.

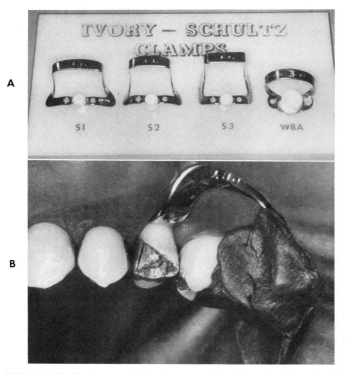

Fig. 7-13. A, Schultz clamps. **B,** Application and stabilization of a Schultz clamp.

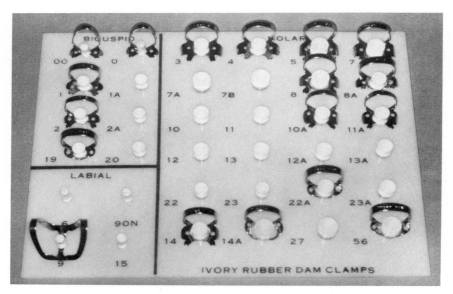

Fig. 7-14. Clamp board for convenient selection in the operatory.

coverage restorations for incisor teeth and the Class V amalgam restorations for the bicuspids and cuspids (Fig. 7-13). The Schultz clamps have very narrow, slanted jaws that make it possible to stabilize the dam by grasping only a small portion of the tooth structure such as a small root surface. The slant of the jaw provides tissue retraction and rubber dam reflection, which makes the clamp helpful in restoring Class V cavities. These clamps are used as a group with the No. W8A clamp and have a wide application in operative dentistry. When they are seated, they must be secured with impression compound because they are not stable.

Clamp boards are useful for storing and categorizing rubber dam clamps (Fig. 7-14). Manufacturers have specifically designed boards for their own clamps and each pedestal has a number that corresponds to the number of the clamp. Because the board makes it possible to see all the clamps that are available, it is excellent for storage. The clamp board should be kept in a place where dust and debris do not collect but which is still accessible to the operator. The choice of a clamp is critical for the application of the rubber dam, and the comparison afforded by the clamp board is helpful in selecting the correct one.

Saliva ejectors

In many cases the saliva ejector helps to allay the apprehension of the patient. Whenever possible, if the ejector is not directly in the way of the working area, the beginning student should use it to prevent the saliva from leaking from the patient's mouth or from running down his throat, which provokes coughing during the operation. The saliva ejector should be inserted through the rubber dam to rest freely in the sublingual space. Depending on the size, the ejector is allowed to pass through a punched hole in the dam that is made to correspond to the size of the bicuspid. This hole will be small enough that the dam will grip the ejector and prevent too much saliva from working its way up around the side of the ejector. To prevent tissue irritation the ejector should not touch the lips directly and should rest over the rubber dam itself or on the napkin that is used to protect the soft tissues.

Numerous types of saliva ejectors are available. The disposable and readily adjustable ejectors are helpful because they can be adapted to any dimension. Some ejectors have rubber tips that minimize the damage to the soft tissues, but they have limited application in that they are composed of metal and cannot be adapted freely to prevent tissue impingement. The ejector is adjusted so as to rest on the incisor teeth, with the uptake end reaching into the sublingual space. The tip should not be in direct contact with the tissue because of the possibility of causing ischemia. The tissue can block the ejector and prevent the elimination of saliva from the mouth. If the mandible is parallel to the floor, the saliva will accumulate around the tip of the ejector and be drained away. The ejector is not placed in the working area until the rubber dam is applied, because the manipulation of the dam could push the object down into the floor of the mouth.

APPLICATION OF THE RUBBER DAM

The method of applying the rubber dam is organized into a logical and concise sequence. The application is accomplished in steps, and the objective of each step must be satisfied before proceeding to the next. The application method can vary with the number of teeth and the type of retaining apparatus used, but this can be better achieved after the ideal technique is mastered.

If desired, the necessary anesthetic should be given prior to the application. Special anesthetics are ordinarily used in cases in which the buccal tissue in the lower jaw and the palatal tissue are impinged by the clamp. When a tooth is either partially erupted and carious or is fractured below the gingival tissue level, the tissue over the area should be anesthetized to prevent a painful clamp application. After anesthesia is obtained, the application of the rubber dam is initiated. When a good rubber dam application has been completed but full anesthesia has not been achieved, it is exasperating to have to remove the gear and reinject the patient. The operator should be certain that the desired degree of anesthesia is present before he begins. It has been noticed that painful clamp placement is practically eliminated when the adjusted No. W8A clamp is used.

The teeth that are to be isolated are scaled and polished in order to remove the stain and calculus that would otherwise prevent a good application by tearing the punched holes (Fig. 7-15). Also calculus may be responsible for false cavity margins if not removed. A better seal is obtained when a clean tooth is in apposition to the punched hole.

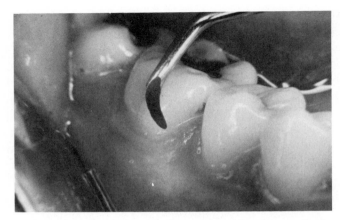

Fig. 7-15. Scaling calculus deposits prior to rubber dam application.

After the teeth are cleaned, the proximal contact sizes and smoothness are tested with dental floss. A 12-inch length of waxed floss should be wrapped around both index fingers and gently placed on the bias through all the contact points. If any of the contacts are overly tight and rough, the floss should be used repeatedly. This procedure produces a small amount of mechanical separation and in some cases smooths the involved restorations and tooth surfaces. In extremely rough contact areas, finishing strips and disks are used to allow proper insertion of the interseptal rubber. When grossly fractured restorations exist, removal of the defective restoration is recommended prior to placement of the dam. If this is done, the proximal areas will not interfere with the interproximal rubber.

Most of the armamentarium is placed on top of the instrument cabinet for easy selection. The armamentarium is arranged in a systematic way and the items are selected from left to right, a procedure that reduces the time involved. First the latex and the rubber punch are placed, then the forceps and clamp, and finally any additional aids can be placed in the order favored by the operator. All of these preliminary procedures can be completed while waiting for the anesthetic to take effect. At this time also, the rubber dam and the steps in its application are explained to the patient. Most patients will not mind the application but will be pleased with the care and concern shown by the dentist. These preliminary steps should be followed at each appointment since they will disclose details, such as tooth interdigitation, that are not in the record. The actual application is performed in the following sequence:

1. The rubber dam is selected according to size and weight. Most dentists routinely use only one or two different weights of rubber dam. A trend has developed toward using the heavier weight rubber dams. Ordinarily a heavyweight dam is used because it provides additional retraction and protection of the tissues. This weight is most helpful in all of the restorative procedures, particularly

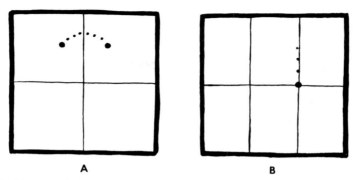

Fig. 7-16. A, Diagram of dimensions for punching the rubber dam for a maxillary application 1½ inches from the border. **B,** Diagram for punching the rubber dam for a mandibular application.

when multiple restorations are being placed, because it does not tear or move as readily as the lighter weight materials. When Class V restorations, particularly the gold foil type, are being placed, the extra heavy rubber dam is helpful because it provides additional retraction of the tissue. Another advantage of the heavier weight dams is that they are not torn as easily with burs and hand instruments during cavity preparation as are the lighter weight dams. This extra protection is afforded by the actual thickness of the heavyweight rubber.

2. The clamp needed to retain the rubber dam is selected. Some clamps, particularly the wing type, should be placed on the tooth and tested for its adaptation at this time. The experienced operator will not have to test clamps often, but occasionally this procedure is helpful. The clamp selected should be held in the forceps on the bracket table until it is placed on the tooth. To facilitate handling, the forceps handle is placed over the edge of the bracket table so that the device can be grasped quickly and accurately. Some operators prefer that the dental assistant hold the forceps containing the clamp.

3. The rubber dam is punched to include the teeth selected for the surgical field. The rules for punching the rubber dam prescribe that the holes be positioned so that the 6 × 6 inch dam can be squared over the patient's face. There should be enough rubber to completely cover the upper lip and fall directly between the lip line and the ala of the patient's nose. Positioning is important in order to distribute the rubber dam equally on both sides of the patient's face, which produces a neat application when the retainer is attached. The key to punching each rubber dam properly is to accurately locate the first hole on the latex sheet. The first molar is the first hole punched in mandibular applications and the upper incisors are the first in maxillary applications. This procedure, as shown in Fig. 7-16, will properly locate each dam and should be followed and used as a guide in each punching procedure.

Another rule for punching is that the rubber must be punched to approximate the center of the tooth being isolated. The selection of the size of the punch should range from the large holes, which are used for the molars, down to the small holes, which are used for the lower incisors. The teeth are punched in the center so as to provide ample rubber for retracting the interseptal tissue and for ready adaptation to the cervical areas of the isolated teeth. The problem associated with this phase of rubber dam application arises from having an inadequate amount of interseptal rubber, which is caused by punching the holes too close together. Proper punching is essential for an acceptable application because a hermetic seal is needed to block the salivary seepage.

The number of teeth that should be isolated in the surgical field has been standardized. It is desirable to have at least two teeth isolated on the mesial and one to the distal of the teeth being restored. This is not possible when the tooth being restored is the most distal one in the arch; in this case only two or three teeth need be isolated anterior to the distalmost tooth. There will be times when isolation of half of the arch will be indicated. When the problem is related to the anterior segment of teeth, it is expected that all anterior teeth will be isolated, and at times this should include the first premolars. According to early teaching, three fourths of the arch should be isolated in the surgical field, but this procedure is no longer used to any extent. With the exception of the occlusal restoration, two or more teeth should be included in the surgical field to provide relationships and guides for replacing the anatomy in the restoration. The anatomic grooves and configurations should correspond or blend with the adjacent teeth, and the exposed surfaces in the field will help to establish desirable contours and functioning components.

Problems arise when the surgical field ends with a tooth that has small bell-shaped surfaces or limited undercuts. Since this is customary in cuspid teeth, the field should go beyond or fall short of the canine tooth in most cases. An infrabulge area is needed to hold the dam in place, and the teeth are observed prior to the punching in order to determine the exact number of teeth that should be included in the field and those that are designated as terminal teeth to hold the application.

Templates have been designed to locate the holes for all deciduous and permanent teeth. The templates merely imprint the dental arch on the rubber to serve as a guide for locating the holes. These are average dimensions and are quite helpful in centering the dam. The tooth positions are stamped on the rubber with ink. After the application technique, which is fundamental to all operative procedures, has been mastered, the dentist will want to discard the template and eliminate this extra step.

4. The punched rubber dam is lubricated so that it will slip between the contacting surfaces (Fig. 7-17). The lubricant is spread thoroughly over and around the punched holes. To ensure that the lubricant does not become dehydrated the assistant should lubricate the dam while the clamp is being seated.

5. The clamp is seated on the tooth or inserted in the rubber dam (Fig. 7-18). The wingless clamps are seated on the tooth and the dam is passed around the

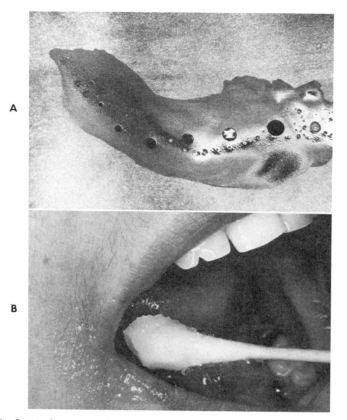

Fig. 7-17. A, Surgical soap is placed on the rubber dam for lubrication. **B,** Cocoa butter is applied at the corner of the mouth to lubricate the tissue.

metal when it is placed in its final position. This method of seating the clamp is advocated because it enables all the gingival tissue to be observed when the jaws are in the recommended position. When using clamps with wings and when working with most second molars (where vision is impaired), the dam is carried into the mouth by the clamp. The clamp is placed into the most distal hole and is held in the rubber by the two notches on the wings. The clamp is seated first and a plastic instrument is then employed to move the rubber off the wings to cover the cervical area of the tooth. These methods will anchor the dam. The other steps in isolation are initiated after the clamp is positioned. Seating the clamp alone is preferred because direct observation results in more gingival retraction and less discomfort.

Prior to seating the clamp the tooth should be dried with air and the depth of the sulcus investigated. This can be accomplished with an explorer or plastic instrument, and the amount of possible displacement of the clamp can be estimated. In seating the clamp the tooth should once again be dried, and regardless

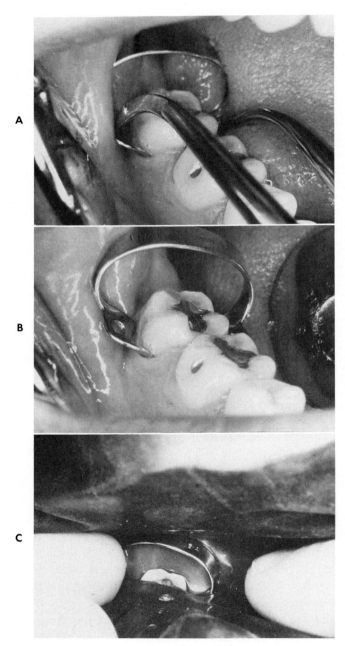

Fig. 7-18. A, Firm engagement of the forceps in seating the clamp. **B,** No. W8A clamp in position. There is 1.5 mm. of tissue retraction. **C,** Punched rubber dam is placed over the seated clamp.

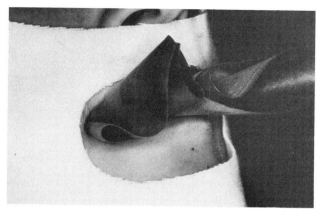

Fig. 7-19. Rubber dam napkin is placed around the projecting rubber and on the facial tissue.

of the design, the jaws of the clamp should be carried into the infrabulge area and below the height of the gingival margin. The rubber will then be in the proper position. The clamp is not seated below the gingival attachment since this would strip the attachment from the cementum surface, causing hemorrhage and destruction in the area. Careful observation of the free gingiva is always necessary.

6. After the dam is secured to the teeth by the clamp, the next step is to place the face napkin on the patient (Fig. 7-19). The napkin is squared on the patient's face and the rubber dam is then drawn through the aperture in the napkin. To keep the corners in position the top right-hand side, which is the first area to be grasped by the retainer, is punched. When this corner is secured, the other fasteners on the retainer are attached to the dam, making it square for proper application to the anatomic dimensions of the patient. The dam will be stabilized and the dentist can proceed to pass the punched holes through the necessary contacts and invert the rubber where it is possible. The retainer and the napkin should be adapted properly at this time, and when this is accomplished, these structures will need no adjustment for the remainder of the appointment.

7. The hole for the terminal tooth or for the tooth distalmost to the opposite end of the clamp is placed over the tooth (Fig. 7-20). This tooth will anchor the dam when the interseptal rubber is passed between the contacting surfaces. This procedure is simplified by stretching the interseptal rubber buccolingually in order to thin it interseptally, and it is then passed on the bias through the contact points. When the terminal hole is secured, the rubber is restretched and passed through the next contact until all of the interproximal rubber is below these structures to compress the gingiva.

8. The inversion of the surgical field is begun by drying the teeth with a sponge. The teeth are then redried with warm blasts of air from the syringe,

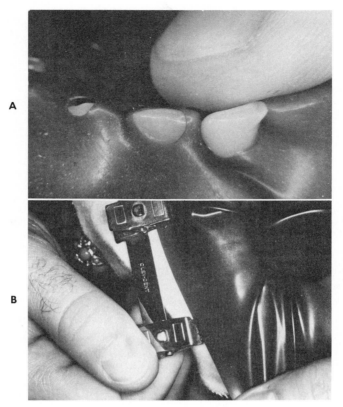

Fig. 7-20. A, Terminal portion of the dam is slipped between the teeth. **B,** Borders of the rubber dam are attached to the retaining apparatus.

which facilitates inversion of the rubber around the necks of the teeth (Fig. 7-21). The rubber dam is not sealed until the dam is inverted. This procedure is extremely critical to the surgical environment. The inversion of the rubber is accomplished with a blunt cement instrument, followed by use of the air syringe around all the teeth. When the rubber dam is not placed far enough into an infrabulge area, the dental floss can be used to tease the interproximal rubber in a gingival direction. The air syringe is trained upon the tucking instrument until all of the punched holes are inverted on the cervical area of the tooth. The teeth are then sprayed to ensure a clean area and dried once again. The best possible operating field has now been produced in the oral cavity (Fig. 7-22).

It was recently thought that ligation of teeth was necessary for the rubber dam application. However, ligation with dental floss is painful and should be avoided. The epithelial and gingival attachment of the tooth does not form a straight line, and the placement of ligatures drawn tautly around the cervical area strips the attachment. This is conducive to hemorrhage and pocket formation around the ligated teeth. The only exceptions are incisor teeth and those

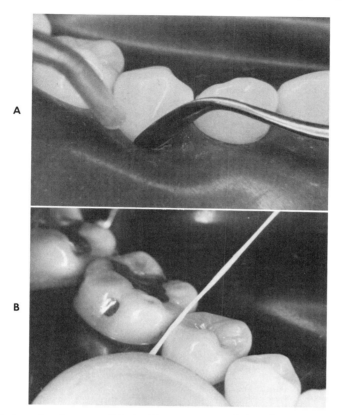

Fig. 7-21. A, Inversion is accomplished with warm air and the plastic instrument. B, Working the interseptal rubber down with dental floss.

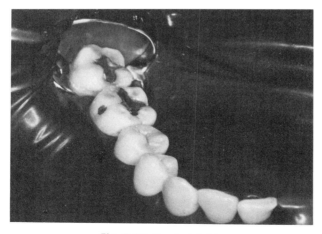

Fig. 7-22. Surgical field.

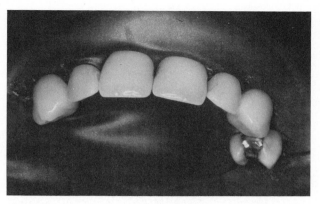

Fig. 7-23. Anterior rubber dam application without clamps or ligations is made possible by the heavyweight rubber material.

areas where a roughened carious lesion or defective restoration produces a tumified gingival papilla. It is occasionally necessary to place a ligature to retract this gingival tissue from the cervical wall of the cavity preparation. Ideally, however, the use of ligatures should be avoided because of the irritation and damage they may cause (Fig. 7-23).

When the procedures just outlined have been accomplished, an ideal type of operating field is achieved. The teeth will be dry, clean, and visible to the dentist, and the operator will be able to work with a minimum of deterrents. The rubber dam is left in place for as much of the restorative procedure as possible. The cavity preparation and restoration of the tooth should be completed in this environment.

REMOVAL OF THE RUBBER DAM

To duplicate the ease of application in the removal of the rubber dam an orderly and logical sequence should be followed. The removal is a separate technique and it is quickly accomplished in order to free the patient and dispose of the soiled materials. Prior to removing the clamp all of the interseptal rubber is clipped with curved collar scissors. This procedure is simplified by stretching the dam buccolingually so that it is thinned out. These small pieces are clipped on the buccal sides of the teeth and then released. The cut pieces are slipped through the teeth from the lingual surfaces and are freed of all the contact points. The forceps is firmly seated in the clamp at this time and is removed from the tooth without touching the tooth surfaces. One side of the rubber dam is then released from the retaining device. The free corners of the dam are held by the operator and slowly pulled from the patient's mouth. The rubber dam and the surplus restorative material that may have collected on the dam are removed in toto. The soiled dam is held up to the light to see if it is intact. If the dam has torn, the rubber pieces are recovered from the patient's mouth. If the rubber dam is intact, it is discarded at this time.

The rubber dam napkin, which remains in contact with the patient's face, is drawn carefully to the corners of the mouth. It is removed and the patient's face is cleaned of ointments and debris or salivary seepage that may have occurred during the appointment. The end of the napkin can be moistened and the soiled areas cleaned.

Attention is then focused on the quadrant that was isolated by the rubber dam. The tissues are immediately irrigated with water in order to clean them and to restore them to a normal condition. In some cases hemorrhage and seepage occur, and these crevices should be flushed of bacteria that could produce untoward tissue reactions. When the rinse is completed, the particular tooth that was restored should be transilluminated or dried. This is accomplished with a mirror and reflection from the dental light and with the air syringe. This will enable the operator to detect certain debris such as amalgam or compound that remains in the gingival sulcus and that must be removed in order to prevent any irritation in the area. When the area is transilluminated, it is helpful to feel around the gingival sulcus with an explorer. This also prevents the operator from overlooking debris that should be removal. Once the area has been surveyed and the restoration checked, with particular regard being given to the type of occlusion and contour, the patient is made ready for dismissal. The area is swabbed with a mild antiseptic solution to further negate the chances of tissue irritation. The antiseptic should be mild and can be a flavored mouthwash that leaves a satisfactory taste.

COTTON ROLLS

A useful procedure for keeping the teeth dry temporarily is the application of cotton rolls. The rolls are made from regular absorbent cotton and are formed in cylinders of different lengths. The rolls are placed over the duct openings of the salivary glands and are useful in the short procedure in which the rubber dam cannot be applied. As it enters the mouth the saliva is absorbed by the cotton. It is necessary to change the rolls at frequent intervals. Saturation time of the cotton rolls varies with each patient and is influenced by salivary flow and viscosity. The saturated cotton roll must be replaced immediately in order to obtain any value from the technique.

Holders or retainers have been designed to help stabilize the cotton rolls over the salivary ducts (Fig. 7-24). Different sizes of holders can be obtained to correspond to the age and development of the patient. The holders retain the rolls on the lingual and buccal surfaces of the mandibular teeth. They are used on only one side of the mouth at a time. Clamping devices retain the holders on the lower border of the mandible. The sublingual and submaxillary glands located in the floor of the mouth and the parotid gland located in the buccal vestibule are the salivary ducts that are to be blocked. Accurate placement and complete blockage is not possible because the rolls move with the muscular activity of the patient.

A delicate technique should be used in placing the cotton rolls. Prior to

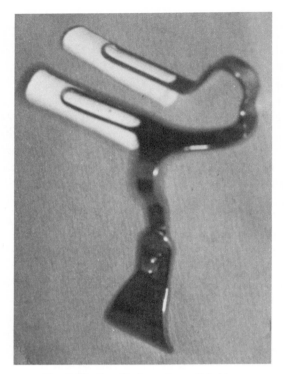

Fig. 7-24. Mandibular cotton roll holders.

placing the rolls the mucosa is dried with warm blasts of air and the roll rotated gently in place with cotton pliers. This rotating procedure seems to keep the cotton roll seated in position more adequately. Different lengths of cotton rolls are available for the buccal application, and separate retainers have been designed to hold the longer sections in place.

The cotton roll technique is an inadequate substitute for the rubber dam. The procedure is used when the rubber dam application is impossible or impractical. The cotton roll retainers provide some tissue deflection, which provides some access in quadrant impression procedures. The tongue and cheek are retracted from the teeth and are more stabilized.

Following are some situations in which cotton rolls are indicated:
1. Procedures of short duration in which the rubber dam cannot be applied
2. Indirect impression procedures using full-arch models for articulation
3. Application of topical fluorides (Caustic drug applications should be made with the protection of the rubber dam.)

The requirements for and preparation of the operating field have been explained. When vision, cleanliness, and dryness are established, optimum operative conditions for tooth restoration exist.

ADDITIONAL READINGS

Allen, C. D.: Keeping cavities dry, Dent. Cosmos **7**:622, 1866.

Barbakow, A. Z.: The rubber dam; a 100 year history, J. Am. Acad. Gold Foil Operators **8**:13, 1965.

Ellsperman, G. A.: Review of operative procedures, J. Canad. Dent. Assoc. **10**:253, 1944.

Hamstrom, F. E.: Evaluation of a rubber dam technique, J. Am. Acad. Gold Foil Operators **5**:15, 1962.

Hollenback, G. M.: Pleas for a more conservative approach in certain dental procedures, J. Alabama Dent. Assoc. **46**:16, 1962.

Ireland, L.: The rubber dam, Texas Dent. J. **80**:6, 1962.

King, E. J.: Inserting the rubber dam, Dent. Cosmos **12**:517, 1870.

Latimer, J. S.: Barnum's rubber dam, Dent. Cosmos **6**:13, 1865.

McAdam, D. B.: Rubber dam, Practical Dental Monographs, Jan., 1964, pp. 3-34.

Medina, J. E.: The rubber dam and incentive for excellence, Dent. Clin. N. Am., Mar., pp. 255-264, 1967.

Modern uses of the rubber dam, Nevada Dent. Soc. **31**:335, 1955.

Murray, M. J.: Value of the rubber dam in operative dentistry, J. Am. Acad. Gold Foil Operators **3**:25, 1960.

Prime, J. M.: Inconsistencies in operative dentistry (fifty reasons for using the rubber dam), Dent. Cosmos **27**:82, 1937.

Stibbs, G. D.: Rubber dam, J. Canad. Dent. Assoc. **17**:311, 1951.

Wolcott, R. B., and Goodman, F.: A survey of the rubber dam. I. Instruction, J. Am. Acad. Gold Foil Operators **7**:28, 1964.

Wolcott, R. B., and Goodman, F.: A survey of the rubber dam. II. Problems in usage, J. Am. Acad. Gold Foil Operators **8**:20, 1965.

Woodbury, C. E.: Operative dentistry, Pacific Dent. Gaz. **38**:484, 1930.

chapter 8

Separation for restoring proximal surfaces and treatment of nonvital teeth

Building the contour of the tooth is one of the most important aspects of the restoration. Special dimensions, shapes, and curvatures are created to provide function and stability to the tooth. Mastication is confined to the occlusal area and to the surfaces surrounding the cusp tips and marginal ridges. Proper dimension and contour of the proximal surface with the adjacent tooth are needed for stability and protection of the periodontium. Convexities in the contact and cervical bulge areas protect the gingival tissue in the concavities around the cervical line of the tooth. Restoration of the contact area and the embrasures is therefore critical for periodontal protection because these areas shunt the food off the tissue while maintaining the arch position of the tooth.

At the beginning of the century the issues discussed most often in operative dentistry were separation and restoration of the contact area. The profession was divided into "separationists" and "contourists." The controversy arose over the merit of contoured fillings. Many dentists routinely filed and disked the contact areas off the teeth to produce a more easily cleaned surface. This group, known as the "separationists," thought that this procedure stimulated gingival tissue and helped minimize recurrent dental caries. At this time the dynamics of occlusion and tooth movement had not been analyzed. Problems occurred as a result of this procedure, but at one time it was widely used. The opposing group, known as the "contourists," was headed by Sanford Perry, and it ultimately gained predominance. The "contourists" placed the original or more ideal curvature in the proximal dental restoration. Within a few years it was apparent to this group and to the profession as a whole that maintaining the proximal contact and anatomy protected and encouraged the health of the periodontium. Tooth drift was not apparent when the integrity of the tooth was maintained. Within a short

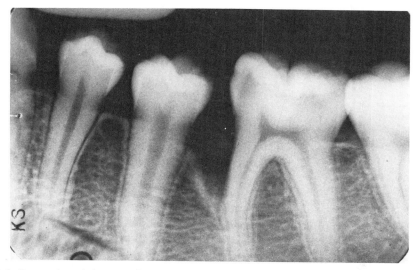

Fig. 8-1. Destruction of the periodontium caused by food impaction that resulted from the open proximal contact area of the first molar.

time a group of mechanical separators appeared and were advocated for use in all restorations involving the proximal surface.

It is now recognized that an equilibrium should exist in the dental arches. Each tooth has its own place and functions both individually and in groups. The muscles of the cheek and tongue help to maintain the buccolingual alignment. Because of the mesial inclination of the teeth an anterior force exists. This anterior force makes it necessary to accurately restore the proximal surfaces in order to maintain tooth position. The dimension of the tooth in the contact area is important but not more significant than the tooth form that affords periodontal protection. Equilibrium is stabilized in an axial direction by multiple, uniform contacts of the teeth when they come together.

A contoured restoration of the proximal surface not only assures tooth position but also protects the periodontal tissues. The firm contacts between the teeth and contours minimize food impaction, which is considered to be the precursor of caries and tissue irritation. A proximal restoration that lacks the proper size and tension with the adjacent tooth potentiates food impaction; when this occurs, detachment of the periodontal membrane, bone destruction, and tooth movement are initiated (Fig. 8-1). An understanding of the anatomy of the proximal surfaces of the anterior and posterior teeth and of suitable restorative techniques and materials prevents this trauma and discomfort from occurring.

PROXIMAL ANATOMY

Research on tooth function is lacking, but certain anatomic structures are considered to be physiologically important because of the protection they afford

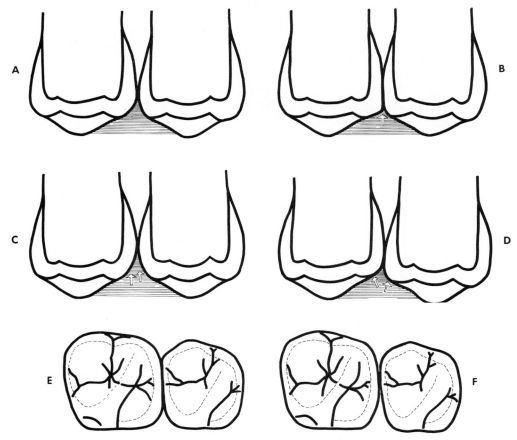

Fig. 8-2. A, An ideal contact and embrasure relationship. **B,** Contacts excessively flat with occlusal embrasure lost. **C,** Contacts too far toward the gingival with enlarged occlusal embrasure. **D,** Marginal ridges not in harmony with each other. **E,** Contacts as expected after teeth have been in position many years. **F,** An inadequately secure contact.

the supporting tissues. Each tooth must maintain its position and physiologic function if it is to be retained in the oral cavity. Ideal replacement of the contact area, interproximal spaces, and embrasures during the operative procedure fulfills this purpose.

Contact area

The contact area is the site of actual contact between two teeth on the mesial and distal surfaces and is sometimes called a "contact point." Some authors describe the contact as a "marble type" of relationship, but this is the case for only a short time following eruption. Attrition causes tooth movement, which results in a flattened contact area of 2 or 3 mm. in posterior teeth and a slightly smaller one in anterior teeth (Fig. 8-2). In ideal conditions a positive relationship exists between the contacts that resists food impaction and protects the gingival tissue. This relationship can be observed and tested by passing dental floss between the teeth and noticing the resistance that occurs when the floss is moved between the contacts in the tooth structure.

The size and shape of the tooth influence the formation of the contact area. Consequently the contacts are of numerous sizes and cause the formation of different types of gingival embrasures. The contact area in the posterior teeth is located nearer the buccal surface, which causes a larger lingual embrasure; and the contact area in anterior teeth is located nearer the lingual surface, which causes a larger labial embrasure. The contact area in an occlusal-cervical direction is located at different heights on the proximal surface and it is usually parallel to the incisal edges of the teeth and to a line drawn through the posterior buccal cusp tips. The tooth formation that is placed in the restoration is influenced by the contact area, meaning that the location and contour of the area are important to function and stability because they in turn influence the other anatomic structures of the tooth. The curvature of the buccal and lingual surfaces and the marginal ridges are influenced by the anatomy of the contact area.

Contacts are classified as being either rounded or broad and flat. The flat contact presents problems in the restoration. It is difficult to carve and form because of limited access and it makes cervical adaptation of the restoration more difficult. The flat contact or the square-shaped tooth is difficult to clean and thus is more prone to caries. Whenever possible the rounded contact with an open embrasure in positive relationship should be produced in the proximal restoration. This artificially treated contact will make hygienic procedures easier. The contact area is a 1 to 2 mm. circle in posterior teeth.

Whenever open contacts or poorly shaped proximal surfaces are discovered, they should be corrected by establishing a more ideal relationship. Food impaction, tooth drift, and periodontal trauma are caused if the condition is allowed to continue. Although the amalgam restoration can be adequately contoured, the inlay is more useful in cases in which the surface involvement is large. The inlays can be waxed and polished to the desirable contour on both the proximal and occlusal surfaces.

Gingival embrasure (interproximal space)

This is a triangular space formed by the contact areas of the two teeth and the supporting bone. The base of the triangle is located on the bone. The entire space should be completely filled with healthy gingival tissue. The size of the embrasure varies with the shape of the contacts and location of the bony support. Restoration of the embrasure should allow only enough room for the gingival papilla, except in cases in which recession has occurred as a result of periodontal disease or surgery.

Home care procedures are designed to encourage the patient to clean the gingival embrasure. Cleaning and massaging this area prevent caries on the tooth surface and stimulate the gingival tissue so as to keep it healthy and capable of filling the triangle. Although the occlusal, buccal, and lingual embrasures are important, they are not filled with tissue.

Proximal caries generally begins directly below the contact area. In some cases hypertrophy of the papilla develops, causing additional food impaction and tenderness. The outline form of the restoration includes this diseased tooth structure and is extended so that the margins are located outside the embrasure on tooth structure that can be easily cleaned.

The contact area and the interproximal space combine to form the labial, lingual, and occlusal embrasures. These openings are much larger on the lingual surfaces of the posterior teeth and serve primarily as food shunts. The food particles that are not crushed between the teeth slide through the embrasures to the tongue and are thrust back onto the occlusal surfaces for mastication. In this way mastication is facilitated by the lingual embrasures and, to a lesser extent, by the buccal embrasures.

Height of contour

The height of contour is the area of greatest bulge on the buccal and lingual surfaces of the tooth. It protects the gingival tissues by forming a survey line around the tooth and preventing food impaction in the buccal and lingual gingival spaces. On posterior teeth the contour is located in the gingival third of the buccal surface and in the middle third of the lingual surface. These contours divert the food over the free gingival margin, and they should be placed in the restoration for the protection of the periodontium.

Tooth contour is very important to the function, stability, and protection of the periodontal tissues. This discussion is presented to make the dentist aware of the importance of the contours and how they function. The value of observing radiographs, tooth arrangement, and masticatory movements cannot be overemphasized in planning the restoration. Ideal forms and contours cannot always be produced, especially if undesirable anatomic features existed in the tooth prior to the damage. The components and purposes of the proximal surface must be understood before a biologic restoration, considered from the standpoint of periodontal protection, can be made.

SEPARATION

Numerous methods are used to separate the teeth in order to accomplish a more ideal dimension and contour of the proximal surface. Tooth movement, made possible by the periodontal membrane, allows separation to be physiologically beneficial when good judgment is used and when kept within the limits of the membrane width. The rapid separation technique is the most common and practical method used for the anterior proximal gold foil restoration. It is usually accomplished with mechanical separators, but when amalgam and tooth-colored materials are used, the wood wedges are also employed.

Table 8-1. Thickness of periodontal membrane of 172 teeth from 15 human jaws*

Age of subjects	Average at alveolar crest (mm.)	Average at midroot (mm.)	Average at apex (mm.)	Average for tooth rmm.)
11 to 16 years (83 teeth from 4 jaws)	0.23	0.17	0.24	0.21
32 to 50 years (36 teeth from 5 jaws)	0.20	0.14	0.19	0.18
51 to 67 years (35 teeth from 5 jaws)	0.17	0.12	0.16	0.15
25 years (18 teeth from 1 jaw)	0.16	0.09	0.15	0.13

*Adapted from Coolidge, E. D.: J. Am. Dent. Assoc. **24:**1260, 1937.

Orthodontic tooth movement results from the application of sustained forces on the supporting tissues. Tension and compression of the periodontal membrane by mild, sustained forces can initiate bone resorption and cause subsequent calcification. The tooth is moved over a period of months at a rate slow enough to form new osseous support along the path of movement. Circulation in the tooth is not altered at this time, and evidence of the movement is usually observed by a thickening of the periodontal membrane. In addition to growth the amount of sustained forces that are needed and the anchorage on the teeth are the primary factors to be considered in orthodontic treatment.

The separation utilized for placing dental restorations is not of the same magnitude as that used in orthodontic procedures. The amount of separation is limited by the width of the periodontal membranes. Thicknesses of the periodontal ligament have been studied and the dimensions indicate that only extremely small tolerances can be sustained without causing some type of severe trauma (Table 8-1). Separation produces compression and tension in each periodontal ligament of the two involved teeth. It has been stated that 0.6 mm. is the maximum movement possible. This dimension was determined by measuring the periodontal membrane in a large number of radiographs. This amount of movement is shared by the two teeth on either side of the space. A space of 0.5 mm. will seldom be needed. To date, no rules to follow in mechanical separation have been established by research.

Excessive or prolonged separation causes damage in the apical pulp vessels. The supporting ligament can be stripped from the periosteum, but tooth vitality is terminated when circulation ceases in the apical vessels. The apex moves against the bone and occludes the vessels.

According to several state dental boards, excessive separation has caused tooth damage (Fig. 8-3). Unnecessary tooth movement and inadequate stability cause the pulp damage and periodontal trauma, which is irreversible in some cases. The gold foil procedure has been blamed for the tooth devitalization, but the condensation of gold has been found to be an atraumatic procedure. Separation is not supposed to provide a simple solution to restorative problems but should

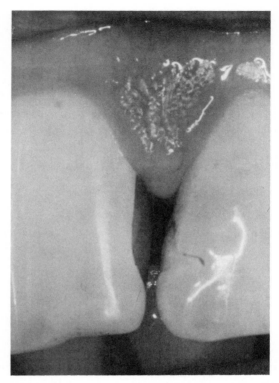

Fig. 8-3. Excessive separation of the teeth by a mechanical device.

serve only as an adjunct to accepted procedures by providing additional access and stability.

Purposes of separation

1. Separation techniques can be used to facilitate the examination of the proximal surfaces of teeth. Lesions may be suspected in areas not readily observable or in places that are impossible to radiograph, such as in malposed, rotated, or overlapped teeth. It is helpful to separate these areas carefully so that the enamel surface can be directly observed. At this time the need for a restoration, the type of material, and the acceptable outline form can be determined.

2. Separation provides more access to the carious lesion, making it possible to use a less extensive cavity outline that will display a minimum of restorative material. Occasionally separation is required with direct gold restorations to produce an acceptable esthetic result. The amount of separation and the type of cavity outline differ with each individual dentist. Because of the longevity of the restoration, careful consideration should be given to the procedure. The extra space is very helpful in polishing the restoration after it is inserted. The addi-

tional space gained with separation (a maximum of 0.5 mm.) does not eliminate the need for an esthetic outline form.

3. Separation helps to restore the tooth to its normal position. In very few cases, however, will it be possible to correct arch position by separation and restoration. Various methods of slow and rapid separation can be used to improve the axial relationship of an individual tooth. This is observed when long-standing caries has destroyed the entire contact area and the tooth has migrated in a mesial direction by tipping. Restoration of the tooth serves to halt the drift rather than to improve tooth position. Separation can make only a small improvement in the tooth inclination.

4. Normal and ideal contours can be restored better when the teeth are separated to make the surfaces accessible. If the underlying gingival tissue needs additional protection, a more positive contact or "plus relationship" can be placed between the teeth. An adequate contact area and embrasure form are produced with less trouble under these conditions.

5. The properly applied separator provides stability for the restorative procedure. When the separator is secured with compound, the covered teeth are splinted and they absorb the forces as an individual unit. This is helpful in direct gold restorations in which the material is compacted into the preparation. The stability alone indicates that the separator should be applied when this type of restoration is used.

Methods of separation

In operative dentistry, separation is divided into two categories. Each type can be used to advantage, but the rapid procedures that are possible with mechanical devices are the most practical.

A. Slow (materials)
  1. Gutta-percha
  2. Brass ligatures
  3. Silk ligatures
  4. Rubber materials

B. Rapid (mechanical devices)
  1. Ferrier separators
  2. Perry separators   } Traction principle
  3. True noninterfering separators }
  4. Ivory separator   } Wedge principle

In slow separation the teeth are forced apart by the expansive properties of materials. The slow method requires more time, which is a disadvantage because two appointments are needed. Rapid separation is produced by devices known as mechanical separators and can be accomplished quickly at the time of inspection or restoration. In some situations both types of separation are utilized to improve the result of the restoration.

The advantages of slow separation are as follows:
1. The procedures do not cause pulp damage if judiciously handled.
2. The chances of damaging the periodontal membrane are not as great because of the gradual tooth movement.
3. When gutta-percha or a similar material is used, hypertrophied gingival tissue can be pushed away from the margins of the cavity preparation if necessary.

The disadvantages of slow separation include discomfort and soft tissue irritation. The separating materials are rough and therefore should not be used for extended periods.

The advantages of rapid separation are as follows:
1. The mechanical separators can be used quickly at the time of the operation.
2. Rapid separation does not damage the gingival tissues.
3. A minimal amount of discomfort is experienced when the mechanical separators are used.

Rapid separation causes trauma only when the devices are injudiciously used. Too much movement crushes and tears the periodontal membrane, causing damage and tenderness in the periodontal ligament. At the same time the pulp circulation is impaired at the root apex and causes subsequent degeneration of the tissue. The size of the periodontal membrane should be surveyed radiographically to guide the application of the separator. In the literature the value of rapid separation has been unfairly challenged because often the judgment employed in tooth movement has been unrealistic and has resulted in irreversible tooth damage.

Materials used for slow separation

Gutta-percha. In teeth in which large carious lesions exist and individual movement has occurred, gutta-percha can be used for slow separation. Sometimes it is used following caries removal during an appointment before the cavity preparation. This separation works better if two adjacent cavities are excavated to retain the gutta-percha.

The space being separated is packed with warm gutta-percha under moderate pressure. Then, between appointments, the applied gutta-percha expands, and occlusion occurs and spreads the teeth apart. The packing is left in place for 24 to 48 hours and is inspected to determine how much movement has occurred. Repacking might be needed in order to gain additional space or gingival compression, but it should not be allowed to remain for long periods of time because trauma occurs.

This procedure always causes trauma to the packed area. The separation that is produced is slow and painful. The forces exerted on the packed gutta-percha cause the tooth movement rather than the properties of the material itself. The intermittent pressures in mastication and in clenching the teeth are the forces employed. Care must be taken to obtain good adaptation between the gutta-percha and the tooth structure because gross amounts of leakage will otherwise result. The leakage allows the saliva to seep under the pack and be forced into the dental tubules when the forces are exerted. This is painful and, if permitted to continue, results in pulp damage and sensitivity. For acceptable adaptation the gutta-percha is placed after being softened with heat. It is helpful to varnish the tooth structure before packing in the still warm and sticky gutta-percha.

Occasionally zinc oxide–eugenol is used for a similar purpose. A packing is made in the same way as gutta-percha to serve as a temporary restoration to minimize tooth drift. The technique is selected more for pulp sedation and gingival treatment in multiple casting procedures. It is helpful to incorporate cotton fibers in the zinc oxide–eugenol to prevent the pack from crumbling.

Either of these materials causes discomfort, and the pack should not be left for prolonged periods. Serious pulp damage and tooth movement are found to occur if this is done. Separation and gingival treatment can be conjointly accomplished with the technique, however, and it is usually indicated for large lesions in posterior teeth when excessive drift and gingival hypertrophy have occurred.

Brass wire ligature (No. 0.020). In some cases, most often in orthodontics or other types of procedures that precede tooth banding, the brass wire ligature is helpful. The wires are inserted through the gingival embrasure and are wrapped around the contact area. The number of turns and the tightness of the wire cause the resultant separation. The procedure is used 48 hours prior to the band adaptation or operative procedure. Separation usually requires only one encirclement of the contact area with the wire. The patient is warned of the discomfort that will result from the brass ligature. The twisted wires are tucked into the gingival embrasure and smoothed to prevent soft tissue damage. Since the ligatures are only in place for a short time, no other instructions are necessary. When the wires are removed, the teeth will be movable, which aids in the construction and cementation of the orthodontic bands.

Silk grassline ligature. In cases in which brass wire cannot be used the silk ligature is helpful. In addition the silk ligature is sometimes needed to provide access for the brass wire ligature. The technique is seldom used because the silk thread is difficult to keep clean and is not too forceful in opening the interproximal space. It is sometimes difficult to pass the silk beneath the contact area. Dental floss can be tied to the silk and forced through the embrasure with a wood wedge. The silk is passed around the contact twice and tightly secured with a surgeon's knot. The string then swells when saturated with saliva and pushes the teeth apart. The silk ligatures are left in place for only 24 hours. If left for longer periods of time the threads will drop out, necessitating the separation to be repeated. At this time the No. 0.020 brass wire ligatures can be applied or the bands adapted. Another reason why the silk ligatures are not often used is because they have an undesirable taste.

*Rubber separators.** Rubber separators are used mainly by orthodontists prior to band adaptation. The rubber wedges are inserted 24 hours prior to the appointment and the teeth are rapidly separated. It is important not to leave the rubber in place longer than this because of the possibility of tissue damage and patient discomfort. The bands are adapted following removal of the separa-

---

*Vulcanite and rubber dam elastics were once used.

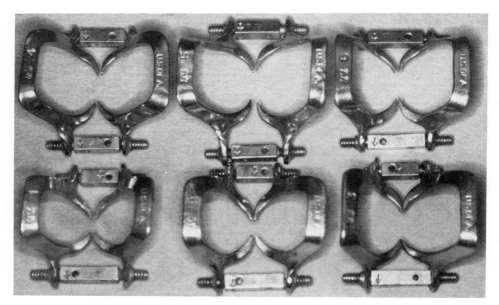

Fig. 8-4. Ferrier separators.

tors, and a thorough examination is made to prevent pieces of the rubber material being left in the gingival sulcus.

Devices used for rapid separation

Any type of separating device must fit the teeth accurately and be stabilized prior to the activation of the forces. The jaws of the separators should have curvatures similar to those of the teeth in the interproximal embrasures. The adaptation of compound prevents movement of the separating device and minimizes tissue damage. Stability is then assured, allowing a uniform force load to move the teeth, which reduces discomfort and irreversible trauma to the pulp and periodontium.

Ferrier separators. The most universally used separating devices are those designed by Ferrier (Fig. 8-4). In the 1930's it became impossible to obtain the Perry separators, which were used extensively at that time. Ferrier redesigned a group of six separators with a pattern similar to the original Perry devices and added many improvements. The bows were widened to produce more access for the operation and the jaw curvature was changed to accommodate different tooth arrangements. Although lack of standardization in their manufacture causes problems, the Ferrier separators are the appliances most widely used by the operative dentist. Priority in the design of these separators was given to minimizing interference in the working space.

The Ferrier separators are numbered from 1 to 6 and the jaw sizes and bows are shaped differently to conform to the typical size and shape of all the

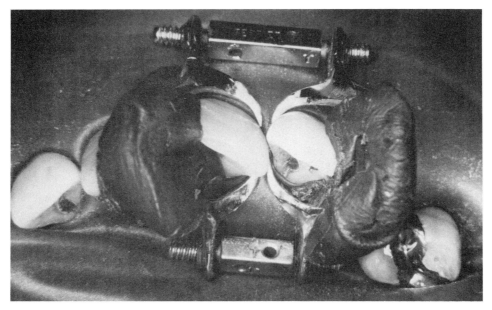

Fig. 8-5. Four jaws of the separator fitting the interproximal surfaces.

embrasures, ranging from the incisors to the molars. The separator that best fits the embrasure is selected. The common choices are the Nos. 1 and 2 separators. So that compound could adhere to the device, Ferrier specified that the separators be made of plated metal. The specific uses of the Ferrior separators are as follows:

No. 1 For all incisors of normal size
No. 2 For cases in which the No. 1 separator cannot be used, especially when the incisors are large and malposed
No. 3 For separating the cuspid and the first bicuspid
No. 4 For separating bicuspids
No. 5 For separating the second bicuspid and the first molar
No. 6 For separating molars

In all cases the separator that best fits the embrasures of the teeth and the arch position that produces the least amount of operative interference should be selected.

These separators operate on the traction principle and provide more stability than do the other designs. The Ferrier separators have two bows that are conveniently stabilized with stick compound that covers four or five teeth. The traction forces applied to the separator are distributed throughout the four or five teeth instead of just to the individual tooth being restored (Fig. 8-5). The compound makes movement of the separator impossible and therefore gives maximum protection to the tissue in addition to distributing the stresses.

The rules and specifications for the separators were given by Ferrier. "Shake"

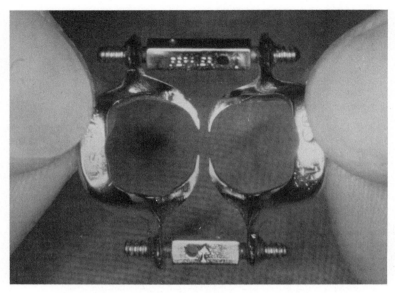

Fig. 8-6. Test for "shake" or looseness of the separator.

or looseness of the devices was an important requirement (Fig. 8-6). Shake is provided by loose attachments and is tested by holding the bows of the separator. The shake simplifies the task of fitting the jaws to the tooth surfaces. This movement can be produced by dry-lapping the labial and lingual screw adjustments on the separator.

The separators may need to be reshaped prior to clinical usage. The bows are routinely too wide and should be reduced with small mounted stones to encourage better adaptation to the teeth. The widths of the jaws are reduced on the tooth side with small carborundum stones and then smoothed with rubber abrasive disks. The height of each separator jaw is also reduced by removing the top or tooth side of the jaw with similar stones and abrasives; the tissue side should not be altered. Thinning the metal will produce more working space in the interproximal embrasure for finishing the gingival margin. Care is taken not to excessively reduce the separator jaws because a weakness will otherwise result in the thin metal. It is helpful, particularly with the Nos. 1 and 2 separators, to make these alterations prior to clinical usage because then the separators will fit the teeth more closely. Occasionally additional adjustments will be required at the time of application, but this can be done rapidly with the mounted stone and rubber abrasive.

For the application the surgical field is isolated with a rubber dam that is wider than the bows of the separator. This will allow the tooth structure to be exposed and dried for securing the compound. The rubber dam application is performed in the regular manner prior to the application of the separator. The separator that most accurately adapts to the teeth is selected. The separator jaws are examined to ensure that all four are similar to the tooth curvature and are in contact all along the metal. The separator is opened to contact the tooth surfaces and the adaptation is determined once again. All four jaws should be in contact and no rock should be detected in the selected separator. If the adaptation is satisfactory, the separator is opened with the wrench while being stabilized with the thumb and index finger. The opening is continued until the device is supported by the initial pressure alone. The position is maintained with the nonworking hand until one of the bows is stabilized with compound to secure the separator jaws against the teeth and in the most gingival position in order to expose the tooth structure and the area in which the cervical border of the preparation will be located.

The same technique is used to place the compound around the separator that is used to stabilize all rubber dam clamps and matrices (Fig. 8-7). A low-fusing compound, usually a green stick type, is selected in order to keep the temperature as low as possible for the stabilization. The operator places the compound on the separator with his free hand while regulating the temperature and the consistency of the material. The stabilization is an efficient and atraumatic procedure for vital teeth and underlying tissue and it enhances the operative procedure.

The stick of compound is passed into the bunsen flame several times until the surface becomes shiny and a change in shape is initiated. The stick is then removed from the flame and rotated to allow the heat to spread and uniformly melt the compound. When softening occurs, the stick is placed in a cup of water to wet the surface; the dentist then pulls the softened portion off the stick with moistened fingers. The compound is balled in the thumb and index finger and passed back into the flame to sear the surface, which promotes good adaptation to the teeth. The prepared compound is then placed under the bow of the separator and is squeezed into the embrasures. The fingers are moistened again and the compound is firmly pressed between the teeth. Air is then applied by the assistant to quickly cool the compound and to stabilize the separator. The same procedure is used to secure the other bow of the separator. The compound is confined more to the teeth and the embrasures rather than extended over the top of the separator bows. Only a thin layer of compound is left over the bows because too thick a layer would interfere with access to the carious lesion (Fig. 8-8).

When the stabilization is completed, the separation can be produced or instrumentation for the preparation can be initiated. If some of the compound was exuded near the tooth being restored or in the labial opening in the separator, the flange can be removed with a warm plastic instrument. The compound should be carved with the warmed instrument to make a neat, smooth appearance. The separator and compound together provide a finger rest, which contributes to stability and to the accuracy of the cavity preparation. When the

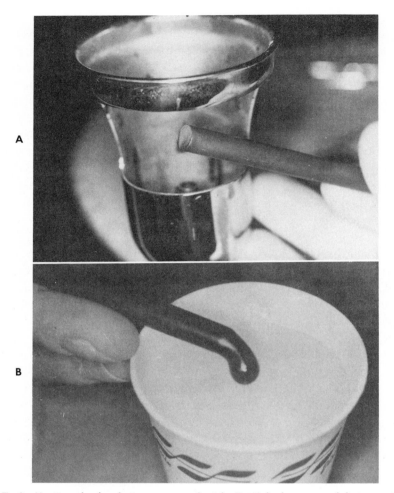

Fig. 8-7. A, Heating the low-fusing compound stick. **B,** Melted compound being moistened on the surface with water. **C,** Detached compound being held with moistened fingers. **D,** Surface of the compound seared for attachment to the teeth. **E,** Direction in which the compound is placed under the separator jaw and pushed into the subjacent embrasures.

separation is completed, the wrench is inserted into the labial and then the lingual bolt (Fig. 8-9). The bolt is turned evenly to produce the same opening and to reduce the torque that might develop in the separator and break the compound assembly. A few minutes should elapse between the turns to give the bone expansion time to react.

Precautions should be taken not to overseparate the teeth. The spring action in the jaw of the separator produces more movement by the pressure applied than is expected near the opening. Therefore slow and judicious opening is the rule for application of the forces, and during the appointment the separator is gradually returned from the opening to prevent overseparation.

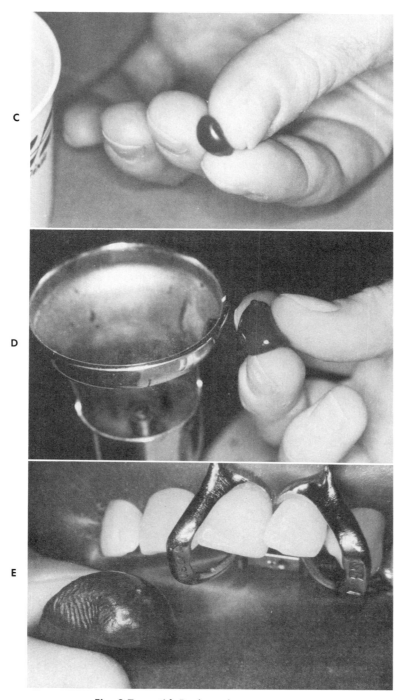

Fig. 8-7, cont'd. For legend see opposite page.

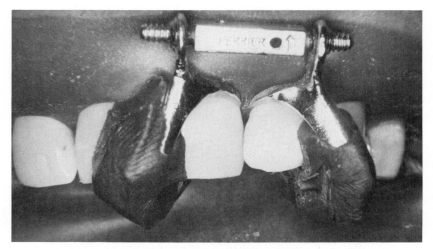

Fig. 8-8. Stabilized Ferrier separator.

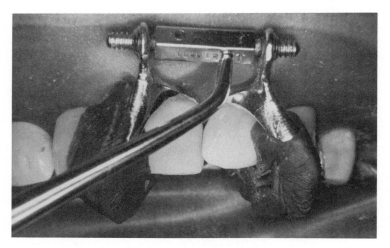

Fig. 8-9. Separator being opened with the wrench.

The Ferrier separator is removed by closing the device completely and by breaking the compound assembly. A small twist of the separator is made, with caution being exercised not to damage the restoration. The compound is removed with the fingers or with a blunt instrument, and it is sterilized by driclaving or by wiping with alcohol. The screw adjustments should be oiled lightly if they are difficult to remove.

The Ferrier separator is optional when condensing gold in the anterior proximal restoration to aid in establishing proper contact. The device is opened only enough to firmly contact the prepared tooth and then it is stabilized to

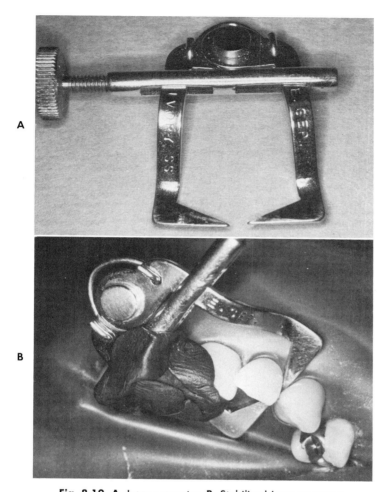

Fig. 8-10. A, Ivory separator. B, Stabilized Ivory separator.

reduce trauma during condensation. The separator is mandatory when strips are being used to finish the contact area. When its only function is to aid in finishing, it is positioned after the lingual, gingival, and labial restorations (if applicable) are partially finished.

The use of Ferrier separators should be mastered for the refined operative practice.

Modified Ferrier separator. This device was designed by Alexander Jeffery to be used with the lingual approach technique in the Class III gold foil restoration. Jeffery modified the shape of the Ferrier No. 1 separator. In addition to reducing the size of the jaws the bows were also made smaller. The modified separator is also made of stainless steel and in general is smaller in all dimensions than the original Ferrier separator. The modified separator can be used in many places. This device, like those previously mentioned, must be reshaped. The same procedure is followed to produce smaller jaws and to permit a more universal application of the separator. The modified No. 1 separator is useful and its inclusion in the armamentarium should be considered if a complete service is to be offered in the direct gold restoration.

Ivory separator. This device can be helpful in simple, quick procedures, and it is particularly useful for the rapid inspection of lesions on the proximal surfaces of incisors and cuspids. The Ivory separator should also be stabilized with stick compound, but even when this is done the device is not adequate for lengthy procedures. However, the insertion of tooth-colored materials and inspection can be accomplished with this separator when the moistened wood wedge cannot be used.

The Ivory separator has only two jaws and is stepped off-angle to clear the incisal edges of the teeth (Fig. 8-10). It contains a two-sided thread to allow right and left quadrant application. The body of the separator should be on the side opposite the proximal surface of the preparation because the separator will be less likely to interfere with the operation in this position. The different applications are made by placing the screw on the side facing the labial surface.

The Ivory separator is seated and opened only enough to contact the two teeth and give support to the jaws. The body is supported and stabilized with compound in the same way as are the Ferrier devices. After stabilization only a few quarter turns of the screw at a time will be necessary for tooth movement, and the degree of opening is accomplished slowly.

True noninterfering separators. These devices, designed by Harry True, are

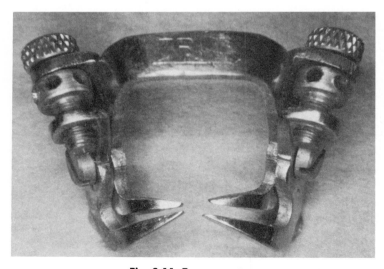

Fig. 8-11. True separator.

manufactured in groups of three. The No. 1 separator is most commonly used (Fig. 8-11). The wedge principle is also employed with this device. The jaws adapt well for a wedge separator, the main reason being that the edge of the jaw has a double extension to provide four contacts for holding the device. The noninterfering separator can be turned to the right or left to avoid the operating field. This device produces good separation but cannot distribute the stress to as many teeth as can the traction type of separator when it is stabilized.

The True instrument is secured differently from the other types in that the compound is placed in the separator prior to the tooth contact. Wedges of compound are produced, warmed, and then placed inside the separator. The entire assembly is placed in the flame and warmed adequately to allow adaptation of the separator. The compound in the separator is cooled with the air syringe and stabilized at this time. The operator then opens the separator with a wrench on the labial and lingual surfaces, observing the same precautions outlined for rapid separation with the other devices.

Summary

1. Restoration of the proximal surface should include an adequately sized and contoured contact area and interproximal space. Health of the gingival tissue and the periodontium is assured by an adequate restoration of the proximal surface that develops a sound relationship between adjacent teeth.

2. The building of ideal proximal forms is not always permissible, but sound conditions should be restored whenever possible even if a poor anatomic relationship existed before preparation of the tooth.

3. Various methods of separation can be used to develop an ideal proximal surface contour. Although a large space and excessive tooth movement are not possible, assistance is provided by proximal openings of 0.5 mm. or less. Stability is a primary reason for employing the mechanical separator.

4. The indications for and accepted procedures of separation should be recognized. Techniques should be used that are suitable for the operation and that will enhance its result. Little scientific information is available to the profession on the biologic effects of mechanical separators.

SPECIAL RESTORATIONS
Endodontically treated teeth

Special procedures are used to restore teeth that have been endodontically treated. In a tooth with a root canal filling the enamel layer becomes dry and brittle within a short time, and when the external surfaces are not intact, the remaining tooth structure must be supported by the restoration. The removal of the pulp tissue and the insertion of an inert canal filling material allows the use of retentive posts in the root chamber of the tooth. The changes resulting from the canal filling include discoloration of the crown of the tooth. Endodontic therapy is valuable in that teeth are retained that are critical for the restorative

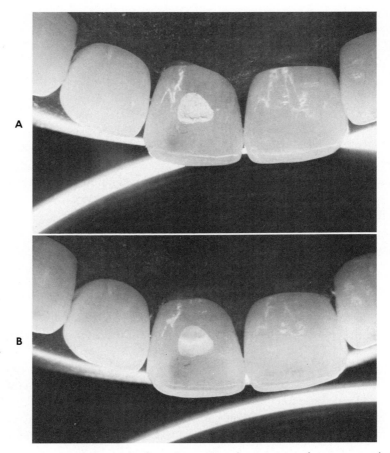

Fig. 8-12. A, Gutta-percha in the lingual opening of an incisor after root canal therapy. **B,** Excavated coronal pulp chamber. **C,** Base of silicate cement that also fills the excavated coronal pulp chamber. **D,** Completed resin restoration.

treatment plan. The dryness and discoloration of the enamel are minor problems in comparison to loss of the tooth.

The methods of restoring endodontically treated teeth are: (1) restoration of a lingual or occlusal opening of an intact tooth; (2) the use of gold casting for replacing cusps and supporting the tooth; (3) full-coverage restorations using metal ceramics; and (4) restoration requiring root canal support.

Lingual opening. The lingual opening occurs in anterior teeth that have been treated. Access is provided by opening into the pulp chamber through the lingual surface to remove the pulp and enlarge the root canal. The opening is made in the center of the lingual concavity with a No. 4 or No. 6 round bur. As the pulp chamber is approached, the coronal dentin is removed to facilitate curettage of all the diseased tissue. The crown of the tooth is opened and

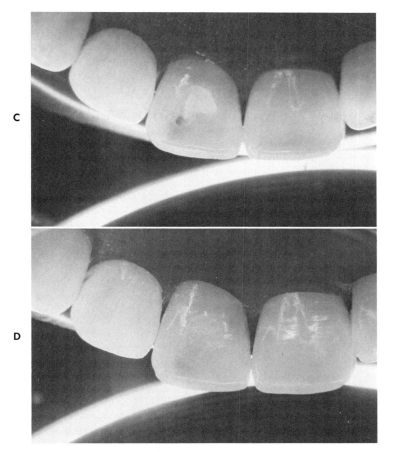

C

D

Fig. 8-12, cont'd. For legend see opposite page.

cleaned down to the level of the root. The root tissue is removed, the canal is enlarged and sterilized in a series of appointments, and the root canal filling is placed.

The simple lingual restoration can be accomplished quickly and in many cases the lingual opening will be the only break in the enamel surface (Fig. 8-12). The temporary cement or gutta-percha, together with all the debris that is present in the coronal pulp chamber, is removed thoroughly with the No. 4 round bur. The bur is revolved slowly to excavate the stained dentin in the crown, including the areas previously occupied by the pulp horns. The excavation is made down to the level of the root canal filling. This level is normally below the margin of the gingival tissue, and the tooth will appear lighter following the excavation. The lingual enamel and intracoronal dentin wall is washed with

3% hydrogen peroxide to remove the remaining debris from tooth grindings. The cavosurface enamel is finished sharply at a right angle if tooth-colored materials are used and beveled slightly if powdered or regular cohesive gold is used.

The lingual opening is restored by first inserting white opaque silicate cement as the base to give the tooth a lighter appearance. A thick mix of silicate is packed through the lingual opening to fill in the excavated pulp chamber. After the cement sets it is trimmed to allow 1 mm. thickness for the covering restoration of the lingual surface.

Only two materials are used to cover the lingual openings in anterior teeth. They are sulfinic acid catalyst resins and direct gold fillings. The new enveloped powdered gold is popular because of the ease with which the gold is inserted, condensed, and polished. Regular cohesive gold pellets are also effective in sealing the lingual opening. Either resin or powdered gold is used for the covering layer because these materials can be smoothed and will not dissolve or discolor the surrounding tooth structure.

The resin is inserted by the brush method and the gold is condensed with special right-angle instruments that can reach the opening. Both materials are built to excess and contoured with round burs, after which they are smoothed with small rubber wheel abrasives and pumiced with the soft rubber cup. The finished restoration and tooth structure are blended smoothly to prevent irritation of the tongue from the incisor teeth. The tongue often rests against these teeth and roughness in this area would be extremely irritating.

The occlusal opening in molars and bicuspids is restored in a similar manner. If the tooth structure is intact or if there is an acceptable supporting inlay, the powdered gold or regular cohesive gold is used. The pulp chamber is excavated with the same instruments, but this time the crater is based with white zinc phosphate cement. The cement for the ideal pulpal wall is reduced and smoothed with a fissure bur.

The preparation is finished with a small cavosurface bevel and the gold is added with a condenser designed especially for the powdered material. The many curvatures on an occlusal surface are finished with the assistance of the cleoid carver prior to disking and smoothing. The gold can serve effectively as both the seal and the restoration of the treated tooth. If the tooth has not been restored previously, the dovetail outline that is regularly used for powdered gold is indicated.

Posterior tooth with limited support. The posterior tooth with limited remaining support is restored effectively with the three-surface inlay that covers the remaining cusps with the gold casting (Fig. 8-13). These are called "onlays" and can be made with or without retention in the enlarged root of the tooth. The onlay commonly relies on only frictional surface retention for holding the casting and supporting the tooth. The full-coverage restoration is commonly seated over a core, the retention of which was achieved by entering the root canal, by anchoring its core with screw-in pins.

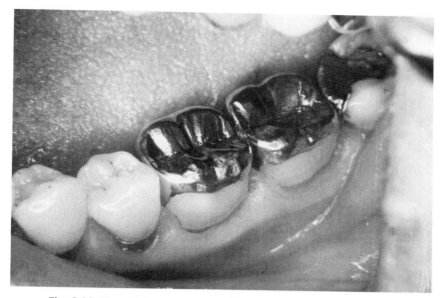

Fig. 8-13. Heavy inlay cusp capping for support of the two molar teeth.

The three-surface onlay casting is an excellent restoration, particularly in the upper bicuspid teeth. To fabricate some partial coverage restoration it is advisable to develop additional support by rebuilding the destroyed portion of the tooth with a pin-supported amalgam or a composite resin. If a thick buccal wall of enamel remains after the restoration is placed, the surface can be masked with white zinc phosphate cement for esthetic purposes. The onlay casting is made to grip and support the nonworking cusps slightly more than the routine casting (Fig. 8-14). If one of the cusps in the bicuspids is short or extensively undermined, the cast core and full-coverage restoration are indicated. The same three-surface inlay casting is used for molars if the buccal and lingual surfaces are intact.

Root canal retention. When it is necessary to use the root canal for retentive purposes, a gold post must be made. This post intrudes into the canal for a length equal to that of the crown. It is expected that the gold post will fit reasonably well, but it is not required to have the same tolerance as a conventional casting unless an external margin is involved. The anterior teeth are most often the subjects for post construction because of convenience. There are times when post formation and final restoration are combined into one operation, but it it a distinct gamble to attempt to seal such a restoration with accuracy and to have the margins be reliable. This will then usually be a two-stage procedure, with the post and core cemented first, followed by the final preparation.

The initial step in constructing a post is to remove the unnecessary occlusal or incisal portion of the tooth. Then a channel is formed up the canal to the

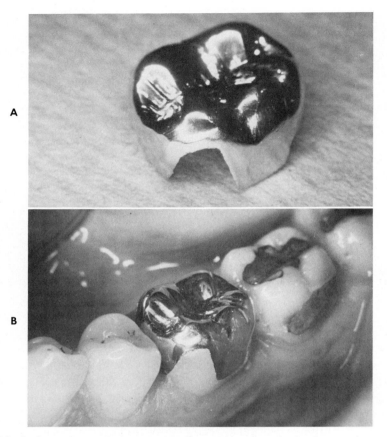

A

B

Fig. 8-14. A, Protective casting to support the weakened tooth. **B,** Cemented casting for retention, tooth support, and function of the first molar.

required depth, using a No. 1 round bur followed by a No. 4 round bur. A round bur will follow the gutta-percha more easily than other burs, which is important in avoiding lateral perforation. As the preparation proceeds it is important to properly study endodontic radiographs to attain accurate orientation.

Sometimes it will be necessary to reduce the size of the shank of the bur to attain the proper post depth. This is done with a heatless stone, and the reduced metal bur shank is polished with a rubber wheel.

The bulk of the preparation is completed using a tapered bur to enlarge the post hole. The final sequence of preparation ensures that the completed post will be seated or keyed into a specific position. This may be done by forming a keyway at the labial or lingual portion of the preparation with a small tapered bur. The depth of the key may approximate 2.0 mm.

This preparation may be reproduced by a rubber impression material, though to prevent distortion the post segment may require reinforcement by incor-

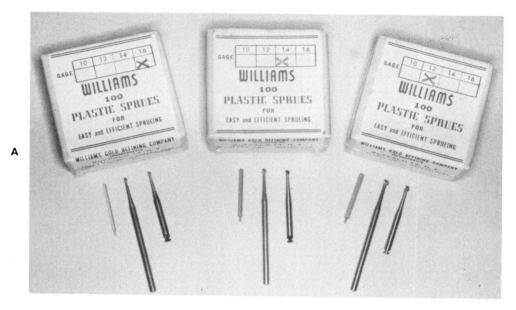

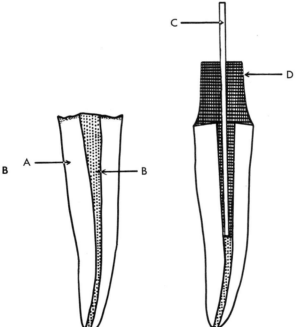

Fig. 8-15. A, Plastic sprue pins the size of the round excavating burs for direct wax carving of the cast core. **B,** Formation of direct pattern with acrylic resin. *A,* Retained devital root. *B,* Root canal filling in position. *C,* Plastic rod or bristle fitted into post preparation. *D,* Acrylic pattern material with preparation partially completed. (**A** courtesy Dr. Samuel Patterson.)

porating a small rigid metal or plastic rod into the impression. From this a stone model may be poured and a conventional wax pattern prepared.

A quicker method of developing a pattern is to form the pattern directly from the preparation using an acrylic pattern material.* Wax is difficult to handle when trying to form a post, since it will not easily reproduce the entire length of the post and is easily damaged.

To form an acrylic pattern, the preparation is lightly moistened and a rod of plastic, which may be improvised or commercially available,* is made the depth of the preparation (Fig. 8-15). This plastic rod is scored to allow retention of the pattern material. The acrylic powder and liquid are combined in a dappen dish and allowed to begin polymerization. An amount sufficient to reproduce the preparation is picked up on the plastic rod, and when the material has a controllable viscosity it is inserted into the moistened preparation. Before polymerization is complete the pattern is partially withdrawn several times so that it is not trapped by undercuts. If upon withdrawal the pattern is not complete, acrylic may be added to complete the pattern. Again additions may be made to have the coronal portion to the desired shape.

Acrylic offers the advantage that it may be tooled by revolving instruments into the final required form. If the original plastic rod has adequate length it may be used as part of the sprue assembly.

The pattern is cast, cemented, and finished for the final impression. As with other types of crown preparation or abutment teeth, the final margins must all be placed on healthy tooth structure (Fig. 8-16).

Some posterior root canals are small in size and must be filled with metal points. This prevents use of the canal for retention and dictates instead the use of the pin-retained amalgam restoration (Fig. 8-17). More pins than usual are placed at greater depths in the nonvital dentin. The amalgam restoration is reduced for the core and the casting is placed over the amalgam and the tooth stump. Small remaining cusps are helpful in placing the amalgam and will prevent dislodgment of the cemented pins. Whenever possible, however, the root canal should be used for retaining the cast gold core.

The gold post core is effective for full-coverage restorations and bridge abutments. It restores the endodontically treated tooth by providing the root with rigidity and strength, which give the tooth additional support. As with the porcelain crown or veneered restoration, the endodontic post maintains excellent esthetics because the labial wall location is regulated to provide an optimum thickness in the full-coverage restoration.

Restoration of the endodontically treated tooth is directed at protecting the remaining brittle enamel, and in some situations measures are taken to retard discoloration.

---

*Duralay by Reliance Dental Manufacturing Co.; Resincap by Lang Dental Manufacturing Co.

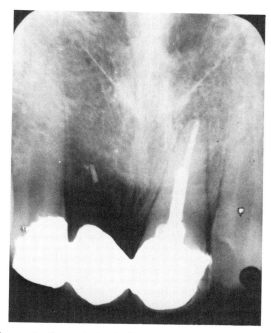

Fig. 8-16. Cast gold core in the endodontically treated tooth to support a three-unit bridge. Note proper length of the post.

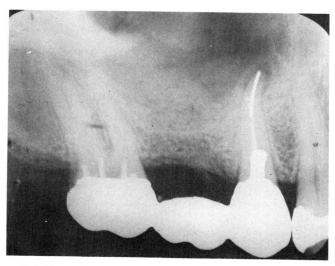

Fig. 8-17. Three-unit bridge with the molar abutment restored with a pin retainer amalgam. The bicuspid has a cast gold core which lacks adequate length and narrowly missed perforation.

Abutment teeth

Restoration of abutment teeth is given special consideration in the treatment plan. When questionable, these teeth are excavated first to determine the pulp conditions and extent of the solid tooth structure. When the abutment teeth have initial caries or recurrent decay around existing restorations, they should be restored first to prevent changes and needless work in the treatment plan. The condition of the tooth and the depth of the caries dictate the type of restoration to be used, and the tooth is prepared in such a way as to limit the depth and surface extension. The extension is limited so that the margins of the casting can be placed on tooth structure. The gold margin should be located some distance from amalgam because of the corrosion that results when the two metals are in contact in the oral cavity.

The deep carious lesion in the prospective abutment is excavated thoroughly, and this includes amalgam restorations that are defective or that were placed by a previous dentist. The dentin surfaces are coated with varnish or are prophylactically lined with calcium hydroxide as usual. If intermediary bases must be used, they are kept to a minimum thickness to reduce thermal conductivity. A thick base produces an amalgam core that is too thin and that will fracture and be lost during the refinement of the cavity preparation.

The extensive surface involvement can be restored with the pin-retained amalgam restoration, as described in Chapter 10, or with the gold casting that has been waxed directly to the tooth. The gold core casting is made with exacting box retention and resistance forms and should include a number of posts. The rubber dam is applied, and the direct waxing method is used to develop an accurate pattern. In mutilated teeth nylon bristles are employed for extra postretentive benefits.

The compound amalgam preparation is altered on the abutment tooth. Since the amalgam will be covered, the proximal outline is more undercut to prevent fracture and loss during rotary surface reduction. The cervical margin, particularly on the surface adjacent to the edentulous space, is not taken below the gingival tissue but is limited so as to provide 1 to 2 mm. of tooth structure for the finishing line. An extensive amalgam restoration is not a desirable core unless pins are used because it is too easily dislodged.

The tooth that has been damaged only superficially by incipient caries or that barely shows a penetration of the surface is disregarded in the preparation. The ideal preparation is made, and if the lesion results in an undercut, it is blocked out with zinc phosphate cement. The cement is then smoothed to become the wall of the preparation, and the need for a regular outline form and amalgam restoration is eliminated.

The restoration of abutment teeth deserves special consideration. The procedure should be done thoroughly because it is part of the foundation of the restoration or bridge. The procedure that is used should protect the pulp tissue, possess extra retentive factors, and provide room for the finished thickness of the casting. The abutment teeth are restored first because of the changes they might otherwise necessitate in the treatment plan.

ADDITIONAL READINGS

Allan, G. S.: The contour filling, a study, Dent. Cosmos 38:321, 1896.

Anderson, G. M.: Practical orthodontics, ed. 9, St. Louis, 1960, The C. V. Mosby Co.

Black, G. V.: A plea for the wider utilization of what is known in filling teeth, Dent. Cosmos 51:1390 (discussion, 1419), 1909.

Black, G. V.: The value of exact methods in operative dentistry, Dent. Cosmos 42:1245, 1900.

Bodecker, C.: Operative dentistry—histology—pathology, J. Dent. Educ. 3:103, 1938.

Coolidge, E. D.: The thickness of the human periodontal membrane, J.A.D.A. 24:1260, 1937.

Ferrier, W. I.: Treatment of cavities in anterior teeth and pit and fissure cavities in the posterior teeth with gold foil, J.A.D.A. 23:355, 1936.

Ferrier, W. I.: Treatment of proximal cavities in the anterior teeth with gold foil, J.A.D.A. 21:571, 1934.

Healey, H. J.: Coronal restoration of the treated pulpless tooth, Dent. Clin. N. Am., Nov., 1957, pp. 885-896.

Healey, H. J.: Restoration of the effectively treated pulpless tooth, J. Prosth. Dent. 4:842, 1954.

Hollenback, G. M.: The most important dimension, J. S. Calif. Dent. Assoc. 29:46, 1961.

Hugo, L. C. F.: Approximal work—the important factor involved, Dent. Cosmos 38:595 (discussion, 599), 1896.

McGehee, W. H., True, H. A., and Inskipp, E. F.: A textbook of operative dentistry, New York, 1956, McGraw-Hill Book Co., Inc., chap. 2.

Perry, S. G.: Additional separators, Dent. Cosmos 30:217, 1888.

Searl, A. C.: A plea for the interproximal space, Dent. Cosmos 42:334, 1900.

Smith, B. B.: A permanent and esthetic anterior restoration, J.A.D.A. 40:326, 1950.

Strange, R. A. W.: A textbook of orthodontia, ed. 3, Philadelphia, 1950, Lea & Febiger.

Wheeler, R. C.: A textbook of dental anatomy and physiology, ed. 4, Philadelphia, 1965, W. B. Saunders Co.

Worsley, W. J.: Separation and restoration of contact, instead of radical extension for prevention, Dent. Cosmos 45:110, 1903.

chapter 9

Amalgam restorations

Silver amalgam is the material most often used to restore teeth; it is estimated that 80% of the restorations placed are made of it. An amalgam is an alloy in which one of the constituents is mercury. The American Dental Association recommended constituents are silver, 65%; tin, 25%; copper, 6%; and zinc, 2%.[1] The controversy produced by the introduction of the amalgam restoration solidified the profession and initiated on-going research in the materials science field. These research efforts have continued to improve the clinical restoration by developing new products and techniques.

The amalgam restoration is produced by a complex setting reaction that basically involves mixing a silver-tin compound with mercury. The reaction is reported to be the following[2]:

$$Y \quad + \quad Hg \longrightarrow Y^1 \quad + \quad Y^2 \quad + \quad Y$$

| Y | | (Silver | | (Tin mercury— | | (Particle— |
| (Particle) | | mercury) | | matrix weakest) | | strongest) |

The unreacted particle (Y) and the Y^1 portions produce the strength, while the Y^2 matrix produces the weakest part of the restoration. It is important to minimize the matrix by using small particle sizes, by controlling the amount of residual mercury, and by minimizing the number of voids in the restoration. The strength of the alloy interface (particle to matrix) is an important factor and is controlled by the trituration and the amount of mercury present in the set amalgam.

The success of the clinical amalgam is attributed to the material's ability to resist leakage. This resistance to leakage improves with time and is attributed to the adaptation of the alloy and the formation of an oxide next to the prepared cavity wall. The good adaptation, compressive strength, economy, and wide usage range are the advantages of using amalgam. The lack of tensile strength, marginal breakdown, and predisposition to corrosion or tarnish are the disadvantages.[3]

Technical variables affecting the success of the restoration include proper

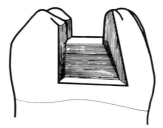

Fig. 9-1. A molar amalgam M.O.D. preparation indicating cavity form for the material.

proportioning of the alloy and mercury, triturating the parts, condensing the mixed alloy, carving the surfaces and marginal areas, and polishing. If careful detail is given to each, an excellent clinical restoration is produced that will provide many years of service.

Many studies have analyzed the problems of the clinical amalgam restoration. A classic survey[4] included 1,521 defective clinical restorations—56% of the failures were the result of cavity preparation and 40% the result of manipulation. Others report that marginal breakdown and the residual mercury content reduce the value of the restoration. It is accepted that errors in cavity preparation produce more problems for the restoration than errors in manipulation of the material.

Recurrent caries and fracture produce a majority of the defective amalgam restorations.[5] It has been reported that 42% of the amalgams become defective. A clinical study of 9,291 surfaces of amalgam restorations revealed that 9.2% of the surfaces contained recurrent caries. The properties of amalgam dictate that bulk be provided in the cavity form and that conservation of the tooth structure be exercised to minimize failures (Fig. 9-1). This chapter examines the amalgam restoration from the aspects of manipulation and cavity preparation.

MANIPULATION
Selection

There are a large number of commercial amalgam products available. The alloy selected should appear on the list of Certified Dental Materials of the American Dental Association to ensure that its physical properties meet the specifications recommended by the Council on Dental Research of the A.D.A.[6] If the directions outlined by the manufacturer are followed, the optimum properties will be developed.

The commercial alloy selected should have the working qualities desired by the individual operator. The setting time, consistency and appearance vary with different products, and the individual should select the alloy that pleases him. The amalgam should be conducive to an efficient procedure and be easy for the assistant to dispense, mix, and carry to the cavity preparation. Standardization and consistency within the limits of acceptable physical properties are the two main criteria for selection.

There are a number of secondary qualities that should be considered, however. The carving and polishing properties of amalgam are important, and these attributes, together with surface smoothness, are influenced by the particle size of the alloy. Personal manipulative habits such as the use of a special condenser or techniques regulating consistency will dictate the selection of one material over another. The selection should be made only after a number of materials have been mixed and compared. In this way the manipulative characteristics can be observed to determine which alloy satisfies the demands of the individual. A different alloy should not be selected merely for the sake of change but only to improve the office procedure and the quality of the clinical restoration.

Certain types of amalgam alloys can be evaluated to aid the selection. The variation in particle size or type and the amount of mercury required are the main variables.[7,8]

Particle size. The size of the particle influences the manipulation and final properties of the amalgam restoration.[9] The small particle alloys should be employed since they have improved handling characteristics and produce greater strengths and smoother carved surfaces. The production of small particles (10 to 50μ) has likely been the most helpful development in amalgam materials.[10,11] The small particle makes it possible to pack more alloy into the cavity preparation to leave less matrix (Y^2) exposed for breakdown, corrosion, and polishing difficulties.

Particle type. The composition of the various alloys is not significantly different, but the type of particle can influence the office procedure.

Regular (conventional). Ingots of the alloy are lathe cut and pulverized to produce particle sizes that are blended for mixing properties. The grains are annealed to relieve the stress of lathe cutting. This annealing develops a sensitivity of the particle to mercury. The annealed grains are compressed into pellets for convenience of dispensing.

The annealing time is varied to divide the regular lathe-cut types into high- or low-mercury ratio alloys. If the amalgam restoration contains 54% or less residual mercury, it is considered successful.

The regular particles are usually mixed at 7:5 or 1:1 alloy-mercury ratio. The high-mercury technique involves "wringing down" the fresh mix to eliminate the 5% to 10% excess mercury required for amalgamation. This regulates the consistency of the amalgam as it is being condensed into the cavity preparation. The low-mercury procedure reduces this hazard, but it also requires minimal mercury to maintain a workable mixture. Results with either system, when properly controlled, are clinically acceptable.

Spherical. Molten alloy is sprayed into an inert gaseous atmosphere and solidified into spheres. The sizes are blended to produce the manipulative properties, and so annealing is not necessary. This produces a low recommended alloy-mercury ratio. The low surface area and the sphere not fracturing during trituration develop restorations with a 35% to 38% residual mercury content. The

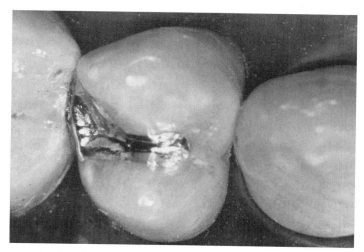

Fig. 9-2. Spherical alloy Class II restoration on the bicuspid.

spherical materials are selected for their strength values and because they require less condensing force to control the mercury and adaptation of the restoration[12,13] (Fig. 9-2).

Dispersion systems. A mixture of regular and spherical particles is advocated to reduce the Y^2 matrix. In addition to increasing the copper content, this is reported to increase the early strength of the restoration.[14,15] This needs additional investigation, particularly the report of the ability of the material to resist corrosion. Resistance to dynamic creep is listed as an advantage of using the dispersion alloy.[16] Preliminary studies have been conducted by adding 10% gold to the alloy for suppressing matrix formation. The data are promising but the cost of producing the alloy is very high.[17]

Residual mercury content

In the area of manipulation, the key to success is controlling the residual mercury content of the restoration. The acceptable percentage is related to the type of particle employed. The problems caused by excessive residual mercury include increased marginal breakdown, susceptibility to tarnish and corrosion, and the general degradation of the restoration. The mercury-rich restoration fails in only a few years and is the result of careless procedure. To prevent mercury-rich restorations, it is mandatory to accurately proportion the alloy and mercury and to use adequate forces for the condensation.

The residual mercury content for different areas of the restoration has been determined. It was reported that the marginal and thin areas of the restoration contained the highest mercury content.[18] For this reason, flaring and beveling of the cavity wall are harmful for the amalgam preparation.

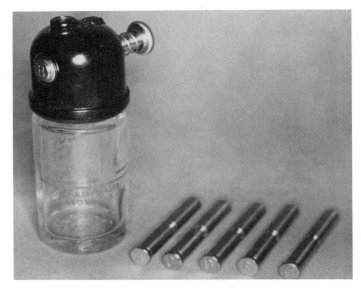

Fig. 9-3. Commercial mercury dispenser that can be used to measure different ratios.

Dispensing

To avoid the problems of inaccurate alloy-mercury ratios and contamination of the working area, it is advisable to use an automatic dispensing device (Fig. 9-3). Mercury presents most of the problems in accurate measurement, since amalgam can be obtained in pellets (4 to 5 grains). Mercury dispensers must be accurate, must prevent contamination, and must be convenient for dispensing prior to the mixing procedure. There should be no contact between the alloy and the mercury prior to amalgamation, since the fresh mix will assure the working qualities expected from the material.

Standardization is better achieved with preloaded alloy capsules that are protected by the manufacturer. One or two pellet mixes can be obtained in disposable capsules that produce consistency. Reports indicate less mercury contamination of the operatory when preloaded capsules are used. These capsules markedly improve the efficiency of the dental practice and are strongly recommended.[19]

Trituration

Trituration of the amalgam is necessary to thoroughly coat the particles of alloy with mercury. Each alloy should be adequately triturated for as long as required to produce a uniform setting reaction. There are numerous ways to produce amalgamation, but the high-speed devices with a capsule and pestle are the accepted method for dental practice (Fig. 9-4). Inadequate trituration results in a reduction of strength and an expansion of the alloy. The resultant

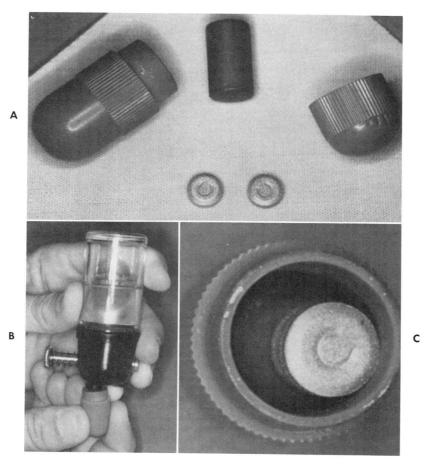

Continued.

Fig. 9-4. A, Equipment needed for trituration includes a capsule, pestle, alloy pellets, and squeeze cloth. **B,** Mercury is dispensed into the capsule. **C,** Pellets of alloy are placed at a right angle to the pestle. **D,** Automatic triturator for amalgam. **E,** The loaded capsule is securely placed into the triturator. **F,** The low-mercury alloy mix is rolled into a rope inside the squeeze cloth. **G,** The amalgam rope is divided into segments and carried to the cavity preparation.

consistency does not lend itself to thorough condensation and often produces a laminated restoration. For adequate trituration a mixing time of 15 to 20 seconds is required, though some preloaded capsules need to be mixed for only 10 seconds. Mixing at an accelerated speed can also be accomplished without a pestle in the capsule.

When each mix is properly measured, the mercury is placed in the bottom of the capsule. One or two pellets are placed at right angles to the pestle. No more than two pellets of alloy should be mixed because of the time required to condense this amount of amalgam into the preparation. Overtrituration pro-

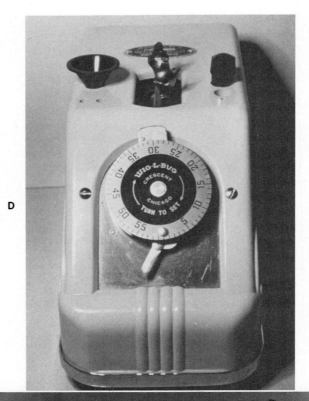

D

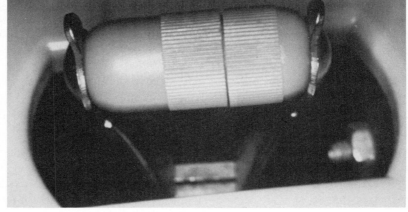

E

Fig. 9-4, cont'd. For legend see p. 273.

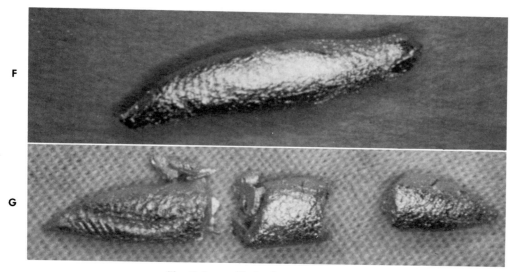

Fig. 9-4, cont'd. For legend see p. 273.

duces shrinkage upon setting, but this is not considered to be a problem with the clinical restoration.[20]

After the trituration, the contents of the capsule are emptied on the squeeze cloth and gathered. The mass is placed back into the capsule without the pestle and mixed for 5 seconds. This combines the mix and cleans the capsule. The contents are placed on a fresh squeeze cloth and rolled into a rope for insertion into the cavity preparation by the assistant.

Condensation

The condensation of the amalgam is another important aspect of manipulation. Condensation should adapt the material to the cavity, regulate the mercury content, and produce a homogeneous mass of metal that can be carved and polished. This procedure must be well controlled if the desired result is to be achieved. A number of factors influence condensation. In general the effectiveness of condensation is related to the diameter of the nib and to the direction and amount of force that is exerted on the condenser.[21] Condensers contain a nib or face, a shaft, and a handle. Some of the handles are flat or have finger stalls for developing force on the nib. Numerous types of condensers are not required for building an acceptable restoration, indicating that the amount of pressure and lines of force are the critical factors.

It is recognized that the smaller condensers are more effective for compacting the dense amalgam restoration. As the diameter of the nib increases, the force required to condense the amalgam exceeds the strength of most operators. The small condensers, less than 1 mm. in diameter, are used to adapt the restoration in the retentions, but they will puncture the amalgam if used for the entire building procedure. The most common amalgam condensers are Black's Nos. 1, 2, and 3. They are round and are 1, 2, and 3 mm. in diameter. They were originally advocated for starting, building, and burnishing the amalgam restoration; however, only the Nos. 1 and 2 condensers are now used for building up the restoration because the No. 3 is too large to be effective.

The role of serrations on the nib of the condenser has long been in question. When used with amalgam, they increase the surface area of the nib and are helpful in carrying the mixed alloy into the cavity preparation. The serrations themselves do not assure a lower residual mercury content or better adaptation to the tooth, but they are advocated as a method of carrying the amalgam. If they become filled with alloy and coat the condenser, the serrations should be reduced in height or removed with a small stone. They are advocated only as a convenience and are not required for an amalgam condenser. If an amalgam carrier is used, the serrations provide no real service in the building of the restoration.

The direction of the force exerted on the condenser is most important. The rule is to initiate condensation in the most distal area of the preparation and to direct the forces so that they bisect or trisect the angles formed by the cavity walls. This establishes a shelf at right angles to the condenser. This shelf is helpful for developing the pressure on the amalgam that is required for good cavity wall adaptation. This direction is maintained until the overpack is produced and all the cavity walls are banked with amalgam. These force lines direct the surplus mercury toward the surface of the restoration where it can either be removed or incorporated into the next increment of alloy.

The force exerted on the condenser is controlled during the condensation. Steady loads on the condenser develop a mercury-rich surface layer. The rich layer is removed, another increment of alloy is added, and the condensation is repeated. Each bank of alloy must be solid before more alloy is added, and the routine is continued until an overpack of 1 mm. is produced. The forces are applied to the surface of the overpack until it becomes resistant to the indentations of a No. 1 condenser. The overpack is burnished in order to pull the mercury to the surface so that it can be removed by carving. The method just described is used with hand condensation to build the acceptable amalgam restoration. Since it is not known just how much force is required on the condenser for the ideal amalgam restoration, the appearance and the solidity of the surface and the overpack must be used as a guide for the condensation.

Automatic condensers have been designed and are helpful for building amalgam restorations.[22] They are employed only for convenience and do not produce results superior to those achieved with hand condensation. When using the automatic condensers, the same rules for building the restoration are followed except that the force on the condenser is reduced and is supposedly compensated for by an increase in mechanical frequency. A number of cohesive gold condensers that have special amalgam points have been converted for this purpose.

The operator must be careful not to injure the cavosurface margin with the automatic condensers. Since the amalgam does not "cushion" the cavosurface margin as the direct filling golds do, the nib can puncture the material and fracture the tooth. For this reason the vibratory type of condensers are preferred. It should be noted that they must be used in conjunction with pressure to assure the adaptation of the amalgam.

The shape of the condenser nib has been studied to determine what influence the design has on the adaptation to the cavity wall.[23] It was found that condensers shaped to fit the internal angles of the preparation produce better adaptation than the usual circular types. The elliptical, trapezoidal, and triangular condensers actually produce better interlocking of the amalgam to the cavity wall. The additional pressure that is achieved is probably responsible for producing the superior alloy. The condensers fit the cavity wall more closely and work more effectively to wedge the alloy. The condition is similar to a stamp mill process in that more pressure is developed, which produces a more effective interlocking of the amalgam to the cavity wall. These specially shaped condensers are often employed with the automatic condensers.

Sweeney, Miller, and Hollenback have advocated the use of condenser points shaped to fit the dimensions of the cavity preparation. These points are used with automatic condensers, particularly the pneumatically driven devices. This is an excellent method for building the Class V amalgam restoration and others that have large surface coverage. Miller has designed a large rubber point to be used with the same series of condensers for burnishing the overpacked restoration. The burnisher and the repeated blows of the condenser effectively pull the excess mercury to the surface, where it can be removed in the carving.

Building the amalgam restoration is no simple task. The amalgam must be added to the cavity preparation in small increments and condensed thoroughly. Miller has advocated an increased dryness technique for placing the alloy in the tooth. Each increment of alloy is adapted and condensed with enough pressure to develop a mercury-rich surface layer. This layer is partially removed and another increment of alloy is added that has been dried by pressure in the cloth. This process is continued until the cavity preparation is filled to an excess of 1 mm. This technique produces a well-adapted and homogeneous alloy for the high-mercury alloy materials.

A similar forceful and controlled condensation is used for the low-mercury alloys. A mercury-rich layer usually results despite the low ratio of mercury and some of the plashy material is also removed. Low-mercury alloys do have advantages in that good results can be produced without as much stress or bother to the operator. A mercury-rich surface layer that can be incorporated into the next increment prevents lamination in the restoration. Condensation is not complete until the overpack is firm.

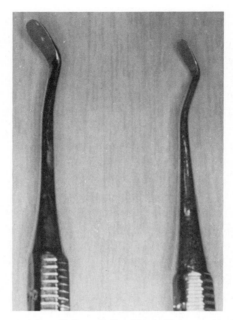

Fig. 9-5. Large and small sizes of discoid amalgam carving instruments.

Carving

This procedure is initiated as soon as the condensed alloy is hard enough to resist the carver (Fig. 9-5). The restoration is shaped to the approximate size required in the final product. The carving should replace the functional anatomy but leave a slight excess of metal to be consumed in the polishing. This is more important in the marginal areas. Some of the surface of the restoration is cut away during the polishing, and this must be watched closely to avoid a negative surface contour.

As soon as the initial set is evident, the overpack is rapidly removed with large discoid carvers. The contour is quickly developed and made to blend with the surrounding tooth structure. The remaining cusps and ridges and the adjacent teeth are utilized as guides in forming the anatomy of the restoration. Well-formed fossae should be developed since this is where most of the functional stresses will occur on the restoration.

The marginal areas are usually the last to be perfected. Smaller discoids, cleoids, or blade carvers may be used as long as they are sharp. A dull, ringing effect is produced when the alloy is being shaped with a sharp carver, and this sound indicates that the surface is not being burnished, which is deleterious to the restoration.

The direction in which the marginal areas should be carved has been a matter of dispute for many years.[24] It was thought that carving from metal to tooth structure caused burnishing to result in a restoration, producing an exceptionally weak margin. However, carving from enamel to metal also causes problems in that a large amount of overhanging metal is left on the cavosurface enamel. A compromise was achieved by moving the carving instrument parallel to the margin with light strokes. This leaves only a minimum of excess metal overhanging the tooth structure and still provides adequate bulk for polishing.

The carved surface should be similar to the contour that is desired in the final restoration. Both primary and secondary grooves are placed to help reproduce the minute detail of the occlusal surface. The surface is smoothed with the carver to provide comfort. The carved restoration should function properly and cause no discomfort in the interval between its insertion and the time when it is polished.

Centric contacts are the most important points on the carved surface. It is helpful to locate the areas on the teeth with articulating paper prior to cavity preparation. The functional marks on the occlusal surfaces are coated with cavity varnish and are either conserved or fixed in mind to guide the reproduction of the new metallic surface.

The final carving can be cleaned lightly with a soft rubber cup and pumice. This is helpful in locating the marginal excess and it smooths the surface. Careful application of the polishing cup is not harmful but rather is helpful to the carved surface. The polishing procedures are simplified by this movement. Care must be exercised, however, to control the pressure of the polishing cup during the smoothing.

The manipulation of amalgam has been emphasized in several areas. The guides for selection and the technical methods are confirmed by research. In the future additional refinement of materials and technique will supplement the existing sound clinical procedure. The manipulative aspects must be mastered by the operating team to gain the qualities and support produced by the cavity preparation.

CAVITY PREPARATION

The prepared cavity is the foundation of the restoration, and it is designed to enhance the physical properties of silver amalgam. The preparation provides a biologic, cleansable outline and contains a mortise form to produce axial-pulpal thickness in the restoration. The tooth is prepared to have the maximum of bulk in the center and at the margin to prevent gross fracture or crumbling of the restoration. The cavity preparation for amalgam is as exacting as the forms employed for other materials and requires the use of definite rotary and hand instrumentations (Fig. 9-6).

General characteristics of amalgam cavity preparations[21]

1. Cavity preparation is extended to the self-cleansing boundaries of the tooth. These are smooth areas that can be cleaned by abrasive foods or by toothbrushing. Self-cleansing boundaries are found on the cusp planes, marginal

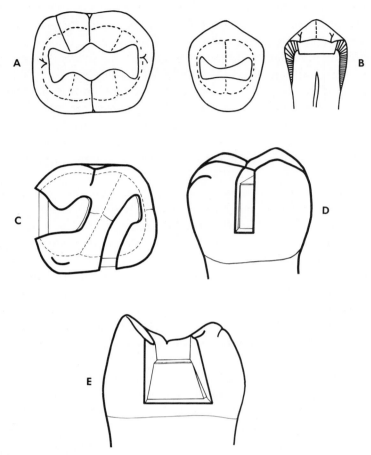

Fig. 9-6. A, Occlusal Class I alloy cavity preparation on a molar. **B,** Occlusal Class I outline for bicuspid. Note the direction of the proximal and marginal ridge enamel rods. **C,** Occlusal view of Class II preparation on upper molar and occlusal view of distal-lingual groove preparation. **D,** Lingual step of distal-lingual groove. **E,** Proximal view of Class II amalgam preparation of upper molar.

ridges, and suprabulge areas of the tooth. When extension is needed below the contour line, an attempt is made to place the cavity wall below healthy gingiva when the tissue exhibits normal contour and height.

2. Bulk is placed in the preparation. To place thickness in a cervical-occlusal dimension, the axial-pulpal walls are located 0.2 mm. within the dentino-enamel junction. No flares or bevels are placed in the cavity walls because they produce feather edges that are susceptible to fracture. The thickness prevents gross fracture of the restoration by enhancing resistance form.

3. The cavosurface margin is made to form a 90-degree or obtuse angle joint. The relationship minimizes marginal breakdown that naturally occurs with

the restoration. The 90-degree seam made of amalgam and tooth structure produces maximum marginal bulk and provides an ideal relationship when working with two brittle materials.

4. The cavity walls are made perpendicular and parallel to each other. The right-angle relationship of the internal walls produces retention and resistance form for the restoration. For a precise cavity preparation the walls should be joined by definite line angles. This angulation will not always be possible, but when adequate tooth structure is present, the design should be used.

5. Accessory retention is used. To support the retentive qualities of the mortise form, small mechanical undercuts are used on the proximal and occasionally the occlusal areas. The interlocking of the filling material with the cavity wall and the small undercuts keep the restoration seated in the tooth.

Preparation of the surgical field

Isolation of the teeth with rubber dam is recommended for placing the amalgam restoration. An absolutely dry field is required because of the reaction produced by the zinc in the alloy and the saliva. The two combine to form hydrogen gas and result in a severe delayed expansion of the restoration. Laboratory data show an expansion of 500μ within 48 hours when the amalgam restoration is contaminated by saliva.[25]

The zinc in amalgam is needed because it acts as a scavenger for the oxides. Theoretically the zinc keeps the amalgam lighter-colored during the manufacturing process and throughout the clinical life of the restoration. Because the zinc alloy is cleaner than other alloys, it merits selection when a dry field can be produced. Supposedly zinc renders the amalgam less susceptible to corrosion and tarnish, and studies conducted in this area do demonstrate this to be a decided advantage.

Where a dry field cannot be maintained, a nonzinc alloy should be selected.[26] The nonzinc alloys have practically the same strengths and manipulative characteristics of the regular alloys, but they do not expand when in contact with moisture. The problems for which the nonzinc alloys are helpful are usually located on teeth that cannot be clamped to retain the dam. This situation usually occurs in large gingival cavities in molars or partially erupted teeth. This slipshod type of operation is not ideal but is the only procedure that can be used when the isolation is impossible. Tissue contouring should be considered prior to the selection of nonzinc amalgam.

Class III amalgam restorations

The need to restore the proximal surface with metal and the ability to hide this specific outline makes the Class III amalgam restoration suitable for lesions on the distal surfaces of cuspids (Fig. 9-7). Ordinarily the lesion is small, with an abundance of surrounding tooth structure to make a small and esthetic outline possible. Direct gold is sometimes selected, but many lesions do not require

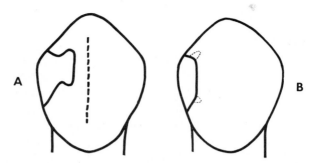

Fig. 9-7. A, Distal view of cuspid Class III amalgam preparation with lingual dovetail. **B,** Distal view of cuspid Class III preparation using proximal grooves for retention.

this fine a material. The tooth-colored restorations are not adequately resistant and allow tooth drift. Gingival irritation from the movement of the first bicuspid and opening of the posterior segment are encountered with tooth-colored materials.

The access to the distal surfaces of cuspids is limited when the contact area is intact and large. To counteract this difficulty a standard cavity preparation and lingual insertion technique is recommended. Naturally the object of the cavity design is to save the enamel in the contact area and thus control tooth drift. The cavity preparation is similar to other Class III outlines. The instrumentation is accomplished from the lingual surface, with the exception of a few movements. The outline on the labial surface is a straight line paralleling the distal lobe of the tooth. The labial wall is kept behind the line angle and below the gingival tissue to end in a square corner. The gingival wall is perpendicular to the long axis of the tooth and is located below the soft tissue. The lingual outline is curved to include half the marginal ridge and is made to join the other portion of the outline. The greatest extension occurs in the center of the lingual outline form so that the instruments can be inserted to finish the inside of the cavity preparation.

A small round bur is used in the contra-angle handpiece to break down the lingual plate and to remove the dentin inside the outline form. This access then accepts a No. 700 bur in the contra-angle handpiece that planes and extends the cavity walls. The side cutters of the bur plane the axial, lingual, and gingival walls. Following this the incisal wall is smoothed with the tip of the bur to make a smooth surface where the labial and lingual enamel join. The labial wall and its labial-axial line angle are cut and smoothed with the end cutters of the No. 700 or a smaller fissure bur to establish all the walls and the outline form.

The retention forms are placed in the dentin in the three corners of the preparation. They are made to undercut the enamel and are placed in a direction away from the pulp. The placement of the No. ½ round bur into the point angle is adequate for interlocking the amalgam. The entrance into the gingival point angles can also be opened and squared with an angle former or marginal trimmer, and the incisal undercut is enlarged with the bibeveled hatchet. These hand instruments are also used to sharpen the inside of the preparation to develop the resistance form of the restoration.

The refinement of the cavosurface margin and the lingual-labial enamel walls is accomplished with the small Wedelstaedt chisel. The mesial and distal cutting edge can be used to reach almost every area of the preparation. The remaining weak enamel is removed with light but definite strokes of the chisel. To aid in the refinement the chisel should occasionally be resharpened. The cavity form is then cleaned with hydrogen peroxide and dried for the final inspection. If the preparation is smoothed, squared, and retentive, the matrix is constructed.

If additional access and retention are needed or if an extensive carious lesion or replacement is present, the lingual lock cavity design is indicated. The lingual lock opens the incisal portion of the cavity preparation and permits better development of the cavity form and better placement of the bases or liners and the amalgam material. The lingual lock cavity design is not noted for weakening the cuspid tooth. If this modification is not adequate, particularly with a proximal lesion or restoration on the mesial surface, the cast gold restoration or full-coverage unit is suggested.

The matrix for the distal surfaces of cuspids must be custom-made. It is called the "S matrix" and is similar in construction to other anatomic matrices. One inch of regular strip matrix, 0.001 inch thick, is used and the matrix is preformed in the area of the contact with the No. 112 pliers. The strip is contoured to the desired form for the restoration and is placed interproximally and stabilized to resist the condensation.

The mirror handle is used to produce the **S** shape in the strip. The band is contoured over the labial surface of the cuspid and pushed lingually toward the bicuspid. The band is wedged firmly below the cervical wall and covered with green stick compound for stability. If the lingual opening to the cavity preparation is blocked, the compound can be removed with a warm instrument. To assure contour in the band a burnisher is heated, placed inside the matrix, and pushed toward the mesial surface of the bicuspid tooth. This produces a stable and anatomically contoured matrix. The only opening to the preparation is on the lingual surface, and the labial wall is adapted by forcefully condensing the alloy against the band.

The amalgam is mixed in a conventional manner and inserted into the lingual opening. Small condensers are used to force the alloy into the retention forms and to pack the material solidly against the labial wall. The next increments of alloy are condensed with the No. 2 condenser to further wedge and adapt the alloy. The condensation is continued until the customary overpack is produced.

The lingual surface is carved first to simplify removal of the matrix. The marginal ridge is formed with the explorer, and when the alloy becomes firm after the initial set, the wedge and matrix band are removed. The band is slowly rotated over the contact area to prevent the partially set amalgam from being

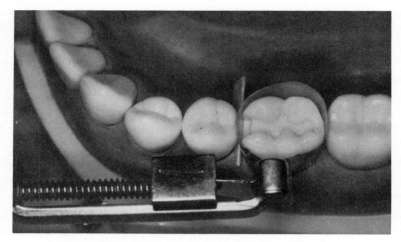

Fig. 9-8. Tofflemire mechanical matrix retainer in place.

shaved off. When the restoration is uncovered, the carving is finished with a sharp explorer. The gingival and labial walls are trimmed and contoured to form the embrasures. The restoration is slowly smoothed with dental floss to produce a better cervical marginal relationship.

The distal amalgam restoration provides a stable and esthetic restoration. Polishing is accomplished with a ⅜ inch sandpaper disk. The disks should be made of cuttlefish grit and directed from the amalgam toward the tooth structure. Other abrasives are used to brighten and smooth the surface of the metal, and finishing strips are used to smooth the inaccessible metal. Less discoloration of the cuspid results when the restoration is polished.

Matrices

A matrix is defined as a metal form that restrains the missing cavity wall and provides contour for the restoration (Fig. 9-8). The matrix holds the plastic materials until they have hardened to produce the missing anatomic surface. The construction and application of the matrix influence the anatomic form and the protective qualities of the restoration.[26-28] The Class II amalgam restoration is the service in which the matrix is used most often. Many types of matrices are advocated and the desirable characteristics include:

1. The matrix must be easy to apply and remove without damaging the restoration or tooth structure. The procedure should also not be time-consuming.
2. The matrix metal must produce the necessary contour for the restoration or furnish the shape of an ideal proximal surface.
3. The matrix assembly must be rigid and not be displaced while the restoration is condensed, and it must remain stable during the setting of the amalgam.

4. The matrix must be contoured or festooned to restrain the gingival tissue and the rubber dam while it is in place. The contour of the band should help to keep the prepared cavity isolated and to prevent injury to gingival tissue.

5. Because of the large number of matrices needed in the operative practice the technique must not be costly.

Mechanical matrix retainers are widely used because they can be easily applied to secure the band and to conserve time. The designs of the commonly used retainers are similar, but they do not produce perfect contour and have limitations with the complex cavity designs. The Tofflemire and Ivory No. 8 are retainers that work well for the regular two- and three-surface amalgam restorations. Properly applied and often stabilized, they secure the band to resist the force of condensation. They need also to be shaped and contoured prior to the insertion of the amalgam.

The matrix bands made for the retainers come in different shapes and sizes. The stainless steel metal is 0.001 to 0.002 inch thick and is curved or lipped to fit bicuspid and molar teeth. A thin band is desirable because it requires less separation to place the amalgam in the contact area in the restoration. Certain bands have holes in the center of the strip for restoring the large gingival lesions in posterior teeth.

Careless application is responsible for many of the disadvantages attributed to mechanical retainers. The overuse and excessive tightening of the stainless steel bands cause inadequate proximal contour. A negative contour or flat area is found against the buccal, lingual, and gingival walls of the restoration. When the bands are overtightened, inadequate space is left interproximally for embrasure development. The same conditions occur when the matrix bands are over-used. The bands can be applied only several times before they become strain-hardened, after which they can no longer be adapted or shaped to accurately fit the tooth. Matrix bands that are stiff and crimped should not be used.

Mechanical retainers and universal matrix bands can be used if the cavity preparation is of normal size. An ideal extension of the proximal preparation provides some foundation for the band to rest upon. A technique of precontouring the bands has been advocated and is useful in replacing the proximal anatomic form. The No. 112 pliers is used to form metal and to shape the band to fit below the cervical margin of the tooth.

The mechanical retainer merely holds the matrix band around the tooth. The force applied should be minimal since this must be offset by the pressure of condensation to produce the interproximal contour. Buccal location of the retainer is helpful to allow placement of the wedge and the compound for stability.

The amalgam matrices must be wedged against the cervical wall of the preparation and stabilized with compound (Fig. 9-9). This augments resistance in the band and also prevents excess amalgam from being pushed over the cervical wall

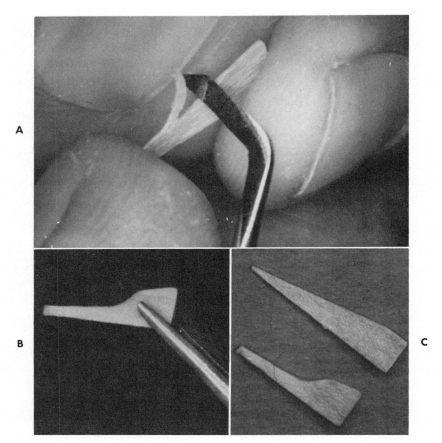

Fig. 9-9. Hardwood wedge for the Class II restoration. **A,** The upper portion of the wedge is excised with the sharp blade. **B,** The carved wedge is moistened to encourage sticking between the teeth. **C,** The finished wedge (bottom) that will stabilize the band allows good contour and will not injure the tissue.

to develop an irritating gingival overhang. The wedges that are used should be made of hickory wood or some other hard material that will hold the band firmly against the tooth. The wedge is trimmed to fit the lingual embrasure and is located on the structure below the cervical wall. The wedge is soaked in water to prevent slippage and is inserted tightly between the teeth. The wedging should produce enough separation to accommodate the thickness of the band, and only the wet wedge will remain against the tooth structure. Even though the band is firmly wedged, the gingival wall of the restoration must still be carved. Discrepancies occur as small bits of alloy flash over the cervical margin. The projections are removed with the explorer and polished with dental floss. The wedge only prevents the occurrence of a large periodontal overhang and does not guarantee the formation of a smooth, exact cervical margin. These areas must always be carved.

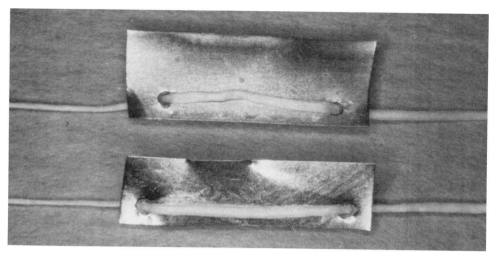

Fig. 9-10. Black's tie-band matrices.

The green stick compound or a similar low-fusing compound is used to stabilize the band.[29] The same sequential procedure is utilized with the compound as for stabilizing the clamps and separators. The adhesiveness of the compound is helpful because it sticks to the band and teeth at temperatures low enough to prevent injury to the soft tissue or teeth. The compound is melted and submerged in a cup of warm water. The operator moistens his fingers and pulls the softened compound off the stick. He holds the compound with his thumb and first two fingers and passes it through the flame. This sears the surface, and the ball of compound is then placed quickly over the band and wedge. The cold air syringe is directed over the compound to quickly solidify and stabilize the assembly. The compound is never heated in the flame and then applied directly to the teeth. This is painful and could cause pulp damage because of the prolonged application of heat.

A useful technique has been developed for adapting matrix bands to teeth. Zolnowiski has advocated that the twist band be used with the matrix retainer.[30] Three widths of strip matrix, $\frac{3}{16}$, $\frac{1}{4}$, and $\frac{5}{16}$ inch, are bent over a template. This adjustment produces a twisted matrix that is placed on the lingual surface of the tooth to provide a more desirable angulation in the band. This refinement produces a suitable contour for the proximal amalgam matrix.

The custom matrix. The best type of proximal amalgam matrix is one that has been anatomically contoured and custom-fitted to the tooth. The technique was first advocated by Black and later refined by Miller (Fig. 9-10). Ordinary steel strip matrix (0.001 inch thick) is used. The strips are cut long enough to pass the line angles of the tooth or the proximal walls of the cavity preparation. The strip is curved with the mirror handle to produce the necessary buccolingual line. The band is placed between the teeth to determine the bulge that is needed

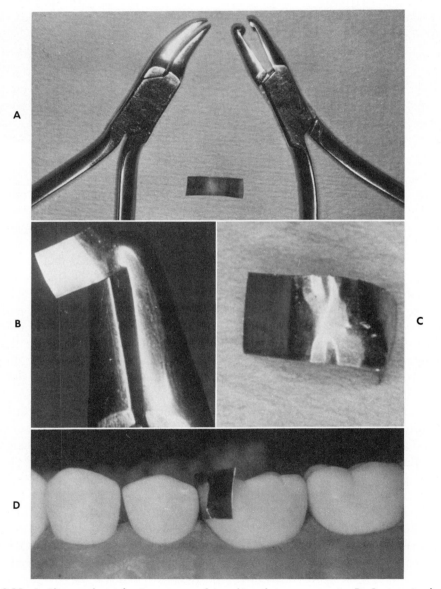

Fig. 9-11. A, Pliers and metal strip necessary for making the custom matrix. **B,** Contour is placed with the No. 112 ball-and-socket pliers. **C,** Contoured metal strip. **D,** Preliminary trial for interproximal contour.

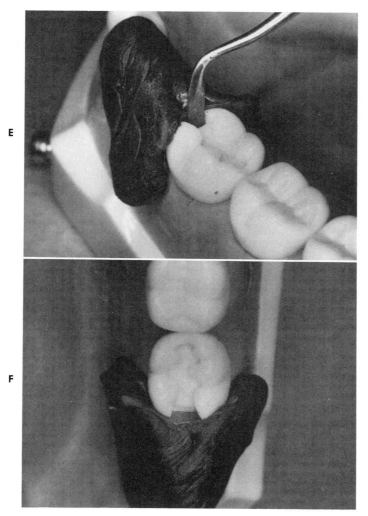

Fig. 9-11, cont'd. E, The matrix is supported with low-fusing compound and the bulge in the band is developed by pushing out with a warmed instrument. **F,** The completed Class II amalgam custom matrix.

in the contact and embrasure areas. The strip matrix is then contoured with the No. 112 and collar pliers (Fig. 9-11). The convexity in the contact area is produced with these pliers in addition to the accurate adaptation for the cervical wall. The band is removed and the contoured metal is smoothed on a soft surface with a ball burnisher. The shape of the band is then checked prior to stabilization.

There are a number of ways to adapt the band to the tooth. The corners of the band can be perforated with the rubber dam punch and tied around the tooth with dental floss. The floss can also be attached by cutting slits in the band

and folding the metal over on the corners of the matrix. Some bands have such accurate contour that they can be held with only the wedge and the compound. These adjustments are used only to hold the band around the preparation until the wedge and compound are applied.

As described previously, the wedge is inserted to separate the teeth and hold the band in place. The low-fusing compound is wrapped around the matrix and teeth and quickly cooled to prevent trauma. When the anatomic matrix is used, the buccal and lingual portions of compound are sometimes held together by a metal clip. A staple is warmed and inserted into the two blocks to prevent the matrix from being broken or moved during condensation. This is an extra precaution that produces the same degree of stability that was afforded by the matrix retainer in the previous technique.

The type of proximal contour that should be used and the way in which it is related to the amalgam matrix have been studied. It was determined that the best contours are produced by the custom-made anatomic matrix. Problems in contour occurred more often in square and ovoid teeth, but sound technique resulted in properly contoured restorations.

Construction of the matrix for the Class II amalgam restoration must be satisfactory. The technique is selected on the basis of contour and not convenience. The matrix should provide a contour that protects the periodontium, and there is no available procedure that does not involve precontouring the band.

Band removal. The matrix band must be removed without breaking the restoration. For this reason an interval of a few seconds is allowed following condensation before removing the overpack on the occlusal surface and forming the marginal ridge. The compound splint is broken and the flash around the proximal wall margins is trimmed with an explorer. This timing allows the initial set of the alloy to take place and produces a harder surface. After the alloy has hardened, the wedge is removed and the band is freed. The band is grasped with the thumb and index finger and tipped toward the tooth being restored. It is then lifted in an occlusal direction and rotated around the contact area. This movement disengages the band without shaving metal off the contact area.

As soon as the band is removed the proximal surface is carved. The margins are all quickly established with the sharpened explorer in order to remove the metallic flash. The proximal surface can be slowly smoothed with dental floss. If the embrasure needs additional enlargement, the carving knives must be used. The last contact of the proximal surface is made with the dental floss in order to smooth the metal until the restoration is somewhat polished. After the contour of the proximal surface has been developed, the occlusal margins and contour of the surface are located. Because of the difficulty of observing the gingival margin the operator must sometimes rely on touch. In order to facilitate this procedure the proximal surface is carved before the amalgam sets. The contact area and gingival embrasure are smoothed at this time because these areas are difficult to reach during polishing.

Class I amalgam restorations

Class I amalgam restorations are used to restore pit and fissure cavities in bicuspids and molars. The occlusal amalgam restoration is classified as a simple cavity preparation and restoration and because of the common occurrence and relatively easy access of these lesions they do not present many problems for the operative dentist, but there are definite rules to be followed in order to achieve the desirable qualities of the restoration.[31] The characteristics of the tooth structure on the occlusal surface and the degree of caries and developmental defects in the pits and fissures furnish an unlimited number of designs for the occlusal amalgam restoration. Amalgam is considered a versatile material in that, within limits, the size of the lesion does not contraindicate its use.

The shape of the occlusal outline is dictated by a number of factors.[32] The unsupported enamel on the surface is removed first. This provides access so that the caries can be removed and the actual size of the lesion can be determined. In the pit and fissure lesion the extension is dictated primarily by the spread of caries at the dentinoenamel junction. The occlusal surfaces are cleaned readily by mastication, which limits the degree of surface damage resulting from decalcification. This protection produces some degree of undermined enamel and the actual outline cannot be determined until the brittle material is excised.

Extension of the faulty areas is advocated for occlusal amalgam preparations (Fig. 9-12). This means that all the pre-carious areas on the occlusal surface that are in contact with the initial excavation are removed. Extension involves excision of all the poorly coalesced primary and secondary grooves on the occlusal surface. The outline is then developed into a gentle, sweeping curve and ends on the cusp planes and marginal ridges where the tooth structure is clean and smooth. The margin of the restoration will then rest in areas that are readily cleaned by mastication or toothbrushing, which prevents the development of secondary caries. Often rough enamel is removed by smoothing rather than extending the cavity wall. This permits a conservative development of the outline form and is called enameloplasty.

The extension of the occlusal surface is regulated by the caries and by the anatomy of the tooth. Certain anatomic properties regulate the degree of cutting necessary to reach the immune areas. The number, length, and amount of coalescence of the occlusal grooves also regulate the extension. The outline should include all pre-carious areas or anything that encourages food entrapment on the occlusal surface.

The groove extremities and the cavity margins abutting the marginal and oblique ridges are given special attention. The marginal ridge is preserved whenever possible to absorb stress and to keep the tooth intact. In addition the curvature of the rods in these areas is compensated for by flaring the wall of the cavity preparation. The wall flare necessitated by the abrupt inclination prevents the ridges from being undercut and produces a desirable bank on which condensation is started. Only the walls on the occlusal-proximal surface are flared.

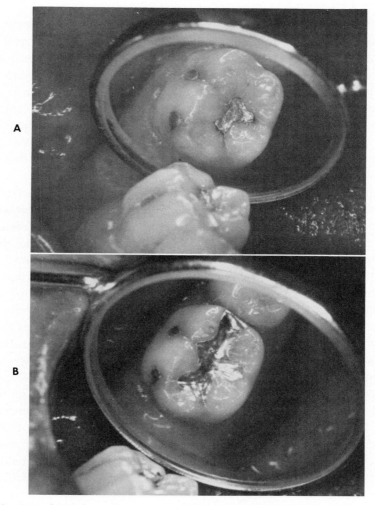

Fig. 9-12. A, Failure of amalgam restoration because of inadequate occlusal extension. **B,** Adequately extended occlusal surface to establish self-cleansing margins on the metal.

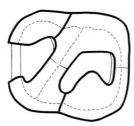

Fig. 9-13. Occlusal view of distal-occlusal amalgam preparation of upper second molar, with occlusal outline of mesial Class I preparation.

Whenever an oblique or marginal ridge crosses the occlusal surface, it is left intact unless it has been undermined by caries or contains a poorly coalesced groove (Fig. 9-13). The ridges will support masticatory forces better than an amalgam restoration, and the conservation of these structures is always attempted. The terminal portions of the occlusal outline are made parallel to the marginal ridges to prevent unnecessary cutting and to increase the retention of the restoration. A similar rule is followed for buccal and lingual pit or groove extensions. Whenever possible these enamel defects should be restored as pits rather than as grooves. If the defect is restored as a groove, a portion of the marginal ridge would be eliminated, which would weaken the remaining cusps of the tooth.

Variations in outline form are caused primarily by the difference in size of the caries. The extension of the outline into sound tooth structure to satisfy the rules of cavity preparation develops a similar pattern in cavity appearance. The appearances of the outline form differ with the shape and configuration of the tooth, but the rule is to conserve all possible sound tooth structure. The outline form for amalgam restorations is made to prevent caries from recurring and to simultaneously place the margin where it is protected from most of the forces of occlusion. The protected margin minimizes marginal breakdown.

The cavity walls are placed at certain depths and angulations to prevent fracture and dislodgment of the restoration. This resistance is achieved by a flat pulpal wall located 0.2 mm. within the dentin. The surrounding cavity walls, with the exception of the groove and dovetail extremities, are parallel to each other and perpendicular to the pulpal wall. Together with placing sharp definite line angles, this technique produces a resistance form that is capable of supporting the amalgam restoration. The thickness achieved produces an occlusal bulk that resists fracture caused by normal function.

Additional refinements are made on the occlusal surface for retention of the restoration. Small mechanical undercuts are sometimes placed in the groove extremities and dovetails at the level of the cavity floor. In addition the roughness of the surrounding walls produces a favorable surface for interlocking the amalgam particles. These two factors provide adequate retention for the occlusal restoration.

Finish of the enamel wall is important because it sets the final angulation and smoothes the enamel wall. Since the enamel margin is unprotected by the amalgam, all brittle and unsupported material must be removed. The enamel should ideally form a 90-degree angle at the point where it meets the amalgam. Theoretically the enamel on the margin should be supported by sound dentin so as not to become brittle after the tooth is restored. The lower two thirds of the cavity wall should remain rough to facilitate the interlocking of the amalgam. Many situations result in an obtuse angle being formed on the enamel cavosurface margin. There should not be an acute enamel cavosurface margin by amalgam.

The preparation of the occlusal cavity for amalgam fits into a pattern. Adequate vision of the occlusal surface and removal of the caries help the operator prejudge the outline form. The other factors of cavity depth and basing procedures are uniform. The local factors dictate the design, and to develop a biologic restoration it is necessary to understand how they vary. The outline in bicuspids and molars is "butterfly shaped" to encompass the caries and caries-susceptible areas.

Class II amalgam restorations

Class II restorations are used for cavities on the proximal surfaces of the posterior teeth. The rules governing restoration of the occlusal surface also apply to the preparation of the proximal surface. It is not often that the proximal surface is restored without an occlusal extension. Ordinarily either occlusal caries occurs in conjunction with the smooth surface lesion or the excision of the overlying fossa is necessary to provide access to the proximal surface. When this is done, the occlusal surface must be extended as previously described so that all margins will be located on sound tooth structure except in the case of teeth with perfectly coalesced grooves.

The proximal lesion differs from the occlusal lesion in that most of the damage is caused by surface involvement. The initial damage results from the difficulty of cleaning the proximal surface, and the lesion begins just gingival to the contact point. The damage is somewhat limited to this area because the adjacent enamel is self-cleansing and prevents the spread of caries on the enamel surface. Because of this the proximal outline has become standardized and rules have been established for the extension required in the embrasure area.

The areas of liability are determined by local anatomic factors, the extent of the caries, and the location of the adjacent tooth. To produce access in the preparation and to place the margins in sound tooth structure the proximal cavity walls must be at least out of contact with the adjacent tooth. Therefore, all three determinants for the outline form dictate the actual design. The proximal walls should be opened adequately to allow the explorer to be passed between the cavity margin and the tooth. When this degree of opening has been established, the cavity wall may need to be extended even more in order to reach the cleansable tooth structure.

Black discussed the areas of liability on the proximal surface as being related to the line angles. In 10,000 clinical cases examined at Northwestern University only nine lesions extended across one of the line angles.[32] Therefore, Black stated that the proximal walls should not be extended past the line angle but that the margin should be taken far enough out of the embrasure to be subjected to the abrasiveness of food that is passed down off the occlusal surface during mastication. This means that the direction of the proximal walls will be parallel or slightly undercut. This angulation is necessary in preventing feather edges in the restoration.

Several factors influence the degree of extension of the proximal walls, particularly in cases where the adjacent tooth is rotated. The shape of the tooth

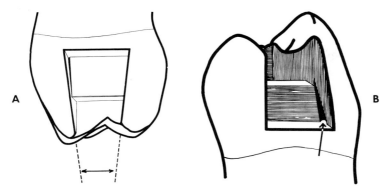

Fig. 9-14. A, Proximal outline for Class II amalgam preparation for upper posterior segment. Note convergence of proximal walls. B, Proximal view of Class II amalgam preparation of lower posterior segment. Note retention form.

creates variations in the outline form. Square and ovoid shapes require the removal of more tooth structure to reach immune areas. The proximal outline is also related to the size and shape of the contact area and the type of embrasures formed from the contour. The contacts are located more toward the buccal surface in posterior teeth so that the lingual embrasure is wider and more effective as a food shunt and provides a cleansable surface. In many outline forms the embrasure opening results in a slight undercut in the lingual wall of the preparation. The proximal outline form is primarily dictated by the adjacent tooth.

The location of the gingival wall does not markedly differ. The rule is to protect the wall by placing it below healthy gingival tissue except in cases in which there has been recession or periodontal surgery. Most preparations permit the wall to be placed below the soft tissue, which is found to influence the gingival papilla. When the crest of the tissue is far below the cementoenamel junction, it is not practical to locate the cervical wall this far down. The area under the tissue is not a self-cleansing area, but it is protective in that food accumulation does not occur on the cervical margin of the restoration.[33] For this reason Black's outline form is preferred for the proximal Class II cavity preparation.

The proximal portion of the Class II amalgam restoration must have independent retention. This relieves the stress in the isthmus of the restoration and creates more retention and resistance form (Fig. 9-14). The proximal depth is prepared in such a way as to attain bulk with a uniform thickness of material. The retention is created primarily by the angulation of the buccal and lingual walls, and if the proper outline is produced, some of the retentive qualities are automatically produced. Early papers advocated double-surfaced walls in the proximal design for retention to prevent the cold flowing of the amalgam restoration. The flow is considered a problem, and the full, smooth wall with uniform depth and angulation appears to adequately support the proximal restoration.

Supplementary retention is also gained by proximal locks. These locks are line angle undercuts in the dentin that converge toward the occlusal surface. The locks serve to complement resistance form because they divert the stresses that occur in the isthmus of the restoration. The proximal retention is obtained primarily by the angulation of the walls, but when wide extensions exist in the walls, the supplementary grooves are essential. The isthmus area is where the occlusal and proximal portions of the restoration join; it is in this area that gross fracture is likely to occur if there is a lack of resistance and retention.

The angulation of the gingival wall must also be considered. This wall is ideally placed perpendicular to the axial lines of the tooth or in directions in which the major forces occur. In most cases the enamel on the gingival wall will need to be smoothed to develop an inclination. This removes the unsupported rods that are commonly present. An undercut for retention is not placed in the gingival wall of the amalgam preparation because it would weaken the tooth structure. Research is needed concerning the effects of angulating the cervical wall.

The isthmus of the preparation is the area on the occlusal surface where the two parts of the restoration are joined. This area has been subject to much discussion and study because in the early days of dentistry isthmus fracture of the amalgam restoration was considered a problem. Many types of stresses occur in the isthmus area and from this standpoint it is the most critical area of the preparation. Black advocated that the isthmus of the Class II amalgam preparation occupy the middle third of the intercuspal distance on the occlusal surface. This dimension and others for assuring depth in the axial-pulpal walls were used to develop bulk in the isthmus so that it could withstand fracture.

Clinical studies have determined that isthmus fracture of the amalgam is not a problem unless a severe traumatic relationship exists.[34] These studies concerned Class II amalgam restorations having high mercury contents and previously determined low strengths. The clinical restorations were found to deteriorate at the margins and on the surface because of the excess mercury, but gross fracture of the restoration took place only when a plunger cusp functioned directly on the isthmus. The incidence of gross fracture in deciduous teeth was also studied and the results corroborated that of the previous study. It was stated that the critical area of the restoration is the buccal-occlusal margin where it joins the proximal surface. Fracture occurs most commonly in the mesial-buccal wall of the proximal preparation.[35] A flare in this wall produces a feather edge of amalgam, which causes a weak and mercury-rich restoration at this location. A reverse curve is used to provide the bulk in the metal that is necessary to prevent a mesial-buccal fracture. The reverse curve assures a 90-degree amalgam joint at the junction of the occlusal and proximal surfaces (Fig. 9-15). Only thirteen cases of fracture occurred in 1,009 controlled Class II restorations in deciduous teeth.

Research utilizing photoelastics further demonstrated the amount of stress present in the isthmus area around the axial-pulpal line angle and in areas where

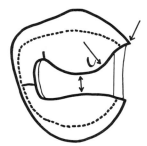

Fig. 9-15. Occlusal view of a two-surface amalgam for upper bicuspid emphasizing the reverse curve and conservative isthmus.

sharp corners or line angles were placed in the Class II preparation.[36,37] From these data the procedure of rounding axial-pulpal line angles and all the other junctions formed by the internal cavity walls developed. It was found that utilizing the engineering principles of flat walls and rounded internal line angles prevented the development of stress. However, rounded line angles present difficulties in the preparation of permanent teeth because they reduce the exactness of the cavity preparation. The Black system of creating a resistance form with line angles and precisioned cavity walls is preferred since gross fracture of the restoration is no longer considered a problem.[34] Analysis of the occlusal patterns, properly located axial-pulpal depth, and acceptable condensation prevent gross fracture of the amalgam restoration.

The Class II preparation for deciduous teeth should utilize rounded line angles and other methods of producing bulk in the amalgam restoration.[38] The deciduous tooth is smaller and the restoration results in a smaller occlusal-cervical dimension. The auxiliaries for retention and resistance as advocated by pedodontists are rounded axial-pulpal and other types of line angles, gross proximal undercuts, and grooves in the pulpal wall. The restorations seldom fracture when these auxiliaries are placed in deciduous teeth. Intermediary bases are not placed as far back as the original dentin location in order to aid in obtaining amalgam thickness.

Restoration of the proximal surface varies with individual teeth. Margins must be located in immune or protected areas. Black advocated separation for access and esthetics and cutting widely in broad and susceptible teeth. He further stated that each tooth requires an individual outline that is dictated by the factors discussed in relation to the occlusal and proximal restorations.

The characteristics of Black's Class II amalgam preparation are as follows:

1. The occlusal outline forms a gentle sweeping curve, the margins of which are located on clean and smooth enamel. The occlusal outline is ordinarily "butterfly shaped."
2. The cavosurface margin forms a 90-degree angle with the restoration. The seam that is produced provides the best support for the amalgam and the

tooth, both of which are brittle structures. Obtuse enamel margins, however, often result.

3. The buccal surface of the isthmus must include a reverse curve to provide bulk at the buccal-proximal margins. The lingual wall is only slightly curved and sometimes is straight with the large lingual embrasure.

4. The terminal portions of the occlusal dovetails and grooves are flared to follow the abruptly turning enamel. When the cervical wall ends in enamel, it is flared for the same reason. The cervical wall is not flared when it is located in cementum.

5. Dovetails are made parallel to the marginal and oblique ridges in order to prevent weakening these stress-bearing structures.

6. The proximal outline is parallel and slightly undercut on the internal walls for self-retentive purposes. This technique also prevents bevels and flares in the proximal preparation.

7. The axial-pulpal walls are located 0.2 mm. within the dentinoenamel junction. These walls are made perpendicular and parallel to the predicted forces or axial lines of the tooth. Some beveling of this line angle is necessary to prevent isthmus fracture of the restoration.

The Class II amalgam restoration is commonly used. The accurate design of the preparation is supported by clinical research and many years of patient service. How well the restoration furnishes internal and marginal bulk and conserves the functional parts of the tooth is the main criterion for amalgam cavity preparations.

Instrumentation for Class I and Class II amalgam preparations

Many instruments have been advocated for the Class I and Class II amalgam preparations. For the sake of efficiency and standardization a minimum number of instruments are used. Consequently only the instruments recommended by Black and the burs used with the air turbine are given. The instrumentation advocated by Black for posterior teeth includes the sequence of round bur, inverted cone bur, and fissure bur series. This systematic approach removes tooth structure or caries and permits access for each additional bur (Fig. 9-16).

Ultraspeed reduction with air turbines has simplified the instrumentation by requiring only one or two burs for the gross cavity form. Since this method of reduction is widely accepted, it is necessary to present it in addition to the standard instrumentation in the regular-speed range. Refinement of the cavity preparation with hand-cutting instruments is still necessary, however, and the same instruments are employed regardless of which rotary device is used. The occlusal preparation is included with the Class II instrumentation.

Occlusal outline form. With regular speeds the deepest pit or the most involved fossa can be penetrated with the No. ½ round bur. The tooth structure that is penetrated is undermined by removing some caries. The pit is gradually enlarged to create access for reaching the dentin. The No. 34 inverted cone bur

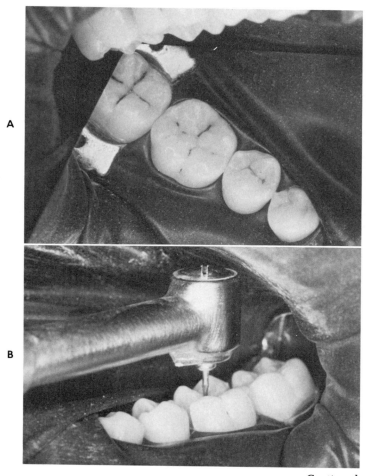

Continued.

Fig. 9-16. A, Surgical field for amalgam restorations. **B,** The air turbine handpiece and bur are used to produce an occlusal outline form.

is used to undermine and fracture the enamel to produce the outline form. The end cutters are placed in the dentin, and the bur is slowly revolved to bring the bur up through the enamel and remove it. After the enamel in the carious area is removed, the bur is pushed through the center of the primary occlusal groove to extend the preparation. After the bulk of tooth structure has been removed, the No. 557 or No. 558 fissure bur is used to finish the extension in the walls and set the angulation. The outline is completed with these three burs and includes the four surrounding walls and the pulpal wall. The side and end cutters of the bur are used to square and flare the walls and to establish the line angles.

In teeth with extensive caries that are characterized by a diamond-shaped lesion surrounding the central fossa, the enamel hatchets are used to expedite

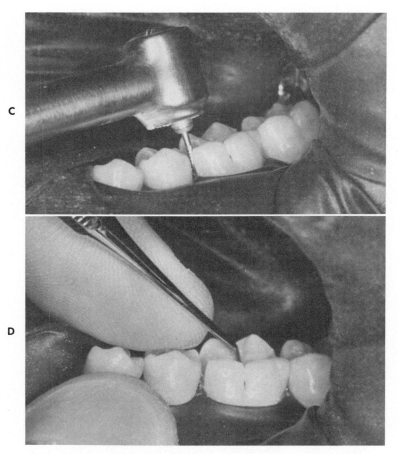

C

D

Fig. 9-16, cont'd. C, The proximal outline form is cut with the air turbine bur. **D,** The monangle is used to smooth the pulpal wall and form the line angles.

the preparation. The No. 15 or No. 20 enamel hatchets are used to break down the grossly undermined enamel in the center of the occlusal surface. Then the large spoon excavators are used to rapidly remove the caries and to determine the best excavation and basing procedures after the actual dentin depth has been established. Following excavation the inverted cone bur is used to extend the grooves that abut the crater, and the final outline form is established with the fissure bur in the same manner. The use of hand instruments to remove unsupported enamel is a time-saving device and is employed to greater advantage in the large carious lesion.

Proximal outline form. With the regular speeds a number of techniques can be used to open the proximal surface. A No. 34 inverted cone bur is pushed from the occlusal outline through the marginal ridge. When the ridge is removed at the level of the pulpal wall, the proximal lesion can sometimes be observed, which facilitates the selection of the proximal instruments.

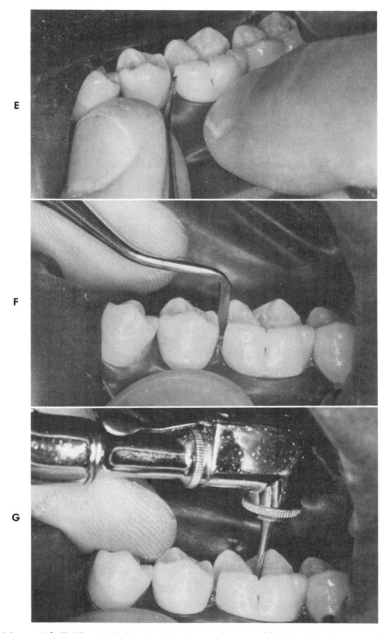

Fig. 9-16, cont'd. E, The Wedelstaedt chisel is used to establish the final proximal extension. **F,** The small enamel hatchet is used to remove the dentin inside the outline to produce the proximal box form. **G,** The regular-speed fissure bur is used to form the acute cavosurface margin and to smooth the cavity walls.

A welling technique is used to undermine the caries in the incipient lesion. The No. ½ round bur is placed at the dentinoenamel junction on both sides of the lesion and the proximal enamel plate is undermined. The hatchets are placed inside the walls and are turned to fracture and cleave the proximal enamel that was undermined to provide access for the bur. The opened surface is then extended with a No. 34 inverted cone bur. The end cutters are used to locate and square the cervical wall. Some undermining and thinning of the proximal enamel plates is accomplished with the side cutters of the inverted cone bur. The final location of the proximal walls is obtained with the small Wedelstaedt chisel or with the enamel hatchet if access is limited. The weak enamel on the buccal surface is punctured and the opening between the adjacent tooth and the tooth being restored is checked with a curved explorer.

With ultraspeed cutting the entire outline is established with one or two small burs. The lesion is the first area to be penetrated and the efficiency of air turbine cutting enables the wall to be squared in the same movement. Small-diameter burs are used with the air turbines to prevent damaging surface temperatures from developing. The No. 700 or No. 557 bur is selected for the occlusal outline and also for the proximal outline if multiple teeth are being restored. The No. 34 or No. 330 bur is indicated when the adjacent tooth has a sound proximal enamel surface or restoration. The shank of the bur can rest against the adjacent tooth structure while the cervical wall is being prepared. If a fissure bur is used, the contact area adjacent to the preparation is occasionally roughened.

The air turbine is considered a gross cutting handpiece, and there is an inherent danger of overextending the preparation when it is used. The Class II outline is underextended for this reason, meaning that the final outline form is produced with the No. 557 tungsten carbide steel bur in the regular-speed range. In setting up the proximal outline, hand instruments must be used for refinement following any type of rotary reduction. For this reason rotary instruments operated at regular speed and hand-cutting instruments are used to finish the cavity preparations.

Resistance form. The bulk in the mortise form is first produced in the proximal preparation. The enamel hatchets (No. 15 for molars and No. 10 for bicuspids) are used to excise the dentin inside the buccal and lingual proximal walls. The hatchets are rotated toward the center of the tooth and are moved toward the cervical wall. This movement produces full-length, smooth walls and locates the square line angles with the axial wall. Square angles are produced with the cervical wall by gradually moving the hatchet into the corners. The cervical wall is then planed and smoothed by pulling the cutting edge of the hatchet from the buccal to the lingual surface. A short bevel is placed on the cervical wall by tilting the hatchet toward the gingival tissue and repeating the movements. The bevel is only needed when the cervical wall is located in enamel because the enamel inclination turns abruptly in this area.

The resistance form on the occlusal surface is established with the fissure bur at the time the outline is completed. The final support and precision will be accomplished while finishing the occlusal enamel wall. If the pulpal wall is rough, it should be smoothed and flattened with the end cutter of the bur or with the No. 15 monangle hoe. The line angles of the pulpal wall are refined at this time with the same instruments.

Retention form. A No. 33½ bur is used in the contra-angle handpiece for the undercut areas. The undercuts are located in the corners of the occlusal preparation and include the groove extremities and the dovetails. They are placed in the dentin by moving the bur laterally at the depth of the side cutters. Excessive cutting for retention results in undermined ridges, and this should be avoided. Moreover, most retention is developed by the angulation of the preparation walls.

The need for proximal retention is determined at this time. The buccal and lingual location of the walls, the length of the tooth, and the type of occlusion are the determining factors. Accessory retention is placed by cutting small grooves in the dentin with the No. 33½ bur; these grooves converge toward the occlusal surface. This undercutting produces locks that will supplement the retention afforded by the angulation and thickness of the buccal and lingual walls. Smoothing of these retention forms can be done with a No. 700 bur if the upper half of the occlusal enamel or margin is not notched. The undercuts should gradually become thinner as they approach the occlusal surface, making the gingival half of the proximal preparation the most retentive area. The mechanical retention forms are located only in dentin and are not made excessively deep since this would cause the enamel to be undermined also. Accessory retention on the proximal surface should not be achieved at the sacrifice of proper cavity design.

Finish of the enamel wall. The finished wall should be smooth in the upper portion and rough in the other areas. The smooth, exact margin removes the fragile enamel and produces a sound footing for carving and polishing the amalgam restoration. The right-angle refinement of the wall provides a smooth knife-edged metallic junction that can be located again when the amalgam is polished.

The enamel cavosurface is smoothed with a plane fissure bur (No. 56 or No. 57) at 2,000 rpm. The bur is used with light pressure and at the lowest speed while being moved perpendicular to the occlusal enamel surface. The entire occlusal outline, the most critical area of the restoration, is slowly encircled with the bur, and this combats breakdown of the restoration. After the refinement the reverse curve on the buccal wall of the proximal preparation is checked. The final reverse curve is enlarged and smoothed if the design made previously with other instruments has been inadequate. This prevents fracture of the most critical area of the restoration. Sharp hand instrumentation finishes the smoothing.

The lower portion of the occlusal cavity walls are roughened at the time the cavity is excised. The rough walls of the restoration produce a better seal for the tooth either because of better interlocking of the amalgam or because of an increase in the surface area of the cavity wall. The crosscut fissure burs are employed for extension to produce the desired roughness. The walls are roughened with the air turbine handpiece to approximate the contour of the blade of the bur. Studies in cavity wall texture have shown this roughness to be a desirable feature of the amalgam preparation.[39]

Toilet of the cavity. The cavity is dried with warm air, and the outline, depth, and refinement are inspected. If the cavosurface is satisfactory, the tooth is washed with 3% hydrogen peroxide. This solution cleans the cavity form of any sediment that might have seeped into the area under the rubber dam. After a few seconds the 2 × 2 inch sponges are used to absorb the excess hydrogen peroxide and water and the cavity is dried with air. The dried preparation is inspected for the last time. A small, sharp explorer is used to clean the line angles and test the cavosurface margin. If the cavity has been properly prepared, two applications of cavity varnish are placed on the walls of the preparation, including the margin. The residue of organic gum that results from the varnish application improves the seal of the amalgam restoration and the varnish is therefore routinely used with amalgam.[40] The varnish dries quickly, and while it is drying arrangements are made to insert the restorative material.

All necessary instruments are assembled at this time. The matrix is applied to the prepared tooth, the condensers and carvers are arranged on the bracket, and the amalgam is mixed. The successful amalgam restoration is accomplished only by meticulously following the accepted techniques mentioned in this chapter.

Pedodontic considerations. The Class II amalgam form for deciduous teeth is prepared in such a way as to increase the resistance form. Many studies of stress analysis in children have been conducted by utilizing the photoelastics method. The methods of increasing retention and resistance that were previously discussed are utilized in the deciduous tooth because of the decreased occlusal-cervical thickness of the restoration. The lack of bulk causes fracture to occur more often, making it necessary to use these methods in the preparation of deciduous teeth. Bulk is increased by rounding the internal line angles, beveling the axial-pulpal line angle, and grooving the pulpal wall. When these dimensions are properly placed, there is no problem of pulpal damage. The outline form of the deciduous preparation is established by following the methods advocated by Black. A change in the direction of the enamel rods causes the occlusal walls to be more constricted and the proximal outline to be more undercut. The increased size of the restoration in a permanent tooth eliminates the need of these additional retentions.

Modern amalgam restorations

Within the last few years the popularity of the modern amalgam preparation has mounted (Fig. 9-17). Basically it is more conservative than the Black design, but it has the same general properties and principles.[41] The main difference between the two is that the modern amalgam preparation has a limited buc-

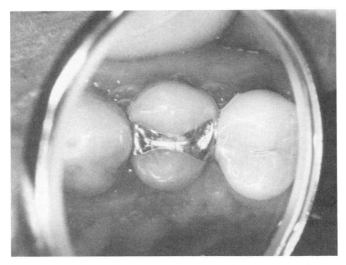

Fig. 9-17. A modern amalgam restoration that has been functional for 6 years.

cal to lingual extension on the occlusal surface. The initial reasons for using the conservative design were largely empirical, but its workability has now been substantiated by several years of excellent clinical performance. Although there are several reasons for using the modern amalgam restoration, the design is used mainly for the conservation of tooth structure it affords. The amalgam restoration does not possess properties that serve to strengthen the remaining tooth structure; therefore, saving the unaffected and clean enamel is critical.

The difference between the Black preparation and the modern amalgam preparation is the width of the isthmus (Fig. 9-18). Black advocated that the "occlusal keyway" occupy the middle third of the distance between the buccal and lingual cusps. This was advocated because 70 years ago isthmus fracture was considered a problem. Also, the amalgam alloys being used at the time exhibited lower strength values when compared to the materials now being used. Another reason for using the wide isthmus was the diameter of the burs that were being employed with the foot engines and initial electric units. To increase the linear surface speed of the rotary reduction instruments, the diameters of the burs were increased to 1.5 to 2 mm. burs. Vibration and efficiency were increased, and by applying these burs once or twice through the isthmus the middle one-third dimension advocated by Black was achieved.

For three quarters of a century Black's dimension remained a classic concept. Rather than evaluate the individual characteristics of each tooth the dentist customarily places a stereotyped one-third extension in the isthmus area. The depth is more critical than the width to increase strength in the isthmus area of the restoration.

Research by Vale indicates that the strength of the remaining cusps is signif-

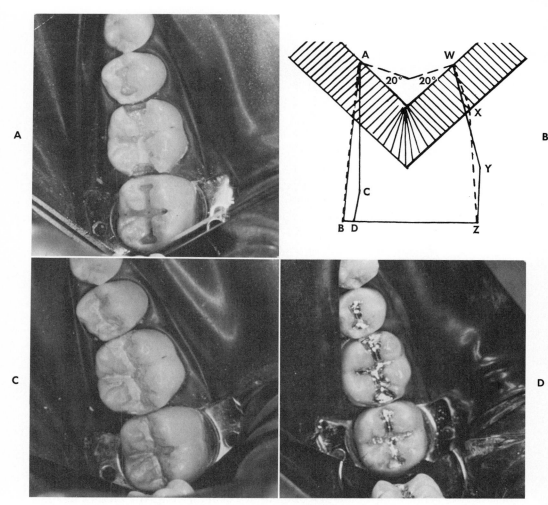

Fig. 9-18. A, Conservative or modern amalgam cavity preparations. **B,** Overcontoured occlusal carving that is necessary with modern alloys. to develop a 90-degree metal seam at the cavo-surface. **C,** Carved amalgam restorations. **D,** Polished conservative amalgam restorations. (**B** from Knight, T.: J. Dent. Assoc. So. Africa **17:**342, 1962.)

icantly influenced by the width of the isthmus (Table 9-1). This investigator used extracted teeth to determine the cusp strength after different extensions were prepared in the isthmus.[42,43] The dimensions of the isthmuses were one third and one fourth of the intercuspal distance. The data indicate the value of the conservative design. The teeth were prepared and forces were applied to the cusps tips at right angles to the occlusal surface. The strength value was recorded at the level at which the cusp fractured, and this record was used to assess the remaining strength of the tooth. The one-third isthmus preparation

Table 9-1. Force required to fracture teeth with M.O.D. cavities of different widths*

Cavity width (proportion of distance between cusp)	Average force required (arbitrary units)	
	Prepared tooth	Sound tooth
One-fourth	133	136
One-third	87	125

*From Vale, W. A.: Irish Dent. Rev. 2:33, 1956.

reduced the strength of the tooth by a value of one-third less than the control. This indicates that the Black preparation weakens the tooth when amalgam is used. The one-fourth isthmus preparations with the modern design did not reduce the strength of the cusps but displayed values similar to those of sound, unprepared teeth. For this reason the conservative preparation should be used for the restoration whenever possible. This rule should apply to all intracoronal Class II restorations.

With the modern amalgam restoration a cavity design is produced that has a buccolingual extension of one fourth of the intercuspal distance or less. The extension of the outline is still governed by the amount of caries and the occlusal groove integrity. When the self-cleansing boundaries are reached, the isthmus should be widened only enough to accept the small amalgam condensers. This method results in a much more constricted outline than those observed in the early publications concerning the use of silver amalgam.[44]

For the narrow outline the average width for intercuspal distances in bicuspids and molars should be 1 mm. or less on bicuspids and 1.5 mm. or less on molars (Table 9-2). According to Vale's data, this type of outline will not reduce the strength of the cusps and the design should be used whenever possible.

The beneficial aspects of preventive dentistry are resulting in lesions that are more suitable to conservative management. Fluorides limit the size of the caries, which causes less undermining of the enamel. Routine brushing around the adequately placed conservative restoration prevents caries from recurring at the margins. The carious lesion in the future will allow greater conservation of tooth structure in the cavity preparation.

Because the cavity is limited, smaller diameter burs are used to produce the outline form and for gross cutting. The No. 34, 330, 699, or 700 is used because the tips of these burs are less than 0.75 mm. in diameter (Fig. 9-19). These burs can be taken through the occlusal grooves several times before the recommended extension is completed. Burs that are smaller than this are fragile and are broken much sooner than the series just mentioned. The outline is slowly produced by moving the bur in the isthmus area at the level of the dentino-enamel junction.

Table 9-2. Average measurements of teeth for cavity preparation*

	Buccal-lingual diameter (mm.)	Intercuspal distance (mm.)	Black's one-third isthmus (mm.)	Conservative one-fourth isthmus (mm.)
Maxillary				
First bicuspid	9.0	4.5	1.5	1.1
Second bicuspid	9.0	5.0	1.7	1.2
First molar	11.0	5.5-6.0	2.0	1.5
Second molar	11.0	5.5	1.8	1.4
Mandibular				
First bicuspid	7.5	3.5	1.2	0.9
Second bicuspid	8.0	4.0	1.3	1.0
First molar	10.5	5.0-5.5	1.8	1.4
Second molar	10.0	5.0	1.7	1.2

*From Wheeler, R. C.: A textbook of dental anatomy and physiology, ed. 4, Philadelphia, 1965, W. B. Saunders Co.

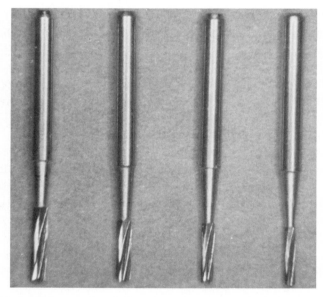

Fig. 9-19. Small-diameter bur (0.75 mm.) used to prepare the limited outline form.

The occlusal preparation is then refined and squared with smaller fissure burs and hand instruments. The outline is taken past the uncoalesced secondary grooves where clean, smooth enamel is located. This satisfies the self-cleansing requirements. The cavosurface will contain depressions where the grooves ended on the cusp planes and these will have to be placed in the carving and the occlusal anatomy of the restoration.

In the modern amalgam restoration a difference will be noted in the reverse

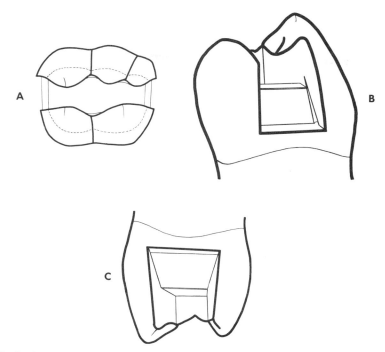

Fig. 9-20. A, Conservative occlusal outline for M.O.D. amalgam preparation on lower molar. **B,** Conservative proximal and isthmus preparation for amalgam. **C,** Proximal amalgam preparation with excessive proximal and isthmus width.

curve that joins the proximal and occlusal walls (Fig. 9-20). Since the isthmus is more constricted, the curve will be exaggerated. The curve is more critical in this preparation since more bulk will be needed in this portion of the modern restoration. The reverse curve elongates the buccal cusp plane, which is the main advantage gained by limiting the extension.

The proximal portion of the preparation is identical to that of Black's preparation because the extension of the proximal walls is dictated by the adjacent tooth. The walls are made out of contact with the adjacent tooth and the same bulk and cervical extension are necessary. The same instrumentation and matrix procedures that were previously described are used. Accessory retention with proximal grooves is used more often because of the limited occlusal width and the need for diverting stress in this area.

A clinical study was conducted to compare the effectiveness of these two types of Class II restorations. Uniform cavity preparations were made and differed only in that the width of the isthmus varied from one fourth to one third of the intercuspal distance. Three observers checked the restorations by magnification and models made from Thiokol impressions. The restorations, 192 in all, did not exhibit a noticeable clinical difference. The marginal breakdown

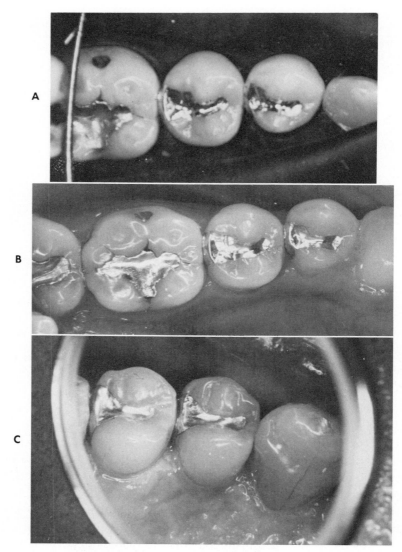

Fig. 9-21. A, Polished conservative restorations. **B,** Appearance of conservative restorations 6 months postoperatively. **C,** Postoperative result of two conservative restorations after 6 years of clinical service.

occurred at the same rate around both types of cavity forms. From these data the benefit of the modern restoration appears to be its ability to conserve the natural tooth structure. Although the limited outline places the metal in a more protected area, this does not seem to prevent the marginal deterioration that is inherent with amalgam. The conservative restoration usually includes more tooth anatomy in the occlusal carving, which is thought to increase the surface area and to improve the masticatory ability of the tooth.

The use of the modern amalgam restoration is advocated for numerous reasons (Fig. 9-21). The design should be used whenever possible because the service it affords is superior to the routine Black preparation, However, extensive caries on the occlusal surface will prohibit the use of the constricted outline, especially when the lesion in a proximal fossa communicates with the proximal surface. In this case the undermined enamel must be removed to produce a sound foundation for the restoration, and this results in a wide isthmus. The difference in time involved in placing the two types of preparations is negligible, which is an additional recommendation for the modern amalgam restoration.

The modern restoration requires closer observation of the lesion and the occlusal anatomy because the difference in extension between the two preparations is small. The advantages of the modern amalgam restoration are as follows:

1. Less tooth structure is removed in the preparation and thus minimizes the pulpal response and conserves the functional tooth structure.
2. The strength of the remaining cusps is not reduced when a one-fourth occlusal isthmus is used in the preparation. This could prevent cusp fracture in later life and add to the permanency of the amalgam restoration.
3. Even though the occurrence of marginal breakdown is not noticeably reduced in the conservative restoration, the metal is more protected.
4. Preventive dentistry has limited the size of the caries and increased the longevity of the restoration, factors that encourage the use of the modern amalgam restoration.
5. The modern restoration has elevated the level of patient care, and additional research and development of this preparation should be conducted. The conservative restoration should reduce the replacement rate of the amalgam restoration.

Class V amalgam restorations

The gingival lesion is difficult to restore because of the difficulties involved in isolating the tooth and gaining access in the molar regions.[45] The Class V amalgam restoration is used almost exclusively for the gingival lesions in molars. The techniques and problems associated with this category merit discussion.

The physical properties of amalgam, mainly its surface roughness and its proneness to expand in moisture, do not always permit an adequate cervical restoration to be placed. If the cavity preparation cannot be isolated and fully observed, the use of nonzinc alloy is indicated to salvage the tooth until conditions can be improved. This service sometimes results in patchwork restorations but is better than the other methods for large molar lesions. Recurrent caries is common in the distal second molar area because of the difficulty in cleaning this area.

Proper isolation of the gingival lesion with the rubber dam, Schultz clamps,

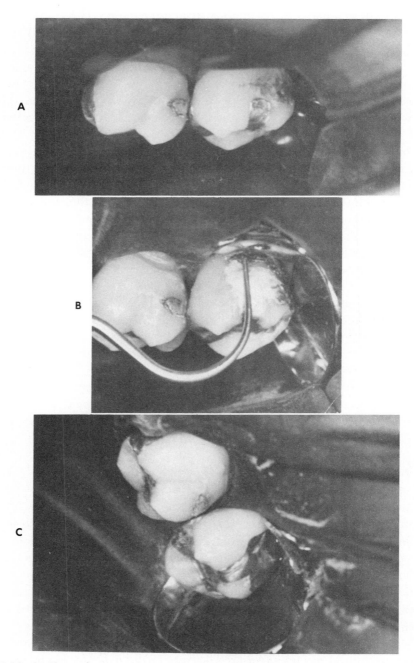

Fig. 9-22. A, Class V lesion on the second molar. Isolation is achieved with the No. W8A clamp. **B,** Carving the Class V restoration with an explorer. **C,** The restoration after it has been polished at a subsequent appointment.

and No. W8A clamps enables a sound amalgam restoration to be placed. These restorations can be polished to produce a satisfactory surface to abut the gingival tissue. As in the other cavity classifications, an exacting procedure is used for the preparation of the tooth and condensation of the amalgam (Fig. 9-22).

The outline form of the preparation conforms to the lines advocated by Black for molar teeth. This oval or kidney-bean form, which requires a minimum of tooth removal, is satisfactory since the restorations are usually not visible. The preparation places the margins in immune and protected areas on the cervical third of the buccal and lingual surfaces of the molars. In some cases the outline form can be made to appear uniform with the restorations in other teeth. If access to the molars is adequate and the caries rate is low, the direct gold restoration should be considered.

The restorations in bicuspid teeth can occasionally be observed and because of this the Ferrier trapezoidal outline is used. The occlusal margin forms a neat, straight line that blends well with the quadrant whether it appears in single or multiple restorations. The instrumentation is similar to that used in the gold preparation except that more rounded undercut retentions are placed in the corners of the form. The amalgam restoration should not be used in anterior teeth except in cases in which inadequate salivation has caused rampant caries.

Instrumentation. When only a small amount of tooth structure is removed, the slow regular-speed rotary instrument is employed. The gingival lesion has less remaining dentin in the cavity floor, which means that the depth of the restoration must be conservative and that it is better regulated with the slower rotary instruments. The sequence and outline for the preparation is that advocated by Black.

1. A small round bur (No. 1 or No. 2) is used to remove the decay or hypoplastic enamel and expose the dentin tissue. This includes the soft tooth tissue inside the lesion.

2. The No. 34 inverted cone bur is used to extend the preparation by undermining and proliferating the sound enamel. The occlusal wall is placed at the height of contour on the buccal surface. The mesial, distal, and gingival walls are located below gingival tissue, which means that the proximal walls are extended slightly past the line angles of the tooth. An oval-shaped outline form is produced with the gingival wall, which should be at a uniform depth and covered by tissue.

3. The No. 557 bur is used to square and flare the cavity walls. The end cutters of the bur smooth the axial wall to produce the same contour as the external surface of the tooth and to locate the wall 0.5 mm. within the dentinoenamel junction. The fissure bur is used to flare the mesial, distal, and gingival walls in the direction of the abruptly inclined enamel. The cavosurface margin is made at a right angle, which helps to guide the angulation of the walls. The occlusal wall is not flared but is made perpendicular to the axial wall with the fissure bur. The internal line angles are made to develop a mortise form prepara-

tion so that the alloy can be condensed. The enamel walls are finished at this time by smoothing them with the fissure bur.

4. The undercut retentions are placed in the four corners with a No. 33½ bur. The bur is moved laterally to undercut the dentin. This technique will retain the restoration in the normal-sized cavity. If the tooth is more extensively involved, pins are considered as auxiliary retentions. The pins are placed mesially and distally in order to avoid the pulp.

5. The cavosurface margin is perfected with a sharp chisel. The instrument is moved lightly across the enamel to remove the loose tooth structure. After smoothness has been achieved, the cavity is cleansed and the amalgam is prepared in a conventional manner.

The insertion of the amalgam can be a problem in the widely extended cavity. A number of special matrices are used when the proximal walls are extended past the line angles. The Nystrom matrix can be applied, and the contoured strip matrix is also useful and sometimes more effective. The strip is placed around the tooth and only the buccal surface remains open. The proximal walls are both wedged and stabilized with compound. The additional confinement of the amalgam is useful in developing the overpacked layer.

The gingival restoration is more difficult to condense because the preparation does not contain the normal boxlike mortise form. The condensation is augmented by the special curved condenser designed by Sweeney and Miller. This condenser acts as a tamp and confines the metal to the cavity better than the regular hand condenser does. The blades of the cement instruments are also useful in tamping in the alloy or producing the burnished overpack.

The carving of the gingival restoration is important to the protection of the gingival tissue. The cervical bulge must be reproduced to create the food shunt that serves as a protective contour. Reproducing the original bulge in the tooth is all that is necessary, and the bulge is usually carved with the curved explorer. The surface is smoothed and the margins are located with the explorer.

The Class V amalgam restoration is useful in those cases in which other materials cannot be used in molars. The location and access of the gingival caries produce conditions that can be alleviated only by the special techniques mentioned.

SUMMARY

The amalgam restoration is widely used and is responsible for preserving more teeth than any other material.[46] The techniques of manipulation and cavity preparation have been refined during this century to produce a nearly permanent restoration. Meticulous attention to the details of all facets of the technique assures the dentist of certain results. Although an extensive amount of literature on the amalgam restoration has been compiled, only the salient work related to the methods that are currently being employed is presented in this chapter.

REFERENCES

1. Boucher, C. O.: Current clinical dental terminology, St. Louis, 1963, The C. V. Mosby Co., p. 13.
2. Wing, G.: Modern concepts for the amalgam restoration, Dent. Clin. N. Am. **15**:43, 1971.
3. Hollenback, G. M., and Villanyi, A.: The physical properties of dental amalgam, J. S. Calif. Dent. Assoc. **33**:422, 1965.
4. Healey, H. J., and Phillips, R. W.: A clinical study of amalgam failures, J. Dent. Res. **28**: 439, 1949.
5. Nadal, R.: Amalgam restorations: cavity preparation, condensing and finishing, J.A.D.A. **65**:66, 1962.
6. Mosteller, J. H.: An evaluation of the A.D.A. specification for amalgam alloy in relation to particle size, Ann. Dent. **12**:19, 1933.
7. Eames, W. B.: Preparation and condensation of amalgam with a low mercury alloy ratio, J.A.D.A. **58**:78, 1959.
8. Miller, E. C.: Clinical factors in the use of amalgam, J.A.D.A. **34**:820, 1947.
9. Crandall, W. G.: Standardizing the amalgam filling, Cleveland, 1915, Cleveland Dental Manufacturing Co.
10. Demaree, N. C., and Taylor, D. F.: Properties of dental amalgams from spherical alloy particles, J. Dent. Res. **41**:890, 1962.
11. Nagai, K., and others: Studies on spherical amalgam alloy in the light of dental technology, Tokyo, 1966, Department of Dental Technology, Nihon University.
12. Wing, G.: Clinical use of spherical particle amalgams, Aust. Dent. J. **15**:185, 1970.
13. Pires, J. A., Hodson, J. T., Scott, W. D., and Stibb, G. D.: Compaction and microstructure of spherical alloy; dental amalgam, J. Prosth. Dent. **22**:234, 1969.
14. Mahler, D. B.: Relationship between mechanical properties and clinical behavior, presented at 50th Anniversary Symposium on Dental Materials, National Bureau of Standards, Gaithersburg, Md., 1969.
15. Mitchem, J. C., and Mahler, D. B.: Influence of alloy type on marginal adaptation and final residual mercury, J.A.D.A. **78**:96, 1969.
16. Mahler, D. B., and Van Eysdan, J.: Dynamic creep of dental amalgam, J. Dent. Res. **48**:501, 1969.
17. Johnson, L. B.: Unpublished data.
18. Swartz, M. L., and Phillips, R. W.: Residual mercury content of amalgam restorations and its influence on compressive strength, J. Dent. Res. **34**:458, 1956.
19. Rupp, N. W., and Paffenbarger, G. C.: Significance to health of mercury used in dental practice: a review, Council on Dental Materials and Devices, Council on Research, J. Am. Dent. Assoc. **82**:1401, 1971.
20. Phillips, R. W.: Research on dental amalgam and its application to dental practice, J.A.D.A. **54**:309, 1957.
21. Blackwell, R. E.: Black's operative dentistry, ed. 9, Milwaukee, 1955, Medico-Dental Publishing Co.
22. Phillips, R. W.: Physical properties of amalgam as influenced by the mechanical amalgamator and pneumatic condenser, J.A.D.A. **31**:1308, 1944.
23. McHugh, W. D.: Experiments on the hardness and adaptation of dental amalgam as affected by various condensation techniques, Brit. Dent. J. **99**:44, 1955.
24. Markley, M. R.: Restorations of silver amalgam, J.A.D.A. **43**:133, 1951.
25. Schoonover, I. C., Souder, W., and Beall, J. R.: Excessive expansion of dental amalgam, J.A.D.A. **29**:1825, 1942.
26. Phillips, R. W., Swartz, M. L., and Boozayaangool, R.: Effect of moisture contamination on compressive strength of amalgam, J.A.D.A. **49**:436, 1954.
27. Castaldi, C., Phillips, R. W., and Clark, R. J.: Further studies on the contour of Class II restorations with various matrix techniques, J. Dent. Res. **36**:462, 1957.
28. Ingraham, R., and Koser, J. R.: The anatomic matrix, J.A.D.A. **51**:590, 1955.
29. Stibbs, G. D.: Cavity preparation and matrixes for amalgam restorations, J.A.D.A. **56**: 471, 1958.

30. Ryge, G.: A fresh look at dental materials; dental amalgam, J. Tennessee Dent. Assoc. **43**:1, 1963.
31. Green, R. O., Lundberg, G. W., and Simon, W. J.: Some fundamentals of cavity preparation, J.A.D.A. **29**:1408, 1942.
32. Black, G. V: Operative dentistry, ed. 3, Chicago, 1917, Medico-Dental Publishing Co.
33. Bronner, F. J.: Engineering principles applied to Class II cavities, J. Dent. Res. **10**:115, 1930.
34. Nadal, R.: A clinical investigation on the strength requirements of amalgam and the influence of residual mercury upon this type of restoration, M.S.D. thesis, Indianapolis, 1959, Indiana University School of Dentistry.
35. MacRae, P. D., Zacherl, W., and Castaldi, C. R.: A study of defects in Class II dental amalgam restorations in deciduous molars, J. Canad. Dent. Assoc. **28**:491, 1962.
36. Guard, W. F., Haack, D. C., and Ireland, R. L.: Photoelastic stress analysis of bucco-lingual sections of Class II cavity restorations, J.A.D.A. **57**:631, 1958.
37. Mahler, D. B.: An analysis of stresses in a dental amalgam restoration, J. Dent. Res. **37**:516, 1958.
38. Ireland, R. L.: Class II cavity preparation for primary teeth and its restoration with silver amalgam, Dent. Pract. **11**:208, 1961.
39. Menegale, C.: The influence of surface texture of the cavity walls on the adaptation of restorative materials and a method of quantitatively measuring marginal leakage, M.S.D. thesis, Indianapolis, 1960, Indiana University School of Dentistry.
40. Phillips, R. W., and Swartz, M. L.: Adaptation of restorations in vivo as assessed by Ca[45], J.A.D.A. **62**:9, 1961.
41. Gilmore, H. W.: New concepts for the amalgam restoration, Practical Dental Monographs, Nov., 1964, pp. 5-31.
42. Vale, W. A.: Cavity preparation and further thoughts on high speed, Brit. Dent. J. **107**:333, 1959.
43. Vale, W. A.: Cavity preparation, Irish Dent. Rev. **2**:33, 1956.
44. Eames, W. B.: A sequence of related amalgam procedures, Practical Dental Monographs, Sept., 1966, pp. 3-39.
45. Markley, M. R.: Amalgam restorations for Class V cavities, J.A.D.A. **50**:301, 1955.
46. Brekhus, P. J., and Armstrong, W. D.: Civilization—a disease, J.A.D.A. **23**:1459, 1936.

chapter 10

Pin-retained amalgam restorations

The problem of amalgam fracture has concerned the profession for many years. Because of the low tensile strength the extensive amalgam restoration often fractures. Fracture failures are attributed to inadequate retention and resistance form and are recognized as a problem in the large restoration. When the cusps, ridges, and broad surface restorations are placed, it is necessary to use pins and bulky preparations to prevent loss of the restoration or fracture of the parts.

Many techniques for supporting amalgam have been recorded in the literature. Initially, small pieces of silver were placed on the floor of the preparation and inside the restoration to provide additional strength. Black advocated the use of wires and staples that were cemented to dentin for accessory support. Small iridioplatinum wires were used to support lost cusps and were cemented in the dentin at the corners of the tooth. Papers were written presenting other techniques for supporting the amalgam restoration. Brennan was one of the first to refine the procedure of providing the amalgam restoration with a pin foundation.

The concept of a pin-retained amalgam restoration was derived from engineering principles. Silver alloy is brittle and crumbles like concrete, and techniques were originally advocated to strengthen the metal with pins by using methods similar to those used in engineering. The value of using stainless steel pin supports is accepted, but the specific mechanism that works to greatest advantage in the amalgam restoration is questioned.

The strength of reinforced amalgam specimens has been studied. In general the results have demonstrated a reduction in compressive strength when the pins are incorporated in the material. These data suggest that the term "reinforcement" could be a misnomer in describing the beneficial aspects of the pins. Engineers use steel rods in concrete to improve the tensile strength of the material and thus reduce its tendency to fracture. This indicates that the term

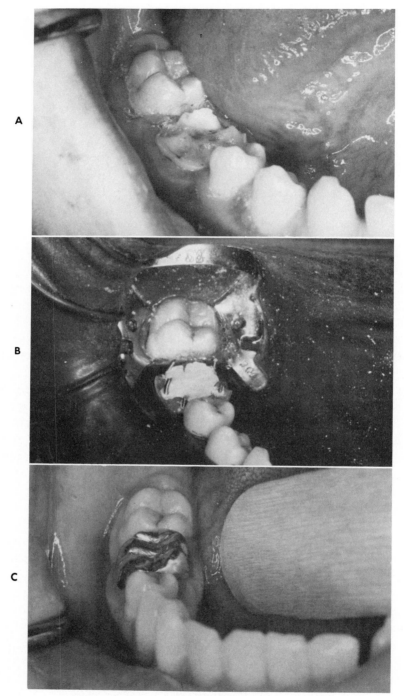

Fig. 10-1. A, Mandibular first molar multilated by caries but still vital, showing no signs or symptoms of degeneration. **B,** Capped and insulated tooth with cemented wire foundations. **C,** Completed pin-retained amalgam restoration.

"pin-retained" amalgam restoration is more accurate in describing the nature of the technique. The pins are thought to improve the retention and resistance properties of the amalgam restoration.

The wide acceptance of the pin-retained amalgam restoration can be attributed to the refined procedure advocated by Markley. By using the prescribed armamentarium it is possible to place from one to eight pins in the dentin at a depth of 1.5 to 2 mm. Kits containing the necessary materials have been prepared to simplify the procurement of the supplies, and they have alleviated difficulties in placing the pins. The increased utilization of pin supports has resulted in the manufacture of other types of wires and mechanisms for this technique. There are merits to the use of pin supports, and the procedure requires only a few additional minutes.

The improved interest in dental health care and the development of workable preventive measures have resulted in increased ability to salvage grossly carious teeth (Fig. 10-1). Economic problems do not prohibit the use of amalgam since the unit cost and time required for placement are minimal when compared to the cast gold restoration. Progress has been made in the management of acute caries and in pulp protection, and these conditions, together with the other factors discussed, create a distinct place for the pin-retained amalgam restoration in practice. Fracture, new caries, and tooth breakdown require the use of the pin-retained amalgam restoration.

Clinical longevity can be achieved in the pin-retained amalgam restoration just as in any other amalgam restoration. Placing a pin-retained restoration is much more practical than removing the tooth and replacing it with a prosthodontic device. As the need and demand for amalgam increases, the use of pins for auxiliary retention will become a routine procedure and a valuable adjunct for saving mutilated teeth. The restorations can also be covered later with gold castings.

INDICATIONS FOR PIN SUPPORT

The greater the size of the preparation or the trauma to the tooth, the more the use of pins should be considered. Numerous clinical conditions provide precise indications for employing the pin-retained amalgam restoration. Following are the common indications.

Gross mutilation from caries or trauma (Fig. 10-2). Many grossly mutilated teeth have only a negligible amount of remaining vital tooth structure. Although most of these problems are caused by caries, accidents produce some fractures that closely resemble the condition caused by a large lesion. Customarily the caries is removed to find the solid tooth foundation level with or below the gingival tissue. The restoration that is placed needs to be firmly attached to the vital root stump because of the excessive forces that will be placed on the retention forms when function is restored.

When the excavation is completed, the existence of a pulp exposure may

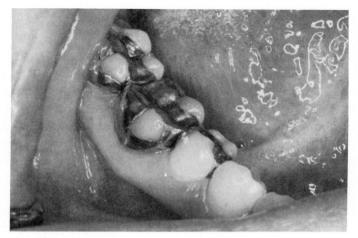

Fig. 10-2. Three molar teeth restored with pin-retained alloys; 6-year postoperative appearance.

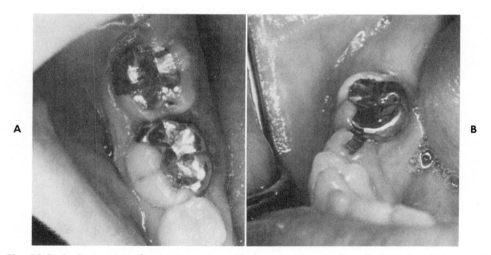

Fig. 10-3. A, Restoration of extensive caries with the pin-retained alloy. **B,** Tipped and fractured mandibular second molar supported by three pins.

be questionable. It is possible to have a minute undetected exposure that would subsequently initiate the degeneration of pulp tissue and loss of the tooth. The excavation is dried and sedated, or if caries removal is complete at this time, an indirect pulp capping with calcium hydroxide is used. This treatment does not negate the use of pins but encourages the pulp to recover if any damage has been caused (Fig. 10-3).

Occasionally the pulp will degenerate when an indirect capping has been employed. However, even when this occurs, the patient and the dentist have

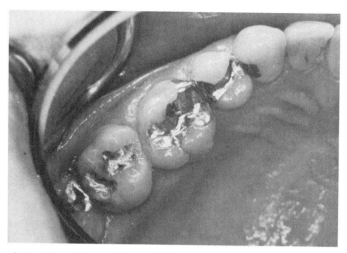

Fig. 10-4. The first molar with excessive mesial extension is supported with one cemented pin.

benefited because the restoration has served as a space maintainer and will be useful as a core during endodontic therapy. The canal entrance is made in the center of the crown and the surrounding pin restoration eliminates the need for banding the tooth during endodontic therapy. The pin foundation then can serve as a subsequent foundation for the restoration of the endodontically treated tooth.

Problems of retention arise in the dish-shaped cavity form. This condition, in which the remaining roots are the only vital parts of the tooth, cannot usually be restored with a casting unless the root canal is used for auxiliary retention. It is not possible to cast and fit the number of pins as accurately as it is in the restoration using multiple cemented pins. Although the use of nylon bristles and parallel pins has improved retention in gold castings, it does not exceed the retention that is possible with the threaded wire in the amalgam restoration.

Widely extended preparations (Fig. 10-4). Lesions develop that require or have extended preparations beyond recommended limits. The cavity walls are extended beyond the line angles, near the cusp tips, and past other stress-bearing ridges. In the extended area one or two pins help to keep the amalgam in the tooth.

The ultraspeed cutting devices and repeated restoration of teeth sometimes produce overextended cavity preparations. Commonly this occurs on the buccal and lingual walls of the proximal form in the Class II preparation. When extra tooth structure is removed, an additional amount of the embrasure and contact area is replaced with metal. A single pin is used to support the overextended amalgam when the proximal wall extends past the line angle of the tooth.

Large amalgam restorations in patients scheduled for orthodontic therapy are placed in the category of overextended preparations. A preventive program is first initiated to control the development of additional lesions. Then the defective restorations and caries are removed to enable the mortise cavity form to be produced. The pins are useful in keeping the alloy in the teeth during the adaptation and removal of the bands and necessary tooth movement. When pins are employed in this situation, less fracture of the amalgam is observed following orthodontic therapy.

The cusp supportive value of the gold casting is not questioned, but there are situations in which this service cannot be offered. All patients do not desire the placement of gold inlays because of either economic or educational reasons. When the dentition is not in good enough condition to use the casting but there are large lesions or fractured areas present, the pin-retained amalgam restoration is effective.

Some fractures occurring in teeth are not caused by trauma but are the result of function. Many times cusps break, leaving only a minimal amount of tooth structure. This can occur on either the working or idling cusps, and the fracture is commonly associated with a widely extended, complex cavity preparation. Over a period of years the restoration undergoes abrasion, which causes the tooth to overerupt in attempting to achieve a centric contact relationship. Premature balancing contacts then develop on the brittle remaining cusps, which can cause the tooth to fracture. Many of the cusp fractures occur below the gingival tissue and do not involve the pulp. Restoration of the remaining tooth can be accomplished with pins and the restoration can be either functional or reduced to serve as a core for a casting. This problem of fracture often occurs in aged patients, and the pins are a valuable reparative service.

The large gingival lesion presents restorative problems primarily in molars that have been previously restored and that are involved with secondary caries. The walls of the cavity preparations are usually obtuse and do not provide the amalgam with much support. The lesions are commonly extended halfway up the buccal surface and beyond the line angles of the tooth. Retention of the gingival restorations should be supplemented with smaller L-shaped pins. Markley states that the technique is necessary because the thermal expansion of amalgam as compared to tooth structure is 2.6:1. It is reported that when the pins are not used, the thermal dimensional change causes either leakage around the large gingival restoration or the complete displacement from the cavity preparation.

Questionable teeth with large lesions (Fig. 10-5). Questionable teeth with large lesions should be restored with pin-retained amalgam. In deep excavations the pulpal prognosis cannot always be accurately determined. The excavation appears sound, the remaining tooth pulp tests are favorable, and the radiographs are acceptable. Occasionally painful symptoms are present prior to the appointment and persist during the time the sedative dressing is in place. Since these teeth are deemed questionable, an expensive or lengthy restorative procedure

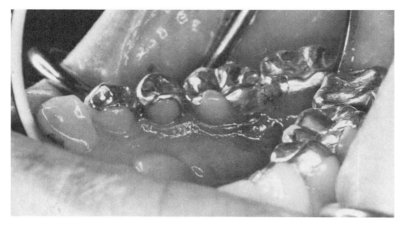

Fig. 10-5. Pain developed in the first molar as a result of recurrent caries around an inlay. Amalgam was placed to retain the tooth until a prognosis was made.

is not risked. After the teeth are restored the symptoms may persist, and eventually the degeneration necessitates endodontic therapy. Occasionally the symptoms disappear and the restorations are then left intact for extended periods before any other service is performed. In these cases pin foundations remain functional for years and can either be covered with a cast restoration or left uncovered to function for a longer period of time.

Teeth that are selected for endodontic treatment are sometimes restored prior to the sequence of appointments in which the endodontic treatment is given. This makes it possible to clamp the tooth being treated and to seal the pulp chamber in order to enhance the canal sterilization. Teeth can then be endodontically treated that could not otherwise undergo such treatment because the complications involved in adapting the copper band or temporary crown form over the questionable tooth.

Problems develop following some root canal treatments as a result of the type of filling placed in the enlarged chamber. Points can slip through the apex, the sealing cement can leak into the medullary spaces, or an incomplete filling can result. Such accidents occur infrequently, but when they do, they require a waiting period following the treatment. To restore function to the tooth and maintain the arch dimension, the pin-retained amalgam restoration can be used (Fig. 10-6). The copper band application may occasionally result in food impaction and irritation of the gingival tissue; these problems are eliminated when this restoration is used.

Advanced periodontal disease causes mobility in teeth because of the loss of bone support. If a periodontist diagnoses the problem and removes the etiologic defects, the mobile teeth can be retained for a number of years. In some of these cases the teeth will remain functional for 5 to 10 years if regular periodontal care is maintained. If caries or fracture occurs in this type of

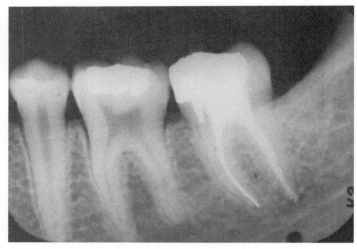

Fig. 10-6. Two mesial pins support the alloy restoration until the postoperative radiograph indicates that the overfilled distal root canal has improved.

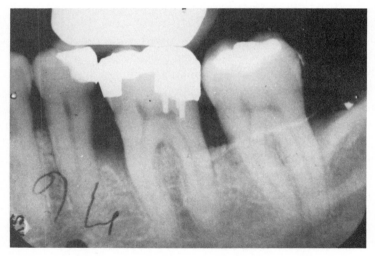

Fig. 10-7. Teeth with questionable periodontal prognoses and extensive lesions are restored with pin-retained alloy.

dentition, the teeth should be restored with pin-retained amalgam because the periodontal prognosis is questionable (Fig. 10-7). Many teeth in this condition contain large amalgam restorations. It is possible that rough edges and overhanging margins contributed to the periodontal condition. Occasionally a number of amalgam restorations must be placed to support temporary acrylic appliances. This service will keep the dentition in working condition and lengthen the prognosis for the natural teeth.

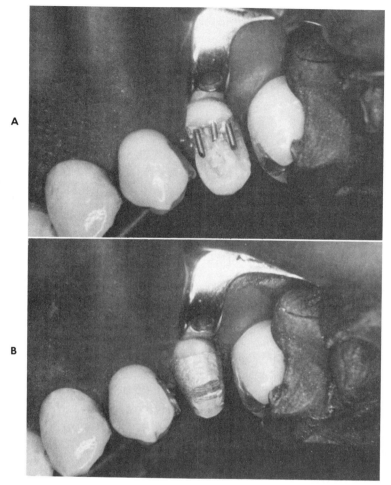

Fig. 10-8. A, Three pins are cemented after the preparation is completed. **B,** Pin foundation amalgam core. Observe the isolation provided by the Schultz clamp.

Cores for crown and bridge procedures (Fig. 10-8). The retention of castings, particularly the full- or partial-coverage types, sometimes necessitates the use of a core. The core fills the excavation and gives form to the preparation over which the casting is cemented. Pin-retained amalgam is often used for the core because it requires less time and provides a more efficient seal. Cast gold cores must be cemented in place, and the resultant restoration has two cement liners and requires two appointments. The amalgam can be inserted and reduced following the initial set of the alloy. This eliminates one appointment and reduces the cost of the cast unit. Some clinicians feel that for these reasons the pin-retained amalgam should be used whenever possible.

It is desirable to restore endodontically treated teeth with a cast core that is placed in the root canal for retention. Because these teeth become dehydrated and brittle, they require optimum support. The root canal core, however, is not always possible. Some small canals can only be filled with silver metal points, meaning that the canal cannot be used for retention. When this occurs, the pin foundation is used as the core. More surface area in the grooves and dovetails provides valuable retentions in addition to the pins. However, the pins are not substitutes for the principles of retention and resistance.

CAVITY PREPARATION

Attention is given to two distinct areas in the cavity preparation. The damaged area needing the pins should be excavated to determine the condition of the dentin floor. The ledge directly inside the dentinoenamel junction is then prepared for pin placement. After all the caries has been removed and the basing is accomplished, the rim of the preparation is squared to resemble a shoulder finish line. The squaring is done to create room in the dentin for placing the pins, to conserve the cervical enamel, and to facilitate placing the amalgam matrix.

The crater previously occupied by caries should be examined closely to be certain that the dentin floor is solid and that the excavation is thorough. The dentin tissue, which will also be part of the foundation of the restoration, is examined to detect pulp tissue. The cavity depth is observed to determine the type of intermediary base that should be employed.

The basing procedure should not interfere with the condensation of the amalgam around the pins. The base is not built back as far as the original dentin thickness to assure amalgam bulk. The cement is placed at the bottom and flattened to allow amalgam thickness in an occlusal-cervical direction and around the pins. If the cavity is deep and a minute exposure is suspected, the walls should be lined with a thin layer of calcium hydroxide. Following this the material is further protected by applying a thin layer of zinc phosphate cement to prevent any breakdown during condensation of the amalgam. The bases and the cavity wall are lined with cavity varnish to improve the seal of the restoration. The protection provided by the thin bases will reduce the thermal transfer to the pulp.

The size of the restoration and the number of pins needed are estimated at the time of complete excavation. The need for additional extension and mechanical retention in the surrounding tooth structure will also be determined at this time.

The rules for extension of the pre-carious areas are executed according to the principles of regular cavity preparations (Fig. 10-9). The poorly coalesced grooves abutting the lesion are excised and the outline is extended onto smooth cleansable enamel. The extension should not be made larger than normal and it should be conservative to save as much sound tooth structure as possible. Occasionally it will be necessary to change the outline to increase the retention

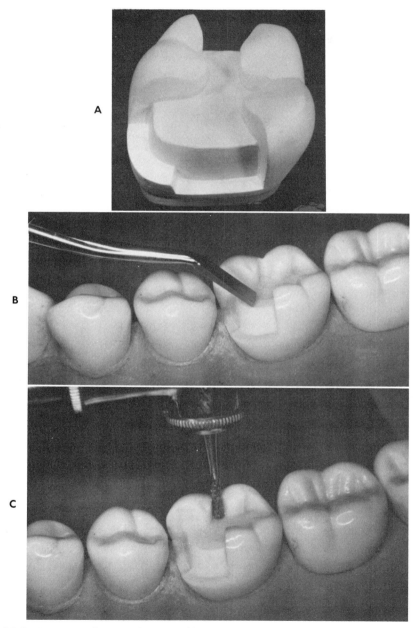

Fig. 10-9. A, Prepared cavity form suitable for the pin restoration. **B** and **C,** The principles of cavity preparation are fulfilled by placing exact and sharp walls in the form.

and resistance form. The terminal end of the dovetails can be increased or made parallel to the ridges or pulpal wall. Accessory undercuts can be made in the cavity walls to lock and assist the retention afforded by the pins.

The cervical walls are extended to the areas advocated by Black. The cervical walls of the pin-retained amalgam restoration should be protected by a healthy gingiva except in cases in which the tissue has receded. The inadequate cleansing of the proximal portion of the restoration makes this necessary. The wall should be out of contact with the adjacent tooth to allow for cleaning with dental floss and for adequate formation of the embrasure and contact area.

The shoulder, which was discussed previously, should not be taken below the soft tissue. This would only complicate adaptation of the matrix, and such extension is considered unnecessary on the buccal or lingual surfaces. Limiting this extension also preserves sound tooth structure on which the finish line of full-coverage restoration is located. The casting should not terminate in amalgam, which means that the actual adaptation of the gold margin will be with tooth structure and be at least 1 mm. beyond the amalgam core.

The depth of the preparation, wall angulation, and location of the internal line angles aid in supporting the extensive amalgam restorations.

PIN ARMAMENTARIUM

In the previous discussion it was pointed out that different types of pins are available. Access for placement, retention needs, and preferred technique are the criteria for selecting the pin type.

TMS system. These pins are threaded to enable the wire to be screwed down into the posthole. Small nontapering burs are used to place the postholes in the dentin. The pins are screwed into the dentin with a wrench or handpiece, which provides the interlocking and retention of the wire. The method requires a straight and therefore a shorter pin. Extra room is needed at the top of the pin to permit placement. Various pin sizes are available.

Friction lock. The wire employed in this technique is larger than the posthole by 0.001 inch. The same type of nontapering posthole is made with a Spirec bur. The steel wire is tapped in place, which creates frictional retention in the tooth. Small taps fit over the end of the wire and are shaped like long-handled gold foil condensers to receive the mallet.

The problem involved in using tap pins is that straight wires must be used. Furthermore, they cannot be removed readily after they are seated in the tooth. Bending the wire in the tooth results in fracture of the shouldered portion of the tooth, which then creates a subgingival margin. Therefore, the wire must not be bent because of the danger of losing the tooth. The stress that accumulates around the tap pins sometimes causes enamel fracture if careless malleting is employed.

Cemented pins. This kit utilizes Spirec burs for the nontapered posthole and

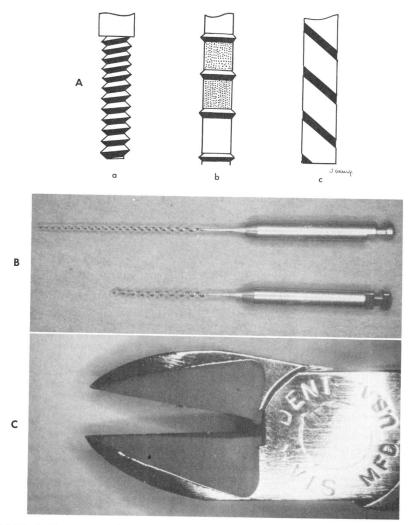

Fig. 10-10. A, Three types of pins: *a,* screw pin; *b,* cemented pin; *c,* friction pin. **B,** The Lentulo spiral is cut in half to eliminate the whip in the instrument during cementation. **C,** Wire cutters are used to hold the wire after the estimated length is cut.

an undersized wire, 0.001 inch, that is cemented for retention (Fig. 10-10). The wires projecting into the restoration can be bent, contoured, or cemented at vertical or horizontal angles. The curved wire allows uniform bulk of the amalgam around the wires and the restoration is not weakened by thin metal.

The Spirec burs are accurate cutters because of the positive, sharp rake angle on the burs. They are made of soft steel, which means they become dull rapidly and should not be used on enamel. The postholes should be located entirely in dentin. To facilitate the proper location of the burs in dentin the lip of the posthole is started with a small round bur. This enables the Spirec bur to be seated and to start cutting at the desired angulation.

The wire used is stainless steel and is threaded to provide interlocking with the cement. The wire has a small clearance on the sides of the posthole, but it must seat firmly on the tooth structure before cementation. The wire can be shaped before cementation to fit any location in the restoration.

The cement is placed in the postholes with a Lentulo spiral instrument. This small spiral wire fits in the right-angle handpiece and picks up and holds the mixed cement. As soon as the rheostat is turned the revolving bur drives the cement down the spiral and into the posthole. Special wire cutters, cotton pliers, and condensers can be obtained to simplify cementing the wires in the tooth structure. They all add to the convenience of the technique and should be considered when procuring supplies.

COPPER BAND MATRIX

The larger the restoration, the more complicated the construction of the matrix becomes. With large buccal and lingual extensions it is necessary to employ the anatomically contoured band. Not only must the desired anatomy be shaped but the assembly must be rigid to withstand the forces of condensation.

The anatomic matrix is desirable because of the contour that results on the proximal surfaces of the restoration. Anatomic matrices may be made from strip matrix that has been prestamped or shaped with universal bands and retainers. Careful application of the materials and controlled condensation permit many different kinds of matrices to be used when some tooth structure is remaining. The stabilization of the matrix and gingival wedge is always necessary because this produces stability and prevents the cervical overhang of amalgam.

When large mutilated lesions are being restored, a contoured copper band is used (Fig. 10-11). This requires additional time and accurate contouring, but it is the only procedure that can be used for mutilated teeth. The thin seamless copper bands, 0.001 inch thick, are used and a technique similar to that used in the anatomic Class II custom matrix is employed to shape the band. A copper band is selected that barely clears the diameter of the tooth in the cervical area. The band is heated in the bunsen flame until it becomes light red; it is then withdrawn and allowed to cool slowly. This softens the band for easier handling and is an aid in the construction of the matrix. The curved scissors are used to festoon the band to correspond to the gingival curvature at the cementoenamel junction. The band is then smoothed with carborundum stones and rubber abrasives to remove the barbs and rough edges. This permits the band to be seated without altering the gingival attachment.

The band is contoured with the No. 112 pliers to produce the bulge and contour in the contact areas and on the buccal and lingual surfaces. The proximal

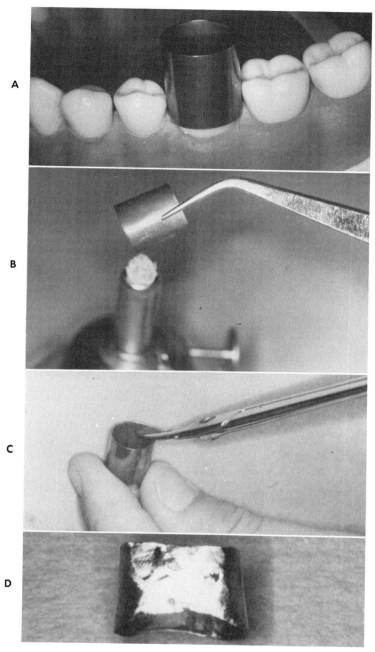

Continued.

Fig. 10-11. A, A copper band that is barely larger than the circumference of the tooth is selected. **B,** It is held in the flame and heated to soften the copper, which enhances the contouring. **C,** The band is festooned with the scissors so that it has the same curvature as the gingival tissue. **D,** Appearance of band after contoured being with the pliers and after the contact area has been thinned with the sandpaper disk.

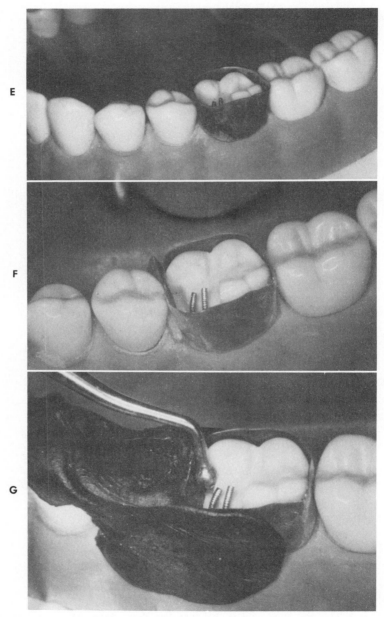

Fig. 10-11, cont'd. E, Fitted copper band. **F,** The band is wedged securely below the cervical wall of the preparation. **G,** The band is stabilized with low-fusing compound and pushed against the adjacent tooth with a warm burnisher to assure contour.

portion of the band is formed to correspond to the contour that is desired in the carved restoration. If the band is expanded, it might be necessary to crimp the cervical portion of the metal to reproduce the contact with the tooth. The band is then placed on the tooth stump and all its dimensions are checked. To facilitate removal of the band and assure contact, the proximal portion of the band is reduced in thickness in the contact areas. A large garnet sandpaper disk is used to thin the contact area until the band bends readily and can be torn off the packed amalgam. This completes the fabrication of the matrix, and the pins and cavity form should be checked before it is applied.

To stabilize the band and prevent a cervical flash of amalgam, wood wedges are placed tightly on the outside of the band and on the tooth below the cervical wall. The entire application is covered with compound to stabilize the matrix. Low-fusing green stick compound is applied in the same way as for the rubber dam clamps and separators. This method assures a good adaptation and does not injure the tooth or the fingers of the dentist during the application.

The ball burnisher is used to force the band out toward the adjacent tooth after the compound has hardened. The areas of concern are the contacts and embrasures where the band has been thinned. The ball burnisher or curved blade instrument is warmed in the flame and then placed against the inside of the band. This melts the compound on the outside of the metal and then forces are applied to push the matrix against the adjacent tooth. The compound is cooled with the air syringe and the cavity preparation is cleaned thoroughly before inserting the amalgam. The technique of contouring and stabilizing the copper band satisfies the requirements of the anatomic matrix.

When cores are being placed for crowns and bridges, accurate contour in the band is usually not needed. The amalgam will only have to be reduced enough so that it contains no undercuts and the stock copper band can be used without shaping. Only stability is required for building the core, and this is provided by the compound blocking procedure.

Because of the problems of food impaction the pin-retained amalgam core should be reduced and the remainder of the tooth prepared and protected with an anatomic temporary crown. After the initial set of the alloy the restoration can be reduced with fissure burs in the air turbine handpiece. Extremely light pressure should be applied to the handpiece and care should be taken to avoid touching the top of the pins. The vibration of a pin results in fracture and in loss of small pieces of the amalgam core. Small carborundum and diamond stones are used to smooth the core and the tooth. Once again light pressure is used and the milling devices are moved from the metal to the reduced tooth surface.

The copper band is removed following condensation and the superficial carving. The thinned areas are easily torn after the initial set of the alloy. The band is gripped with two cotton pliers and is twisted in opposite directions. When the band is completely torn, it is rotated around the contact areas

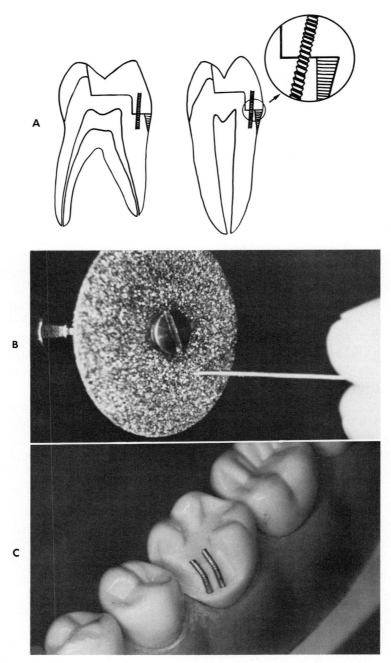

Fig. 10-12. A, Indication of pin direction, depth of 1.5 to 2.0 mm. penetration into dentin and an extension of 2.0 mm. **B,** The end of the threaded wire that is inserted into the posthole is squared on a separating disk. **C,** The wires are curved and adjusted for height to ensure uniform amalgam bulk.

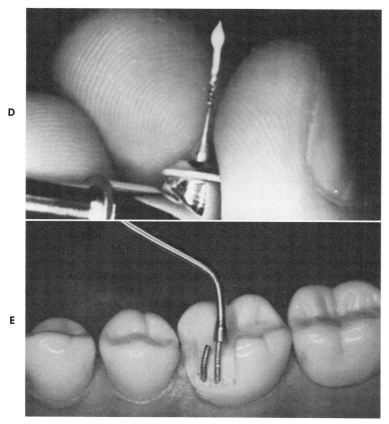

Fig. 10-12, cont'd. D, Cement is picked off the slab with the Lentulo spiral and buttered between the fingers. **E,** The curved pins are forced into the postholes with the amalgam condenser.

one proximal surface at a time. The band may also be split with the air turbine bur.

PIN PLACEMENT FOR CEMENTED PIN

Placing the pins does not require much time. Certain rules must be followed and with the help of the assistant the pins can be placed in 5 to 8 minutes, regardless of the number of wires cemented (Fig. 10-12).

The pins are located in areas where stress will occur in the restoration. Because these areas usually contain most of the tooth structure, bulk is available for the pins. These areas are located under marginal ridges, cusp tips, and line angles. Care is exercised to avoid dropping the pins out of the tooth or into the pulp when the postholes are made. The pins are not placed over bifurcations or in the center of the dentin crater because of these dangers. They are placed instead in a circle around the excavated dentin.

The depth to which the pin is placed is regulated by the length of the metal projecting into the restoration. The postholes are placed to a depth of 1.5 to 2 mm. and are always located in dentin to stabilize the wires. The wires are curved to follow the contour of the restoration and to produce a 2 mm. thickness of alloy on the top and side of the pin in the final restoration.

The pins provide more retention if they are not parallel. Because the external curvatures of the tooth act as a guide for the direction of the postholes, the pins will seldom be parallel. Also the base of the pins should be placed at different levels in the tooth. This will provide support and prevent a fracture line from developing at the level of the base of the pins.

Determining the angulation of the postholes is not complicated; they are made parallel to the surface of the tooth or root. The drill of the flat-bladed instrument is held tangentially to the external surface directly outside the tooth in which the pin will be located. The bur is moved into the dentin 0.5 mm. and the posthole is placed to a depth of 1.5 mm. The radiograph is also helpful in determining the depth of the postholes and the location of the pulp. Following these rules will prevent perforation of the tooth or pulp exposure.

The number of pins to be used is influenced by the surface area of the restoration. From one to six pins can be used for the support. A minimum distance of 1 mm. is needed between the pins to permit condensation and adaptation of the amalgam to the threaded wire. An excessive number of pins weakens the tooth structure and amalgam in which they are placed.

Horizontal pins are useful in large two- or three-surface lesions (Fig. 10-13). The pins are placed in the dentin to the depth of the enamel. The pins can be made L shaped and can be rotated into the mass of the preparation when they are cemented. These pins can serve as a splint in holding the remaining cusps together. At times, however, it is difficult to find dentin under the cusp tips that will hold the pins. In addition the problem of pulp involvement exists, and these two considerations limit the use of horizontal pins.

Procedure

The procedure to be followed in placing the pins is as follows:

1. After the location and angulation of the pins for the tooth have been determined, the posthole is started in the dentin with a No. ½ round bur to minimize dulling the Spirec bur. Then the Spirec bur is placed in the posthole and the dentin tissue is cut to a depth of 1.5 to 2 mm. The bur is not moved laterally because the posthole would then be oversized, causing the pins to fit loosely.

2. The threaded wire is cut and the end is squared with a separating disk, and then it is placed in the tooth structure. The height and curvature of the pins are adjusted with the wire cutters and the pliers. All the wires are placed in the tooth at one time to determine the degree of retention being developed and the need for additional wires.

3. A small diagram of the preparation is drawn on the bracket cover. The

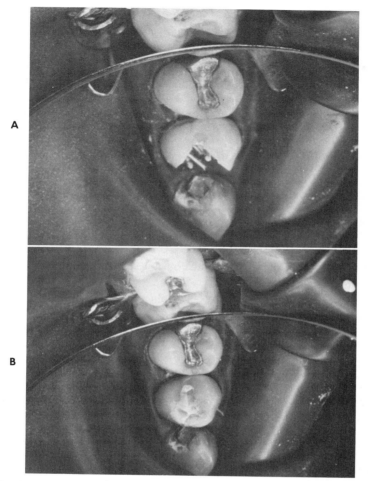

A

B

Fig. 10-13. A, Example of vertical and horizontal pins. This technique is not often possible due to lack of dentin in the areas underlying the cusps. **B,** Carved amalgam restoration on the first bicuspid.

wires are removed from the preparation and placed on the drawing to prevent them from being switched during the cementation. Carrying the wires in and out of the postholes is facilitated by grooving the inside of the beaks of the cotton pliers. Two angulations are made in the beaks with the separating disk, or some of the kits can be purchased with grooved cotton pliers.

4. Cavity varnish is applied to the preparation, including the cavosurface margin. Some clinicians place the varnish inside the postholes to minimize forcing the cement into the dentin when the wires are cemented.

5. A retarded mix of zinc phosphate cement is made for cementing the pins. The slab is chilled. Some individuals place small amounts of powder into the liquid before mixing. A large area of the slab is used and the mix is slowly made

until the cement has a creamy consistency but still glistens on the surface. This will enable any number of pins to be cemented without necessitating an additional mix of material.

6. The Lentulo spiral is cut in half to prevent whipping of the small metal tip. The cement is picked up in the spiral and the excess is removed by buttering the point between the thumb and index finger. The loaded Lentulo spiral in the handpiece is then placed in the posthole and the rheostat is quickly opened to produce a few revolutions that spin the cement to the bottom of the posthole.

7. The pin is taken from the bracket drawing and placed into the filled posthole. An amalgam condenser is placed on top of the pin and force is applied to fully seat the pin in the tooth.

8. If cementation has been complete, a small ring of cement will form around each pin. In approximately 2 minutes the set will permit removal of the excess cement with a sharp explorer. After this has been accomplished the matrix is applied and the amalgam is inserted. The assistant does much of the manipulation during the cementation. A rhythmic routine prevents the complications that could occur during pin placement.

9. If the TMS or friction lock pins are selected, a similar procedure is used. The postholes are made the same way and the pin size is selected. The armamentarium that is furnished with the pin is employed to seat the pin to the full depth of the posthole. Directions are afforded with each pin type.

PLACING THE ALLOY

Numerous mixes will be required for the large pin-retained restoration. The capsules should be loaded with two pellets and the additional amalgamations can be requested anytime during the building procedure. The assistant should be trained to mix and carry the amalgam efficiently so that the condensation is not interrupted.

A slow-setting alloy is selected for the large pin-retained restoration (Fig. 10-14). The alloys that are mixed in a 1:1 ratio usually permit some extra working time and are helpful when developing a well-adapted restoration. Condensation is achieved with the normal pressure and direction, being certain that a mercury-rich layer is present on the surface before each increment is added. This will minimize lamination of the restoration. The dense packing will be appreciated when carving is initiated.

Special condensers are helpful in beginning the condensation and adapting the metal around the pins. The Mortonson and Wesco "O" condensers have small diameters and fit well between the wires. The amalgam is packed against the floor of the preparation and moved laterally to adapt to the pins. Metallurgic studies have demonstrated adequate adaptation to the threaded wires when this method is used. These special condensers are placed in the kits that contain the other material for the armamentarium.

When the alloy has been adapted around and over the tops of the pins, the

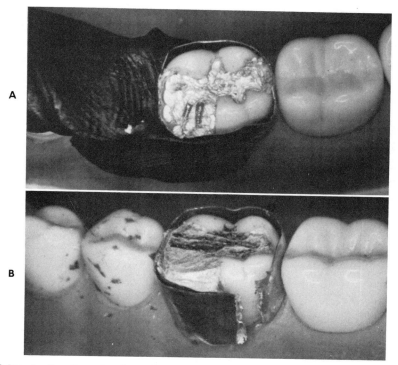

A

B

Fig. 10-14. A, The first mix of amalgam condensed into the cavity preparation and around the pins. **B,** Condensed and burnished amalgam with the copper band torn for removal.

overpack can be started. A larger condenser, preferably Black's No. 2, is used to compress the amalgam on top of the pins. The building is continued until an overpack of 1 mm. is produced. This layer is excessively condensed to pull up the residual mercury so that it can be removed during the carving. The overpack will appear to be burnished because of the excess mercury, but this will be no problem since the mercury is removed during the carving.

Carving can be initiated after the initial set. The material need only be hard enough to resist the carver. The instrument should be sharp and should produce a dull ringing sound when the anatomy is being formed. Carving is not important when cores are placed because they will later be reduced and covered with a gold casting. More metal must be shaped in the regular pin-retained restoration prior to the removal of the rubber dam and the establishment of a good working occlusion. The functional anatomic components should be placed during the carving to aid in mastication.

The blade-shaped carvers are helpful because they can be used to rapidly contour the buccal and lingual surfaces and form the embrasures. Timing the set of the amalgam will allow the dentist to quickly shape the extended surface surrounding the pins. When the core is being carved, the contour is purposely flattened to reduce the amount of rotary reduction that will be needed.

Many techniques can be developed to aid in placing the alloy once the procedure becomes common practice. The use of the rubber dam is almost always necessary and in certain cases special clamps are helpful. The adjusted No. W8A and No. 14A clamps facilitate placement of the matrix. The divided or individual No. 212 clamps and the Schultz series are helpful in restoring bicuspids that have fractured and can be grasped only below the gingival tissue. All these clamps must be stabilized with compound to prevent movement and dislodgment of the dam or damage to the tissues.

The pin-retained restoration has gained popularity and is a useful method of restoring extensive lesions. Precise indications exist for the pin-retained amalgam restoration, and several types of pins can be selected for the advantage of technique and retention.

POLISHING

Because amalgam is extensively used, the polishing procedure is often neglected. A polished surface is one that is smooth and exact, and it is important in all types of restorations. Any rough surface in the oral cavity acts as a constant irritant to the soft tissues. Food collection, which accelerates recurrent caries on the adjacent enamel surface, is more prone to occur on the unpolished surface. When these facts are realized, it becomes apparent that all amalgam restorations should be polished. The weak margin of the amalgam restoration produces a special need for polishing. Some of the permanency and success are sacrificed by improper finishing. To minimize the breakdown the restoration should end in a right-angle joint with the cavosurface enamel. This procedure removes the overhanging material that often fractures and sharply demarcates the edge of the restoration with the tooth.

The surface of silver alloy is susceptible to tarnish and corrosion. Because amalgam is not a noble metal, the formation of surface oxides becomes apparent shortly after insertion. Abrasives are used to condition the surface of the amalgam during the polishing to produce an amorphous layer. This type of surface is more resistant to the attack of corrosive products.

The amalgam can be damaged if improperly polished. The mercury is attracted to the surface layer if the polishing is done before 24 hours after the condensation or if temperatures above 140° F. are developed. The presence of extra mercury causes the surface to be more susceptible to tarnish. A period of 3 days following insertion allows the setting reaction to be terminated and is the ideal waiting period for amalgam polishing. To minimize temperature elevations the rotary abrasives are applied with light pressure, particularly when the rubber wheels are used.

The polishing instruments should be limited in number and used in an order of descending abrasiveness (Fig. 10-15). Also when the restoration is being marginated, excellent vision is needed. For this reason the application of the rubber dam has proved to be quite helpful and economical, especially when a number of

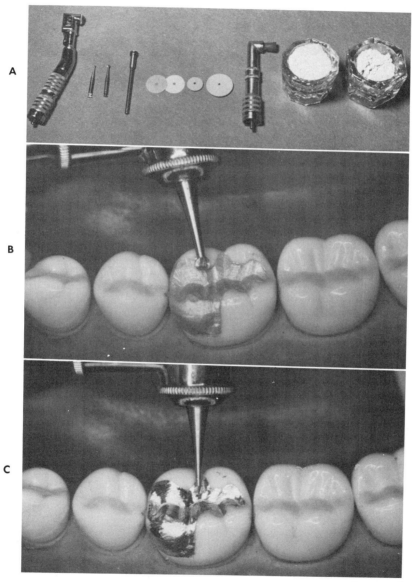

Continued.

Fig. 10-15. A, Armamentarium for polishing the amalgam restoration. The equipment from left to right includes the No. 1 and No. 4 round burs, cuttlefish sandpaper disks, rubber abrasive wheel, and polishing angle filled with silica and whiting. **B,** The No. 4 round bur is used to initiate the polishing procedure. Margination of the metal is the first objective of the technique. **C,** The No. 1 round bur is used to clean the oxides from the grooves.

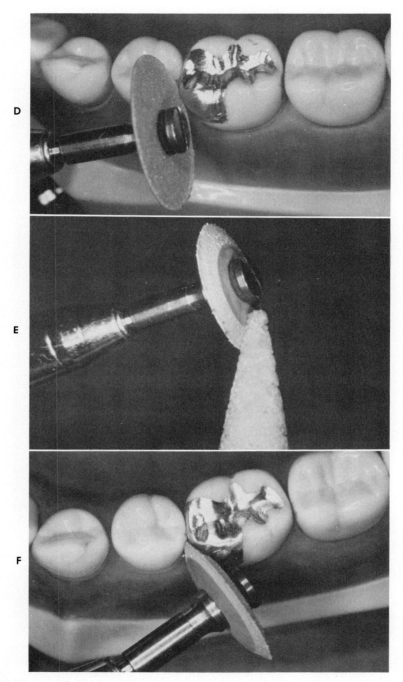

Fig. 10-15, cont'd. D, Smoothing the metal with a cuttlefish sandpaper disk. **E,** Placing a sharp edge on the rubber wheel. This procedure is helpful in each restoration. **F,** Proximal surface application of the rubber abrasive wheel.

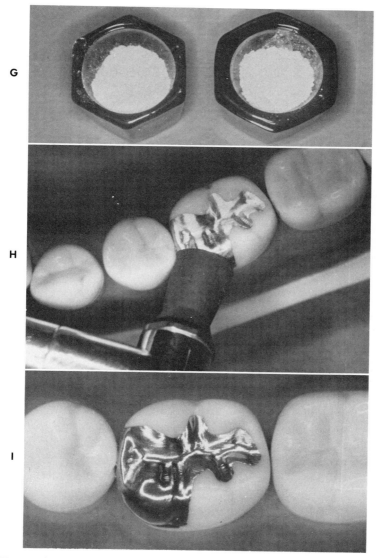

Fig. 10-15, cont'd. G, Dishes containing silica and whiting, materials used for the surface luster of the restoration. **H,** Application of the polishing powders or slurry with the soft rubber cup. **I,** Completed pin-retained amalgam restoration.

restorations are being refined. The polishing is accomplished at low speeds and with 1 to 2 pounds of pressure to prevent painful responses. Following is an orderly procedure that can be used with some efficiency to polish all types of amalgam restorations. The instruments are used to locate the margin, reshape the anatomy, or smooth the surface. Each step must be accomplished for polishing any restoration in the oral cavity.

1. No. 4 round bur (favorite steel finishing burs can be substituted). A steel bur is used to mill the amalgam. In most cases the bur will not damage the tooth structure as do finishing stones or diamonds, and this minimizes small enamel defects or roughness around the metal. The round bur is used both to find the final margin and to create the contour and direction of the cusp planes. The bur produces a smooth surface in a very short time.

2. No. 1 round bur. This bur is used to clean the oxides that have been deposited on the carved surface out of the grooves. The bur should not burrow the groove but should be directed only enough to provide a hint of a demarcation between the cusp planes. A nidus for bacteria is formed by grooves that are too deep to be cleaned during mastication. Adequate grooves are necessary to aid the grinding during mastication and to place harmony in the restoration. Conservative restorations will usually have secondary grooves that blend with the depressions in the outline. A No. 700 bur can also be well used for this purpose.

3. One-half inch cuttlefish sandpaper disks. These disks are used on the buccal and lingual margins of the proximal portions of the restorations. The disks can be mounted in a straight mandrel and rotated in or out to finish the mesial and distal surfaces. The cuttlefish grit requires only a few revolutions to marginate the alloy. The proximal margin is aligned with the occlusal outline and the marginal ridge is rounded with the disk. The flattened disk is then brushed over the occlusal surface.

4. Small Burlew wheels. These disks are utilized to rapidly smooth the accessible surfaces of the restoration. The wheel can be manipulated and flexed to reach the grooves and cusp planes. A sharp edge should be maintained on the rubber disk at all times. This edge enhances the access of the disk in the groove areas, and it can be pointed with large abrasive stones. A rise in temperature, which can be deleterious if excessive, is miminized by using only light pressure on the handpiece. This abrasive actually produces the amorphous surface layer, which is considered from a metallurgical standpoint as being polished.

5. Silica and whiting. These materials are applied to enhance the surface luster of the restoration. They are placed on the restoration with a soft rubber polishing cup, and caution is again exercised to minimize temperature elevations. A mirrorlike finish is produced on the surfaces of the restoration, and the powders should be moistened to encourage surface apposition.

6. Dental floss. To facilitate cleaning with dental floss, the interproximal surface should be polished or smoothed. This is accomplished with separation whereby the contact is barely polished to remove the metal projections that tear dental floss. Following this, the separator is removed and the extrafine finishing strip is used to smooth the cervical half of the proximal restoration. The interproximal portion can then be more satisfactorily cleansed by the patient.

This completes the polishing procedure, and the restoration is inspected before removing the rubber dam. The polished amalgam restoration is an object of pride to both the dentist and the patient. Whenever possible the polishing procedure should be employed. When a number of restorations have been placed, a separate appointment should be made for polishing. If only one or two restorations have been placed, they are best polished during the periodic recall appointment.

SUMMARY

1. For patient comfort and tissue health the amalgam restoration should be polished.

2. Amalgam must be marginated because of the low edge strength of the material. This technique retards marginal fracture because thin layers of the material are removed.

3. The armamentarium for polishing should not be difficult because the procedure requires use of only a few instruments in an order of descending abrasiveness.

4. Patient education is enhanced by the polishing procedure and concern for saving the teeth results.

ADDITIONAL READINGS

Bell, B. H., and Grainger, D. A.: Basic operative procedures, Philedelphia, 1971, Lea and Febiger.

Courtade, G. L.: A simplified procedure for creating artificial dentin, Dent. Clin. N. Am., Nov., 1963, pp. 805-822.

Courtade, G. L., and Timmermans, J. J.: Pins in restorative dentistry, St. Louis, 1971, The C. V. Mosby Co.

Duperon, D. F., and Kasloff, Z.: Effects of three types of pins on compressive strength of dental amalgam, J. Canad. Dent. Assoc. 11:422-428, 1971.

Going, R. E.: Pin-retained amalgam, J.A.D.A. 73:619, 1966.

Going, R. E., Moffa, J. P., Nostrand, G. W., and Johnson, B. E.: The strength of dental amalgam as influenced by pins, J. Am. Dent. Assoc. 77:1331, 1968.

Goldstein, P. M.: Retention pins are friction locked without use of cement, J.A.D.A. 73:1103, 1966.

Manderson, R. D.: Accessory pin retention for large amalgam restorations, University of Durham Med. Gaz. 56:77, 1966.

Markley, M. R.: Pin reinforcement and retention of amalgam foundations and restorations, J.A.D.A. 56:675, 1958.

Moffa, J. P., and Phillips, R. W.: Retentive properties of parallel pin restorations, J. Prosth. Dent. 17:387-400, 1967.

Moffa, J. P., Rozanno, N. R., and Doyle, M. G.: Pins—a comparison of their retentive properties, J. Am. Dent. Assoc. 78:529, 1969.

Resnick, C. R., and Shaeffer, R. L.: Pin-reinforced restorations, Practical Dental Monographs, Mar., 1966, pp. 36-38.

Roberts, E. W.: Pin reinforced alloy restorations, Texas Dent. J. 79:4, 1961.

Walter, M.: Pin reinforcement for amalgam restorations, Brit. Dent. J. 108:194, 1961.

Watson, P. A., and Gilmore, H. W.: Use of pins for retaining amalgam restorations: a synopsis, J. Canad. Dent. Assoc. 36:30-31, 1970.

Welk, D. A., and Dilts, W. E.: Influence of pins on the compressive and transverse strength of dental amalgam and retention pins in amalgam, J. Am. Dent. Assoc. 78:101, 1969.

Wing, G.: Pin retention amalgam restorations, Aust. Dent. J. 10:6, 1965.

Wright, R. W.: Use of stainless steel pins to strengthen amalgam restorations, Aust. Dent. J. 3:369, 1958.

Youngs, R. S., and Schmitt, F. M.: Technique for reinforcing amalgam restorations, Dent. Dig. 67:282, 1961.

chapter 11

Silicate cement restorations

Silicate cement is a commonly used tooth-colored restorate material. A simple but exacting technique of mixing a liquid acid and powder is used to prepare silicate cement for insertion into the tooth. The silicate can be mixed on the slab or more conveniently triturated in a preproportioned capsule. Upon mixing the powder and liquid acid a gel structure is formed that is sensitive to the oral environment (Fig. 11-1). The cement produces a tooth-colored restoration that has some degree of esthetics and that serves a useful purpose in restorative dentistry.[1]

A survey of the use of silicate cement was first made by Paffenbarger in 1940. At that time 115 dentists were questioned concerning the use of the material.[2] It was determined from the questionnaires that 11 million silicate restorations were being placed per year and that the average life of the silicate restoration was 4½ years. This was one of the first studies conducted concerning silicate cement restorations and it included the powder-liquid ratio, the setting time, and other manipulative variables of the material. The figures concerning the life of the silicate restoration were determined from the survey and are still quoted.

Some interesting observations can be made on the clinical appearance of the silicate restoration. Initially the results are excellent; the esthetics appear to be good since many shades are available and blend adequately with the tooth. The restorations are finished directly to the enamel at a subsequent appointment and appear to blend with the shading and anatomy if the procedure has been followed properly. Within a few months, however, most silicate restorations become rough on the surface because of the solubility of the cement in the oral fluids.[3] When the gel structure of the restoration begins to dissolve, stains collect from the diet or from microorganisms in the oral cavity. These stains make the silicate restoration noticeable and, after the dissolution has progressed, the tooth margins also become exposed, causing poor adaptation of the material to tooth structure. The longer the restoration ages the darker it becomes, and a line usually appears around the restoration, indicating an open and stained margin. In some cases the restorations dissolve completely, leaving bare enamel and dentin; this condition must be corrected in order to prevent tooth drift

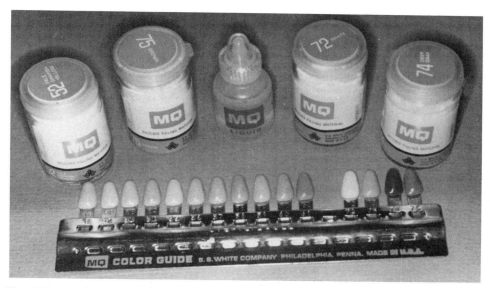

Fig. 11-1. Powder, liquid, and shade guide needed for placing the silicate cement restoration.

and hypertrophy or destruction of the gingival tissue. Dissolution of the silicate restoration commonly occurs below the contact area.

Although the immediate esthetic result of silicate cement restorations is good, the restorations need to be replaced frequently. The dissolution of the silicate could be advantageous because in the process fluorine is leached from the restoration and is deposited in the tooth structure.[4] Even though the restoration requires continual replacement, the occurrence of secondary caries in the surrounding enamel and dentin is controlled by the fluoride transfer. Recurrent caries seldom occurs but if each restoration does become larger, the enlargement is caused by extending the new cavity preparation. The infrequent recurrence of caries around the silicate restoration is the greatest advantage of the material other than its esthetic qualities.

It is helpful to place the silicate cement in a dry cavity, which means the rubber dam must be used if an ideal result is to be achieved. The presence of moisture in the cavity preparation produces a weakened gel structure where the material contacts the tooth structure. If any stain or debris is present in the cavity preparation, it causes discoloration of the restoration a very short time after the insertion. Toilet of the cavity and a dry preparation are important to the successful use of silicate cement. All measures are taken in this regard to alleviate the undesirable properties of silicate cement.

MANIPULATION AND PROPERTIES

To use silicate cement properly it becomes necessary to understand the physical and chemical properties. A powder and liquid are used to produce the mix.

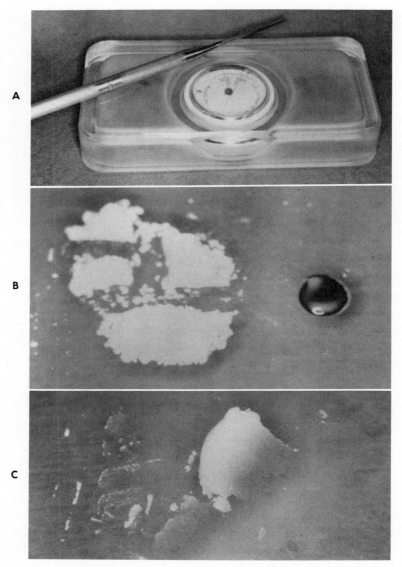

Fig. 11-2. A, Mixing slab with thermometer that is manufactured for use with silicate cement. **B,** Powder and liquid dispensed on the slab. **C,** Ideal mix of silicate cement has a "puttylike" consistency and shines on the surface.

The restoration is a silicic acid gel (acid-soluble glass) that is made by dissolving the surface of the powder particle in liquid. The powder is a mixture of silica, alumina, and fluoride that serves to hold the powder constituents together during the manufacturing process. A cake containing these constituents is formed at high temperatures (1,400° C.) and is plunged into cold water to produce cracking and crazing, which simplifies the milling procedures.[1] These cakes are ball-milled or crushed and sorted into uniform particle sizes.

The liquid is phosphoric acid that is buffered with aluminum and zinc phosphate.[5] Approximately half of the acid is distilled water and the liquid should be mixed before it is dispensed for mixing with the powder. The acids have pH values ranging from 0.8 to 1.5, and when mixed with the powder, they dissolve the surface of the particles to form the gel structure. The reaction is termed "condensation polymerization." The acid is usually present on the surface of the mix for 24 hours and eventually reaches a pH of 6. Research on altering the constituents of the powder has been conducted, but for the most part the silicate cements are similar in composition and manipulation. The liquid should be discarded when the bottle is only one-fourth full because of the danger of altering the pH of the acid by having too much distilled water in the solution.

The matrix of the silicate restoration is the gel structure. This material comprises approximately 25% of the restoration and is minimized as much as possible because of its sensitivity.[5] The technique of mixing and finishing the silicate cement is designed to minimize and protect the gel structure. The gel portion is susceptible to high temperatures and dehydration, and it will dissolve in acid. Once the gel is effected, the undissolved portion of the particle simply drops out and a rough surface is produced that is conducive to staining.

It is important to use the proper powder-liquid ratio in the mixing procedure (Fig. 11-2). A number of variables that are critical for developing an acceptable silicate restoration are related to this ratio.[6] The setting time is influenced both by the powder-liquid ratio and by the temperature at which the material is mixed. Solubility and strength are also dependent upon the powder-liquid ratio, and for this reason manufacturers have packaged accurate measuring devices for the two constituents.

The scoop for the powder usually has a large and a small end. To achieve a successful mix two drops of liquid should be mixed with two large scoops and one small scoop of powder. The powder should be completely in corporated within 1 minute and the mix should have a "puttylike" consistency and exhibit some shine on the surface. The proper ratios are given by the manufactures. The type of mix specified is developed and a bulk of the material is packed into the tooth and held under pressure. The measured powder is required to produce a consistency that helps to control the solubility of the silicate.

To facilitate mixing the slab is cooled and then warmed slightly above the dew point or to the temperature at which moisture does not form on the glass. Slabs can be purchased with thermometers in order to regulate the temperature of the glass before the mix is begun. Also the mixing surfaces of some slabs are etched to facilitate incorporating the powder into the liquid. Numerous types of spatulas have been designed for mixing silicate cement. Some are made of agate but the most popular seem to be the stellite metal and diamond-shaped spatulas. These are used to develop large amounts of pressure during the mixing, which also aids in incorporating the powder into the mix. The diamond-shaped spatula is used to fold the powder into the liquid with pressure. These slabs and spatulas should be used for mixing the silicate because the design makes it easier to develop the proper mix.

The object of the mixing technique is to incorporate as much of the powder into the liquid as possible within 1 minute. The thick mix is placed into the cavity preparation under pressure. Problems arise when too thick a mix is produced. A dry mix adapts poorly to tooth structure and is characterized by an inferior gel. This means that problems concerning solubility and staining of the restoration will arise and that the restoration will last for only a short time. Experience is needed in mixing silicates to recognize the optimum working conditions of the material. Because of its influence on the physical properties, the proper consistency should be achieved in each restoration.

The greatest weakness of silicate cement is its susceptibility to dissolution in acid.[7] When a thin mix is used, the solubility is greater because more gel structure is contained by the restoration. The silicates are extremely vulnerable to dilute organic acids, many of which are ingested in the diet or are formed by the metabolism of microorganisms. A.D.A. Specification No. 9 concerning silicate cements states that only 1.4% of the silicate by weight should dissolve in a 24-hour period after it has been placed in a medium of distilled water.[8] Most of the silicates meet this specification, but solubility is apt to proceed at a greater rate in the oral environment because of the presence of more acids. Solubility is associated with staining of the restoration. The surface becomes darkened by sodium and tin fluoride that is a noticeable black or brown stain.

The advantage of using silicate cement is that the fluoride is released from the restoration after it is placed in the tooth. When the surface dissolves, the fluoride that is used as a flux deposits 500 parts per million into the surrounding tooth structure to produce a fluorapatite. The solubility of the affected enamel is reduced 25%, which discourages recurrent caries around silicate restorations (Table 11-1). So much fluoride is absorbed by the surrounding enamel that the tooth structure becomes hard[10] and brittle to complicate replacing the restoration. It is difficult to remove the unsupported enamel and weakened tooth structure in the marginal areas because of the brittleness associated with the fluorapatite.

The compressive strength of silicate cement is ordinarily 28,000 to 32,000 pounds per square inch. This is considered too low to withstand the forces of occlusion but hard enough to produce a brittle restoration. This means that silicates should neither be used to replace missing incisal angles nor be rein-

Table 11-1. Average change in solubility of intact enamel surfaces induced by silicate cements after 2 weeks[*]

Silicate	Average change in calcium solubility (%)
S. S. White	−27.5
deTrey's	−22.8
Ames' Berylite	+20.4

[*]From Phillips, R. W., and Swartz, M. L.: J.A.D.A. **54**:623, 1957.

forced with pins and other techniques. Fillers added to silicate cement have caused a slight reduction in solubility and an increase in strength, but the values have proved to be of limited clinical significance. The strength and brittleness of silicate cement indicate that the material is best suited to the Class III preparation in which a minimal amount of functional force is developed.

The acidity associated with silicate cements necessitates pulp protection whenever the material is used. Phosphoric acid is present on the surface of the freshly inserted silicate for 24 hours and the pH is elevated from 1 to 6 during this period.[1] If the cavity preparation is deep or if very little dentin remains between the restoration and the pulp, some response in the tissue occurs. It has been shown recently that 600μ of sound dentin are needed to prevent a pulpal reaction with silicate cement.[11] Because of the danger of small undetected exposures all deep cavities are lined with calcium hydroxide. The calcium ions protect the pulp and serve as a base to allow the formation of reparative dentin on the pulpal side of the dentin.[12] On the side of the restoration the calcium ions will neutralize the acid and prevent it from causing any damage.

Cavity preparations that are not too deep or that do not have adequate space axially to employ the calcium hydroxide base should be lined with cavity varnish. The cavity varnish will block a portion of the free acid by serving as a semipermeable membrane on the dentin. Also part of the fluoride that is released from the restoration will be blocked by the cavity varnish, which means that the varnish must be confined to the dentinal surfaces.[13] The accepted procedure for pulp protection is to either use varnish alone on the dentin or to employ calcium hydroxide as an intermediary base when there is a deep cavity. Pulpal protection is an important consideration when silicate cement is used because of the free phosphoric acid.

The importance of developing a thick consistency of silicate cement has stimulated the development of mechanical mixing techniques. It is possible to use an amalgamator for mixing silicate cement (Fig. 11-3). The mechanical mix is accomplished by using capsules into which the powder and liquid are placed.[14] The capsule is mixed in a high-speed amalgamator for 10 seconds. Following this the mix is spooned out of the capsule and placed in the tooth. Studies of this technique have determined that some compounds can be manipulated by

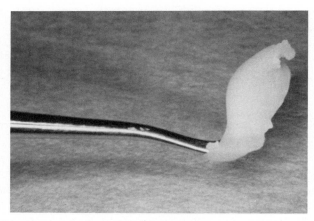

Fig. 11-3. Consistent mix produced by triturating the preproportioned capsule.

this method. The advantages of the technique appear to be the standardization and ease of mixing. The data reported no superior benefits derived from using the mechanical mixer since the physical properties of silicate were not improved.

One of the disadvantages of the mechanical mixing technique is that the setting time is accelerated and the available working time is thereby reduced. Also this technique requires more material and produces some waste. There are, however, some compounds commercially designed to be used specifically with mechanical mixing. As a result of standardization and the development of optimum properties, the trituration method is recommended.

INDICATIONS FOR SILICATE CEMENT

The silicate restoration is indicated only for small and incipient lesions because of the physical qualities; with the anticariogenic properties of silicate, the ideal lesions and cavity preparations should involve a minimum of tooth structure. This will conserve the enamel and make it possible to surround the restoration with an abundance of tooth structure. The material is therefore limited mostly to Class III cavities or to small anterior proximal lesions that do not involve the angle of the tooth. Occasionally small pits caused by developmental defects or small carious lesions on the smooth enamel surfaces can be restored. Toothbrushing readily abrades the silicate restoration, which results in a rough and stained surface. This roughness is detrimental to tissue health, and silicates should not be placed in Class V or cervical cavities when the outline is extended below the gingival tissue.

An excellent indication for silicate cement is in caries-susceptible patients. When many restorations need to be placed quickly, silicate cement is an ideal restorative to control the caries (Fig. 11-4). The material is helpful in gross caries removal and for acute caries when the existing lesions are excavated and Z-O-E is placed in the posterior teeth. For an immediate esthetic result silicate

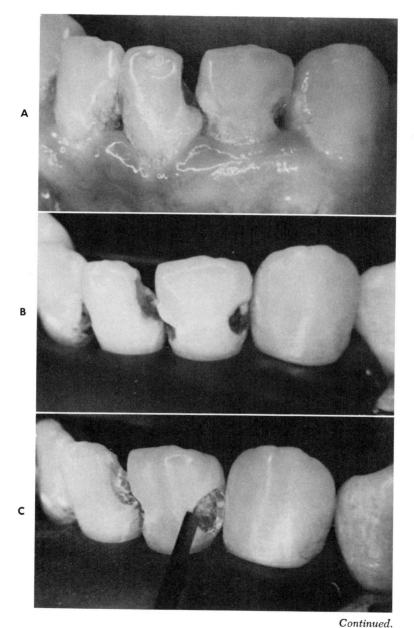

Continued.

Fig. 11-4. A, A practical example of an excellent indication for silicate cement. Note the defective restorations, caries, and plaque. **B,** The teeth are isolated following prophylaxis. **C,** Removal of brittle and chalky enamel with the small Wedelstaedt chisel.

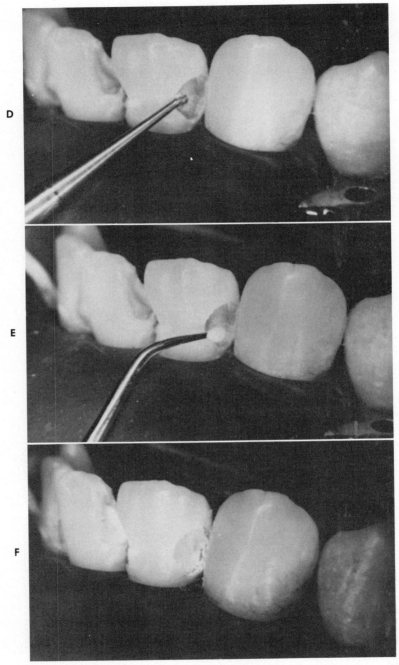

Fig. 11-4, cont'd. D, Thorough excavation of the caries with the slow-turning No. 2 round bur. **E,** Prophylactic pulp capping with calcium hydroxide on the excavated dentin. **F,** Pulp protection afforded by the calcium hydroxide compound.

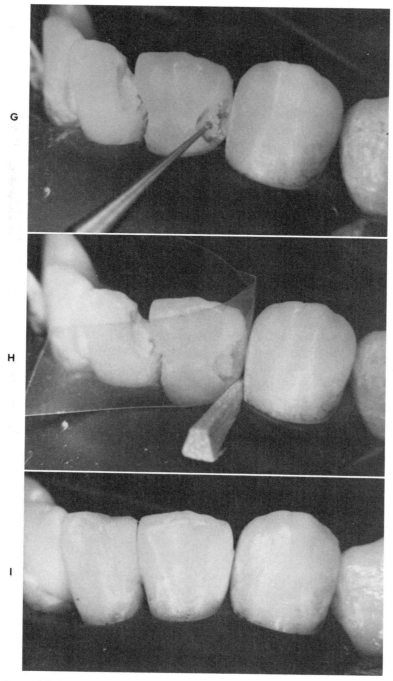

Fig. 11-4, cont'd. G, Cleaning the enamel walls and placing the retention forms with the No. ½ round bur. **H,** Strip and wedge prior to the insertion of the mixed silicate. **I,** Polished silicate restorations 24 hours after placement.

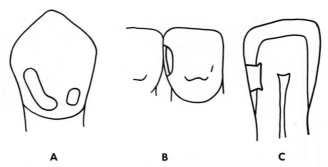

Fig. 11-5. A, Labial silicate outlines maintaining as much intact labial enamel as possible. **B,** Recommended lingual opening for silicate. **C,** Axial penetration and retention for silicate.

cement is placed in the anterior teeth. There is more chance of success with the silicate than with the acrylic resin materials when moisture contamination is a problem. The direct restorative resins have catalysts that are water soluble, and the materials will not polymerize in the presence of moisture. Silicate cement should be used whenever this situation occurs.

CAVITY PREPARATION

The cavity preparations for silicate cement fall into two basic categories. The first is used to restore the incipient or limited lesion and the other is used to replace a restoration or to restore a large lesion. The incipient lesion is conservatively prepared by maintaining the labial enamel plate of the incisor tooth in the cavity form (Fig. 11-5). In the maxillary teeth it is advisable to preserve the labial enamel plate, and in the mandibular teeth the lingual enamel ridge is occasionally preserved for the purpose of access. The mixed silicate is inserted through either the labial or lingual embrasure.

In the replacement type of restoration and the large restoration only the defective material or caries is removed. The stained dentin and faulty silicate remnants are then excavated, after which the walls are squared and the retentions are freshened in the tooth structure. This procedure produces a larger cavity preparation, which results in a shorter clinical life for the silicate restoration because of the lesser amount of protection.

The basic rules to be followed in silicate cavity preparations are as follows:

1. The tooth structure surrounding the area being restored is conserved. Extension is not important in preparing the tooth because of the fluoride transfer and the reduction is solubility that are associated with the silicate. This means that the self-cleansing areas are not reached and that the outline of the cavity preparation is minimized. The opening in the preparation should be only large enough to provide access for preparing the internal portion of the preparation and the retention forms. This access should also allow for the insertion of the mixed silicate.

As mentioned previously, the labial enamel is preserved whenever possible in order to protect and maintain the contact point. If the contact area is replaced with silicate cement, then once the dissolving process begins the tooth will drift, causing a discrepancy in the involved arch. A conservative outline should be used to keep the preparation above the gingival tissue because of the reaction caused when epithelial tissue contacts the rough surface.

2. A mortise form is produced in the internal cavity preparation. The cavity walls are placed as nearly parallel and perpendicular to each other as possible. This will produce the resistance form and assist in holding the material in the tooth when it is placed by the pressure technique.

3. The retentions in the silicate cavity preparation are larger than those used in other types of preparations. Because the thick material has a low viscosity it is difficult to fill the retention forms adequately. The retentive areas are filled with silicate cement to lock the material in the tooth structure and prevent its dislodgment. Small grooves produce excellent retentions.

4. A right-angle cavosurface relationship is produced on the enamel. The strength of the cement results in a brittle restoration, and thin layers of the material over the enamel will fracture and produce noticeable discrepancies in the restoration. The smooth, sharp cavosurface allows for accurate finishing, which in itself helps to minimize the amount of overhanging material. If a feather edge of silicate exists over the enamel, the restoration will exhibit a halo stain within a short time. These areas stain faster or can be detected sooner than corresponding areas in the well-marginated restoration. When the cavosurface is finished for the silicate preparation, the loose enamel should be removed and perfected in a way comparable to other types of cavity preparations.

Before starting the cavity preparation the heavyweight rubber dam is applied. Special mention should be made here of the hypertrophied gingival papilla that is sometimes associated with rough, defective silicate restorations. When in contact with a rough restoration for extended periods, the papillae can become edematous and swollen and hemorrhage upon being displaced. In this situation the heavyweight rubber dam is useful because of the extra tissue compression it provides. Some teeth need to be ligated with dental floss, but this is the exception rather than the rule. If the rubber does not displace the tissue satisfactorily, the ligations should be applied snugly in the gingival crevice over the dam to retract the enlarged papilla. The ligations are damaging and should not be left on the tooth for long periods of time because the attachment will be torn. The cavity preparation is then restored and coated with a protective film, usually cocoa butter. The ligation is removed by cutting the dental floss with the gold finishing knife, but this is not done until the silicate restoration is grossly finished.

Only a few instruments are employed for the incipient lesion (Fig. 11-6). The enamel plate covering the caries is removed with a hatchet or chisel for access, depending on whether the lingual or labial approach is being used.

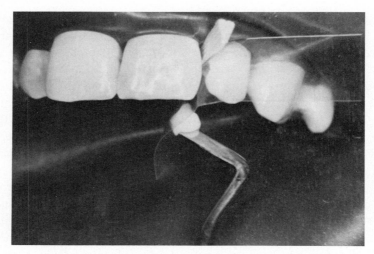

Fig. 11-6. Bulk packing the silicate from the lingual into the wedged matrix.

When the caries and dentin are observed, a round bur (No. 2 to No. 4) is selected according to the actual size of the lesion. The bur is inserted and revolved slowly to remove the caries and any dentin that did not feel solid when examined. When all of the involved tooth structure is removed, the depth of the crater and the degree of access is observed to determine the need for a base and the path to follow in packing in the cement. The opening only needs to be large enough to insert the round bur without damaging the adjacent proximal surface. When the excavating bur is in the cavity, the closed cavity wall is smoothed and extended to an area just visible in the embrasure. This small opening or wall is refined by using the thin No. 10 Wedelstaedt chisel with sharp delicate strokes to remove any remaining frail enamel. The silicate can then abut a sound cavity wall, and the acute cavosurface that is produced will enhance the marginal relationship of the material.

The outline of the incipient cavity preparation is then refined on the surface through which the material is to be inserted. Two undercut grooves are placed with a No. ½ round bur to hold the material in the preparation. The bur is placed in the top and bottom of the crater, usually on the dentin of the incisal and cervical walls, and slowly withdrawn from the cavity preparation. This will produce two divergent undercut grooves that adequately serve to mechanically lock the silicate into the tooth structure. A lingual approach is generally used to hide the cement and the cavosurface enamel is smoothed with a No. 700 bur in the contra-angle handpiece. The finished cavity preparation is washed thoroughly with hydrogen peroxide and dried prior to the insertion of the material.

The large Class III preparation or the one used for replacement differs from the preparation just described. If the caries or the defective silicate does not provide access, the unsupported labial or lingual plate is removed with the sharp hatchet or chisel. Often these lesions can be excavated quickly with a No. 4 round bur to remove the old material and any caries that might be present in the dentin. A deep preparation in an axial direction commonly results, which requires the use of calcium hydroxide as an intermediary base.

After the internal portion of the preparation has been excavated and formed, the retentions are located with point angles in the cervical and incisal corners of the form. These retentions all diverge in order to lock the material into the cavity preparation. In some lesions the angle formers should be used to establish definite line angles and walls because these also produce access for placing the silicate in the point angles. Placing the cavosurface is the last phase of the cavity preparation, and after the marginal areas have been extended and opened, the refinement is completed with small sharp chisels.

A mylar matrix is needed with the Class III cavity preparation to exert pressure on the restoration and force it into the cavity preparation. The matrix is wedged firmly below the cervical wall of the cavity preparation and a suitable length of the material projects onto the labial and lingual surface to enable it to be grasped for holding the cement under pressure. The mylar is thick to produce the toughness required for pressure. The wedge is inserted far enough into the embrasure to separate the teeth, which enables the proper contour to be established in the proximal restoration.

The wood wedges must be custom-made for the tooth. They are placed below the cervical wall and trimmed similar to the amalgam wedge so as not to project or interfere with the contour of the restoration. The wedges are moistened for the stable matrix procedure. The wedge holds the mylar matrix while the cement is being prepared and minimizes the cervical flash when the material is inserted. For these reasons wedging the silicate restoration is as critical as the wedging procedures used with amalgam.

Silicate cement has limited applications in the Class V or gingival lesions and other smooth surface cavities. The silicate restorations in these areas cause disturbances in the gingival tissue and are abraded readily by toothbrushing. Because of these factors the extension of the preparation in a gingival direction is limited. The rule is to restore the labial or buccal lesion as a pit rather than to use the classic outline. Silicate is used in small hypoplastic areas located above the height of contour and in small lesions or defects that do not need to be placed below the healthy gingival tissue in caries-susceptible patients. In large Class V lesions other restorative materials are more suitable. Extension is limited so that a small area of natural tooth structure will remain between the restoration and the gingival tissue.

Smooth surface preparations present complications because of the inadequate matrices that are utilized to hold the silicate under pressure. Clamping devices and matrix retainers can be made of impression compound, but for the most part the result is not exceptional and the procedure is time-consuming. Class IV cavities that combine with gingival cavities are sometimes restored with a double right-angle mylar matrix, but because of the extensive surface exposure the silicate restoration has a limited clinical life. The blade of the cement instrument is commonly used for inserting the labial silicate restoration, and pressure is exerted with a cotton roll coated with cocoa butter. The method is inaccurate but is the only one that is not excessively time-consuming.

MIXING AND INSERTION

To obtain optimum physical properties as much powder as possible is incorporated into the silicate mix. This is accomplished by proportioning the powder, chilling the slab, using pressure during the mix, and confining the mixing to a small area of the slab. A mix with a "dough" consistency and a glistening surface is desired.

The slab is cooled by placing it under the cold water tap or by storing it in the refrigerator. The slab is dried and is continually wiped with a tissue until moisture no longer forms on the glass. A chilled, dry slab makes it possible to incorporate more powder into the acid. Two drops of acid are placed on the slab with the dropper after the solution has been agitated in order to mix the distilled water. The drops are placed near the center of the slab to allow the leverage to be placed and to prevent them from rolling off the glass. The powder is dispensed onto the slab. The portions are calibrated to blend with one drop, but extra powder should be available if it is possible to get it into the mix. The powder is placed into mounds by the dispenser. The second mound is divided and then quartered because these portions will be dropped into the liquid as they are needed.

The mix is made quickly and with pressure in the center of the slab. The mixing should be completed within 1 minute, inserted into the cavity during the following minute, and held under pressure during the initial setting for 5 minutes. The proportions of powder, starting with the largest first, are added to the liquid and mixed by a folding motion. The mixing is continued with each portion until the particles appear to be coated with acid. The remaining portions are placed into the mix and are folded over rapidly to develop the thick consistency and to incorporate most of the powder within 1 minute.

The silicate cement is picked up from the slab with the blade of the Tarno instrument and placed into the opening of the cavity preparation. The instrument is used to push the initial increment of cement against the axial wall and the next increment fills the cavity preparation. The matrix is then held on the lingual surface and the labial portion of the strip is pulled to better adapt the silicate and to exude the majority of the excess onto the labial surface.[15] The thumb and index finger are used to stabilize the matrix and to apply pressure for a period of 5 minutes. Clamping devices are sometimes used for this purpose, but the economy is questionable and the stability is not as satisfactory.

The strip and wedge are removed at the proper time and the silicate restoration is coated with cocoa butter. This prevents dehydration of the surface,

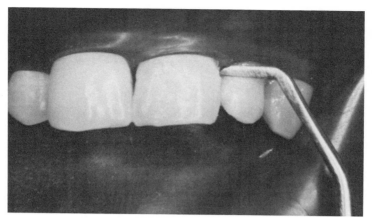

Fig. 11-7. Initial finishing of the silicate restoration is accomplished with the small gold knife.

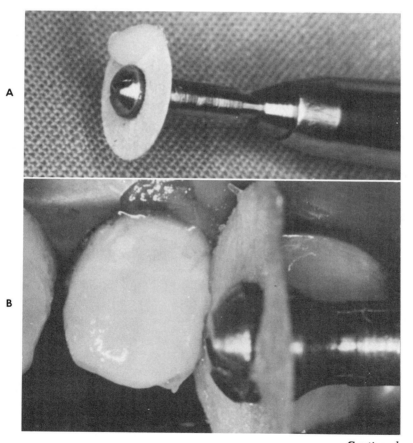

Continued.

Fig. 11-8. A, Cuttlefish finishing disk lubricated with cocoa butter. **B,** Smoothing the silicate restoration. Note the rounded mandrel head that is used for additional access. **C,** Finished silicate restoration on the distal surface of the lateral incisor. **D,** Silicate restoration 3 months postoperatively.

C 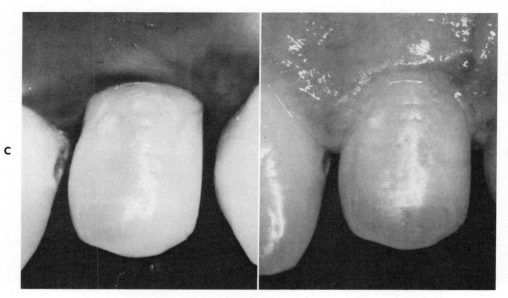 D

Fig. 11-8, cont'd. For legend see p. 361.

which is deleterious to the gel structure of the restoration. The restoration is kept covered with the protective coating for the remainder of the appointment.

FINISHING

The silicate restoration is delicate to finish in that the gel structure must not be damaged by excessive temperatures or dehydration.[16] If it is damaged, the restoration will stain and dissolve readily. It is necessary to refrain from polishing the restoration for at least 24 hours following insertion so that the gel structure will not be disturbed. After this interval has elapsed, the restoration is kept coated with cocoa butter and mild abrasives are used with light pressure. The initial finishing is done immediately after the strip is removed. The sharpened gold finishing knife is used to clear the excess out of the embrasures and roughly finish the restoration (Fig. 11-7). The cleoid carver can be used to shape the surface where the excess exists, taking care not to uncover a margin or a surface area that will appear in the restoration. The trimmed restoration is coated with cocoa butter or cavity varnish and the patient is dismissed after being told to protect the silicate from stress for a number of hours.

The silicate is smoothed at a subsequent appointment (Fig. 11-8). Only as much polishing as is necessary is done to produce the smooth surface, and it will not actually appear polished. The final contour in the embrasure and the surface is produced with the proximal gold knife and the cleoid instrument. The margins are located by using the ½ inch fine cuttlefish sandpaper disk in the straight mandrel. The disk is lubricated with cocoa butter, and the polishing is done with the assistance of the air coolants. The margins and smooth surface are slowly developed by carefully applying the sandpaper disks.

SUMMARY

1. The silicate restoration is a commonly used anterior restorative material. It is indicated when esthetics are involved because it is tooth-colored. It is also helpful in preventing recurrent caries because fluoride seeps into the tooth structure. These are the main reasons for the extensive use of the material.

2. Silicate cement is difficult to manipulate in that the gel structure is minimized by proper proportioning and mixing. This sound technique serves to check the solubility and staining of the restoration. Trituration of the silicate is recommended as a result of the mixing difficulties.

3. Finishing procedures for the restoration protect the gel structure by minimizing the temperature and preventing dehydration.

4. The complete dental practice must include a suitable silicate cement restorative service. Indications for use of the material include caries problems, replacements, and moisture complications.

REFERENCES

1. Skinner, E., and Phillips, R. W.: The science of dental materials, ed. 6, Philadelphia, 1967, W. B. Saunders Co.
2. Paffenbarger, G. C.: Silicate cement: an investigation by a group of practicing dentists under the direction of the A.D.A. research fellowship at the National Bureau of Standards, J.A.D.A. 27:1611, 1940.
3. Henschel, C. J.: Observations concerning in vivo disintegration of silicate cement restorations, J. Dent. Res. 28:528, 1947.
4. Phillips, R. W., and Swartz, M. L.: Effect of certain restorative materials on the solubility of enamel, J.A.D.A. 54:632, 1957.
5. Paffenbarger, G. C., Schoonover, I. C., and Souder, W.: Dental silicate cements: physical and chemical properties and a specification, J.A.D.A. 25:32, 1938.
6. Paffenbarger, G. C., and Stanford, J.: Zinc phosphate and silicate cement, Dent. Clin. N. Am., Nov., 1958, pp. 561-569.
7. Norman, R. D., Swartz, M. L., and Phillips, R. W.: Studies on the solubility of certain dental materials, J. Dent. Res. 36:977, 1957.
8. Specification No. 9 for dental silicate cement, guide to dental materials, ed. 3, Chicago, 1966, American Dental Association.
9. Hine, J. F., Swartz, M. L., and Phillips, R. W.: Staining of resin and silicate restorations by topically applied solutions of stannous fluoride, J. Periodont. 28:138, 1957.
10. Phillips, R. W., and Swartz, M. L.: Effect of fluorides on hardness of tooth enamel, J.A.D.A. 37:1, 1948.
11. Mitchell, D. F., Buonocore, M. G., and Shazer, S.: Pulp reaction to silicate cement and other materials: relation to cavity depth, J. Dent. Res. 41:591, 1962.
12. Hassan, E. H., Van Huysen, G., and Gilmore, H. W.: Deep cavity preparation and the tooth pulp, J. Prosth. Dent. 16:751, 1966.
13. Swartz, M. L., Phillips, R. W., and Chamberlain, N.: Continued studies on the permeability of cavity liners, J. Dent. Res. 41:66, 1962.
14. Phillips, R. W., Swartz, M. L., and Chong, W. F.: Properties of silicate cements mixed by hand and mechanical means, J. S. Calif. Dent. Assoc. 33:239, 1965.

15. Charbeneau, G. T.: The silicate restoration, a practical approach to serviceability, New York J. Dent. 31:231, 1961.
16. MacPherson, W. G., and Charbeneau, G. T.: Influence of surface finishing procedures upon solubility of silicate cement, J. Michigan Dent. Assoc. 44:306, 1962.

ADDITIONAL READINGS

Brannstrom, M., and Nyborg, H.: The presence of bacteria in cavities filled with silicate cement and composite resin materials, Sven. Tandlak. T. 64:149-155, 1971.

Habu, H., Fisher, T. E., and Appleton, J. H.: Dimensional changes of silicate cements, J. Nihon Univ. School Dent., vol. 12, no. 2, 1970.

Kent, E. B., Lewis, B. G., and Wilson, A. D.: Dental silicate cements: XIII. The crazing and dulling of the surface, J. Dent. Res. 50:393, 1971.

Norman, R. D., Swartz, M. L., and Phillips, R. W.: Studies on film thickness, solubility and marginal leakage of dental cements, J. Dent. Res. 42:950, 1963.

Wilson, A. D., Kent, B. E., Clinton, D., and Miller, R. P.: The formation and microstructure of dental silicate cements, J. Mater. Sci. 7:220, 1972.

chapter 12

Resin restorations

A new and controversial restorative material in operative dentistry is the direct-curing resin. Resins can produce esthetic restorations and serve many useful purposes. The physical properties of the material limit its use to areas of low stress, and the resin restorations should be protected by sound tooth structure whenever possible. Acrylic resins were first used in Europe and have been a subject of controversy since their introduction in the United States in 1946. Reports that resin can produce an altered relationship with tooth structure gave rise to speculation on the possibility of developing a chemical bond that would result in a perfectly sealed restoration.[1] In the past few years there has been much interest in the development of an adhesive restorative material, and various types of resins have been evaluated for this purpose.

The esthetic quality of the resin restoration is its greatest attribute (Fig. 12-1). Many other desirable properties of the material have not been adequately explored, but the extensive clinical use of resin and postoperative observations provide a means of further evaluation. Resin restorations are found to last longer than the silicate cement restorations and to produce a smoother surface and better margin. There are indications that recurrent caries is not as prevalent with resin as was previously suspected. However, long-term, well-controlled studies must be conducted to determine the clinical efficacy of the resin restoration.

The introduction of the acrylic resin restoration resulted in rapid and widespread use of the material. At first the resins were considered a panacea for operative dentistry, and many restorations were placed before the material was fully evaluated. This led to an abuse of resin restorations and resulted in slipshod operating methods according to present-day standards. The resin materials used at that time were not sensitive to moisture and were slow setting, resulting in poorly adapted restorations. The initial materials were slow-setting, benzoyl peroxide catalyst compounds. Although these compounds polymerized, they did not adapt to tooth structure. The resulting polymerization shrinkage and dietary temperature changes caused gross discrepancies and a prevalence of

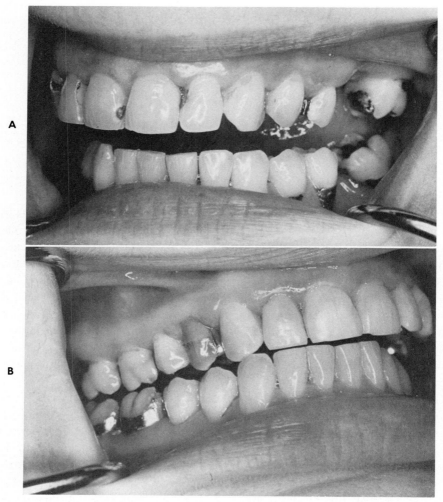

Fig. 12-1. A, Defective silicate restorations and recurrent caries. **B,** Six-month postoperative appearance of sulfinic catalyst resins.

recurrent caries.[2] The leaking restorations severely damaged the teeth and resulted in a need for replacement. The clinical result of this procedure was that the restoration commonly lasted only for a period of 5 years, which gave the acrylic restoration a bad reputation that still persists. The issue concerning the use of resin has been paramount in the field, and the misunderstanding should be resolved because of the value of the material in the practice of operative dentistry.

Hedegard[3] documented the behavior of the acrylic restoration when undesirable operating conditions were used. In his survey of the use of acrylic resins he observed numerous operators in the Scandinavian countries who placed approximately 400 restorations. Within 2 years the restorations were removed and the presence of recurrent caries or odorous dentin was recorded. Hedegard pointed out how the material was being abused.

Directions for manipulating the different compounds have been formulated and they must be followed carefully. The resins require a sensitive technique, with attention being directed to the timing of the polymerization. Adjusting the timing of mixing and insertion to the condition of the cavity preparation is considered essential when using acrylic resin. The new resin materials that polymerize rapidly enable the operator to completely finish and polish the restoration at the time it is inserted. It is then possible to evaluate the result and be certain that the marginal relationships necessary for a good restoration exist.

Several types of resins are used for an individual tooth restoration. According to the literature, resins are similar to the polymethyl methacrylate compounds used in prosthetic dentistry. The main difference is in the catalyst systems; the compounds employed in operative dentistry polymerize much faster than the denture base materials. The use of heat-cured acrylic inlays cemented into the preparation were advocated during the early years. This procedure failed because of the low strength of the acrylic inlay; therefore it is no longer considered acceptable except as a temporary restoration for a gold casting.

The resins selected for operative procedures are classified into three groups according to their catalyst systems. The quick-curing compound has a monomer and polymer that are dispensed as a powder and a liquid. The powder is polymethyl methacrylate, which has some acceleratory, inhibitory, and caries-preventive agents. The liquid is also methyl methacrylate and it possesses the catalyst agent that initiates polymerization. The composite resins are different; they are discussed as a group later in the chapter. The three resin compounds referred to are the sulfinic acid and benzoyl peroxide catalysts and the composite resins.

The compounds are classified into slow- and fast-setting materials according to their catalyst systems. Benzoyl peroxide is used as the catalyst in the slow-setting materials, which have a polymerization time of 24 hours.[4] These compounds do not develop good marginal adaptation, which means they are best suited for temporary coverage. Temporary jacket crowns can be made by confining the slow-setting material in celluloid crown forms and placing it on the tooth. After the initial polymerization the crown is removed, trimmed to contour, and cemented over the preparation with zinc oxide–eugenol cement. The acrylic bridge temporary restorations are the benzoyl peroxide catalyst resins that have been plasticized to provide a stretchable material. These also must be trimmed and retained with a sedative cement because of the undesirable marginal relationship that results from polymerization. Temporary acrylic restorations can provide an esthetic service and fulfill other purposes of interim restorations.

The resin that is advocated for restoring the tooth is the compound activated

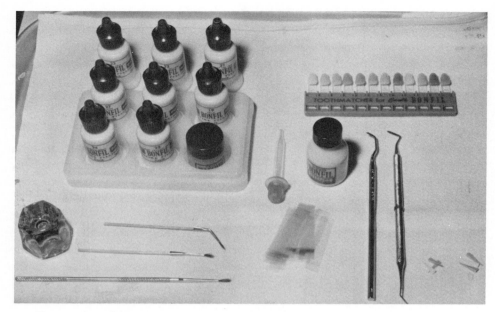

Fig. 12-2. Armamentarium for sulfinic acid resin—monomer, polymer, brushes, and shade guide.

by sulfinic acid (Fig. 12-2). The polymerization time is between 5 and 12 minutes.[5] The rapid curing makes it possible to produce an adapted resin restoration that can be directly finished and polished. The chemical and physical properties of the sulfinic acid resins are similar to those of the other resins, the main difference being the rapid polymerization. These resins are tooth-colored and can be finished immediately after insertion without disturbing the material. Although the composite resins are also finished directly, they have limited use as compared to the sulfinic catalyst materials.

PHYSICAL PROPERTIES

A textbook on dental materials should be consulted to study the physical properties of resin materials.[6] However, a few properties that manifest the necessary characteristics of and indications for using the material will be discussed here. Most of the physical properties of the resin materials are undesirable, the greatest problem being their low strength. Their degree of hardness (18 to 20 Knoop) is very low when compared to metal restorative materials and to tooth structure. The strength value is too low to resist the forces of mastication, and the restorations must therefore be protected from functional forces.

Another undesirable property of acrylic resins is their low resistance to abrasion. Improper toothbrushing and use of abrasives will quickly wear down the restoration, resulting in a faulty contour and tooth sensitivity. The lack of resistance to abrasive particles in the diet is demonstrated by the worn appearance of larger restorations that have been in service for a period of time.

Modulus of elasticity values, a measure of stiffness, are low as compared to other materials. Its low modulus of elasticity indicates that resin will bend under stress more readily than will other restorative materials. When the Class IV resin restoration is used to replace a missing tooth angle, it will become displaced because of the low modulus of elasticity. When force is placed on the Class IV restoration, the material bends away from the tooth structure and is dislodged.

The dimensional stability of resin restorations has been the subject of much discussion and research. During polymerization there is a linear shrinkage of 7% to 15%, which if not controlled alters the adaptation of the material to the tooth.[7] Also water sorption in the oral cavity causes a dimensional change in the restoration. Although measurements indicate that the expansion from water sorption is only 0.5%, it is an additional dimensional change associated with acrylic resins that must be considered. Water sorption in itself has been termed clinically insignificant since the slight expansion is completed within 24 hours.

Much discussion centers on the dimensional change associated with temperature variations. The coefficient of expansion of resin is established as seven times greater than that of tooth structure. The term "marginal percolation" was applied to resin materials because of the gross discrepancies caused by the slow-polymerizing compounds.[2] In one study teeth with resin restorations were extracted and 200μ spaces were observed between the restoration and tooth structure. The results of this study naturally served to decrease the popularity of the resins.

All factors influencing dimensional change should affect marginal adaptation. As previously discussed, the leakage around restorations can be studied in many ways. The use of radioactive isotopes, which appears to be the most critical approach, does not demonstrate a poor adaptation with the sulfinic acid compounds.[8] Studies on the influence of temperature changes on these resins have not shown an additional amount of leakage, a fact that favors the clinical use of resin. When the adaptation produced by resin is compared to that produced by other types of materials, the resins should not be condemned on the basis that they cannot seal the cavity preparation adequately.

Clinical leakage around the sulfinic acid resin restoration is difficult to detect. Thin black or brown stain lines attributed to fluoride applications can be found, but gross leakage, characterized by discoloration of the tooth, is not often observed. Quick-setting resin restorations that have been in service for as long as 5 years do not often exhibit recurrent caries, which is another indication that a relatively good seal is maintained with the enamel and dentin. These findings indicate that thermal dimensional change is not as great a problem as was originally thought.

The sealing ability of the resin restoration is assisted by the wettability of

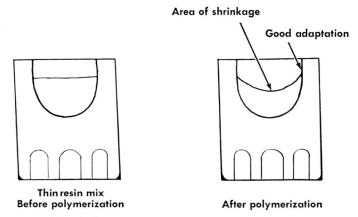

Fig. 12-3. Diagram illustrating adaptation mechanism with thin resin flow mix. (Courtesy Dr. D. A. Boyd.)

the mix (Fig. 12-3). A thin mix allows good interlocking of the resin with the roughened cavity wall and the retentive undercuts. The material is quickly inserted to wet the cavity wall. When recurrent caries occurs, it does so where loose restorations or open margins exist. Although the resin restoration is an unstable material with many undesirable properties, an acceptable result can be obtained when the restoration is protected from stress and temperature changes.

A desirable property of the "plastics" is their insolubility in oral fluids. This is a serious problem with silicate cement, but the resins are soluble only in solutions of ether and acetone. This makes the material resistant to the attacks of acids and other ingested solutions that tend to dissolve or stain the cements.

Because they are insoluble and have a short polymerization time, the resin restorations do not change chemically to any extent following the curing cycle. Some resins have 2% sodium fluoride added to the polymer to reduce the enamel solubility. The fluoride acts as a caries-preventive agent in this manner. The fluoride is deposited in the first few seconds after contacting the cavity wall and causes a 25% reduction in the solubility of the tooth, which is close to the value obtained with silicate cement.[9] The fluoride additive and the improved adaptation undoubtedly act to prevent secondary caries.

The effect of moisture on the resins is considered another undesirable property of the material.[10] The sulfinic acid resin is soluble in water, which makes it necessary to place the material in a dry cavity. Any moisture from saliva interferes with the polymerization and produces a soft surface on the restoration. Moisture contamination results in insufficient adaptation, which makes it necessary to use a hermetic rubber dam for the insertion.

One outstanding feature of the resin restoration is the esthetic service it provides. Many shades are possible because of the translucency of the resin materials. The various shades are produced by placing metallic oxides (tin and iron oxides) on the polymer particles by a ball-milling process. Many shades are included in kits, but the operator will find that only a few are used to mix and match many variations of tooth color. The shades vary according to their saturation of gray, brown, or yellow. Shades are selected similar to the selection of prosthetic teeth. The tooth should be wet and viewed in natural daylight when comparing it with the shade guide. Proper esthetics in shade selection can also be obtained by combining the polymers to make up individual differences. The size of the tooth, the extent of the restoration, the angulation of the tooth, and the location of the cavity preparation will influence the desirable shade of the restoration.

A property worthy of mention is the smooth surface obtainable with resin restorations. The polish produced by the use of abrasives is an additional aid to esthetics because a smooth surface and accurate margin make the tooth less susceptible to staining and discoloration. A smooth surface, which remains for the life of the restoration, also enhances patient comfort.

INDICATIONS FOR RESIN

Large Class III lesions and defective proximal restorations. The extent of damage to the labial wall of the cavity preparation dictates the needed esthetics. The use of gold materials is not feasible in extensive lesions with open labial walls. Resin can be used if care is taken to prevent excessive stress on the material.

Small Class III lesions. When caries is not a problem, resin can be used to make the restoration, especially if the use of gold foil is not indicated and appearance is a consideration.

Gingival lesions. Resin is the material of choice when esthetics is important and when a deep axial lesion exists because tooth-colored material must be used and the restoration must be placed under soft tissue. Unlike silicate cements, the smooth surface provided by resin restorations is compatible with gingival health.

Class IV lesions. Restoration with resin is indicated in Class IV lesions when no other material can be used. Incisal edges should be shaped for esthetics only and not for functional purposes. Stresses from the incisal guidance will dislodge the restoration or abrade the corner. It is possible to retain the restoration by stainless steel wires, but even when this technique is employed, the restoration and the opposing tooth should be adjusted so that they will not collide.

Castings and crown forms. Castings and crown forms can be veneered with resin material, but in some cases proper shading is difficult. In instances of extensive labial and incisal damage a gold casting is used with an acrylic veneer. In a few years after restoration with an acrylic veneer crown the resin will require replacement because of discoloration. Short-lived esthetic results are produced by using resin as a veneer on inlays.

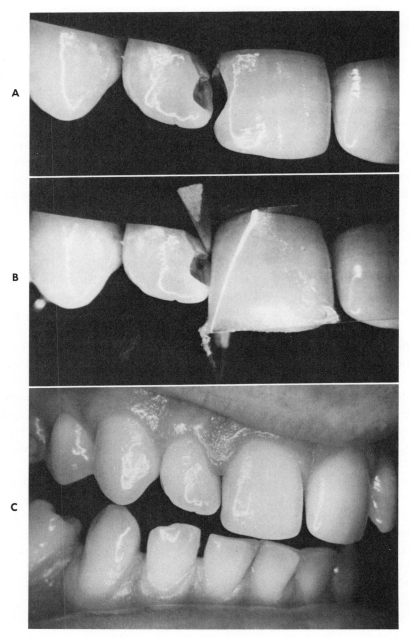

Fig. 12-4. A, Cavity preparations, showing Black's outline, squared walls, acute margins, and bulky point angles. **B,** Polymerized flow mix in the central incisor. Note position of the wood wedge. **C,** Postoperative appearance after 1½ years.

Small enamel defects or hypoplastic areas. These defects sometimes occur above the height of contour near the incisal or occlusal surface. If the defect is not directly visible or is in an area of stress, resin can be used as a restorative, but it may need to be replaced occasionally.

Different types of temporary restorative procedures. The use of different types of acrylic crown and bridge temporary restorations can produce immediate esthetic results. Teeth of questionable prognosis are best restored with these procedures because of pulpal or periodontal considerations. Numerous applications of resin are helpful in cases of vital fractured permanent incisor teeth.

CAVITY PREPARATION

Cavity preparations are designed to complement the physical properties of resins. The weak, soft resin material requires support from surrounding tooth structure. Proper access to the preparation is necessary to insert the restoration and to finish the margins. The cavity preparation should be made with the exacting techniques employed for other types of restorations; however, certain phases are not as important because of the lack of stress on the surface of the restoration.

Outline form. The outline form is not as critical as when gold restoratives are used because the tooth-colored resin is inconspicuous. The extension of the outline is dictated by the location of immune areas on the tooth. Although fluoride additives are beneficial in reducing enamel solubility, it is desirable to place the margins where they can be easily cleaned. The margins must be visible because of the flash that develops from the wet compound and because it is difficult to trim the material from the tooth.

The preferred outline for anterior proximal restorations is the design advocated by Black (Fig. 12-4). The labial margin is curved slightly to permit some degree of opening. The lingual margin is usually extended to one half of the marginal ridge to allow for insertion of the resin. The gingival margin should be extended to an area not in contact with the adjacent tooth and should be accessible for finishing. In cases of gingival recession the preparation should not be unduly extended to locate the gingival wall under the soft tissue.

The outline form of the gingival cavity has similar characteristics, and the oval shape designed by Black[11] is used. Limited but adequate extension should be used to place the margins in protected areas. The No. 212 gingival rubber dam clamp is applied and stabilized with impression compound. The location of the gingival tissue should be noted before isolation in order to judge the amount of extension required. The walls in contact with the gingiva are located according to the contour and are placed under the tissue (mesial, distal, and gingival walls). The occlusal margin is placed just above the height of contour and the occlusal wall becomes a gentle curve to blend in with the other walls. The outline form is rounded to prevent formation of thin layers of plastic that may fracture during finishing.

Outline forms are planned and located with exacting movements. A smooth, straight enamel margin is obtained by removing the enamel projections. This procedure is necessary to guide the enamel wall finishing.

Resistance form. The depth of the preparations should extend to the dentin to provide retention, to assure a thickness of the restorative material, and to protect the pulp tissue. The cavity wall should be uniform in thickness and extension to produce the bulk in the mortise form needed for the resistance form. Whenever possible the surrounding enamel walls should be perpendicular to the axial dentin to provide additional resistance form.

To produce a smooth preparation the enamel wall is refined to a uniform thickness. The cavosurface is also smoothed and finished to an acute sharp angle that eliminates the bevels. A definite junction is then produced with the resin, and it facilitates the finishing and produces a satisfactory margin.

Retention form. Retention is accomplished by mechanical undercuts. Retention forms should be located in an area of the tooth where the pulp will not be damaged; usually the corners of the preparation are suitable locations. All undercuts and retention forms should be located in dentin. Since retention of the restoration cannot be accomplished by the use of mechanical undercuts only, it is necessary to place adequate resistance forms by properly designing the cavity walls.

The retentive undercuts are termed point angles. They should be slightly enlarged to allow proper flow of the resin. The retentions need not be as refined as the convenience points for direct gold restorations, but they should be placed in strategic locations and must be of adequate size to allow good retention.

Toilet of the cavity. Of equal importance is the cleanliness of the cavity preparation. The deleterious effect of moisture has been discussed, but it is necessary to consider the effects of other debris that might have seeped inside the preparation. Soilage occurs with the use of the rubber dam and in some cases results in accumulation of blood, saliva, and tooth grindings inside the cavity preparation. This debris must be removed prior to insertion of the resin because it contributes to discoloration of the restoration. The reduction of hemoglobin in the blood produces a black stain on the cavity walls, which can be noticed following the appointment as a dark halo around the margin of the restoration.

A cotton pellet moistened with water is suitable for cleaning the cavity preparation and tooth surfaces immediately surrounding the area. Caustic drugs and solutions or oil-based medicaments should not be used because of possible pulp irritation and interference with the catalyst of the resin. After the preparation is washed, it should be dried with blasts of warm air. The retention forms are cleaned out with a sharp explorer. The cavity preparation should be closely inspected to make certain all contaminates have been removed. Hydrogen peroxide can be used as a cleaning agent if excessive seepage has occurred.

• • •

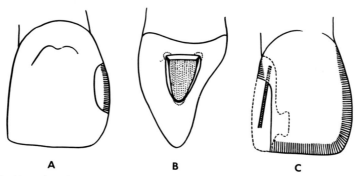

Fig. 12-5. A, Lingual outline for Class III resin preparation. **B,** Proximal view of Class III resin preparation with emphasis on retention. **C,** Class IV resin preparation with pin support.

In summary, the following points concerning cavity preparation should be remembered.

1. The outline form is limited in extension but must be placed in immune areas of the tooth. The design of the outline form is not demanding because resin is tooth-colored. Rounded outlines are preferred to eliminate formation of thin edges of the material.
2. For the resistance form, cavity walls should be made uniform in thickness and placed at angles to develop a preparation with "boxlike" qualities. The cavosurface should form a precise, acute angle on the enamel.
3. Retention is accomplished by bulky undercuts placed in the corner of the preparation in the dentin.
4. In the toilet of the cavity the preparation should be cleaned with water and dried with warm air. The cavity preparation must be dry to allow polymerization of the resin (Fig. 12-5).

Instrumentation

Class III cavity preparation

1. For initial opening of the tooth the unsupported enamel is removed from the labial surface with a small chisel and from the lingual surface with a small hatchet. Excavation of caries or defective restorations is accomplished with a round bur in a contra-angle handpiece through the lingual access. A No. 2 or No. 4 round bur is selected for the excavation, depending on the size of the axial wall damage.

2. A No. 15 Wedelstaedt chisel is used to remove the unsupported enamel to establish a rough outline form. The mesial and distal cutting edges are reversed and used on the labial and lingual surface, depending on the surface exposure of the lesion.

3. A No. 33½ inverted cone bur in a straight handpiece is used to establish the final outline form. The bur is inserted from both the labial and lingual sur-

face to prepare each side of the preparation. The end cutters of the bur are used to cut and square the gingival wall. The side cutters are used to plane the labial and lingual walls and to establish the angulation of these structures. A moistened wood wedge may be needed to mechanically depress the rubber dam and tissue away from the desired extension in the gingival wall.

4. Retention forms are placed in the three corners of the preparation with a No. ½ round bur in a contra-angle handpiece. Each point angle is made to the depth of the head of the bur and diverges from the center of the axial walls. The direction of this cutting is away from the pulp, which places the undercuts lateral to the enamel plates.

5. A small angle former (No. 2½-7-9) is used to enlarge the entrance of the point angle, providing access for the resin to flow into the point angle. Pyramidal forms should not be produced, but an adequate size is established in the retention. The point angle is left rounded to form the mechanical locks.

6. The refinement of the cavity preparation is accomplished with a resharpened No. 15 Wedelstaedt chisel. The enamel wall and the cavosurface margin are smoothed with the instrument.

Class V cavity preparation

1. The No. 212 rubber dam clamp is stabilized to retain the rubber dam and to deflect the gingiva. The lesion or defective restoration is excavated with a No. 2 or No. 4 round bur to determine the extent of the carious damage. If grossly undermined plates are present, they should be removed with a small Wedelstaedt chisel. This will provide access for the bur to remove the caries.

2. Cavity extension is completed with a No. 557 bur. A straight handpiece should be used whenever possible for added control in cutting the tooth. The bur is turned on the gingival, mesial, and distal walls to flare the preparation in order to compensate for the abrupt turning of the enamel inclination. Well-supported enamel will be prepared by mastering these movements.

3. A No. 33½ bur is used to place lateral undercuts in the four corners of the preparation. Only a lateral movement of the bur is employed to undercut the dentin to the depth of the side cutters. This retention is adequate and nothing else is done to undermine the enamel walls. Additional movements produce sensitivity and weaken tooth structure.

4. A No. 15 Wedelstaedt chisel is employed to finish the enamel walls and to establish the cavosurface relationship. Rounding and smoothing of the axial wall can be accomplished with the distal cutting edge of the instrument. This provides definite line angles (not undercut) and sets the angulation of the walls to complement resistance form of the restoration. The preparation is cleaned in the usual manner.

5. Small pit cavities, hypoplastic areas, enamel defects, and soft white spots can be prepared almost entirely with the No. 557 bur. The same rules apply to these preparations in that the cavosurface must be sharp and the enamel walls

must have definite angles and possess slight undercuts for retention. The refinement of these small preparations is done with a slowly revolving fissure bur and a very light load on the handpiece.

Pulp protection

Cavity preparations with axial walls deeper than 0.5 mm. inside the dentinoenamel junction should receive a protective base. The material of choice is calcium hydroxide and it is used to cover the small, undetected exposures and present a firm wall to abut the restoration. The base need not extend back to the desired axial depth but must thoroughly coat and protect the dentin in the excavation. The capping material should not be left on the enamel wall or in the retention forms. A calcium hydroxide compound that does not contain oil should be used because of the danger of inhibiting polymerization of the resin.

Other types of bases and liners do not serve as adequately as calcium hydroxide. Varnish is dissolved by the monomer and polymerization is altered. Zinc phosphate cement can cause pulp irritation in the deep cavity. For these reasons calcium hydroxide is preferred when an intermediary base is indicated with the resin restoration.

Matrices

The high degree of flow associated with resins complicates the matrix technique in proximal restorations. The material must be confined to produce the bulk to compensate for the polymerization shrinkage and to prevent movement from the cavity wall during the curing. Pressure cannot be exerted on the matrix because of the negative contour and excessive flash that develops. A thin, pliable matrix that can be stabilized is required for the sulfinic catalyst resins.

Plastic strips provided commercially with each compound are advocated for the matrix technique. They should be curved and cut in half to prevent excessive material from complicating proper closing of the matrix. The strips are inserted below the gingival wall and wedged firmly against sound tooth structure. A moistened wood wedge, previously trimmed to shape, will secure the strip and serve to slightly separate the teeth. Separation also helps to compensate for polymerization shrinkage and assures an adequate amount of restorative material in the contact area. The strip and matrix should not be removed until the recommended curing time is completed.

This procedure is used for Class III and some Class IV restorations. Extremely large Class IV restorations require plastic crown forms, which will be described later in this chapter.

The Class V restoration is placed without a matrix because it is almost impossible to apply an acceptable matrix in a cervical preparation. The brush technique or multiple flow mixes are used for the gingival restoration. These techniques are executed successfully without the use of a matrix.

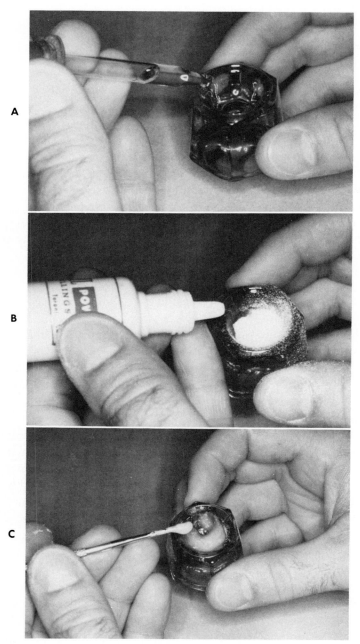

Fig. 12-6. A, To make the flow mix, 5 drops of monomer are placed in the small end of the dappen dish. **B,** The solution is saturated with polymer and the excess powder is discarded. **C,** The shade guide flow mix is made by adding 2 more drops of monomer and stirring the solution with the sable brush.

MIXING PROCEDURES

Techniques have been devised to quickly place the resin into the cavity preparation before polymerization begins. The flow mix method and the brush method are used for the sulfinic acid compounds. Both techniques require rapid insertion to obtain acceptable adaptation. The wettability of the mixes used in both methods encourages good interlocking of the resin to the cavity wall, and when this occurs, the polymerization shrinkage takes place on the surface of the restoration instead of away from the cavity walls. This is referred to as the directional path for curing and is only accomplished by a flow mix or brush application of the resin.

Flow mix method. The quick-setting resins must be mixed in a dappen dish (Fig. 12-6). The saturation method is used to estimate the amount of polymer needed. Five drops of liquid are placed in a dappen dish and the polymer powder is quickly saturated with the solution. The dish is continually tapped as the powder is dispensed to incorporate as much polymer as possible. Upon saturation the excess polymer is dumped off the top of the dish, two more drops of monomer are added, and the solution is stirred for a few seconds to develop a homogeneous consistency. The small end of the dappen dish is used to facilitate picking up the resin for insertion.

The mix is completed and standardized in 30 seconds by using this procedure. The resin must be placed into the preparation and the strip pulled down onto the margin before polymerization advances past the flow stage. This must be done within 1 minute of the start of the mix.[11] A brush is used to carry the mixed resin to the tooth. The material is picked up in the brush bristles and rotated into the cavity preparation to minimize air being trapped inside the preparation. Proper timing and strip closure produces a restoration with an acceptable adaptation.

The flow properties of the sulfinic catalyst resin produces a material that cannot be bulk-packed into the cavity preparation. This consistency requires that a nonpressure technique be used for the flow mix or the restoration will be displaced from the preparation and result in faulty contour. In the preferred method the thin, pliable matrix with the wood wedge placed to separate the teeth and to hold the strip is employed. An excessive amount of mixed resin is placed through the labial opening to overfill the cavity form. The lingual strip is closed and is held in place by the index finger in the lingual concavity of the tooth. The labial strip is slowly and carefully pulled down onto the margin so that a minimum excessive contour will result. This prevents air entrapment and allows enough material to remain so that the preparation will not be undercontoured after polymerization shrinkage.

The strip is held in a fixed position for 2 minutes. This is done so as not to disturb the adaptation by moving the resin away from the cavity wall. After 2 minutes the strip will not require additional support because the setting will hold the matrix on the surface of the tooth. At the end of a 5- to 6-minute period the strip is removed and the restoration can be finished.

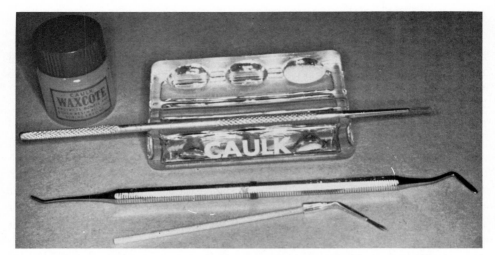

Fig. 12-7. Tray and instruments necessary for Nealon technique. The tray has two places for monomer and one for polymer.

Brush method (Nealon technique). This procedure was designed for the slow-setting benzoyl peroxide catalyst resins.[12] Originally better adaptation was attributed to this method when the slow-setting compounds were used, but the technique is also applicable with the fast-setting compounds. In the Nealon technique a sable brush is passed from monomer to polymer and applied to the cavity preparation (Fig. 12-7). Beads of resin formed on the pointed bristles are repeatedly placed on the cavity walls to replace the volumetric loss by polymerization with each successive increment. Numerous applications are needed to complete the restoration.

The brush technique is used when it is difficult to apply a matrix. The cervical lesion is usually restored with this procedure (Fig. 12-8). Large Class IV restorations are placed by stabilizing a clear plastic crown form that has had the labial surface excised. The form is filled with resin using the brush technique because of the difficulty of applying the regular strip matrix around the missing incisal angle.

With the brush method the surface of the restoration is excessively contoured. The resin is then coated with a protective film, which is usually supplied by the manufacturer, to prevent evaporation of the monomer. This ensures adequate polymerization on the surface of the restoration.

The brush method necessitates the use of a special tray with three depressions, or several dappen dishes can be used. Two sections of the tray are filled with monomer and the third is filled with the selected polymer. Plain monomer is placed into the preparation to wet the tooth structure. The brush is cleaned in the first monomer solution and passed on to the second monomer to pick up the necessary drops. The brush is then touched to the polymer and a bead forms that

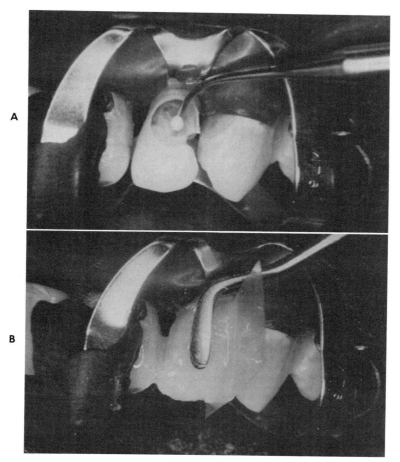

Fig. 12-8. A, Applying calcium hydroxide to the axial dentin wall. **B,** Adding wax coating to the surface of the brushed-in resin.

is placed into the cavity preparation. Every few seconds the procedure is repeated until an excess contour is produced. When the building process is finished, the surface is coated. After 5 to 8 minutes the polymerization is complete and the restoration can be finished. This is also a nonpressure method and each increment replaces the volume lost on the surface from the polymerization.

Large Class IV and V restorations can be placed by using multiple flow mixes. Each successive mix is applied after the surface of the buildup loses its shine. Two or three mixes can be used for extremely large restorations. The last mix is not covered with a matrix and therefore must be coated with the protective film employed with the brush method.

The matrix employed for the large Class IV restoration or the fractured incisor is the clear plastic crown form. The labial wall of the crown form is partly removed with curved scissors and is then placed interproximally in the preparation and wedged for stability and the recommended separation. The matrix is shaped closely to the desired form for the resin restoration.

The brush method is used to insert the resin through the labial opening in the crown form. The beads of resin are first placed in the lingual-cervical area to fill in the retentions and to coat the support wire. The contour is developed gradually in the restoration and the results should produce an excess and overlapping of the material in the labial margin of the cavity preparation. The protective coating is applied over the exposed surface. After a required setting time of 5 to 8 minutes, the restoration is finished in the conventional manner.

CLASS IV RESIN RESTORATIONS

As previously mentioned, it is not ideal to restore the Class IV lesion with resin restorations, but there are instances when no other material can be used to repair the tooth. The dental profession has always desired an enamel-colored material strong enough to rebuild the incisal corner on the tooth. The resin restoration is not capable of withstanding the stresses placed on these areas; therefore, adjustments must be made in the restoration to lessen or completely prevent stress on the resin. Caries often occurs on the proximal surfaces of anterior teeth, undermining the incisal edge of the tooth. When stress is placed on the undermined enamel, the edge fractures and the corner must be restored to maintain the mesial-distal dimension of the tooth and to improve esthetics.

Many times anterior teeth are fractured by accident. Particularly in young patients, these teeth cannot be restored with full-coverage restorations unless endodontic procedures are performed for the vital remaining tooth structure. It is impossible to place full-coverage restorations and jacket or veneer crowns on all fractured angle teeth. Economic factors, pulp conditions, and growth factors may also prevent the use of this type of restoration. Since the very young patient has a large labial and lingual extension of the pulp chamber because the tooth has not been in function for a long period, a full-coverage restoration would damage the vital pulp. As a stop-gap measure and as a means of providing good esthetics the Class IV resin restoration is applicable in these cases. The resin restoration can be used alone or in conjunction with wires retained by the tooth that serve to enhance the retention and resistance form. The material also can be used to veneer gold castings of different types or it can be placed inside stainless steel crowns, which are useful in pedodontic procedures for teeth that have been traumatically injured. These methods produce esthetic resin restorations that can remain in use until the pulp recedes or until vitality is established in injured teeth.

When resin is used entirely as the restorative material, the cavity preparation is not too different from the procedure for Class III restorations. The gingival two thirds of the preparation is the same, with the exception of increasing retention forms to give some added support to the restoration. The incisal portion is cleaned and smoothed to remove unsupported and weak enamel. The incisal portion is cleaved until sound dentin is found supporting the incisal edge of enamel. Usually the labial outline form of this preparation is made into a straight line so that the restoration is unnoticeable after the restoration is finished. Difficulties often arise in placing adequate incisal retention. Because of the type of fracture line or the lack of sound dentin, the point angle might be included as for the Class III preparation. There will not be as much undercut in the incisal point angle because the incisal enamel is more undermined and in some cases a support wire is employed. Smooth complete rods are required in this cavity preparation and all of the other principles previously described must be applied to the Class IV cavity preparation.

The Class IV restoration can be contoured on the labial and incisal surfaces to conform to the arch and fulfill the anatomic needs of the individual tooth. Correct incisal guidance requires that the lingual surface of the restoration be shaved adequately and taken out of contact with the teeth in the opposing arch during the movements of the mandible. This will prevent wear on the incisal edge of the restoration as well as prevent dislodgment of the restoration from the cavity preparation. All the adjustments are made on the lingual surface and therefore will not be visible.

Auxiliary supports

Different types of pins can be used to aid the Class IV resin restoration. Most pins are made of stainless steel and are secured in the dentin inside the cervical wall. The pins are hidden in the mass of the restoration by being placed more to the lingual half of the tooth. This is done by making the pin parallel to the lingual surface of the incisor tooth and locating the pinhole just in front of the lingual-gingival point angle. Different types of pins are employed and in some cases the wires are shaped at right angles to support portions of the incisal edge where extensive trauma has occurred.

However, the pins do not enhance the strength of the resin restorative material. It is believed that they do improve the retention and resistance forms of the restoration, thereby preventing dislodgment of the material from the cavity preparation. Pins can also be used in large gingival restorations but are more commonly applied to the Class IV restoration. The procedure to place the pins is relatively simple and can be accomplished in a short period of time. The use of pins should be considered in an extensive Class IV restoration in order to improve the effectiveness of the service and to add support to sulfinic catalyst resins.

The wire employed for the grossly fractured incisor is that advocated by Markley, which is also used for amalgam restorations (Fig. 12-9). This technique requires a definite armamentarium and procedure, which were previously described in the discussion of the large amalgam restoration. The most critical pinhole is located in the cervical wall and must be placed in dentin tissue at a depth of 1.5 mm. This is as deep as the pinholes for posterior teeth. The

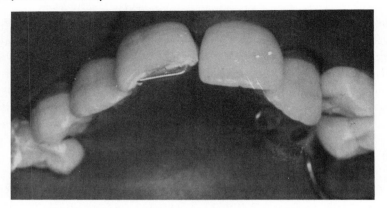

Fig. 12-9. Cemented wire on proximal and incisal surfaces.

anterior posthole is more difficult because there is less tooth structure. The stainless steel wire can be shaped at angles and also cemented on the incisal surface. This procedure is not possible with curved pins because the tooth can be fractured. The wires can be made to bend around the missing angle and can be stabilized at both ends.

The initial pinhole is made with a No. ½ round bur in the dentinal tissue just labial to the lingual-gingival point angle. This small hole is made only 0.5 mm. in depth, which guides the twist drill that cuts the nontapering pinhole. This pinhole is made to a depth of 1.5 mm. and the wire, which is threaded for retentive purposes, is adjusted for the proper length and stability in the posthole. Adjustments of the wire can be made with pliers or separating disks and should be perfected prior to the cementation.

Zinc phosphate is used for cementation and the mix should be made to be consistent with the seating of castings. The Lentulo spiral used for endodontic purposes is placed in the cement and then into the posthole and turned abruptly to spin the cement into the retention for holding the wire. The wire is then inserted, and as soon as the cement sets, the tooth is prepared according to the principles previously outlined. It is important not to bend the wire after it has been secured in tooth structure. This is especially true in the Class IV restoration because the cervical enamel is quite weak and fractures readily under small amounts of pressure. If force is exerted on the wire, the enamel will chip, necessitating repreparation of the tooth, which is not always successful. This points out the necessity of properly adjusting the wire prior to cementation.

The friction-lock pin (manufactured by the Unitek Corporation) is another stainless steel wire that is used for the smaller Class IV restorations with the limited and straight labial outline form. The armamentarium is similar to that described previously, but the procedure differs in that the pins are tapped into place instead of being cemented (Fig. 12-10). The spiral drills are slightly smaller than the orthodontic steel wire, which makes it possible to drive the wire into

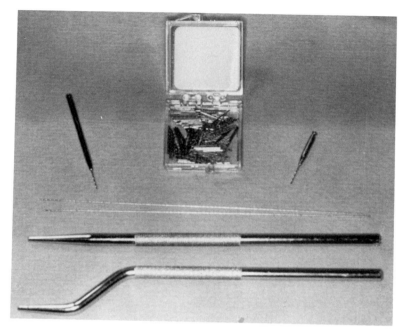

Fig. 12-10. Friction pin kit.

the dentin so that it will be retained for prolonged periods. These wires are placed to the same depth (1.5 mm.) and serve to support the resin restoration. In anterior teeth it is possible to use the tap pin successfully because access allows the wire to be tapped in a direction parallel to the long axis of the tooth. Also in the small Class IV restoration it is not necessary to bend the wires, making it ideal to use this procedure. As with other pins, the ones used in this procedure should not be altered by bending after they have been placed into the tooth because of the danger of splitting the surrounding enamel. Whenever possible, the friction-lock pin should be used to support the Class IV resin restoration in order to simplify the technique (Fig. 12-11).

The advantage of using the friction-lock pins is that they save time. The use of cement is not necessary to secure the restoration because good retention is provided by the straight pin. Another advantage is that the smaller pin used with this technique is not as visible as are others for the Class IV resin restoration.

Although thermoconductivity may present a problem with the use of these pins, it has not been proved that they produce trauma or that they are annoying to the patient. It has been stated that these pins can be reduced in height with the air turbine drill after they are seated. Although this procedure is not recommended, it might be necessary to reduce a tap pin after it is fully seated if the pin is too long or projects from the resin restoration. All pins should be placed

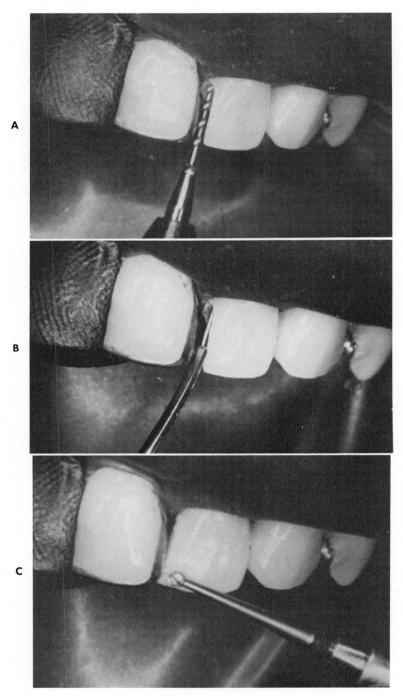

Fig. 12-11. A, Posthole is made in the cervical dentin parallel to the external surface of the tooth. **B,** Punch is seated on the wire in the proper direction. **C,** Gross finishing of the restoration with the No. 4 round bur.

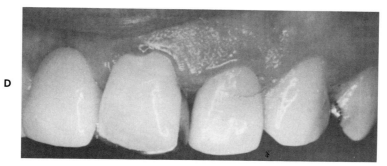

D

Fig. 12-11, cont'd. D, Completed Class IV resin resoration.

at least 1 mm. below the final contour of the labial and incisal surfaces of the restoration.

Certain types of pins that do not have application for the Class IV resin restoration can be screwed into tooth structure. Although these pins are not as easy to use as others, the armamentarium could work well in some operators' hands. The rules applying to the depth and location of the pins are identical to those used for other types. The main difference in procedure is that the pins are screwed into the postholes with a special apparatus. If this particular technique is appealing to a dentist, it should be evaluated, but from the standpoint of time it is doubtful that this armamentarium will be routinely employed for the retention of the resin restoration.

Class IV resin veneer inlays

The resin restoration is useful as a veneer material over castings. This technique is often used to restore large Class IV lesions that would otherwise require an inlay and display a large amount of gold on the labial surface of the tooth. Because an excessive display of gold is objectionable, the further the casting passes the line angle of the incisor tooth, the greater the indication for this procedure. The technique is to remove the labial portion of the casting and to restore the area with a resin to match the shading of the tooth. The brush procedure appears to be the most useful for placing the resin in the castings. The main indication for use of the veneer inlay is the large carious lesion involving the angle in anterior teeth with large healthy pulps. This type of lesion often occurs in young patients and is difficult to restore without damaging the large pulp or placing an unsightly restoration. Pulp size and growth factors in the young patient usually contraindicate the full-coverage preparation. In endodontically treated teeth the veneer inlay is used to improve the appearance until premaxillary growth is completed and eruption has occurred. Grossly fractured vital teeth can be restored satisfactorily with the resin veneer inlay. The procedure should be used in teeth that have good healthy pulps. If there are questions as to the health of the pulp

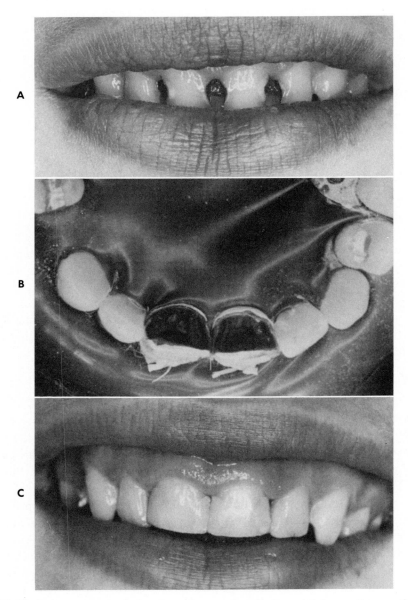

Fig. 12-12. A, Large anterior lesions in a young patient. **B,** Two pinledge castings on the central incisors. **C,** Sulfinic catalyst resins painted over the castings to produce an esthetic veneer.

or if the tooth is not responding normally to testing, the wire technique should be used because it is more temporary and does not involve the time and expense associated with the veneer casting. Even when there are many indications for using this restoration, it should be remembered that this is one of the most difficult procedures in operative dentistry.

Difficulties arise during the inlay procedure when the retention is altered on the casting. When the gold material is removed for the window, there is less frictional retention for the casting. This makes the restoration more vulnerable to the torsional forces or shearing forces that exist on the incisal edges of teeth. The possibility of dislodging the restoration makes retention and fit critical for the resin veneer inlay.

Many types of inlays can be used (Fig. 12-12). The governing factor in the outline form is the amount of retention required. The outline form is judged by the extent of labial, incisal, and proximal surface damage. Castings used for this procedure must have at least two postholes and one groove for the retention. This amount is needed because the surface apposition of the casting is minimized by removal of the gold for the resin window.

Parallel pin castings are useful because of the accuracy produced on the gold posts of the casting. Because of the added retention supplied by the pin casting, not as much surface coverage or reduction is required. The rules for retention are the same as elsewhere, but in this case retention dictates the selection of the type of preparation and the outline form that is necessary. The use of parallel pins still requires two postholes for stability of the casting in addition to the groove because they serve as guides for cementation.

Basically the same preparations are used for the veneer inlay as for other anterior castings. As previously mentioned, it is sometimes necessary to increase the lingual extension for surface coverage to develop more retention. The lesions are excavated and the proximal crater is blocked out with zinc phosphate cement to facilitate withdrawal of the pattern and seating of the gold casting. The labial wall is also smoothed into an area containing sound tooth structure and all the undercuts in this area are removed. The conventional two- or three-surface inlay anterior preparations are utilized. The incisal edge preparations are terminated with postholes on both the incisal and the cervical areas. In the conventional three-surface inlays the postholes are placed only on the gingival walls of the cavity preparation. The lingual dovetail retention inlay is not used for the veneer casting.

If the conventional preparation is not satisfactory, the lingual surface is covered to serve as the vantage point for the pinledge and partial veneer retainers. The extra surface coverage can be complemented with grooves, ledges, and postholes to increase retention. In such cases additional postholes are helpful, and when this type of preparation is used in conjunction with parallel pins, the casting will have adequate retention for almost any clinical situation.

The direct method is advocated for anterior inlays in order to produce the wax pattern. Access to the anterior teeth is excellent when the rubber dam is used. The wax pattern is fabricated as if the procedure were being accomplished with a die. Proper amounts of pressure applied to the wax and proper carving result in an accurately adapted marginated wax pattern.

Direct carving is also helpful in that the window can be made on the pattern while it is on the tooth. The wax is removed from the labial surface and is made so that it does not include the proximal groove. The window is made to minimize the display of gold. Careful judgment is needed to carve the pattern on the tooth in order to remove enough of the wax but still provide adequate incisal-lingual bulk for the casting. Most adjustments are made on the pattern, but the final undercuts and details can be made on the casting. The casting is finished and cemented by ordinary methods to obtain the proper margination on the casting not involved with the acrylic window.

The veneer should be 1 mm. thick to be certain of developing the proper shade in the plastic. If minimum space is available inside the casting, the wall can be masked with zinc phosphate cement or some of the commercially prepared opaque acrylics designed for this purpose. The rubber dam should be in place. The resin is brushed in the preparation after the casting is checked following cementation. Caution is needed when finishing the plastic to be certain that no feather edges of material are present on the tooth structure or the casting. Finishing procedures should be regulated so as not to scratch the gold casting because of the difficulties associated with finishing the casting and smoothing the surface after the resin has been placed.

With this type of restoration the incisal edge is supported by the gold casting and the veneer is used only for esthetics. When plastic is used as a veneer, discoloration soon develops. In some cases the veneers have to be replaced; this should be done without disturbing the casting or removing additional tooth structure. When replacement is necessary, the veneer should be removed with excavating burs, the cavity margin and cavosurface refreshened, and the resin inserted in the same manner as before. Microleakage behind the veneers causes gross discoloration and should be corrected immediately.

Additional uses of the sulfinic catalyst resins have been advocated in pedodontics. Techniques have been devised for the restoration of permanent and deciduous teeth. The resin materials can be used in conjunction with stainless steel crowns as a masking material, similar to the method employed with gold castings. There are also other procedures that utilize the resin restoration alone, sometimes employing supportive wires.

A novel approach for using resin material is the restoration of permanent incisors that have undergone vital pulpotomies.[13] As soon as the pulpotomy has been determined to be successful, the temporary cement is removed above the calcified bridge. A core is constructed above the calcific bridge by placing an orthodontic band in the coronal pulp chamber. The contour is built up around the metallic tubing with the restorative resin, which is later finished to a contour satisfactory for a full-coverage core. After the core has been built up the remainder of the tooth structure is prepared in a manner acceptable for the full-coverage preparation. The tooth and the core are smoothed and the crown constructed in the usual manner. This procedure is a quick, relatively simple method of building up a permanent incisor tooth that utilizes the coronal pulp chamber and the quick-curing resin for retentive purposes.

FINISHING

The soft resin restoration is easy to finish. The contours and margins are quickly obtained with rotary cutting instruments. One advantage of using the resin restoration is that a smooth surface can be developed. There are two separate polishing procedures for proximal and gingival restorations, and they will be explained in detail.

Proximal restorations

In proximal restorations (Class III and Class IV restorations) the matrix or protective film is removed and the restoration is inspected to find whether any voids or faulty contour resulted from the insertion. The initial finishing is done with a No. 4 round bur. The bur is revolved slowly between 1,000 to 2,000 rpm while it is cooled with a stream of air. The surface is cut down initially with a sharp bur, and when the margins are approximated, the pressure is lessened and the finishing is accomplished as slowly as possible. Most of the contour will be produced with the No. 4 round bur; when the resin becomes thin, the cavosurface margin will be visible. The margin is located with light pressure in order not to overreduce the restoration or abrade the tooth structure. The labial and lingual margins are established with the bur. The surface contour must be established without damage to the adjacent tooth.

The thin gold knife (No. 28 Ferrier) is used to complete the contour and form the embrasure. The knife is controlled with short, light cutting strokes. If the instrument is sharp and properly directed, there will be no danger of dislodging the material from the cavity preparation. The knife is used by pulling it from the restoration to the tooth so as not to disturb the adaptation of the resin. However, this procedure is not possible on the gingival wall, emphasizing the need for an extremely sharp gold knife. Some dentists select scalpels for this particular area of the restoration, but because of the difficulties in controlling these instruments a gold knife is preferred.

The incisal resin is removed and the labial and lingual embrasures are shaped with the gold knife. Good form results from proper use of the gold knife, and only a small amount of finishing is necessary following the application. These first two steps in finishing require only a few seconds if the excess resin on the tooth surfaces has been controlled by the strip matrix.

The surface and margins of the restoration are then smoothed with a cuttlefish finishing strip. A light abrasive is used so that the surface inside the embrasure will not be flattened. Pressure is applied with short strokes on the strip rather than pulling it quickly through the embrasure. Only minimal finishing is required in this area to reduce gingival irritation and to prevent overcutting of the soft surface of the restoration. The surface and marginal areas will be noticeably improved following application of the finishing strip.

The final polishing is accomplished with silica or pumice mixed to a thick consistency. This polishing compound is applied with a white rubber cup to avoid discoloring the surface of the resin. The cup should be revolved slowly and used with soft pressure. Only a few movements across the surface are needed for this polishing procedure. The tooth is then dried with warm air and dental floss is used to clean out the embrasure. When the restoration has been cleaned off with the abrasives, the margins and contour should be inspected. The rubber dam is then removed and hydrogen peroxide is applied to the embrasure area to clean the gingiva. The patient is then instructed to rinse his mouth to remove the debris that may remain from the polishing. When large restorations have been placed or when the marginal ridge has been altered and reproduced to a large extent, the occlusion should be checked. The centric relationship is tested with blue paper as the patient makes the protrusive movements. If any blue marks are detected on the lingual surface, these contact areas should be removed to eliminate the stress on the restoration.

Gingival restorations

Gingival restorations (Class V restorations and pits) are more difficult to finish because more flash and excess contour are accumulated by the brush method. Basically the same instrumentation is used, but all the finishing is accomplished with rotary instruments. The surface location does not permit the use of the gold knife and strips. The use of sandpaper disks is discouraged because it removes needless amounts of tooth structure and roughens the enamel surface. If not controlled, the sandpaper disks will damage the gingiva and score the cementum of the tooth.

A No. 4 round bur is selected to produce the contour of the restoration. The bur is moved quickly at first to eliminate the flash of material. As the margin and approximate contour are approached the bur is revolved slowly and with the same light pressure. It is advisable to sweep the bur uniformly from the mesial and distal surface of the restoration to produce uniform reduction. The margins are usually established with this bur and much of the contour is finished at this time.

The final contour and surface smoothing are accomplished on the large gingival restoration with a No. 700 bur. It is used in the same manner as the round bur in that it is moved back and forth across the surface of the restoration to produce a uniform contour. It is ideal to replace the contour that was present in the tooth before the attack of caries or erosion. An attempt should be made to avoid the margin because of the danger of trenching the restoration with this bur. The No. 700 bur is used only to create the protective gingival contour of the restoration.

The final polishing is accomplished with the white cup, using moistened silica or pumice. Extra caution should be exercised not to touch the cementum with the rubber cup and to confine the polishing activity to the restoration because the cementum is abraded by the cup and the tooth becomes sensitive. Also a nidus may be created for bacteria and the development of secondary caries by the ditched area. Minimum pressure is used at all times in the final polishing procedures. When the polishing is finished, air is used to remove the abrasives and a sharp explorer is placed in the rubber dam crevice to remove the debris. It is much easier to remove the polishing compounds at this time rather than to rely on the rinsing following the rubber dam removal.

Polishing of the resin restoration is of major importance for the technique and is performed 5 to 8 minutes following the insertion of the material. The resulting smooth surface does not collect debris or stain faster than the tooth enamel. A successful polish contributes much to the esthetic attributes of the resin restoration.

COMPOSITE RESINS

The dental profession and the associated industries became acutely interested in developing an adhesive restorative material as a result of an interdisciplinary conference.[14] Investigators from various fields discussed the restorative problems associated with tooth structure and the compounds that could be used to develop a chemical and mechanical bond with the cavity preparation. The only inroads to the problem of bonding and the development of new compounds has been the composite resins. The deterrents in bonding caused by tooth structure are listed as the inherent moisture of apatite, the monomolecular surface layer of the tooth, and the endless configuration and tissue differences in the cavity wall.[15,16]

It is accepted that the composite resins are not a panacea to the problems associated with filling materials. The value of the composite resins is the simplification of manipulation and an improvement in compressive strength and resistance to abrasion as compared to the sulfinic catalyst compounds. Other factors such as surface roughness and brittleness limit the selection and use of these materials to the small, protected anterior proximal restoration. Studies on microleakage of composite resins show that the material adapts well to the cavity wall but does not hermetically seal the tooth. It would appear that the actual value of the composite materials to the dental profession is the eventual development of new and better resins because this material is thought to be the only compound available that has the capability of producing a chemical bond to tooth structure.

The composite resins are "filled" compounds in that they have 70% to 80% inert fillers present by weight. The compound often employed has 80% ether of Bisphenol A and some acrylic monomers that form an epoxide molecule. It is a cross-linking co-monomer that forms an adduct resin for the restoration. The composite resin is activated by benzoyl peroxide for polymerization and results in a restoration with a high molecular weight.[17,18]

The fillers influence manipulative and physical properties. The materials used as fillers are glass, silica, or tricalcium phosphate, commonly referred to as artificial apatite. The particles are treated with vinyl silane that eliminates surface moisture and encourages a molecular attraction to the resin. Small glass rods or beads and other fillers are visible on the surface of the restoration and produce the roughness and staining tendencies of the composite resin. Because of the properties of the various fillers, the selection of shades is limited when using the new resins.

The indications for using a composite resin will be based on personal preference and, perhaps, convenience. It is not necessary to have a wide variation of shades for a composite restoration as compared to silicate or unfilled resins, since the composite will effectively borrow the color from its environment. When needed, the color may be varied by using supplied modifiers. They are effective for the small lesions but also can be used where it is required to utilize pins for retention. The composites are of marginal benefit when used for posterior interproximal lesions. The resistance to abrasion is not as dependable as with metallic restorations. Proper morphology and finish for the completed posterior restoration are difficult to accomplish, and as result quality control is difficult to maintain.

When caries is poorly controlled and extensive, the composite resins are not the best solution, since it will be necessary to first bring caries into control. An intermediate filling will be useful as an initial step, and following its success one may use the composite material.

Preparation. Composite resins should be placed in the mortise form preparation in bulk.[19,20] In small lesions that require restoring, enamel penetration should be accomplished by high speed from the lingual direction. This maintains as much of the labial enamel as possible for esthetic purposes. When possible, it is preferred that as much of the restorative activity as possible take place from the lingual angle (Fig. 12-13).

The preparation is developed mostly by burs, with a very minimum use of hand instruments. A No. 1 or No. 2 round bur is the usual choice for determining the outline and axial penetration. When the preparation is completed, the enamel should have good dentin support.

When it is feasible to use hand instruments, curved chisels or margin trimmers are easiest to use.

Retention is gained by using a No. ½ or No. ¼ round bur and placing it 0.5 mm. from the enamel in dentin. It will be located at the lingual and labial extension of the gingival wall, which, at times, will be a slight channel between the labial and lingual with the remaining retention at the incisal.

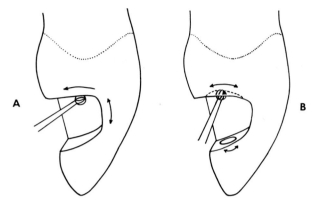

Fig. 12-13. A, Lingual opening for Class III composite preparation. **B,** Location of retention for composite Class III preparation.

When the preparation is enlarged, it is essential to support it by using threaded pins placed to a depth of 2.0 mm. in the dentin. The length of the pin as it protrudes from the dentin should approximate 2.0 mm. With a resin restoration there are times when it is essential to allow the pin to extend further than 2.0 mm.

Composite resin is dispensed as a liquid and a paste (Fig. 12-14). It may also be utilized in a powder and liquid form. The envelope containing the paste is opened and a concavity is formed in the middle of the material. Usually 2 drops of the liquid are placed in the center of this crater and the plastic is mixed for 30 seconds to thoroughly incorporate the two elements. Only 1 minute is allowed for the insertion of the mixed composite resin. The thick consistency of the material resembles a thin, poorly mixed silicate cement. The advantages of composite resin are ease of mixing and quick polymerization, which takes place 5 minutes after the material is inserted into the tooth. The composite resin should be mixed and handled with nonmetallic instruments, for the abrasiveness of the composite material will corrode metal instruments, which may influence the color of the restoration. There are nonmetallic instruments available for handling this material.

The composite must be inserted from a bulk mixture, and a matrix for form development is essential. For most interproximal restorations a closely adapted plastic strip will provide an acceptable matrix. For restorations involving an incisal edge, a contoured crown may be used to provide the general form. A Class V restoration offers considerable difficulty in using a matrix, so many will be manipulated without one.

A syringe may be used to transport the material into the preparation. This does closely control the amount used, which is a convenience.

A weakness with the composite is the difficulty that exists in providing

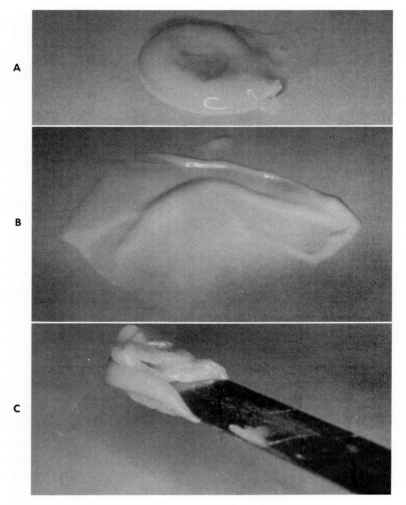

Fig. 12-14. A, Composite paste with a concavity formed in the middle to receive the liquid monomer. **B,** Mixed composite resin with a working time of 30 seconds. **C,** Appearance at 1½ minutes, demonstrating the rapid setting reaction.

a smooth surface. A matrix finish is the best, but it is rarely obtained. Gross adjustment is accomplished by ultrafine diamonds or twelve fluted carbide burs. Any routine steel instrument will leave gray marks on the surface, so it will have limited use. Final polish may be obtained by using lubricated strips or fine disks. A plastic disk with fine diamond particles bonded to the surface is useful in final finishing to help produce a smooth surface. The twelve or more fluted carbide burs are also used to produce the final contour and smoothness. Levigated aluminum in a white cusp may be useful as a final polishing agent. Future research in this area will produce many changes and improvements in the tech-

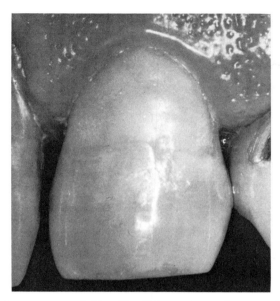

Fig. 12-15. Marginal appearance of Class V sulfinic catalyst resin restoration after 5 years of service.

nique and the clinical restoration. Teachers and practicing dentists will need to constantly evaluate the work conducted with the restorative resins and must understand the clinical significance of the properties being altered. At the present time the dental profession does not have access to a resin that produces a chemical bond with tooth structure and has the strength necessary to resist the functional forces (Fig. 12-15).

ACID ETCHING

Much interest has developed with acid etching and the resin restoration. The procedure involves treating the enamel with 50% unbuffered phosphoric acid and keeping it moist for 30 seconds, to clean and prepare the surface for attachment of the resin. The procedure should be accurately timed and controlled, with the acid removed by syringe water. Data have shown that by using a primer on the etched surface, the bond strength at the resin-tooth interface exceeds the tensile strength of the material.[21] Clinical procedures are outlined for acid etching and data show that the resin material penetrates the area of the enamel that is conditioned by the acid.[22,23]

Several type acids can be employed to produce the etching.[24,25] Selection should be made of an acid that can be controlled on the enamel surface, in order not to etch the dentin or irritate the gingival tissue. The minimum time should be used for acid application, since the technique is advocated for all types of resin materials and restoration types. The 50% unbuffered phosphoric acid

Table 12-1. Average change in calcium solubility of enamel surfaces after a 2-week treatment with resin cements*

Resin	Average change in Ca solubility (%)
Resin and 5% NaF	−17.4
Resin and 2% NaF	−22.9
Resin and 2% SnF₂	−24.0
FluorOn	−53.3
Kadon	+18.5

*From Phillips, R. W., and Swartz, M.L.: J.A.D.A. **54:**623, 1957.

is recommended at this time and can be purchased from the chemical supply or dental dealer.

PIT AND FISSURE SEALANTS

Certain resins are now being advocated for sealing the pits and fissures of teeth as a preventive measure. The products were designed to be effective for these areas, since the fluorides act mainly to protect the smooth surfaces. The initial data look promising, and one system includes the use of an ultraviolet light to initiate polymerization.[26-28] The actual success will be determined only after long-term clinical studies are conducted, but the materials could serve a useful purpose in the preventive and highly controlled practice.

The success of the resin in sealing the enamel would depend upon the cleanliness of the fissure area and the viscosity of the resin. The effects of enamel maturation produced by fissure sealants are questioned, but there appear to be applications of the concepts in public health programs.[29] Isolation and etching of the fissure must be accomplished before application of the resin. The concept has enough promise to include the treatment in the modern practice.[30]

SUMMARY

Although there are many undesirable physical properties associated with the restorative resins, this chapter explains how they can be successfully used in certain situations. Permanent results cannot be achieved with the material, but in comparison with cements, the resins have more lasting qualities that produce greater clinical success (Table 12-1). A controversy over the value of resin restorative materials has existed for many years, but research and conjecture indicate a promising future for these compounds.

Precise operative procedures are required. The cavity preparation must be dry and exacting to allow polymerization of the resin in the tooth. Standard techniques are critical because proper consistency and correct timing are necessary for acceptable adaptation. The restoration is successful only when delicate finishing procedures are employed. The resin restoration must be placed quickly;

therefore, the recommendations of the manufacturers must be followed exactly.

Conservative measures must be followed with the use of resin because the restorations must be protected. Existing tooth structure should be left whenever possible in order to compensate for the numerous undesirable physical properties of resins. Caries does not appear to be a problem, but it is advocated that margins be placed in areas that ensure protection and proper access for cleaning.

In the future a resin compound that bonds to tooth structure will undoubtedly be produced. The principles for using the resins must be mastered by the operative dentist so the compounds of the future can be evaluated. Research on microleakage indicates that only sulfinic catalyst and composite resin compounds should be used as restorative materials.

REFERENCES

1. Buonocore, M., Wileman, W., and Brudevold, F.: A report on a resin composition capable of bonding to human dentin surfaces, J. Dent. Res. 35:846, 1956.
2. Nelson, R. J., Wolcott, R. B., and Paffenbarger, G. C.: Fluid exchange at the margins of dental restorations, J.A.D.A. 44:288, 1952.
3. Hedegard, B.: Cold-polymerizing resins as restorative materials: a clinical evaluation, Int. Dent. J. 65:173, 1957.
4. Coy, H. D., Bear, D. M., and Kreshover, S. J.: Auto-polymerizing resin fillings, J.A.D.A. 44:251, 1952.
5. Manning, J. E.: A clinical assessment of the unlined Sevriton filling, Brit. Dent. J. 106:308, 1959.
6. Skinner, E., and Phillips, R. W.: The science of dental materials, Philadelphia, 1960, W. B. Saunders Co.
7. Smith, D. L., and Schoonover, I. C.: Direct filling resins: dimensional changes resulting from polymerization shrinkage and water sorption, J.A.D.A. 46:540, 1953.
8. Swartz, M. L., and Phillips, R. W.: Influence of manipulative variables on the marginal adaptation of certain restorative materials, J. Prosth. Dent. 12:172, 1962.
9. Phillips, R. W., and Swartz, M. L.: Effect of certain restorative materials on solubility of enamel, J.A.D.A. 54:623, 1957.
10. Phillips, R. W.: Some current observations on restorative materials, Aust. Dent. J. 9:258, 1964.
11. Boyd, D. A.: The direct self-curing resin restoration, Dent. Clin. N. Am., Mar., 1957, pp. 107-122.
12. Nealon, F. H.: Acrylic restorations by the operative non-pressure procedure, J. Prosth. Dent. 2:513, 1952.
13. Castaldi, C. R.: The management of some pedodontic problems, J. Canad. Dent. Assoc. 28:80, 1962.
14. Phillips, R. W., and Ryge, G.: Adhesive dental materials, proceedings from a workshop, Spencer, Ind., 1961, Owen Litho Service.
15. Phillips, R. W.: Certain biological considerations in the use of restorative materials, New York Dent. J. 28:397, 1962.
16. Adhesive restorative materials, requirements and test methods, U. S. Public Health Service Publication No. 1433, Washington, D. C., 1966, U. S. Government Printing Office.
17. Phillips, R. W.: Recent improvements in dental materials the operative dentist should know, J.A.D.A. 73:84, 1966.
18. Bowen, R. L.: Effect of particle shape and size distribution in a reinforced polymer, J.A.D.A. 69:481, 1964.
19. Hollenback, G. M., Villanyi, A. A., and Shell, J. S.: A report on the physical properties of a new restorative material (Addent), J. S. Calif. Dent. Assoc. 34:250, 1966.

20. Petersen, E. A., Phillips, R. W., and Swartz, M. L.: A comparison of the physical properties of four restorative resins, J.A.D.A. **73:**1324, 1966.
21. Lee, B. D., Phillips, R. W., and Swartz, M. L.: The influence of phosphoric acid on retention of acrylic resin to bovine enamel, J. Am. Dent. Assoc. **82:**1381-1386, 1971.
22. Laswell, H. R., Welk, D. A., and Regenos, J. W.: Attachment of resin restorations to acid pretreated enamel, J. Am. Dent. Assoc. **82:**558-563, 1971.
23. Sharp, E. C., and Grenoble, D. E.: Dental resin penetration into acid etched subsurface enamel, J. S. Calif. Dent. Assoc. **39:**741-746, 1971.
24. Abert, M., and Grenoble, D. E.: An invivo study of enamel remineralization after acid etching, J. S. Calif. Dent. Assoc. **39:**747-751, 1971.
25. Gwinnett, A. J.: Histologic changes in human enamel following treatment with acidic adhesive conditioning agents, Arch. Oral Biol. **16:**731-738, 1971.
26. Buonocore, M. G.: Cares prevention in pits and fissures sealed with an adhesive resin polymerized with an ultraviolet light: a two-year study of a single adhesive application, J. Am. Dent. Assoc. **82:**1090-1093, 1971.
27. McCune, R. J., and Cvar, J. F.: Pit and fissure sealants: preliminary results, IADR Abstracts **745:**239, 1971.
28. Gwinnett, A. J.: Caries prevention through sealing of pits and fissures, J. Canad. Dent. Assoc. **37:**458, 1971.
29. Reports of councils and bureaus: pit and fissure sealants, J. Am. Dent. Assoc. **82:**1101-1103, 1971.
30. Phillips, R. W.: Report of the committee on scientific investigation of the American Academy of Restorative Dentistry, J. Prosth. Dent. **28:**82-108, 1972.

ADDITIONAL READINGS

Bowen, R. L.: Properties of a silica-reinforced polymer for dental restorations, J. Am. Dent. Assoc. **66:**57, 1963.
Chandler, H. H., Bowen, R. L., and Paffenbarger, G. C.: Method for finishing composite restorative materials, J. Am. Dent. Assoc. **83:**344-348, 1971.
Langeland, L. K., and others: Histologic and clinical comparison of Addent with silicate cements and cold curing materials, J. Am. Dent. Assoc. **72:**373-385, 1966.
Lee, H. L., Swartz, M. L., and Smith, F. F.: Physical properties of four thermosetting dental restorative resins, J. Dent. Res. **48:**526, 1969.
Johnson, L. N., Jordan, R. E., and Lynn, J. A.: Effects of various finishing devices on resin surfaces, J. Am. Dent. Assoc. **83:**321-331, 1971.
Phillips, R. W., Swartz, M. L., and Norman, R. D.: Materials for the practicing dentist, St. Louis, 1969, The C. V. Mosby Co., chaps. 4 and 11.
Stanley, H. R., and others: A comparison of the biological effects of filling materials with recommendations for pulp protection, J. Am. Acad. Gold. Foil. Operators **12:**56-62, 1969.

chapter 13

Erosion

Erosion is a pathologic condition of individual teeth. As with dental caries, many factors are responsible for erosion, a widespread condition. Erosion is classified as attrition and is a chemical-mechanical wearing away of tooth substance in the absence of specific bacteria (Fig. 13-1). Erosion is common in the adult patient, and its occurrence is thought to increase with age. When first discovered, the lesions are characteristically sensitive and are found adjacent to normal gingival tissue. Diagnosis of erosion is confirmed when healthy gingival tissues are found to be in contact with the eroded area on the tooth structure.[1]

Restoration of all areas of erosion is not feasible; many lesions do not require restorative treatment. The process should be controlled to limit growth of the erosion because pulp exposure and tooth loss sometimes occur. Some dentin protection occurs with most lesions. The formation of secondary dentin with dead tracts has been reported under the eroded areas, pointing out the need for lesion control and measures to protect the pulp.[1]

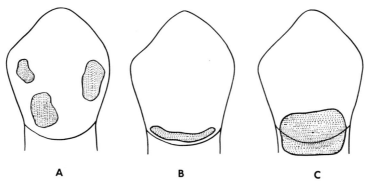

A   B   C

Fig. 13-1. Various types of erosion lesions. **A,** Random erosion location; **B,** V or wedge-shaped lesion; **C,** dished-out erosion lesion.

Lesions caused by erosion have typical shapes and characteristics. Ordinarily only the labial and buccal surfaces are attacked, but proximal and lingual erosions can occur. A crater is formed in the affected tooth, exposing the dentin; the floor of the lesion is smooth and appears to be polished. Tooth sensitivity and lack of gingival irritation are associated with each lesion. The edges of the lesion are smooth and present no demarcation with the external tooth surface when examined with an explorer. The enamel, cementum, and dentin seem to have the same vulnerability to the attritional process.

Early it was reported that the occurrence of erosion is greater in the maxillary arch than in the mandibular arch.[2] The most prominent teeth in the quadrant are often the most severely affected. Incidence of erosion is reported to differ among patients according to income levels and racial groups. In addition, erosion is associated with systemic diseases, but studies conducted on the subject have not provided conclusive evidence. It is common to discover erosion in all types of patients. Methods should be used to minimize the damaging effects produced on the dentition. Dental caries rarely occurs in the eroded tooth substance.

Sognaes[3] studied 10,827 teeth with a dissecting microscope and reported that 1,700 teeth, or 18% of the sample, had typical patterns of erosion-like lesions. Also, 500 of these lesions were found in the presence of other conditions such as calculus, dental caries, and various types of restorations.

The same group[4] used profile studies to determine the advancement of erosion lesions. It was reported that the process continued at 1μ per day, regardless of whether the surface had been treated with sodium fluoride. When restorations were placed, the erosion process decreased to about half the rate. It can be concluded that erosion is a widespread clinical problem and that treatment methods are mostly ineffective. Erosion is perplexing to the dentist because many lesions are discovered that have no obvious reason for development.

The types of lesions and their characteristics are as follows.

Dish-shaped (saucer-shaped) lesions. Dish-shaped lesions are shallow concavities that most commonly occur on the incisor teeth. The deepest part of the lesion is in the center of the concavity and the walls radiate upward to sound tooth structure. The circular outline of the dish-shaped lesion is mainly confined to the gingival half of the tooth, and it is common to discover the border of the lesion in contact with gingival tissue. This lesion does not grow rapidly. Because the lesion has a smooth surface, it will appear glossy when the tooth is dried for inspection. These lesions assume a U shape if their size continues to increase. The outline appears to be the pattern taken by saliva and dietary solutions when flowing over the teeth.

Wedge-shaped (notch-shaped) lesions. These lesions are V shaped and most commonly occur on the mesial aspect of the buccal surfaces of bicuspids and molar teeth. The most prominent tooth in the quadrant (buccal version) usually has the largest lesion. This type of erosion causes pulp stimulation or irritation.

Severe lesions do not usually occur past the mesial surface of the first molar. Tooth sensitivity is often a problem with this type of lesion.

The wedge-shaped lesion begins at the level of the gingival border. Early lesions are difficult to detect. They are characterized by a thin, straight, sharp line. The lesion spreads rapidly and the tooth structure below the gingival tissue becomes involved. The wedge develops along the gingival wall, perpendicular to the surface of the tooth and the buccal wall and at a right angle to the base of the lesion. Sharp angles, tooth sensitivity, and pulp exposure are associated with the wedge-shaped lesion, and depth control is important.

Irregularly shaped lesions. Lesions with irregular shapes occur on the proximal and lingual surfaces and often result from severe systemic or environmental disorders. Restorative measures are difficult in these lesions. Chemical fumes or chronic regurgitation can cause this type of disorder and results in damage to large amounts of tooth structure. The causative factors must be determined to control the lesion and to prevent loss of the dentition. The irregularly shaped lesions do not occur as often as do the types previously discussed.

THEORIES OF EROSION

There were many early reports concerning erosion, and the damage it caused was recognized by a number of scientists. The multiple etiologic factors involved have resulted in a number of theories. Possible contributing factors can be more clearly understood by studying the various hypotheses. The information gained is also valuable in interpreting the results of research conducted on the causes of erosion. Only the established theories will be discussed. Early suppositions concerning developmental defects are not included.

Acids

Of the theories on the etiology of erosion, acids have received the most attention.[2] Dietary acids have been the primary concern, although glandular acid secretions have also been studied.

W. D. Miller,[5] noted for his pioneer work on caries, also investigated the causes of erosion. In his experiments, extracted teeth were placed in contact with cloths saturated with dilute acids. The teeth were then brushed for extended periods with an apparatus driven by an electric engine. Miller believed that toothbrushing was the main offender, but he concluded that acids also play a role in hastening tooth erosion. Miller observed that abrasion causes fillings to wear as fast as teeth, but erosion attacks tooth structure more readily than fillings. From the results of his research and clinical observations he concluded that mechanical wear greatly accelerates erosion.

It is interesting to note that G. V. Black visited Miller's laboratory in Berlin and observed his experiments on erosion. Upon returning to the United States, Black repeated some of Miller's methods in addition to circulating dilute acid over the surfaces of incisor teeth. The teeth exhibited areas identical to clinical erosion, which convinced Black of the role of oral acids in erosion. This investigator described tooth sensitivity as a characteristic symptom of erosion and further concluded that calcific deposits protected the tooth from this condition. Black noted that the deepest areas in the lesions occurred where the acids made abrupt turns on the tooth surface.

The effect of acids present in saliva have been studied as a possible cause of erosion. A study similar to Black's was conducted with citrate and lactate ions. Solutions were circulated over teeth extracted from rats.[6] These solutions were selected because of their frequency in the diet and also because of their presence in caries. Three solutions were used in which the pH ranged from 5.5 to 7.2. These investigators reported a marked local decalcifying action with neutral solutions of calcium citrate. However, the lactate solutions did not prove to be harmful. The researchers suggested further studies utilizing other anions and the calcium citrate complex.

Another study examined the role of salivary citrate in erosion.[7] Determinations of citric acid were made in individuals with and without tooth erosion and ranged from 0.20 to 2.00 mg.%. Citric acid was found to be quite unstable in stimulated salivation, and a positive statistical correlation between the severity of erosion and salivary citrate content was reported.

To test these claims, Shulman and Robinson[8] studied the citrate content of saliva from 1,345 male students with and without tooth erosion. In this group twenty-eight students demonstrated evidence of gross erosion. Analysis of the citrate in saliva showed small and varying amounts and they concluded that no correlation existed between this solution and erosion. Studies on salivary components have declined in number since this research was reported.

The influence of acid secreted by the gingival glands in instances of traumatic occlusion is listed among the acid theories. The secretion is considered to have a local acidic action. Bodecker[9] surveyed 469 teeth by placing red and blue litmus paper in crevicular gingival fluid. More acid was found around eroded teeth. Surveys were conducted to further study the clinical problems of erosion by using teeth treated with an alkaline protective coating. This procedure created much interest, but the treatment was short-lived, probably because the coating was washed away by saliva. The protective film containing oleic acid, lanolin, and alkaline phosphate was placed directly on the eroded area and on the adjacent gingival sulcus.

An early study by Sognaes[10] placed new light on the theory of local acidity. By using microradiography he observed an alteration of the calcium content on the surface of eroded areas. In lesions produced by toothbrushing the surface layer was found to be intact, indicating more than one specific cause for erosion. The study led this investigator to make the following observations:

1. A loss of protective saliva on the tooth is caused by secretions of the local glands.
2. A decalcifying agent drains the tooth of its vital minerals.

3. This process could occur as the result of a change in eating and drinking habits.

4. When a mechanical problem is present, there will be a more rapid loss of tooth structure.

Sognaes suggested that the tooth be fortified with frequent applications of highly concentrated fluoride solutions. The data obtained by use of microradiography support the results of other studies. Fluoride therapy was said to promote tooth protection by surface hardening and reduction in solubility. However, this was not found to be the case in the recent profile studies.[4]

The role of occlusal factors in the secretion of acid has not been adequately studied. Crevicular fluid from the gingiva has not been evaluated from this aspect. Because there is a higher incidence of occlusal disharmonies than true erosion lesions, the examination of these factors has not been extensive. It has been suggested that premolar teeth develop erosion when the dentition does not have prominent protection by the cuspids in lateral movements of the mandible.

When different acids were compared for their decalcification potential, citric acid was found to be the most damaging to tooth structure. This conclusion supports the theory that erosion occurs as a result of dietary factors. It is possible to dissolve much of the tooth structure during prolonged or repeated exposure to citric acid.

The effects of acids on extracted teeth have been compared to determine the factors influencing the action of the acids in diets.[11] Extracted human teeth were uniformly exposed to and regularly immersed in acids. The results indicated that dissolution resulted from specific action of the acids themselves and was more related to the pH of the solution than to the concentration of the acids by weight. Citric acid again proved to be more destructive to tooth structure than other acids.

The erosive action of commercial beverages and other products has been tested in vivo and in vitro (Table 13-1 and Fig. 13-2). Most of the beverages and fruit juices dissolved extensive amounts of tooth structure, pointing out

Table 13-1. Amount of tooth enamel surface (mg./cm.^{2}) eroded in 5 days*

Acid	pH					
	1.5	2.0	2.5	3.0	3.5	3.8 (pH dust)
Hydrochloric	123.6	72.1	23.7	—	18.7	13.7
Nitric	125.6	78.2	17.6	—	10.9	10.0
Sulfuric	26.2	18.4	21.6	—	2.3	19.8
Acetic	121.5	94.5	74.6	56.4	43.4	—
Citric	311.2	189.5	156.3	94.2	80.1	—

*From Elsbury, W. B.: Brit. Dent. J. **93**:177, 1953.

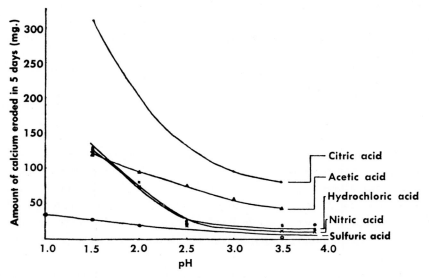

Fig. 13-2. Erosive effect of different types of acids. Graphic representation of data in Table 9. Note the extent of decalcification by citric acid. (From Elsbury, W. B.: Brit. Dent. J. **93:**177, 1952.)

the need for moderation in consuming such products.[12] A combination of 2 parts per million sodium fluoride solution caused a reduction in the dissolving capability of the acids. Results of the study showed that the amount and type of sugar used in the beverages influences the degree of erosion.

When toothbrushing after food consumption is not possible, some investigators have advocated chewing a dental cleaning tablet.[13] A tablet for this purpose has been formulated that combines malic acid (pH 4.5) with calcium and phosphate ions. The erosive properties of the tablet were determined in rats and compared with those of water and fruit beverages. The citric acids contained in fruit juices again proved to be the most harmful.

Fruit juices and carbonated beverages are destructive only when they are consumed in excess. Extensive amounts of tooth structure are dissolved in people who are habitual "lemon suckers." Elderly people may habitually drink warm lemon juice to combat infectious diseases in the winter. Prolonged habits of this nature lead to destruction of the natural dentition by erosion. A normal consumption of citrus fruits and their juices does not increase the occurrence of erosion. A balanced diet should include portions of fruit to maintain good health. The properties of saliva and the cleaning action of mastication serve as natural protective factors against small amounts of citric acid consumed in a well-balanced diet.

In a recent study the acidity of certain foodstuffs was surveyed and it was concluded that overuse of these substances can severely damage the dentition.[14]

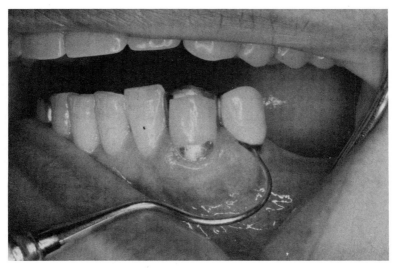

Fig. 13-3. Decalcification under a crown restoration produced by excessive use of "sour mints."

These investigators found that foods or liquids in the pH range of 5.5 to 9.0 are not likely to adversely affect tooth structure. Many commercial breath fresheners have much lower pH values. Certain mouthwashes and mints were found to be potentially hazardous. The volume of acid in relation to the volume of saliva was believed to be the cause of decalcification in this study. The oral clearance of the acid was also considered a determining factor in the occurrence of caries or erosion.

It is the prolonged contact of candy and lozenges to the teeth that makes them a prominent factor in erosion. Sour drops and mints have a pH of 2.5, while other mints such as clove, peppermint, spearmint, and wintergreen have a pH of near 6.0. Therefore, habitual consumption of mints, lozenges, and candy should be discouraged (Fig. 13-3).

Abrasion

The abrasion theory has also been extensively discussed as a cause of erosion. A number of studies not designed specifically to study sources of erosion have yielded significant data on the influence of dentifrices and of toothbrushing. The first thorough study on erosion was conducted by Miller,[5] and he stated that it was possible to produce V-shaped eroded areas on extracted teeth with dentifrices and abrasives. Part of the study employed large calcium carbonate particles, which could cause more abrading of tooth structure than present-day compounds. Early investigators also compared the abrasion caused by various toothpastes and powders. The powders demonstrated more wearing of the tooth structure.

The amount of abrasion is influenced by the particular tooth area. Certain grades of calcium carbonate and calcium phosphate have been found to be 10 times more abrasive to the cementum and dentin than to the enamel surfaces.[15] Early lesions begin on the enamel, but as is the case in attrition, the softer tissues of the cementum and dentin are exposed, resulting in tooth sensitivity and accelerated erosion.

Cementum exposure has been studied in all age groups. The amount of surface area exposed could contribute to the high incidence. Ferrier[16] reported that "20% of the cavities that need to be filled are eroded areas." He measured cementum exposure and the depth of the cut on the exposed surface in 200 individuals. Cervical exposure was observed in 15.5% of the teeth in persons 50 to 59 years of age. The sizes of lesions were found to increase with age. Women were less susceptible to cementum exposure than men, and abrasion was more prevalent in the older patients. According to this study, controlled brushing techniques become more important as the patient ages.

The effects of many types of abrasives were evaluated by Manly and his associates.[15] The extracted teeth were photographed and the contour was measured before and after brushing. All the dentifrices tested produced wear in the cementum and dentin ranging from 0.2 to 2.1 mm. after 86,400 strokes of the brush. According to Manly and co-workers, this would be equivalent to 6 years of brushing under normal conditions. The type of abrasive, the type of bristle in the brush, and the pressure applied during cleaning all influence the rate of wear. Therefore, the method used to clean the teeth over a period of years is a critical factor.

Harrington and Terry[17] studied the abrasive properties of various types of toothbrushes. Many variables were evaluated, including electric toothbrushes, nylon and natural bristles, and restorative materials. It was demonstrated that electric toothbrushes with an arcuate motion produce 160% more abrasion than the reciprocating, short-stroke type. In manual brushing the side-to-side motion produced 80% more abrasion and the up-and-down motion caused 50% less abrasion than the reciprocating, short-stroke electric brush. It would appear that electric toothbrushes hasten abrasion and therefore should be used with caution when cementum exposure is a problem.

These authors believed that the type of dentifrice rather than the type of brush was more influential in abrasion. Natural bristles caused more abrasion than nylon bristles. Small-diameter bristles produced more abrasion because they tended to bend and mat. Large-diameter bristles became more abrasive when tooth powders were used. These observations serve to point out the many variables related to toothbrushing and erosion and abrasion.

Erosion and abrasion have been thought to be related because of the location and appearance of the lesions. The shiny appearance of the lesion could be caused by the highly polished surface produced by phosphate abrasives. Surface changes, remineralization, and characteristic lesions by location and prominence of the teeth could well be attributed to abrasives. Problems occur when there is excess acid along with improper brushing techniques, and decalcification could hasten the removal of tooth structure. The effect of the toothbrush on dentin was evaluated and reported to be insignificant.[18] Abrasion and V-shaped eroded grooves were found to be related to linear crossbrushing movements. As abrasive dentifrices are added, the wear on the dentin increases and becomes a clinical problem that needs to be controlled in the susceptible patient.

Alkalies

Another theory on the cause of erosion is that it results from the action of alkaline materials. The chelation theory of caries is well established, and drugs with chelating agents are used to help soften dentin in endodontic therapy. The process is observed as calcium is removed from apatite when solutions are in the neutral or alkaline pH ranges.

Pyrophosphates present in saliva are effective chelating agents.[19] The accumulation of pyrophosphates results from fermenting oral microbes. This material was obtained from whole saliva, salivary debris, and mixed cultures of microbial flora. Sodium fluoride was added to the mixtures to inhibit pyrophosphatase because this enzyme would prevent most of the pyrophosphate from accumulating. Pyrophosphates from fermentation mixtures reportedly decalcified powdered tooth structure. The saliva obtained from patients with erosion was found to contain pyrophosphates.

The effect of chelation in oral biology is a relatively new concept and not many studies have as yet been conducted. The process involving removal of calcium and the formation of chelating agents could result in an increase in the incidence of clinical erosion. The enzyme-inhibiting action of fluoride could result in more pyrophosphate becoming available to react with tooth structure.

• • •

Investigators have been active for many years studying the problems of erosion. The problems of erosion are similar to those of caries. The condition of the oral cavity, diet, and toothbrushing technique all influence the process. When certain factors appear to be out of balance, damage occurs to the dentition. In some cases diagnosis and treatment must be instituted to save the teeth. A review of the literature has been presented to acquaint the reader with the factors associated with erosion and to furnish material helpful in advising and treating patients.

TREATMENT
Surface hardening

The conservative approach is the best treatment of erosion. This involves making the affected surface resistant to acid dissolution.[20,21] Surface hardening can be accomplished in a number of ways, but the application of fluoride compounds seems to be the most effective method. The treated surface becomes hard, making the tooth structure less soluble in acid. Surface hardening should combat erosion caused by acid in the oral cavity.

A 10% topical application of stannous fluoride solution is suitable for this purpose. Periodic applications of concentrated solutions of topical fluorides are recommended. The teeth are cleaned thoroughly and isolated prior to application of the fluoride to permit maximum uptake by the tooth structure. The recommended application time for 10% stannous fluoride is 30 seconds. The patient must not rinse his mouth or eat for 15 minutes following the treatment if the solution is to be effective. Acidulated phosphate fluorides are also useful for treating the problem of erosion.

Sodium fluoride pastes aid surface hardening. These high-viscosity compounds require longer contact times with tooth structure. The pastes prove effective only when a few teeth are involved. In instances of gross erosion, topical applications are faster and easier to apply. The fluoride paste is tamped gently into the lesion after the eroded area is cleaned. The tooth must be dry to permit better surface contact with the paste. A damp cotton roll may be used to tamp the material into the lesion. The patient should not rinse his mouth after application of the paste. Fluoride pastes are beneficial in reducing tooth sensitivity and can be quickly applied in emergency cases.

The use of desensitizing solutions that do not harden the enamel should not be encouraged. Obtundents and other solutions only serve to stimulate the growth of secondary dentin and do not otherwise benefit the tooth surface. Solutions with a staining potential such as silver nitrate are effective in minimizing erosion but produce unsightly dark stains in the dentin and cementum.

Remineralization is another possible method of preventing destruction of enamel and dentin. The process is of little benefit in the detectable lesion but is helpful in treating the incipient stage of surface decalcification. If applied in acid solutions, the phosphates can combine with the organic matrix and rebuild tooth structure. If the lesion can be reversed, it is beneficial to apply phosphates to the eroded area. Dentifrices and solutions contain phosphates capable of causing surface changes.

Koulourides[21] stated that fluorides may be involved in remineralization and he claimed that the rate of rehardening or remineralization of enamel is accelerated by fluorides containing calcium and phosphate ions. The value of applying fluoride solutions is further supported by evidence of its action on tooth structure and by its possible role in remineralization.

Careful observation and examination are necessary to determine the course of erosion. Surface treatment is indicated whenever possible. All aspects of the patient's history should be explored to discover factors contributing to the process. Restoration of the area should not be attempted until the variables are controlled. If the variables are not controlled, erosion will occur around the restoration.

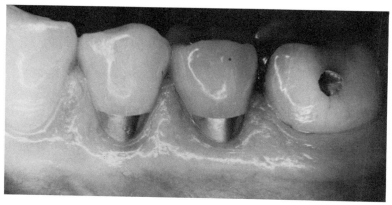

Fig. 13-4. Direct gold restoration of eroded areas.

Restorations

The progress of erosion should be checked regularly. Yearly diagnostic models are helpful in noting changes in the lesion. Although erosion is difficult to observe on a cast, this method provides an evaluation for the treatment. Eroded areas on critical or prominent teeth in the quadrant should be restored to prevent disfigurement and subsequent damage to the pulp.

The sensitivity is determined by drying the tooth and examining it with an explorer. Sensitive areas should be treated to harden the area and to allow the deposit of secondary dentin. The subsequent restoration will then be less liable to leakage and thermal sensitivity. Restoration prevents further damage to the eroded area by the abrasive action of toothbrushes.

Selection of the restorative material is governed by the location and extent of the lesion.[22-24] The less common dish-shaped lesion is usually found on incisor teeth and is best restored with resin or porcelain inlays. The extensive dish-shaped lesion requires a sizable preparation. Restoration is delayed until loss of enamel occurs, necessitating replacement for esthetics.

Wedge-shaped lesions on posterior teeth are best restored with metallic materials. Small lesions are well suited for cohesive gold restoration (Fig. 13-4). Large lesions on molars can be restored with amalgam or pin inlays because this type of restoration resists abrasion caused by toothbrushing and protects gingival tissue in contact with the restoration.

Extension is not a paramount feature of the cavity preparation because erosion usually occurs on clean tooth surfaces and the gingiva around the lesion is in excellent health. The outline form of the restoration includes only the affected area, the tooth structure necessary to establish esthetics, and gingival extension when the lesion abuts or undermines the soft tissue. Gingival margins are ordinarily located below the soft tissue in wedge-shaped lesions.

Procedures for cavity preparation and rubber dam placement are the same as for other gingival restorations. Cavity depth is regulated to provide retention and resistance. Special clamps are necessary to mechanically retract the tissue on the tooth being restored and are described in other chapters.

The application of a protective base is usually not necessary because of the limited depth of the axial wall. However, a protective base is often necessary in caries restorations because the axial wall ordinarily suffers the greatest damage. Protection and treatment of the dentin is accomplished by cavity varnish, which serves to minimize postoperative sensitivity and inflammation by reducing leakage around the restoration. Postoperative obtundents designed specifically to allay pain are usually not necessary and are occasionally harmful.

Restorative measures are not used to arrest erosion. The procedures just outlined serve to protect involved tooth structure and to resist additional mechanical damage. If other possible etiologic factors are not controlled, the margins of the restorations become involved. A thorough case history must be taken to discover the causative factors. Comprehensive treatment of erosion will restore oral health and retard the occurrence of additional erosion. An effective method of treating erosion is still needed.

SUMMARY

1. Erosion, like caries, is a result of multiple etiologic factors. Lesions can cause pulp irritation, surface disfigurement, and tooth loss.

2. Extensive research indicates that acid and abrasion influence the processes of erosion.

3. A thorough case history and examination should be employed to locate lesions and determine the causes.

4. Tooth sensitivity should be controlled and treated without the use of restorations. Diagnostic models are used to record the development of lesions.

5. A normal intake of citrus fruits is not considered to be a factor in tooth erosion. Unusual dietary habits such as sucking lemons and chronic use of lozenges, mouthwashes, and beverages should be discouraged.

6. Improper toothbrushing techniques and the use of toothbrushes with stiff bristles and harsh abrasives should be discouraged because the erosion process appears to be accelerated by mechanical factors.

7. Initial lesions should be treated to harden the surface to arrest the erosion. Applications of topical fluorides and sclerosing pastes have proved to be beneficial in such instances. Surface decalcification is minimized by fluorides, resulting in hardness and reduced solubility of the exposed surface. Remineralization of the eroded surface is possible, but no usable technique has as yet been devised.

8. All of the preceding measures are used as control measures and are not totally effective. Erosion continues to be a severe problem of the aged patient.

9. Restoration procedures are necessary in abnormally large lesions that collect food or plaque and that are subject to abrasion from toothbrushing. Metallic restorations are used whenever possible, and conservative restorative measures are employed for cavity preparation.

REFERENCES

1. Shafer, W. G., Hine, M. K., and Levy, B. M.: A textbook of oral pathology, ed. 2, Philadelphia, 1963, W. B. Saunders Co.
2. Black, G. V.: Operative dentistry, ed. 3, Chicago, 1917, Medico-Dental Publishing Co., vol. 2.
3. Sognaes, R. F., Wolcott, R. B., and Xhonga, F. A.: Dental erosion: 1. Erosion-like patterns occurring in association with other dental conditions, J. Am. Dent. Assoc. **84:**571-576, 1972.
4. Xhonga, F. A., Wolcott, R. B., and Sognaes, R. F.: Dental erosion: 2. Clinical measurements of dental erosion progress, J. Am. Dent. Assoc. **84:**577-582, 1972
5. Miller, W. D.: Experiments and observations on the wasting of tooth tissue variously designated as erosion, abrasion, chemical abrasion, denudation, etc., Dent. Cosmos **49:**109, 1907.
6. Hartles, R. L., and Wagg, B. J.: Erosive effect of drinking fluids on the molar teeth of the rat, Arch. Oral Biol. **7:**308, 1962.
7. Zipkin, I., and McClure, F. J.: Salivary citrate and dental erosion, J. Dent. Res. **28:**613, 1949.
8. Shulman, E. H., and Robinson, H. B. G.: Salivary citrate content and erosion of the teeth, J. Dent. Res. **27:**541, 1948.
9. Bodecker, C. F.: Local acidity: a cause of dental erosion–abrasion, Ann. Dent. **4:**50, 1945.
10. Sognaes, R. F.: Microradiographic observations on demineralization gradients in the pathogenesis of hard tissue destruction, Arch. Oral Biol. **1:**106, 1959.
11. Editorial comments: Occupational hazards to the teeth, Brit. Dent. J. **106:**235, 1959.
12. Holloway, P. J., Mellanby, M., and Stewart, R. J. C.: Fruit drinks and tooth erosion, Brit. Dent. J. **104:**305, 1958.
13. Hay, D. L., Pinsent, B. R. W., Schram, C. J., and Wagg, B. J.: The protective effect of calcium and phosphate ions against acid erosion of dental enamel and dentin, Brit. Dent. J. **112:**283, 1962.
14. Benfield, J. W.: Possible effects of substances commonly used in or taken into the oral cavity, paper presented to the American Academy of Restorative Dentistry, Feb. 2, 1963, Chicago, Ill.
15. Manly, R. S., Wiren, J., Manly, P. J., and Keene, R. C.: A method of measurement of abrasion of dentin by toothbrush and dentifrice, J. Dent. Res. **44:**533, 1965.
16. Ferrier, W. I.: Clinical observations on areas of erosion and their restoration, J.A.D.A. **20:**1150, 1933.
17. Harrington, J. H., and Terry, I. A.: Automatic and hand toothbrushing abrasion studies, J.A.D.A. **68:**343, 1964.
18. Bjorn, H., and Lindhe, J.: Abrasion of dentine by toothbrush and dentifrice, Odont. Rev. **17:**17, 1966.
19. Rapp, G. W., Propuolenis, A, and Madonia, J.: Pyrophosphate: a factor in tooth erosion, J. Dent. Res. **39:**372, 1960.
20. Mannerberg, F.: Changes in the enamel surface in cases of erosion, a replica study, Arch. Oral Biol. **4:**59, 1961.
21. Koulourides, T.: Remineralization of enamel and dentin, Dent. Clin. N. Am., July, 1962, pp. 485-497.
22. Dunworth, F. D.: Class V restorations, Aust. Dent. J. **7:**17, 1962.
23. Kapp, J.: Restoring Class V eroded and abraded areas of teeth, J. Missouri Dent. Assoc. **40:**17, 1960.
24. Knight, T.: Erosion-abrasion, J. Dent. Assoc. S. Afr. **24:**310-316, 1969.

chapter 14

Manipulation and properties of direct restorative golds

The gold foil restoration has been discussed extensively because it was the first dental restoration in which contour development was possible. The direct golds have been used for many years and are still considered to be an outstanding restorative material. When the proper techniques are used, the service of the gold foil restoration is unexcelled; it is the only restorative material that lasts as long as the tooth. Improved gold materials and methods of placing the restorations offer a new and challenging future. Because the gold foil procedures have been partially supplemented by new techniques and gold materials, the term "direct restorative golds" is now commonly used.

The principles of placing the restoration and the mechanisms for cohesion and finishing have not been significantly influenced by the new developments. The gold materials are placed into the prepared cavity and are strain hardened by condensers. Forces are applied to adapt the gold to tooth structure as it hardens. During condensation the strength changes from that of pure gold to that similar to a medium gold inlay. Malleability, the capacity of gold to harden under an impact load, is the property that enables a resistant restoration to be inserted, burnished, and smoothed to seal the preparation.

The gold foil restoration is known for its fine margin. This is attributed to the ductility of pure gold.[1] The metal elongates to intimately interlock with the marginal tooth structure. The restoration is permanent because pure gold is a noble metal that does not readily tarnish or corrode in saliva; therefore, the polished surface and margin remain unchanged for many years of service.

Gold pellets are placed into the prepared cavity one at a time and initially condensed to fill in the retention forms. A building shelf of gold is produced to permit uniform stepping of the condenser and application of forces. This procedure requires discipline and exacting movements to ensure that the gold will compress the dentin tissue. Although compression of dentin was thought to produce perfect adaptation, studies indicated that this only serves to improve

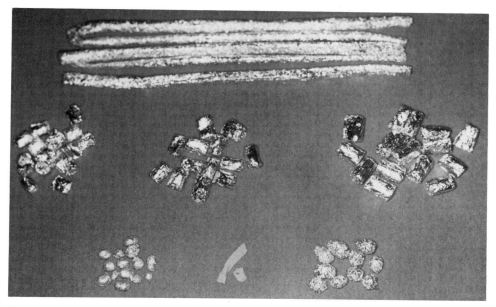

Fig. 14-1. Available direct restorative golds. Top row: regular cohesive ropes. Middle row: commercially made pellets. Bottom row: powdered gold, mat gold, and custom-made pellets.

retention.[2,3] When the manipulation of gold materials is neglected or performed in a slipshod manner, the restoration provides poor service. Each pellet of gold coheres with the material inside the preparation, and it is the objective of the condensation procedure to build a solid block of gold inside the tooth.

Most operations involve the use of more than one type of gold because a combination of different materials can reduce the time involved in building the restoration (Fig. 14-1). Certain classes of restorations require the use of specific types of golds. The handling characteristics of each of the gold materials must be mastered in order to offer a complete and efficient restorative service.[4] The various compounds all contain high percentages of pure gold to ensure cohesion between the different types of pellets. The use of gold combinations is advocated mainly for the convenience of the operative dentist.

The direct gold restoration requires an ideal surgical field, an exacting and conservative cavity preparation, methodical condensation, and systematic polishing.[5] Because of these demanding criteria, the direct gold restorative procedure is used extensively in teaching programs and by examining boards. The valuable service provided by pure gold must not be neglected because of the lengthy and exacting restorative routine. The permanent qualities of the restoration are more important than the ease of manipulation to the operator. Research to make gold less troublesome to manipulate without changing its beneficial properties is now in progress.[6]

INDICATIONS FOR DIRECT GOLDS

The indications for use of direct golds will be discussed briefly.[7]

Incipient carious lesions. The smaller the lesion, the more suitable it is for direct gold restoration. Because of the nature of cohesive gold, it is advisable not to expose the restoration to excessive stresses such as the shear forces that occur during mastication. The classes in which direct golds are commonly used are as follows:

1. Class I lesions in bicuspid teeth and other accessible developmental pits
2. Class V cervical lesions
3. Class III lesions in maxillary and mandibular anterior teeth
4. Class II lesions in bicuspid teeth when the grooves are well coalesced and the lesion is small enough to allow a conservative cavity preparation; some small Class II lesions on the mesial proximal surfaces of molars

Erosions. Direct gold restorations are used in small eroded areas on the buccal surface of bicuspids and cuspids and some eroded areas on incisors. The condition is first arrested and then the tooth is restored in order to prevent food entrapment and abrasion from toothbrushing.

Hypoplasias, white spots, or defective pits. Conservative direct gold restorations are advocated in small circular and irregular areas such as hypoplasias, white spots, or defective pits. Incisal edges, cusp tips, lingual pits of the upper incisors, and defective areas on the labial and buccal surfaces are the usual areas requiring restoration.

Limited extension to maintain esthetics. When there is a choice of using either a cast gold inlay or a direct gold restoration, the latter should be selected because the limited extension of the cavity preparation displays less gold. Another factor is that direct golds can be placed in one appointment, thereby requiring less time for the completed restoration.

Atypical lesions are occasionally restored with direct golds. The conditions just listed constitute the common applications of the restoration.

● ● ●

There are a number of advantages for using gold restorative materials because of the physical properties of gold and the way they can be used to provide function and esthetics.

1. The direct gold restoration is the most permanent method of repairing the individual tooth; it usually lasts as long as the tooth. This degree of permanency is usually not obtained with the other materials.
2. Gold is a noble metal and will not readily tarnish or corrode in the oral cavity.
3. The direct gold restoration is insoluble and has a thermal expansion similar to that of dentin.
4. The cavity preparation, which is small and exacting, is atraumatic to the dental pulp and supporting structures.

Table 14-1. Physical properties of three common direct gold materials*

Material	Speci-men number	Time to prepare specimen (min.)	Specific gravity	Knoop hardness	Standard deviation of hardness	Wear (mm.³/hour)		Ratio (silica/crest)
						Abrasive agent		
						Silica	Crest	
Mat gold	1	120	19.4	71.3	14.2	0.145	0.062	2.3
	2	41	19.2	59.5	16.2	0.143	0.058	2.5
	3	45	18.9	63.1	13.2	0.213	0.049	4.4
	4	43	19.1	77.4	11.2	0.147	0.037	4.0
Average		63	19.2	67.8	13.7	0.162	0.051	3.2
No. 4 gold foil	1	80	19.3	71.8	16.4	0.189	0.054	3.5
	2	55	19.1	64.8	14.8	0.195	0.049	4.0
	3	52	19.4	84.8	7.0	0.145	0.040	3.6
	4	50	19.3	87.8	4.4	0.146	0.036	4.1
Average		59	19.3	77.3	10.7	0.169	0.047	3.6
Goldent	1	105	18.9	65.6	14.2	0.144	0.055	2.6
	2	47	19.0	71.4	13.6	0.172	0.041	4.8
	3	46	18.9	65.5	14.5	0.207	0.034	6.1
	4	45	18.8	71.4	8.0	0.220	0.049	4.5
Average		61	18.9	68.5	12.6	0.186	0.047	4.5

*From Hollenback, G. M.: J. Calif. Dent. Assoc. **42:**9, 1966.

5. Tooth discoloration does not occur around the direct gold restoration because of the adaptation of the material to the cavity wall and because of the noble and inert qualities of gold.

6. The density and hardness of compacted gold enable the restoration to withstand the compressive forces of occlusion (Table 14-1). Severe shear stresses will fracture condensed gold; therefore, the majority of the stress should be absorbed by surrounding tooth structure. The malleability and cohesive properties of gold produce a hard surface. Fracture occurs through the cohesive bonds, not the individual grains of the metal.

7. Direct gold develops good adaptation to the cavity wall. In addition no cementing medium is necessary for the restoration as for the casting.

8. The surface of condensed gold can be effectively polished. The luster and smoothness last indefinitely.

9. Pure gold is ductile, which means that the metal will elongate under a tensile load. This property is useful in producing an accurate margin for the restoration. The gold is pulled over the cavosurface enamel and inter-locked with the configurations of tooth structure.

10. The restoration procedure develops the skill of the operator. The acquired abilities will prove valuable in other procedures, thus improving the quality of the entire service of the dental practice.

As with other materials used in dentistry, there are difficulties associated with the use of gold as a restorative material. The direct gold restoration is not used extensively in dental practice because of some of these difficulties.

1. The yellow color of pure gold is objectionable to most patients. It must be used in a harmonious, well-protected outline in order to minimize the display of gold.
2. Thermal conductivity is a problem in the newly restored tooth. Patient discomfort is reduced within a few weeks because the formation of protective dentin provides insulation for the pulp.
3. The manipulation of gold is regarded as difficult to master. The discipline required for successful gold restorations has discouraged many dentists from offering this service to their patients. Proficiency is developed only by repeated use of the material in placing a number of restorations.[8,9] Clinical study clubs that meet on a regular basis help to develop individual proficiency.

AVAILABLE MATERIALS

As stated previously, there are several types of direct golds that can be selected for the restoration. One gold is better than another in certain situations. All of the gold materials are cohesive and will combine successfully inside the restoration. Manipulation procedures vary with the choice of material; therefore, it is necessary to understand the properties of and indications for each material. The combination techniques are used mainly for convenience and for conservation of time.

Gold foil

These golds are soft and can be used to build the entire restoration. Regular cohesive gold is used as a surface veneer for most direct gold restorations. The noncohesive and starter foils are used to line cavity walls and facilitate starting the restoration. Finishing is simplified by soft gold on the surface and marginal area.

Regular cohesive gold is the original gold foil and the material for which the principles of condensation and finishing were first developed. Regular cohesive gold is commonly supplied in books of 1/10 or 1/20 ounce. Each book contains twelve or six sheets of gold, weighing 4 grains each. The weight of the sheet serves to identify its thickness. The 4-grain sheet is No. 4 foil and will measure 1/20,000 of an inch thick. The sheets are formed into round pellets and noncohesive cylinders by the dentist or the assistant. The No. 4 soft foil is the most commonly used cohesive gold. The gold is hardened during condensation by cold working, a method analogous to processing sheet metal.

The manufacturing of cohesive gold sheets is very interesting.[10] The gold is purchased from the U. S. Assay Office in bars that are 999.9 fine. These bars are melted in a reducing atmosphere and poured into a mold approximately

12 inches long, 1¼ inches wide, and ½ inch thick. The gold is then rolled and hammered to produce very thin sheets of gold. This is the starting point for the different packaging processes.

The gold is first passed through a series of cold rollers until it is 1/1,000 inch thick. The resulting ribbon of gold is then cut into 1¼-inch squares and interleaved with 4-inch squares of very smooth and tear resistant parchment made of ox intestine. Approximately 200 squares of gold are stacked on top of each other and wrapped with the special parchment paper to prevent tearing during the hammering process. The package of gold is then beaten with a 16-pound hammer on a granite shaft. It takes 1½ hours to spread the gold squares to the edge of the parchment.

The squares are then quartered and interleaved with 5-inch pieces of "goldbeater's skin." These squares are again stacked, wrapped with the parchment paper, beaten with 12-pound hammers until they spread to the edge of the parchment, and removed for packaging. The sheets are cut into 4-inch squares for booking. Some of the sheets are heated until they become wrinkled and cohesive and are then smoked in ammonia gas, which acts as a surface protectant. Cylinders are made noncohesive by not removing the ammonia. The gold sheets can also be rendered noncohesive with sulfide gases, but this process is not used for dental materials.

Commercial ropes and cylinders are manufactured from foil sheets that weigh only 2 grains. The thinner sheets are interleaved with pure white tissue paper and then subjected to intense heat in a gas furnace. This gives the gold a wrinkled surface and facilitates the formation of ropes or cylinders after the charred tissue paper has been discarded.

The ropes are placed into cutting machines to form pellets of various sizes and weights. Some dentists prefer to use the ropes because they can be cut into different sizes of pellets as they are needed during condensation.

The gold foil restoration is similar to the sheet metal process in that the metal is hardened by cold working. Regular cohesive gold can be purchased or formed into many different shapes and sizes. The use of the material then becomes unlimited and sizes can be selected for accessibility and convenience in the cavity preparation.

The ideal pellet is produced from No. 4 gold foil and made by the dentist or the assistant (Fig. 14-2). The pellets can be formed into any number of sizes, providing unlimited use of the pellets anytime during condensation. The custom-made pellets are round balls of loosely packed cohesive gold. The pellets are rolled from the sheet, stored in the gold box, and heated prior to placing them in the cavity preparation.

An advantage of custom-made pellets is that the dentist can make different sizes of uniformly shaped pellets that are more cohesive than most other golds because of the loosely rolled spongy mass of gold. The weight of the gold is another advantage. The custom-made pellets are twice as dense as the com-

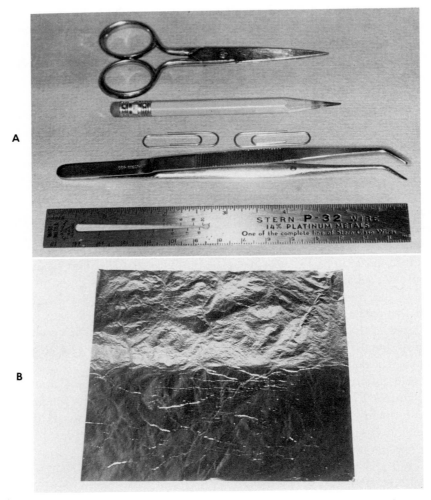

Fig. 14-2. A, Armamentarium for custom-made cohesive round pellets. **B,** Cohesive sheet of gold weighing 4 grains.

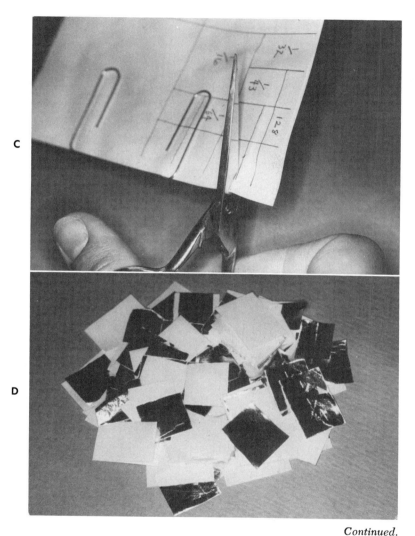

Continued.

Fig. 14-2, cont'd. C, Marked-off paper and the cutting of several sheets of cohesive gold. **D,** Cut pieces of gold and paper.

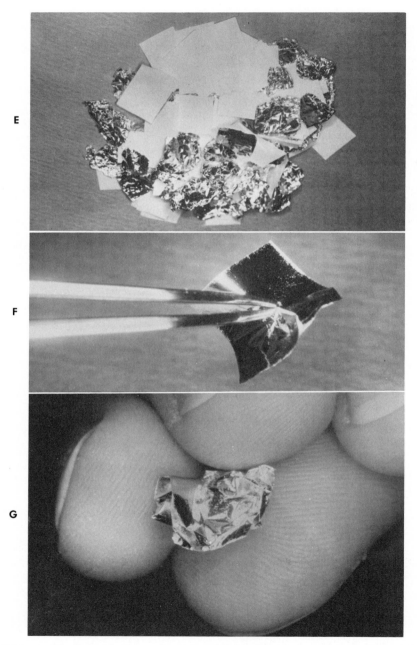

Fig. 14-2, cont'd. E, Gold pieces after being lightly vibrated in a clean cardboard box. This facilitates the rolling of each pellet. **F,** Picking up the piece of gold with cotton pliers. **G,** Rolling the gold pellet with the thumb and first two fingers.

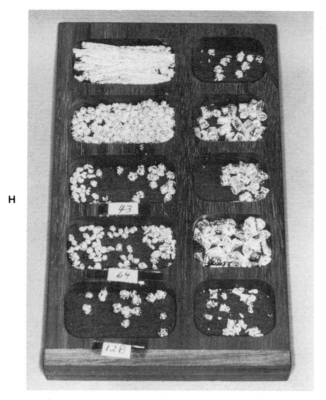

H

Fig. 14-2, cont'd. H, Custom-made round pellets are on the left side of the gold box.

mercial products, which reduces the condensation time by half. The thickness of the pellet is also useful in protecting the cavosurface margin of the restoration. The condenser is more "cushioned," which helps to prevent fracture of the marginal tooth structure. Clinical experience warrants the use of the custommade pellet, and it is the first technique to be mastered in the direct gold restoration.

The No. 4 gold foil labeled "soft and noncohesive" is used to form round pellets and noncohesive cylinders. The cylinders are kept noncohesive by not subjecting the gold to heat. The pellets are made cohesive by heating them immediately before they are placed in the cavity form.

The materials for custom-made pellets and noncohesive cylinders are as follows:

One book (1/10 ounce) No. 4 soft gold foil
Pair of small, straight scissors
Sharp pencil and ruler
Pair of long-nose cotton pliers
Clean towel

Clean, small plaster spatula
One gold box
Three reservoir bottles
18% ammonia

Round pellets. Four or five sheets of foil are removed from the book and the tissue paper covering the gold is lined off with the pencil and ruler to the size of pellet desired for the gold box. The covering paper is quartered and then lined off for round pellets in a 1-grain section of the sheet. The pellets are made into round specimens of $\frac{1}{16}$, $\frac{1}{32}$, $\frac{1}{64}$, $\frac{1}{96}$, and $\frac{1}{128}$ sizes. The respective pellets are made separately for each size to fill the space allocated in the gold box.

The sheets of gold are held together with two paper clips and then marked with the pencil and ruler. After the lines are drawn, the sheets are cut with the straight scissors. The gold sections and the tissue paper are put into a small, clean cardboard box and vibrated until the edges of the gold turn. The contents of the box are placed into a pile and the gold is extirpated with cotton pliers for rolling. The pieces of gold are shaped between the thumb and first two fingers. The gold is then rolled into a loose, round pellet and placed into its respective place in the gold box. Because a loose pellet is more cohesive, the size of the specimen is made uniform to gauge the amount of metal needed during condensation.

The pellets are stored in the gold box until they are needed during the condensation. The compartments of the box should be three-fourths full at all times in order to have an adequate amount of gold available. The most commonly used sizes of pellets ($\frac{1}{64}$ and $\frac{1}{32}$) have two separate storage spaces.

The gold box contains compartments for round pellets and cylinders. The drawer is closely fitted to prevent possible contamination of the gold. For surface protection a small pledget of cotton saturated with 18% ammonia is placed in each compartment. The pledgets are changed weekly to protect the gold and to ensure optimum cohesive properties when the gold is heated.[11]

A number of reservoir bottles are filled in order to maintain a safe supply of pellets. The three most common sizes are placed in tightly stoppered glass bottles. The $\frac{1}{32}$, $\frac{1}{64}$, and $\frac{1}{128}$ pellets are prepared in advance so that they will be available when needed. The reservoir bottles must also contain 18% ammonia, which is changed weekly. The amount of surplus gold in the reservoir bottles and the number of pellets stored in the box are estimated from previous requirements.

An adequate amount of the most desirable gold pellets is ensured by this system. In a practice where direct gold restorations are often used, this system is most efficient. When pellets are made too far in advance and are exposed to the atmosphere for prolonged periods, the gold becomes harsh. Only a small reservoir should be maintained, but there must be enough to fill unexpected needs. The level of the supply and pellet making are responsibilities of the assistant.

Noncohesive cylinders. The cylinders are formed from the same gold as the pellets, but only $\frac{1}{2}$, $\frac{1}{4}$, $\frac{1}{8}$, and $\frac{1}{16}$ sizes are used (Fig. 14-3). The cylinders are used in cavity preparations that have four surrounding walls. They greatly reduce the building time and facilitate starting the gold. The soft metal margins produce an exceptional finish. Supposedly there is no better margin than that established by the noncohesive cylinder.[12] The cylinders are merely wedged into the tooth structure. To preserve the noncohesive properties the gold cylinders are not heated but are placed directly in the preparation. The cylinders are wedged against the walls by large, regular cohesive round pellets. This causes the soft gold of the cylinder to adapt to the cavity walls and to overlap the cavosurface margin. Whenever possible this procedure in used in Class I

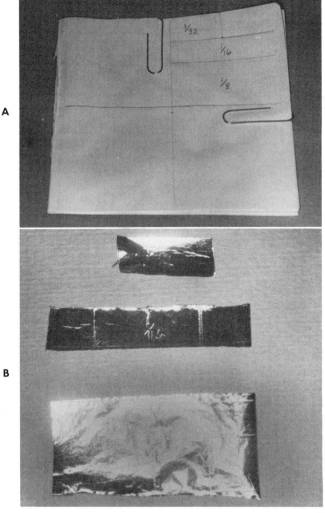

Continued.

Fig. 14-3. A, Marked-off gold book for the sizes of sheets to make noncohesive cylinders. **B,** Three sizes of sheets ordinarily used to make noncohesive cylinders.

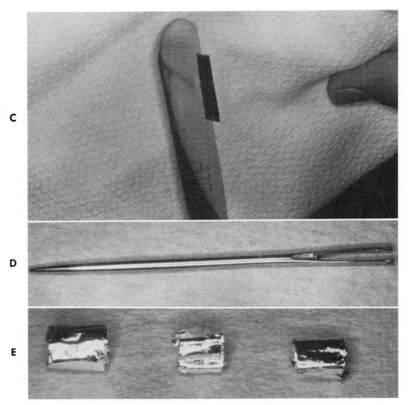

Fig. 14-3, cont'd. C, Cylinder is formed by folding the gold over the blade of a spatula with a clean towel. **D,** The strip of sheet gold is wrapped around the end of an opened No. 2 darning needle or a jeweler's broach. **E,** Three noncohesive cylinders (1/8, 1/16, and 1/32 sizes).

and V restorations. In the past the Class II restoration has been started by placing three noncohesive cylinders on the cervical wall of the cavity preparation.

Commercial ropes and pellets. Ropes and pellets are rolled sheets of No. 2 foil and can be shaped or cut into different sizes as needed. The commercial pellets are available in different sizes and are placed according to the amount of gold needed. The custom-made round pellets have no known advantages over the commercial types, and the various types have arisen as a result of individual preferences. The ropes and pellets have half the density of the custom-made pellets.

Platinized foil. Sheets of platinum are interleaved with regular cohesive gold to produce an alloy with a platinum content of 15% to 30%. The platinum increases the hardness of the finished restoration.[13,14] Therefore, this alloy is used in areas of excessive stress such as the incisal edge of anterior teeth. Platinized

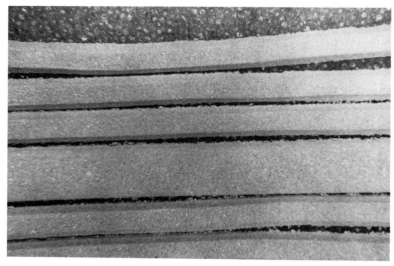

Fig. 14-4. Close-up view of crystalline precipitated mat gold.

gold is difficult to manipulate because of its harsh qualities; therefore, it is best applied by the experienced operator.

Extra pliable gold foil. Extra pliable gold foil was produced to make a more cohesive gold. The "feel" of the gold indicates an improved tendency to cohere. Laminated gold utilizes this principle.[15] This material is produced by wrapping a loosely formed, regular gold rope with an extra sheet of gold foil. The rope is then used as it is or cut into pellets. These pellets, which come in a number of sizes, are sometimes folded two or three times and used as a noncohesive cylinder. The extra pliable gold can also be heated and condensed in the same manner as other golds. These large pellets are best suited for the Class I and V restorations.

There are many types of cohesive gold available. Being pure gold, basically they are handled in the same manner and are selected to fill certain needs in the various types of cavity preparations.

Mat gold

This is another form of pure gold that is often employed as a restorative material.[16] Mat gold is used to form the core of the restoration and also serves to simplify starting the condensation. The mat gold is spongy and adapts well to the wall of the prepared cavity (Fig. 14-4). This and its cohesive quality shorten the time required for placement, thus encouraging the use of this combination technique. Mat gold and regular cohesive gold were the first to be advocated in the combination filling method.

Mat gold is an electrolytic precipitate of pure gold (99.995% pure gold or better). The "pine tree" appearance of the cantle of gold results from the electrolytic process. The mat gold is placed in a mold at room temperature to become compacted and is then sintered in an oven. The density and size of the mat gold sandwich vary, depending upon particle size and the amount of material present when the heating occurs. The sintering process holds the crystalline gold together until it is placed in the cavity.[17] The process is accomplished by heating the gold slightly below the melting point. Partial fusion occurs, causing apposition of the particles until they become condensed in the tooth. Adaptation of mat gold to the cavity wall is influenced by factors regulated by the manufacturer, such as the density and thickness of the ribbon and the sintering temperature.

Although mat foil is similar to regulate mat gold and used in much the same manner, it differs in that the ribbon of mat gold is wrapped with two regular cohesive gold sheets and is then cut to fit the bottom of the cavity form. The cohesive sheath tends to hold the crystalline gold together while it is being condensed into the tooth.

Crystalline gold is limited to use inside the preparation. The material becomes harsh when it is worked and has a higher surface hardness than cohesive gold. The margination, condensation, and polishing procedures are made difficult by the harshness of crystalline gold. Mat gold requires a veneer of regular cohesive gold to facilitate the finishing and surface formation of the restoration.

Active research has been performed that has developed gold alloys for use as direct filling materials. An electrolytic precipitate of gold with small inclusions of calcium has been developed into a workable alloy. For convenience, the alloy is sandwiched between two layers of cohesive foil. This direct filling alloy has been tested in the laboratory and utilized for clinical restorations. The hardness and strength values are superior to those of direct restorative gold. It adapts well to cavity walls, and its ease of handling was comparable to related materials.

A number of preparations lend themselves well to the use of mat gold. Because of the condensation pressure and spreading required, the cavity preparation must have five walls. This is possible in Class I and V cavity forms. The advantage of mat gold is the ease of placing the gold in the retention forms and starting the condensation in addition to reducing the placement time.

Powdered gold

This material has created much interest and more direct gold restorations are actually being placed since it has been on the market.[18-21] Powder metallurgy is now a new process, and powdered gold has been used by the dental profession for a number of years. The manufacturing process is similar to mat gold in that a number of powders are mixed and molded together. The particles are heated below the various melting points or sintered to hold the gold in clumps. The powdered form of some metals has properties similar to a casting made with the same metal. The proximity fuse and light filaments are examples of powder metallurgy in industry.

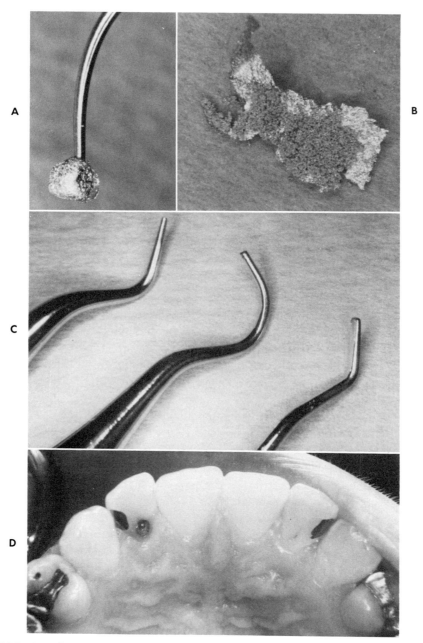

Fig. 14-5. A, Pellet of powdered gold on the end of an explorer. **B,** Encapsulated powdered gold pellet that is ruptured to show the two types of gold. **C,** Special condensers used for powdered gold. Only hand pressure is used. **D,** Two powdered gold restorations on the distal surfaces of the lateral incisors.

Spherical gold particles or clumps of gold are classified as powdered products. They are characterized by an increase in density, which necessitates alterations in cavity preparation, condensation, and finishing. The increased bulk is conducive to bridging, which is a problem in producing acceptable adaptation.

A new powdered gold product was developed by wrapping the material in regular cohesive sheets (Fig. 14-5). An envelop is formed and gold particles of mesh sizes 100, 200, and 325 are wrapped to form a pellet. The ratio is 95% powder to 5% foil.[10] Both of the metals are pure gold and are cohesive. The sheets hold the powdered particles in the preparation during condensation and complement the cohesive properties of the gold. This powdered gold is being used for many types of restorations. The powdered material is not limited to use as a core material. Small incipient lesions of all classifications can be restored with powdered gold. Because of the increased density, this material has changed the basic direct gold preparations and some of the manipulative methods. Hand methods are used to condense both mat and powdered gold.

GOLD CLEANING

For many years the term "annealing gold foil" has been used to refer to the removal of surface contaminants. The actual process involves the use of heat to remove the protective ammonia gas placed on the gold by the manufacturer.[22] Certain gases that would otherwise serve as contaminants, such as sulfur and phosphorus compounds that are picked up from the environment, are also removed at the same time. The gold must be rendered pure to be cohesive enough to build the restoration. The gold is placed directly in the cavity preparation from the heating device.

Most golds are recrystallized by the manufacturer and then coated with ammonia gas. A temperature in excess of 400° F. must be produced on the surface of the gold to volatilize the gas.[23] Two methods can be used—the alcohol flame and the electric annealer. If the surface is not thoroughly cleaned, the cohesive properties are impaired and pitting of the restoration results. Since recrystallization of the gold does not occur at this time, Phillips[22] believes the term "heating" might be more appropriate.

The relation of surface hardness of condensed gold to temperature has been studied. Although results have varied, it is generally accepted that higher temperatures produce greater hardness; this principle is applicable to the clinical restoration. The heating must be below the melting point of gold to prevent the formation of solid pieces of metal on the surface of the pellet because solid particles impair cohesion and condensation.

Heating at high temperatures is best accomplished with the alcohol flame.[23] Absolute or 90% ethyl alcohol is used in the lamp to produce a clean blue flame (Fig. 14-6). The gold is held with the carrying instrument and passed directly through the flame until the metal becomes a dull cherry red. This

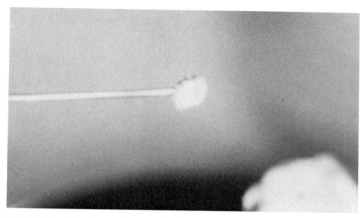

Fig. 14-6. Cleaning the gold over the alcohol flame using a small nichrome wire.

takes only a short time before placing the gold into the cavity preparation. It was found that direct heating in the flame develops a temperature of 1,300° F. on the surface of the gold. Many variables are eliminated with this method and good working qualities are obtained. Only the required amount of gold is prepared.

The heating procedure is enhanced by proper care of the alcohol lamp (Fig. 14-7). The vial should be kept nearly full to avoid running out of solution during the gold placement. The lamp and wick adjustment mechanism should be thoroughly cleaned to remove surface contaminants and waxes. Prior to each heating procedure the wick is trimmed and rounded with the curved scissors to produce a tear-drop flame. This shape produces an inner cone of flame where the gold pellet should be heated. The pellet is placed on the inner line and held momentarily until the gold changes color. If it is difficult to observe the flame, a guard can be used. The guard blocks wind currents and places the flame into a better contrasting background, making it possible to see the inner cone of the flame.

Lighting the lamp deserves attention.[24] Because matches contain sulfur that could adhere to the wick and contaminate several pieces of gold, the wick should be ignited with the stub end of a match or with paper wicks to prevent charring of the wick and crust formation during the gold heating. Cleanliness of the armamentarium for placing the gold is also important.

"Bulk annealing" is the term applied to other heating methods. Mica trays can be used to support the gold above the flame. Many gold pellets can be placed on the tray and heated together to eliminate passing them individually through the open flame. The gold pellets may stick together if the tray is moved. Convection air currents can also cause inadequate heating of the tray and result in gold with poor welding properties. The tray is useful when working alone but is not as reliable as passing the individual pellets through the flame.

A 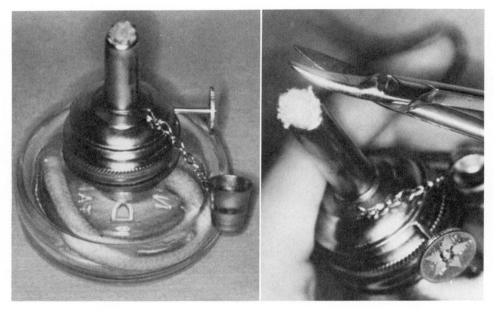 B

Fig. 14-7. A, Properly trimmed, cleaned, and filled alcohol lamp. **B,** Cotton wick of the lamp is trimmed before each operation.

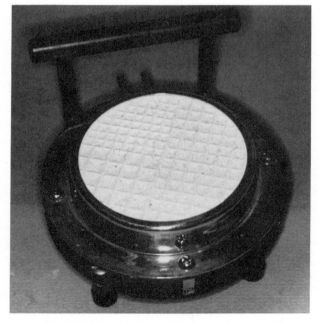

Fig. 14-8. Electric annealer, which is used in many offices.

Electric annealers have been used with success and are popular in offices in which the direct golds are frequently used (Fig. 14-8). The dentist who places more than one direct gold restoration per day can benefit by employing the electric annealer because it holds more gold than the tray. The desired gold is placed in the divided trays in the annealer and the lid is closed. The gold is heated for 10 minutes at 850° F. and then allowed to cool before placing it in the tooth.[25] This takes a few minutes because the metal walls of the annealer increase the temperature quickly. The gold remaining in the tray at the end of the day should be discarded because of possible air contamination. It is difficult to accurately judge the amount of gold needed for each restoration, which results in the heating inadequate or excessive amounts of gold.

The method of flame heating varies according to the type of gold being used. Regular cohesive gold is held in the flame only momentarily until the color changes to dull red. The heating time is brief because of the low density of the gold. Mat gold or other crystalline compounds are passed quickly through the flame to remove moisture from the surface. Mat gold has no surface protectants; therefore, cleaning is not a critical procedure, but overheating can cause surface melting the same as with regular cohesive gold (Fig. 14-9). Powdered gold

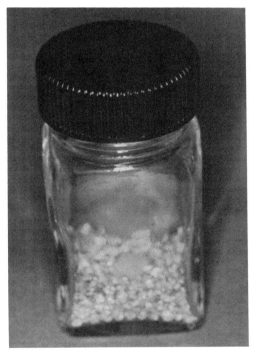

Fig. 14-9. Reservoir bottle of regular cohesive pellets protected from contamination by cotton saturated with 18% ammonia.

pellets receive special attention during flame heating because they must be heated for purification. The pellet is held in the flame until a color change is observed to ensure that the heat reaches all the powdered particles. Caution must be exercised to avoid pulp damage from high temperatures by allowing the pellet to cool before placing it in the cavity preparation.

A suitable carrying instrument is used to hold the gold in the flame. The most desirable is a fine nichrome wire, since it does not interfere with the heat utilized in cleaning the metal. Also, if it is small, it allows for maximum ease in placing the gold accurately during condensation (Fig. 14-6). The metal must not become charred in the flame because this will contaminate the material. The nichrome wires and stainless steel instruments are found to be satisfactory. The gold must be firmly engaged to prevent dropping and to permit accurate placing of the pellet on the building shelf.

Cleaning of the gold is usually performed by the dental assistant. The procedure should be rhythmic and steady so that the dentist is free to concentrate on the procedures for the restoration. While the previously placed pellet is being condensed, the assistant picks up the pellet requested by the operator, passes it through the flame, and holds the pellet until it cools. Therefore, the assistant must stay one step ahead of the dentist. The last movement of the condenser nib locates the spot where the pellet should be placed and it is then seated by the assistant. The assistant is also free to perform the malleting necessary in condensation or to adjust the unit light and instrument tray. The team approach must be efficient to keep the placement time at a minimum and to enable the dentist to place the entire restoration without diverting his eyes from the surgical field.

Working without the aid of an assistant complicates placing the direct gold restoration. If this is the case, the mica tray is used or a number of pellets are heated at one time. The pieces can then be picked up with the condenser and carried directly to the tooth, eliminating one instrument transfer for each pellet of gold.

CONDENSATION

The method for placing and finishing the gold restoration is exacting and requires discipline. Techniques differ with the type of gold selected, but an overall systematic approach is necessary to place the gold into a clean and exacting preparation, develop a building ledge, and produce cohesion and hardness with each pellet. The direct gold preparation must be accurately designed and must have adequate retention to withstand the forces of condensation and to support the restoration.

Condensation is the procedure used to harden the gold inside the preparation. After the pellet is placed in the tooth, it is impacted to develop hardness and to produce adaptation of the material to the cavity wall. When the gold is condensed, slip planes develop between the anatomic structure and restoration and the resultant stress produces the hardness.[6] Each pellet must be thoroughly condensed and hardened because once it is covered there is no method to reach the gold in order to remove the porosity. Thorough condensation will result in a dense, nonporous gold restoration.

The rules for condensation were established for regular cohesive gold. The variables of condensation are the heft of the blow, the angulation and size of the condenser, and the method of stepping the instrument. Mat and powdered gold are hardened with special condensers and different applications, which makes it necessary to initially master the techniques for regular cohesive gold. Adequate condensation requires skill and judgment as well as a knowledge of tooth structure, and these are developed by mastering the techniques for regular cohesive gold.

The effect of the force or heft of the blow on the condenser has been studied by many investigators.[23,26] The force has been calibrated for the diameter of the condenser. The larger the diameter of the nib, the more force will be required to condense the gold. It is also known that, regardless of the type of condensation employed, the force should be at least 15 pounds per square inch. The amount of force is controlled by using only the smaller nibs. The forces employed are well within the physiologic limits of the tooth, and stabilizing the surrounding teeth with compound is a further safeguard.

The direction of the force applied during condensation is called the line of force.[2] If properly applied, the lines of force ensure sound adaption of the gold by harnessing the elasticity of dentin. Black advocated that lines of force on the condenser be directed at an angle of 45 degrees to the cavity walls (Fig. 14-10). This means the nibs are directed to trisect the point angles and to bisect the line angles formed by the cavity walls. The same angulation is maintained for building the entire restoration, with all the forces being directed toward the inside of the cavity form.

The lines of force are also directed at right angles to the surface in seating the gold. A building shelf is produced for proximal restorations and a gold bank is employed for the occlusal and gingival restorations. The shelf and ledge

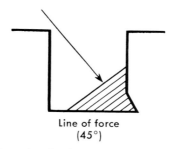

Line of force
(45°)

Fig. 14-10. Illustrating the direction for the proper lines of force.

are kept concave to permit access for the condenser; this relationship causes the gold to be tightly wedged into the tooth structure.

When an improper building shelf is produced, a bridging occurs. The gold bulges out and produces a convexity in the material. The contour of the gold prevents the condenser from reaching the cavity wall, causing porosity. The bridging of the gold prevents the proper lines of force from being applied and poor adaptation results. Bridging is prevented by uniform placement of the material and by adequate condensation of the gold, using the proper lines of force.

For years discussion and research have centered on the elasticity of dentin.[2,27] Supposedly the tightness and adaptation of the gold restoration is increased by compressing the vital dentin tissue. This is the main reason why the axial-pulpal walls and retention forms are located in the dentin. Initially it was thought that the elastic property of dentin produced a hermetically sealed gold foil restoration. The value of this property is now doubtful, but differences in adaptation do occur even when the rules of condensation are precisely followed. The influence of the elasticity of dentin is not fully understood and further research is needed to determine the actual stress distribution and bending of the dentin produced by gold condensation.

Stepping of the condenser is important to be certain of strain hardening the entire pellet. The condenser is uniformly moved over the building shelf, making sure to overlap the working point by one fourth of its diameter (Fig. 14-11). The stepping method can be compared to putting shingles on a roof and it ensures a smooth and even shelf. Uniform stepping not only produces a denser restoration, but it reduces the time required for condensation. When the rule of uniform stepping is followed, it is unlikely that the operator will neglect any of the pellets, as often happens when the condenser is skipped around on the gold. Uniform stepping is as important as any other procedure in placing regular cohesive gold.

Convenience points are placed in the preparation to facilitate starting the gold. These points are refined retention forms placed in the corners of the tooth to accept the first pellets. The convenience points are pyramidal or triangular

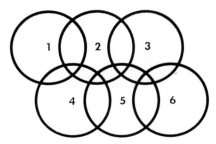

Fig. 14-11. Method of uniform stepping of the condenser.

in shape and prevent slippage of the pellet. They are used in proximal restorations because these preparations do not have four confining walls. The corners are used in gingival and occlusal preparations but do not have as much of an undercut to hold the gold. The gold is wedged into the convenience points and held there until it is condensed. To be effective the convenience points are located in the dentin and undercut below the enamel. The refinement of convenience points is one of the last details of the proximal gold restoration.

In summary, the following rules are observed for the condensation of regular cohesive gold:

1. Fifteen pounds per square inch of force should be exerted on the condenser nib. A condenser with a diameter of less than 1 mm. should be selected.

2. The lines of force on the condenser should be directed at an angle of 45 degrees to the cavity walls. Forces are directed into the preparation in such a manner as to seat the gold in the cavity form, and they should bisect or trisect the line and point angles.

3. Uniform stepping of the condenser should be employed. It is desirable to overlap the nib by one fourth of its diameter. A minimum thickness of pellet of gold is placed between the cavity wall and the nib to prevent crazing the enamel rods.

The method used to evaluate the effectiveness of condensation is to measure the density of the gold. A perfect restoration should be as dense as pure gold and have the same specific gravity. Condensed gold has a specific gravity of 19.30 to 19.35. Research has been conducted to determine the density of the various golds. The values do not differ significantly; therefore, the selection of the material can be made on the basis of its handling characteristics. An increase in density of commercial products complicates condensation and inhibits adaptation of the material to the tooth. To reduce the placement time, dense materials are generally used for the internal core and regular cohesive gold is used to veneer the surface of the restoration.

Methods of condensation

Gold foil condensers differ from other instruments in that they have longer handles and flattened ends for malleting. Long-handled condensers are used with the hand mallet and they have straight shafts designed to help the dentist direct the lines of force. They are made of plated carbon steel and can be cleaned and sterilized like the hand-cutting instruments.

Gold foil condensers are unique because of the serrations on the nib. The serrations are small and pyramidal in shape to increase the surface area of the working point; they serve to interlock each pellet with the previously placed gold and are instrumental in creating cohesion. The serrations are the same size on all condensers; therefore, more projections are present as the diameter of the nib increases.

Cohesion and hardness are improved by the use of small pieces of gold because the actual working pressure and surface contact are improved. The serrations tend to improve these qualities by biting into the foil and permitting a firm application of the working point before the force is applied. The serrations should be kept clean at all times to ensure optimum working qualities. Occasionally they become plugged with small pieces of gold and must be cleaned with a wire brush. Some investigators have advocated removal of the serrations, but this produces a burnishing instrument. Burnishing of the gold is done on the surface layer after condensation, but not on the internal material.

The shape of condenser points varies and numerous investigators have designed a series of instruments for the respective preparations. The Black, Woodbury, and Ferrier instrument sets are frequently used for regular cohesive gold. The common points are of the monangle (circular), foot, parallelogram, and bayonet designs. Each design is serrated and is available in different sizes. Condensers are specifically designed for the various preparations. The purpose of each design is to provide proper access in order to obtain good condensation. Because of the large number of condensers, only a general discussion of the application of basic designs is included.

Monangle condensers are used to start the gold in the convenience points. The proximal restorations are started with one or two monangles because they are small and fit into the convenience points on the cervical wall. They are ideal for developing the building shelf in the Class III restoration and are the most frequently employed condensers in this class. Monangles are small and are capable of producing excellent initial adaptation to the cavity wall. They are used in the Class V restoration to develop the building shelf and to cover the axial wall after the retentions are filled.

Foot condensers are considered to be the most commonly used design. They are available in many sizes and have a wide range of application when the toe and the heel of the instrument are used in combination. Some operators use the foot for the entire gingival restoration. The inclination of the condenser face is appropriate for the forces needed to develop the building shelf for the Class V restoration. Occasionally the Class III restoration, especially the lingual-gingival portion, can be placed by rocking the foot to harden the gold. This is not needed when a lingual-gingival shoulder is restored with the monangle condenser, but not all preparations include this design.

Foot condensers are used to burnish the surface layer of the restoration. Occasionally the serrations are removed from the condenser to facilitate the burnishing procedure. This is used on many types of gold restorations as an initial procedure to hand burnishing.

Parallelogram condensers are helpful in adapting the internal line angles of the restoration. Some preparations are suited for this design because the corner of the preparation is made in the same shape of the parallelogram. The instrument is also used to build up the gold in conditions similar to those in which the monangle round nib is employed.

Bayonet condensers are useful for providing access inside the preparation. It is commonly applied in condensing the incisal point angle in Class III preparations. The bayonet point reaches around the labial wall and hardens the gold in the incisal retention form. Many different sizes of bayonets are available for application to the different thicknesses of incisor and cuspid teeth.

Occasionally the bayonet condenser is used as a holding instrument to start the Class III and IV restorations. The gold is inserted in the lingual retention form and condensed and held with the bayonet point from the lingual side. This keeps the labial portion of the preparation open for manipulation of the gold. Pellets are placed across the cervical wall and into the labial point angle. When the gold hardens, the bayonet is removed after the triangular bars have been produced inside the convenience points.

Only the common applications of the condensers have been described. Many other techniques can be performed with each type of condenser; other designs not mentioned in this discussion are favored by some dentists. The design is selected for the lines of force and the stepping procedure. The purpose of the design is to improve the wedging of the gold inside the cavity preparation and to enable the proper lines of force to be applied. Condensers differ according to the shape and angulation of the working point.

The long-handled condensers are designed to be used with the hand mallet. Many types of mallets are available; the most commonly used mallets are those designed by Prime and Ferrier. The hand mallets are employed by the assistant because the dentist must both set and hold the condenser. Cleaning the gold, placing the pellet, and using the hand mallet are all duties of the assistant.

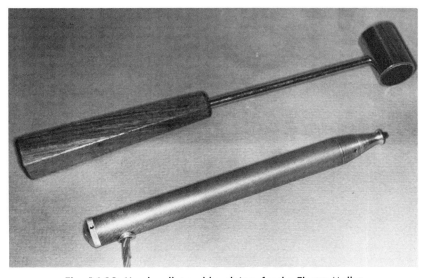

Fig. 14-12. Hand mallet and handpiece for the Electro-Mallet.

The hand mallet is still widely used and considered by some dentists to be the most acceptable method for condensation (Fig. 14-12). A skillful assistant follows a set routine. Rhythmic blows of the mallet are applied after the condenser is set in the gold pellet. Hand pressure is used to position the condenser in the desired place on the pellet before force is applied and before uniform stepping is initiated. The frequency and intensity of the blows are regulated by the dentist because the effectiveness of the malleting can only be determined by holding the condenser. Training of the assistant is part of the responsibility of the study club because these movements require skill and practice.

Through the years a number of automatic gold condensers has been produced.[26] The purpose of the automatic condensers is to produce a more efficient and atraumatic procedure. Some dentists believe that the pulp is better protected with a regulated blow, and this device makes it easier to direct the lines of force. The early automatic condensers included a spring mallet, which was not very effective because slipping resulted when forces were applied.

The pneumatic condenser by Hollenback is driven by a small electric engine and air compressor. The pressure develops from the compressor and is propelled through a small rubber tube to the handpiece. The handpiece can be regulated to adjust the frequency and intensity of the blow. An advantage of using the pneumatic condenser is that a soft, firm blow is produced on the gold surface.

The number of points available for the straight and contra-angle pneumatic handpieces makes it possible to reach any type preparation. The condenser is seated on the gold and the handpiece is pushed. The load is produced by the column of air that travels through the handpiece. Condensation is accomplished at a rapid rate, observing the same rules as in hand malleting. Normally only two blows are directed for each position before overlapping the working point for the next area of the pellet. The Woodbury condenser points are commonly used with the pneumatic condenser.

The Electro-Mallet manufactured by Robert C. McShirley Products is another automatic condenser that is used (Fig. 14-13). This condenser has a frequency range of 0 to 3,200 vibrations per minute. The value of speed condensation is questionable, but the simplification of the building procedure is evident. An electric contact is formed with a rotating ring, which vibrates the working point. The intensity is calibrated with a dial that regulates the force exerted by the condenser.

The Electro-Mallet has three separate condensing speeds. The lowest range is from 0 to 1,600 cpm and is used for starting the restoration. The speed is regulated so that the point impacts twice upon pressing the condenser on the bracket table. This slow speed is necessary for filling the convenience points or for combining the initial gold placed into the retention forms. At this time the monangle points are used to obtain complete condensation in the small areas. The dial is set at 5 or 6 and left there for the entire starting procedure.

The frequency is then raised to 1,600 cpm to build up the restoration. This

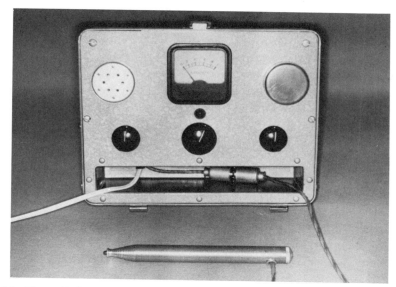

Fig. 14-13. Electro-Mallet—an automatic condenser. (Courtesy Robert C. McShirley Products.)

speed is fast and care must be taken to avoid skipping around on the surface of the gold. Application of forces and overlapping the condenser are continued until the restoration is contoured. This speed range is employed until the full contour is developed, being certain to use the proper size of pellets and prevent bridging of the gold.

The overpack is then burnished or "after condensed" with a speed of 3,200 cpm. The value of this speed in building the restoration is questionable, but the burnishing effect is excellent because it prepares the surface for hand working. The fastest speed on the Electro-Mallet is employed only for burnishing. The face of the condenser is moved over the entire surface and marginal areas until the surface acquires a dull burnished appearance. This procedure hardens the surface for hand burnishing and filing.

The Electro-Mallet must be maintained and cleaned thoroughly for an optimum performance. The straight and contra-angle handpiece attachments are cleaned with an alcohol sponge following each procedure. The ring inside the straight handpiece must also be cleaned. Surface deposits are removed from the ring to permit the electric contact that produces the vibrations. If not kept clean, the condenser will stop when "deal spots" form on the ring.

Studies have been conducted to determine the effectiveness of the various types of condensers. Surface hardness has been measured by numerous investigators and the automatic condensers were found to be effective. Low values are observed when the high frequency of 3,600 cpm is used with the Electro-Mallet.[23] Most of the surface hardness is produced by burnishing, but if properly executed all the methods of condensation adapt the gold to the wall, build the restoration, and produce the initial hardness and cohesion. The final hardness is produced by hand working the restoration with burnishers and files.

The advantage of automatic condensers is that the force of the blow is regulated, leaving the assistant free to concentrate on other aspects of gold placement. The type of condenser employed is influenced by particular schools and study clubs. If used properly, all the types of condensers produce a successful restoration (Table 14-2).

Condensation of mat gold

The condensation of mat gold is different from that of regular cohesive gold.[25] The metal is condensed by hand and spread thoroughly into the retention forms. Mat gold is spongy and thick and requires a rocking motion to obtain adaptation. Special large condensers with fewer serrations are used to place mat gold.

The thickness of the mat gold sandwich creates problems in obtaining cavity wall adaptation. If the gold is too thick, the surface strain hardens, preventing the condensation forces from reaching the material against the tooth. A poorly adapted, leaky restoration results when a thick increment is used. The nature of crystalline mat gold also produces a higher degree of surface hardness than the other types of gold. Even though adaptation is difficult because of the thickness, mat gold is easy to start in the cavity because it is spongy.

This mat gold technique is employed primarily for the Class V restoration. A piece of mat gold approximately the size of the axial wall of the preparation is selected. The gold is quickly heated and placed on the wall. Hand condensation is directed toward the retention forms with a rocking motion. The condenser is then placed in the center of the axial wall and rocked to harden and spread the gold toward the outside walls. The surface is worked until the gold develops a dull shine and is burnished. This type of surface is necessary for cohesion of the regular pellets added for the surface veneer.

Condensation of powdered gold

Powdered gold is also condensed by hand and it is similar to the manipulation of mat gold.[20] The pellets of encapsulated powdered gold are large and dense, which requires more pressure for hardening. If the cavity is not self-confining a stable anatomic matrix is employed. There are special condensers for powdered gold that have smaller working points but the same serrations.

The powdered pellets are placed in the cavity and the envelopes are ruptured with the face of the condenser. The gold is placed in the deepest part of the preparation and the metal is spread into the retention forms and line angles. To develop adequate force the palm and thumb grasp is used; even finger rests are placed on the shafts of the instruments for this purpose. Much pressure is used with a rocking motion to gradually harden the gold. The envelope is ruptured and spread to prevent bridging of the gold before the metal is hardened.

Table 14-2. Relation between diameter, area, and pounds of stress*

Diameter (mm.)	Area (mm.²)	Force required (pounds)
0.5	0.1963	3.75
0.75	0.4417	8.43
1.00	0.7854	15.00
1.25	1.227	23.43
1.5	1.767	33.25
2.0	3.141	60.00
2.5	4.908	93.75

*From Black, G. V.: Operative dentistry, ed. 3, Chicago, 1917, Medico-Dental Publishing Co., vol. 2.

The condensation of powdered gold is more difficult to achieve and to control than the other materials. The pellet is very easy to place and start in the retention forms because of the density and cohesive properties of the powdered gold.

Cohesive and mat gold has been studied metallurgically in respect to hardness. Originally it was conjectured that a pure block of gold was developed inside the cavity preparation. Hodson[28,29] has shown this is not so, either for mat or regular cohesive gold. Specimens were prepared by numerous operators and condensed with standard hand-malleting procedures. Hardness and density varied with the operators, but characteristic metallurgical specimens were developed. Solid pieces of gold were formed around the serrations of the condenser points. Voids were observed around these areas, presenting a spongy looking specimen.

In another study the investigator found similar specimens to be laminated. There were patterns in the gold at right angles to the lines of force. The adaptation of the cavity wall displayed some solid material and the surface of the Class V restorations was covered with a 600μ layer of pure gold. This layer was attributed to burnishing, which points out the importance of this procedure. The dense parts of the restoration were found on the surface and against the cavity walls. This research has contributed much to an understanding of the factors that produce the lasting qualities in the direct gold restoration.

FINISHING

There are other factors of equal importance in producing a successful direct gold restoration. Preparation and condensation are important, but as pointed out, the finishing of the restoration must be done adequately to prepare the metal and protect the tooth.[30] The finishing procedure differs for each class of restoration. Contouring the metal, conditioning the surface, and providing margins are necessary in all classes. The instrumentation differs according to the access available for reaching the restored surface. The tooth structure is not touched or shaped during the polishing; therefore, the instrumentation is confined to the surface of the restoration.

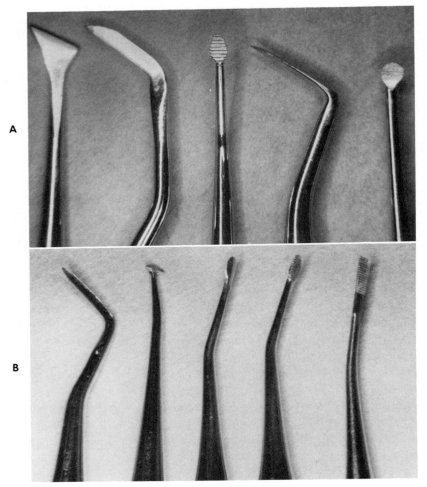

Fig. 14-14. A, Knives and burnishers for the initial finishing procedure. **B,** Files, burnishers, and knives to harden and finish the restoration.

Burnishing is the first procedure in finishing the gold (Fig. 14-14). This pre-pares the surface for filing and requires only a short time. A rounded instrument or small burnisher is pushed across the metal with excessive pressures. The metal is pushed to close the voids and to place the metal down on the enamel margins. The pressure and rubbing cause the gold to shine even though the surface is not smooth. For proximal restorations a blade carver or plastic instru-ment can be used to burnish the gold in the embrasure. Burnishing increases the hardness of the surface.

When hardness is obtained, the filing can be initiated. Many types of files are available and they come in push- and pull-cut designs. The filing is the most important part of the finishing. The final hardness is developed in addition to the margins and the contour. The filing requires forceful but controlled application of the instrument. The gold is pulled out over the tooth and pinched off at the cavosurface margin. More delicate strokes should be used in filing as the contour surface nears completion.

The files contain many small blades that abrade the surface of the restoration. The files must be kept free of gold or they will become ineffective in cutting. The rounded or rectangular files can be cleaned with a wire brush. The blades are turned to be effective for push- or pull-cut forces. Files are selected for the access they provide to the particular surface being finished.

Instruments such as knives, files, and burnishers have been specially designed for finishing the gold and these can be used as necessary. The Spratley burnisher and Jones knife are examples of special designs for contouring the filed restoration. The Spratley burnisher is helpful in marginating the gold. The Jones knife is used to rapidly cut down and contour the surface of the Class V restoration. Usually the surfaces where these instruments are used are reconditioned with files prior to final smoothing. The restoration is then smoothed and polished.

Interproximal finishing strips are made of linen or plastic charged with different types of abrasives for smoothing the metal. They are available in regular and extra-long lengths and are passed between the teeth and over the surface of the gold. The garnet and cuttlefish abrasives are used on the strips in an order of descending abrasiveness. The strips are used only for the proximal restorations.

The final polish is produced with a plain linen strip that is moved across the restoration in the same manner. The strip is moistened to pick up the gold from the surface. The gold in the strip is then pulled across the restoration to produce a "satin finish." This is the most satisfactory finish for all Class II, III, and IV direct gold restorations.

Abrasive disks are used for gingival restorations as well as occlusal and proximal restorations. This disking procedure is discussed more fully in other chapters, but it should be mentioned here. The disks should be small—¼, ⅜, or ½ inch in diameter—to prevent damaging gingival tissue and to allow them to be used inside the special clamps. The abrasives on the disks should be No. 00 or No. 000 cuttlefish because this smoothing procedure is conducted with light pressure over the entire surface of the restoration. The disks are moved from the metal to the tooth. All the irregularities left from the filing are removed at this time to produce a smooth and exacting margin and surface on the restoration. Lubricants and air coolants are used to prevent elevated temperatures in the restoration and the tooth.

With the exception of the Class III and IV restorations, a high surface luster is developed on all restorations. This is done with dry abrasives and is a very short procedure. Silica and pumice can be used for smoothing and then the metallic oxide polishing compounds are used to produce the shine. The compounds are applied with a soft rubber cup, taking care not to elevate the temperature or abrade the surrounding tooth structure. For this procedure the polishing is confined to the surface area. A high luster will develop in a matter of seconds if the preceding finishing steps have been well performed.

Stibbs[11] has reported that compounds 303 and 309W are effective powders for polishing the direct gold restoration. These are available from commercial sources and seem to be more effective in producing the final smoothness and luster for the gingival restoration.

The finishing enhances the qualities of pure gold. The polished gold restoration will not tarnish or corrode in mouth fluids. The smooth surface promotes the health of gingival tissue in contact with the restoration.

The hardness of the polished surface of different types of gold has been studied. Mat and powdered gold produce a slightly greater hardness than regular cohesive gold. If the rules are followed carefully, the hardness of the restoration will be acceptable and stable for many years of clinical service. It is thought that platinum alloys and laminated gold restorations will not flake after many years of service, supposedly because the materials produce a harder or denser surface layer. However, clinical research with the materials and many years of close observation are necessary before this can be verified.

Materials and techniques influence the sealing ability of the gold restoration. The penetration of isotopes around the walls of the direct golds has demonstrated a better cavity seal than most materials.[3,31] The type of gold material used and the method of condensation are important. In general mat and powdered gold are not as effective as regular cohesive gold. It has been found that routinely good results are more difficult to obtain with the materials that have been hand condensed. The cavity seal and adaptation produced by the golds are factors to be considered in selecting a restorative material.

BIOLOGIC PROPERTIES

Extensive studies have been made on the biologic factors of restorative materials. The gingival health and resultant periodontal support are excellent when in contact with the gold restoration.[32] The health of the epithelial tissue is promoted and histologically appears comparable to tissue abutting sound enamel or glazed porcelain.

The periodontal health of the tooth following the placement of the gold foil restoration has been questioned. The trauma of malleting and the damage to the periodontal membrane have been widely discussed. Damage to these structures results if a traumatic method of condensation is used or if the tooth does not receive proper stabilization during the procedure. To combat periodontal injury all restorations must be stabilized with compound or acrylic die prior to condensation. This usually is not a problem because the separator, the gingival clamp, or the contoured matrix is in position. Even if access is limited, these devices are necessary and should be applied and stabilized with compound. The "blocked-out" structures prevent tooth movement and damage to the gingival tissue. When this precaution is taken, it is impossible to damage the supporting

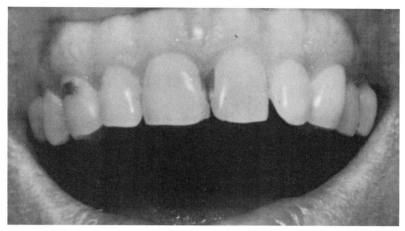

Fig. 14-15. Two Class III cohesive gold restorations that are 45 years old. The result speaks for itself. Such a permanent service is possible only with regular cohesive gold (Courtesy Dr. Emory Laporte.)

structures because four or more teeth absorb the forces rather than just the tooth being restored.

The effect of gold foil procedures on the pulp has been studied. The use of gold material has been challenged because of the supposedly damaging characterists of the material and techniques. Some investigators claim that damage to the pulp results from separating devices and neglect. However, it has been found that the vitality of the tooth is lost primarily by negligence.

The effects of condensation procedures have been studied. Results demonstrate that the placement of regular cohesive foil is an atraumatic procedure.[33] In histologic sections of 120 human teeth the Ferrier Class V procedure was found to produce a pulp response similar to silver amalgam. When secondary dentin was present in the teeth, pulp response to condensation was too small to measure.

These studies indicate that proper technique can eliminate pulp damage produced by gold condensation. Recovery in a 6-week period indicated biologic acceptance. It has been stated that pulp damage as a result of gold foil restoration is conspicuous by its absence. This is partly because the material is placed in incipient carious lesions or cervical erosions where a suitable thickness of dentin is present to protect the pulp tissue in the properly extended cavity preparation.

The gold foil restoration has been used in dentistry for many years. It is apparent that the procedure has been improved, both in available materials and in methods of placement. The gold restoration still provides the most permanent service for the individual restorations.[34] Until the field of operative dentistry changes radically, there will still be a need for the outstanding treatment and service provided by the direct gold materials (Fig. 14-15).

Because the gold foil restoration is emphasized on a number of licensure examinations and in the curriculum of schools of dentistry, it often creates an unfavorable attitude. However, new methods and materials are gaining broader acceptance both in schools and in practice. Because of preventive dental programs, more lesions are suitable for use of direct golds.

The manipulation of gold and the many facets to be considered in placing the direct gold restoration have been discussed. Discipline and close attention to details are important. The skills and techniques involved in direct gold restorations can be transferred to other operative treatments. Optimum conditions must be present to place the gold. A dry surgical field and an accurate preparation are necessary before adaptation and cohesion of the gold can be achieved.

The general rules for selecting and manipulating the direct restorative golds have been presented. Specific applications will be given in the following chapters, including procedures for the classes of cavities that can be restored with direct golds.

REFERENCES

1. Shell, J. S., and Hollenback, G. M.: Tensile strength and elongation of pure gold, J. S. Calif. Dent. Assoc. 34:219, 1966.
2. Black, G. V.: Operative dentistry, ed. 3, Chicago, 1917, Medico-Dental Publishing Co., vol. 2.
3. Taylor, J. B., Stowell, E. C., Murphy, J. F., and Wainwright, W. W.: Microleakage of gold foil fillings, J. Dent. Res. 38:749, 1959.
4. Hollenback, G. M., Lyons, N. C., and Shell, J. S.: A study of some of the physical properties of cohesive gold, J. S. Calif. Dent. Assoc. 42:9, 1966.
5. Hollenback, G. M.: There is no substitute for gold foil in restorative dentistry, J. S. Calif. Dent. Assoc. 6:275, 1965.
6. Wolcott, R. B.: A progress report on gold powder metallurgy, paper presented at the Interin Meeting of the American Academy of Gold Foil Operators, Feb. 24, 1966, Iowa City.
7. McGeehee, W. H., True, H. A., and Inskipp, E. F.: A textbook of operative dentistry, New York, 1956, McGraw-Hill Book Co., Inc.
8. Brass, G. A.: Gold foil—discipline for service, J. Am. Acad. Gold Foil Operators 5:28, 1962.
9. Romnes, A. F.: The place of gold foil in dental education, J. Am. Acad. Gold Foil Operators 2:8, 1959.
10. Smith, W.: Personal communication, 1966.
11. Stibbs, G. D.: Teaching outlines, Seattle, Department of Operative Dentistry, University of Washington.
12. Ferrier, W. I.: Gold foil operations, Seattle, 1959, University of Washington Press.
13. Rule, R. W.: A preliminary report of tests made to determine the physical properties and clinical values of gold and platinum foil, J.A.D.A. 23:93, 1936.
14. Rule, R. W.: Gold foil and platinum centered gold foil; methods of condensation, J.A.D.A. 24:1783, 1937.
15. Hollenback, G. M.: The why and the wherefore of laminated cohesive gold, J. Alabama Dent. Assoc. 47:17, 1963.
16. Hemphill, W. F.: The use of mat gold, J. Am. Acad. Gold Foil Operators 2:75, 1959.
17. Ingersoll, C.: Personal communication, 1967.
18. Xhonga, F. A.: Direct gold alloys, Part II, J. Am. Acad. Gold Foil Operators 14:5, 1971.
19. Wolcott, R. B., and Vernetti; J. P.: Sintered gold alloy for direct restorations, J. Prosth. Dent. 25:662, 1971.

20. Lund, M. R., and Baum, L.: Powdered gold for the Class III restoration, J. S. Calif. Dent. Assoc. 33:262, 1965.
21. Lund, M. R., and Baum, L.: Powdered gold as a restorative material, J. Prosth. Dent. **13**:1151, 1963.
22. Phillips, R. W.: Personal communication, 1967.
23. Hollenback, G. M., and Collard, E. W.: An evaluation of the physical properties of cohesive gold, J. S. Calif. Dent. Assoc. **29**:280, 1961.
24. Rowberry, S. H.: The use of powdered gold in dentistry, Dent. Digest **71**:208, 1965.
25. Ingraham, R., Koser, J. R., and Quint, H.: An atlas of gold foil and rubber dam procedures, Buena Park, Calif., 1961, Uni-Tro College Press.
26. Kramer, W. S., Trandall, T. R., and Diefendorf, W. L.: A comparative study of the physical properties of variously manipulated gold foil materials, J. Am. Acad. Gold Foil Operators 3:8, 1960.
27. Miller, C. H.: Condensing gold foil, J. Am. Acad. Gold Foil Operators 9:6, 1966.
28. Hodson, J. T., and Stibbs, G. D.: Structural density of compacted gold foil and mat gold, J. Dent. Res. **41**:339, 1962.
29. Hodson, J. T.: Structure and properties of gold foil and mat gold, J. Dent. Res. **43**:575, 1963.
30. Stebner, C. M.: Correlation of physical properties and clinical aspects of gold foil as a restorative material, Dent. Clin. N. Am., Nov., 1955, p. 571.
31. Avery, D.: The sealing ability of different type Class V direct gold restorations, Senior paper, Indianapolis, 1966, Indiana University.
32. Waerhaug, J.: Histologic considerations which govern where the margins of restorations should be located in relation to gingiva, Dent. Clin. N. Am., Mar., 1962, p. 161.
33. Thomas, J. J.: The pulpal effects of gold foil condensation procedures, M.S.D. thesis, Indianapolis, 1966, Indiana University School of Dentistry.
34. Knight, T.: Gold foil: a re-appraisal of its properties as a restorative material and its use in general practice, J. Am. Acad. Gold Foil Operators 6:13, 1963.

ADDITIONAL READINGS

Christensen, G.: The practicability of compacted gold foils in general practice—a survey, J. Am. Acad. Gold Foil Operators **14**:57, 1971.
Hodson, J. T.: Compaction properties of various pure gold restorative materials, J. Am. Acad. Gold Foil Operators **12**:52, 1969.
Mahan, J., and Charbeneau, G. T.: A study of certain mechanical properties and the density of condensed specimens made from various forms of pure gold, J. Am. Acad. Gold Foil Operators 8:6, 1965.
Richter, W., and Cantwell, K. R.: A study of cohesive gold, J. Prosth. Dent. **15**:722, 1965.
Thomas, J. J., Stanley, H. R., and Gilmore, H. W.: Effects of gold foil condensation on human dental pulp, J.A.D.A. **78**:788, 1969.
Thye, R. P.: A comparison of the marginal penetration of direct filling golds using Ca[45], J. Am. Acad. Gold Foil Operators **10**:12, 1967.
Virmani, R., Phillips, R. W., and Swartz, M. L.: Displacement of cement bases by condensation of direct gold, J. Am. Acad. Gold Foil Operators **13**:39, 1970.
Welk, D. A.: Physical properties of 24 carat gold restorative materials; a progress report, J. Am. Acad. Gold Foil Operators 9:26, 1966.
Xhonga, F. A.: Direct golds, part I, J. Am. Acad. Gold Foil Operators **13**:17, 1970.

chapter 15

Class V direct gold restorations

Because of the area of the tooth involved, restoration of the gingival cavity entails specific problems. Access and isolation, sensitivity following restoration, and retention are problems encountered in gingival restorations. The gingival tissue usually covers a portion of the restoration; sometimes esthetics is difficult when the lesion is located anterior to the second bicuspid.

Protection of the gingival tissue is essential so that the periodontal support of the tooth will not be altered. This is accomplished by a protective contour or gingival bulge in the restoration that serves as a food shunt and by an exacting marginal relationship that seals the restoration and does not entrap food below the tissue. The condition of the surface of the restoration is also important to the tissue. The surface must be smooth and inert in order to encourage health and circulation in the covering epithelial gingival tissue.

The direct golds fulfill most of the objectives of a gingival restoration. Pure gold can be placed into the tooth and hardened to produce the desired adaptation and contour. The packed gold can be accurately marginated to the tooth structure and then polished to produce a surface conducive to gingival health. This type of restoration causes difficulties in esthetics because of the yellow color; however, the appearance is improved by a neat cavity outline. Direct gold restorations are placed in many cervical lesions, resulting in as near a permanent service as restorative dentistry has to offer.

Improper toothbrushing abrades the gingival restoration. Usually the surface of a large tooth restoration becomes roughened or notched after being subjected to toothbrushing. This trauma produces recession of the gingiva, exposing the cementum, and in long-standing cases the tooth structure is worn away. The surface of the gold restoration is not susceptible to toothbrushing. This factor adds to the effectiveness of the restoration and is an important consideration when selecting a material for the Class V restoration.

The type of caries observed in areas having fluoridated water and also an increase in the number of erosions have stimulated new interests in using gold foil for the gingival lesion. More pathologies are being detected that require restorative service. Preventive measures are reducing the incidence of larger lesions, and this type of restoration is ideal for small lesions. The outline form of the small lesion can be limited, producing less pulp stimulation. As discussed in the previous chapter, these factors make gold placement a relatively atraumatic procedure. The incidence of smooth surface caries has been significantly reduced but some such lesions still occur.

Erosions are becoming more prevalent because of longer retention of the natural dentition. Improper brushing and the increased intake of acids and sugars account for more eroded areas requiring restoration. The active erosion is found to be associated with decalcification; the use of hardening agents and restorations to preserve the gingival third of the tooth are necessary in such conditions. Healthy gingival tissue is ordinarily found around the eroded area and the lesions commonly occur in patients with good oral hygiene, which favors the use of gold foil restorations.

Prominent teeth in the arch are most likely to become eroded. These areas of erosion are commonly observed in cuspids and rotated bicuspids located in crowded or poorly arranged arches. To prevent additional damage to the tooth the diet should be surveyed and the damaged area of the tooth recontoured with a gold foil restoration. Neglect of damaged areas sometimes results in an unsightly notched area or loss of the tooth as a result of pulp exposure. The depth of the cavity is more critical because many eroded areas are not supported by thick amounts of secondary dentin as is observed with caries.

Gold foil is particularly adaptable to the gingival restoration. The contour, marginal relationship, and surface texture promote gingival health, which is essential to the periodontium. As discussed previously, discipline is required for the successful restoration. The sequence of treatment—application of the rubber dam, cavity preparation, gold insertion, and finishing procedures—is planned and discussed with the patient. Each phase must be done with exacting detail before proceeding to the next step.

RUBBER DAM APPLICATION

Complications develop when the gingival cavity cannot be isolated from the saliva. In the gingival restoration access is a problem because of the location of the lesion on the tooth. The gingival tissue must be pushed away mechanically to expose the lesion and boundaries on the tooth where the cavity margin will be placed for protection. For this purpose the rubber dam clamp is used to retract the gingival tissue as well as to retain the dam. The key to placing a Class V direct gold restoration is proper location and stabilization of the No. 212 clamp. This restoration requires more time and stability than the other types of gingival restorations.

Both the clamp and the technique were developed by Ferrier specifically

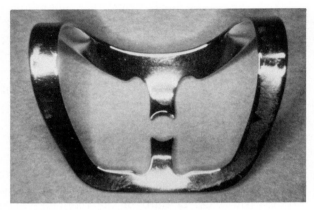

Fig. 15-1. No. 212 Ivory clamp designed by Ferrier for the Class V cohesive gold restoration.

for the Class V gold foil restoration. The No. 212 S. S. White rubber dam clamp is the device used (Fig. 15-1). Multiple jaw retractors and hatch clamps have been advocated, but the efficiency, retraction, and versatility are not as suitable as with the Ferrier clamp. The Ferrier technique includes a special application of the rubber dam in addition to the use and modification of the No. 212 clamp. The rubber dam procedure originated by Ferrier can be mastered in a short time. Although the technique is exacting, it is easy to learn and lends itself well to the isolation of gingival lesions in which gold foil is to be used. The rubber dam must always be left in place for the entire procedure, which necessitates completion in one appointment. Two applications of the dam are not advisable because of the trauma to the tissues that would result.

Rubber dam

The heavy to special heavyweight rubber dam is used for the isolation of gingival lesions. The thicker dam provides more retraction because the resistant rubber causes compression of the tissue. The gingival papillae fill the embrasures on each side of the lesion and subsequently cover the finished restoration. The papilla must be retracted completely past the marginal borders of the cavity preparation. This provides access for the preparation and protection of the papillae. The heavier weight rubber dam materials are selected for these reasons.

Although the Class V restoration technique is different, many of the general rules for punching and applying the rubber dam are followed. The dam is punched to correspond to the location of the teeth to be isolated in the arch and at such a distance that the hole will be in the center of the tooth. The punch plate is rotated to select the proper hole size because adequate sealing is very important. Saliva or other moisture will contaminate the surface and render the gold noncohesive. An ideal application of the dam must be made because the surgical field must be maintained during the long appointment.

Special adjustments are made because the lesion is located on the buccal-cervical surface of the tooth. The hole for the tooth being restored should be located ¼ inch buccally of the normal alignment of the teeth. This provides more rubber to stretch toward the gingival location. The importance of this placement is noted when strangulated gingival tissue and leakage around the tooth are found because of inadequate rubber dam material. Placing the hole buccally provides the necessary coverage.

It is expected that the anterior teeth would always be isolated, and where pertinent an adequate number of posterior teeth included, so as to have at least two teeth distal to the tooth requiring restoration. This at times requires a clamp in addition to the No. 212 for the purpose of securing the rubber dam.

It is of great importance to isolate an adequate number of teeth to facilitate placing the No. 212 clamp. The very minimum suggested is two teeth on either side of the tooth to be restored; however, it is easier to place the clamp if a greater number of teeth are isolated.

Since the dry field is needed for a long period of time, some copalite can be used to seal the area. The application should be completed by inverting the dam with a blunt instrument. The copalite can be placed on the dam and the teeth to prevent the rubber from creeping during the appointment. This procedure is not always necessary with the heavy rubber, but it is useful in problem cases.

All the adjustments of the rubber dam are made to stabilize the armamentarium and to make the patient comfortable. Proper application of the dam provides an ideal operating environment, which must be maintained until the restoration is completed. It is too traumatic to the gingival tissue to polish the restoration without the clamp in place or to reapply the clamp at a subsequent appointment for the finishing.

Surgical intervention

There are times when the location of the lesion is such as to make the retraction of the tissue with the clamp potentially traumatic. In some instances this trauma can be minimized by slowly stretching and relaxing the gingival tissue prior to placing the clamp. This is done by using a blunt instrument like a beaver tail burnisher to apply pressure against the gingival tissue to depress it (Fig. 15-2). This must be done slowly over a period of 2 to 3 minutes to produce any benefits. In conjunction with this, the No. 212 clamp is positioned very slowly to allow a minimum of trauma.

Some believe that these precautions will not be adequate, so as an alternative they execute an incision on each side of tooth in question, which allows a reflection of tissue adjacent to the gingival portion of the preparation.[19] The length of the incision will be 2 mm. The normal placement of the rubber dam and No. 212 clamp is made. At the completion of the operation, when the clamp and the dam have been removed, the wound is refreshened to allow for a normal clot formation. The reflected tissue is then returned to its normal relationship without

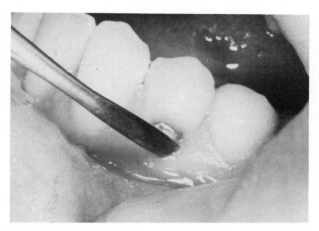

Fig. 15-2. Burnisher is used to stretch gingival tissue before No. 212 clamp application.

any sutures being placed. If preferred, an oral bandage may be used for initial protection.

For a description of selection and modifications of the No. 212 clamp, the reader is referred to Chapter 7.

Clamp placement and stabilization

The No. 212 clamp that has been selected is placed only after the dam has been adapted and sealed around the teeth present in the field. The headstrap and napkin should be adjusted beforehand and the patient made comfortable.

The clamp is placed firmly in the beaks of the forceps and checked for stability. The lingual jaw of the clamp is fully seated and braced with the index finger of the free hand. The labial jaw of the clamp is seated in the predetermined location by forcing back the rubber dam and the free margin of the gingiva. When the labial jaw is firmly seated, the thumb is placed over the center of the clamp and the forceps is removed. The clamp is held in place with the thumb and index finger until the first bow is stabilized with compound. Before the compound is added the isolated teeth can be painted with cavity varnish to encourage adhesion of the material to the enamel.

Green stick (or any low-fusing impression compound) is used to stabilize the clamp. The dental assistant is needed at this time because the seated clamp must be firmly held by the operator. The compound is passed through the bunsen flame several times until the surface glistens. The compound is held over the bracket table until it droops, indicating the temperature has conducted through the material.

The melted compound is inserted into the water to moisten the surface and the solid end is given to the assistant. The warmed compound is removed from the stick and the surface is seared in the flame. Then the fingers are moistened and the compound is placed under the mesial bow of the clamp. The material is packed into the embrasures but confined to the teeth directly below the metal bow. The clamp bow can be overlapped but no compound should project into the opening of the exposed lesion on the tooth.

After the compound is inserted the labial jaw of the clamp is pulled to the gingival border with a hooked instrument. During this time the assistant directs the compressed air on the inserted compound to rapidly cool the material. This enables quick stabilization and eliminates trauma from the temperature of the compound. The clamp is then released with the free hand and its relationship to the gingival tissue is checked before proceeding.

If everything is satisfactory, the distal bow of the clamp is stabilized. The same procedure is used to heat, pass, and insert the compound. This technique is efficient and does not injure the tissue. If needed, the saliva ejector should be inserted. The dam apparatus is also rechecked for the final time.

Attention is then focused on the lesion. This will probably be the first time the entire lesion is observed. The adjacent gingival papillae are compressed further by tucking in the mesial and distal margins of the heavy rubber dam toward the tissue. Debris on the tooth and dam should be removed with warm tap water or hydrogen peroxide. The stabilized clamp can then be used as a finger rest to enhance accuracy of the preparation.

The following are the specific rules for the Class V rubber dam procedure.

1. Because of the long appointment required for the placement of the gold restoration, a stable armamentarium should be used. Proper application of the strap retainers and napkins is necessary.
2. A heavy to special heavyweight rubber dam is selected to produce more compression and retraction of the tissue.
3. An adequate number of teeth are isolated, which facilitates placement and stabilization of the No. 212 clamp.
4. The No. 212 clamp is used for isolation of the lesion and retraction of the tissue. The clamps are modified to fit the basic problem areas and they are selected and adjusted by a specific method.
5. The rubber dam procedure previously described is advocated for the Ferrier preparation and technique. Suitable application of the dam must be made before instrumentation is initiated. The clamp is not disturbed until the restoration is finished because of the possibility of injuring the soft tissue.

CAVITY PREPARATION

Modern techniques require the Ferrier preparation for the Class V direct gold restoration. The preparation is trapezoidal, with the widest dimension on the occlusal wall (Fig. 15-3). It has many advantages over the original preparation designed by Black. The Ferrier preparation has been universally accepted by those operators who frequently employ the Class V restoration because of the features that are provided for both dentist and patient.

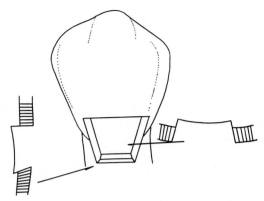

Fig. 15-3. The trapezoidal outline of a Ferrier Class V direct gold preparation. At the left is indicated the angulation of gingival and incisal or occlusal walls; the right gives angulation of mesial and distal walls.

Black's Class V preparation has a kidney-shaped outline and also satisfies the requirements of Class V lesions. The rounded corners are more difficult to prepare and finish, which leads to a less refined preparation. The outline in most cases is not as esthetic as the trapezoid form. The objectionable color of gold is minimized when a neat appearing outline is used.

The Ferrier preparation can be modified for a number of lesion shapes and locations. The trapezoidal preparation is outlined by four straight walls. The occlusal margin is made to parallel the occlusal plane of the posterior teeth and have the same angulation as the gingival wall and labial jaw of the No. 212 clamp. The proximal walls parallel the external surfaces of the tooth, forming the trapezoid. The axial wall joins the other walls at definite angles to form accurate point angles for the retention and adaptation of the gold. This is the basic cavity design, and the variations needed for hypoplasias, decalcification, and esthetics are made from this basic outline.

Variations of the Ferrier outline

Proximal extensions or "panhandle" design. One or both proximal walls can require extension in the line-angle area. The box form is still used in the extension and the outline resembles a "panhandle." Smooth, straight walls are not sacrificed for the modification (Fig. 15-4).

Curved variation. The direction of the occlusal margin is sometimes varied for esthetics· The location of the tooth and the self-cleansing boundaries permit the occlusal margin to be curved to display less gold. This variation can be used on many cuspids, particularly in the maxillary arch when the tooth appears constricted at the gingiva. The cervical portion of the preparation is not altered. The indication for this outline is esthetics.

Ribbon outline. This outline is used to restore the incisor teeth. Esthetics is demanding and room for gingival extension is limited, which makes the ribbon

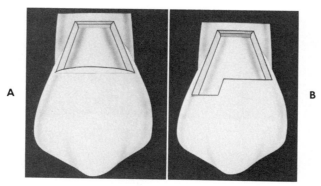

Fig. 15-4. **A,** Curved outline for the Class V preparation. **B,** Extension for the Class V preparation.

outline preferred for these teeth. A thin-line preparation is employed that has the same curvature of the enamel at the cementoenamel junction. There is minimal extension of the incisal margin to an immune area. The cervical portion of the preparation is curved to nearly parallel the incisal margin. When the restorations are large, it is sometimes possible to develop the box form in the cervical portion of the preparation. The mesial and distal corners of the preparation are pointed, resulting in a moon-shaped cavity outline.

The trapezoidal outline, if necessary, can be altered to fit most cases. An understanding of extension and design is important to obtain the desired esthetics and a well-formed preparation.

Advantages of Ferrier trapezoidal preparations

1. The outline for the Ferrier trapezoidal preparation has basic and definite margins. Forming the tooth structure and the restoration in a straight line simplifies the procedure. The instrumentation for forming the cavity is not complicated because definite line and point angles are formed in the corners of the preparation.

2. Esthetics is improved with the outline. The occlusal margin is the only one visible and it blends into the arch when the line is parallel to the occlusal plane of the teeth. When the outline is used in multiples, the appearance is enhanced by the harmonious design.

3. The more precise internal box form lends itself well to gold placement. The retentions are more accessible, which simplifies directing the proper lines of force. Compression of the dentin and adaptation of the gold are more adequate because of the internal form of the preparation.

4. Different types of coring or starting golds can be used with the outline. The form was developed for noncohesive cylinders. The flat walls support the cylinders, allowing rapid starting and insertion of the cohesive gold. Mat and

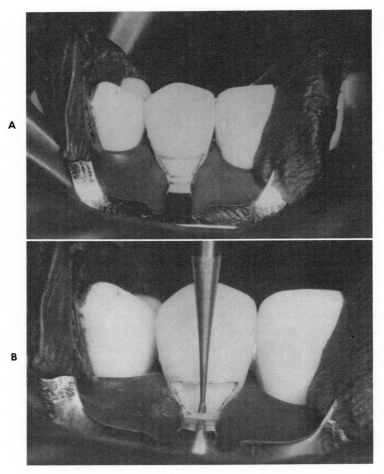

Fig. 15-5. A, Positioned clamp and penciled outline form. **B,** Gingival wall is established with the No. 33½ bur.

powdered gold can also be used in the box form to reduce the building time. The retention form is varied for the different golds and the basic cavity design is not limited to one specific material.

5. The outline facilitates burnishing, margination, and polishing. The marginal perfection and contour are developed by finishing to a straight line.

Instrumentation

Only a few instruments are required to make the preparation, which reduces the time used for tooth reduction and refinement. The recommended instrumentation can be mastered in only a few applications. The use of other favorite instruments complicates the technique and in most cases does not enhance the result. The instrumentation is presented in a logical sequence recommended

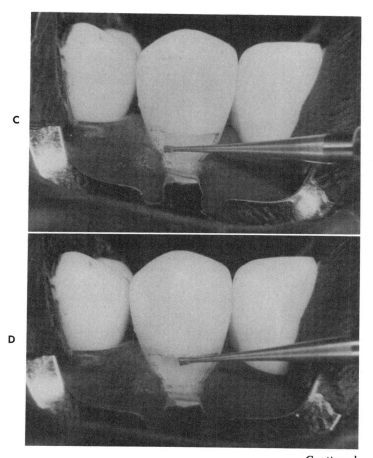

Continued.

Fig. 15-5, cont'd. C, Proximal wall is established with the No. 34 bur. **D,** Occlusal wall is established with the side cutters of the No. 34 bur.

by Ferrier and Stibbs. Difficulties may necessitate altering the steps, but ideally each instrument is used only once in the procedure.

The tooth is prepared with regular rotary speeds and hand instruments (Fig. 15-5). If high-speed instrumentation is preferred, care must be exercised to avoid overcutting the preparation. The preparation does not involve volume reduction; it is mostly refinement. Since postoperative sensitivity is occasionally noted in the gingival restoration, all precautions are taken to ensure sound operating procedures. Compressed air is used at all times to cool the rotating burs and to remove the debris produced by the hand instruments.

1. The lesion is opened and the stock of the tooth inside the outline is removed with a knife-edged stone in a contra-angle handpiece. This is helpful in eroded lesions that require the excision of tooth structure in the enamel. In the

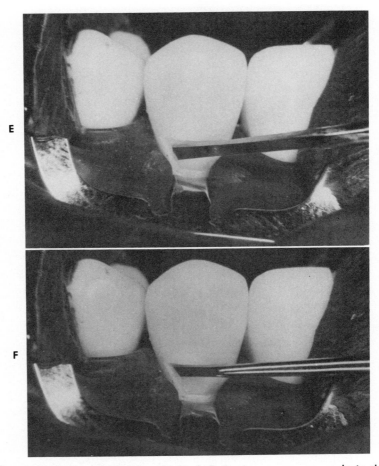

E

F

Fig. 15-5, cont'd. E, Use of Wedelstaedt chisel. **F,** Precise corners are made in the trapezoid preparation with an angle former.

large carious lesion a round bur or a spoon excavator is used to remove the decay and explore the axial dentin wall, which aids in estimating the outline form and the need for a base or insulating materials.

2. The rough cavity outline and extension are accomplished with a No. 33½ or No. 34 bur in a straight handpiece. The side and end cutters of the bur are used in addition to the sharp corner to form the trapezoidal outline and to attain cavity depth. The straight handpiece bur is used because the handpiece turns more centrically and the bur has a longer and thinner shank. A new steel bur is used for each cavity preparation to provide maximum sharpness for cutting efficiency.

First, the gingival wall is placed with the end cutters of the bur. The wall is established 0.5 mm. above the wall of the clamp and is usually located on cementum. The wall should be made slightly deeper than the width of the bur.

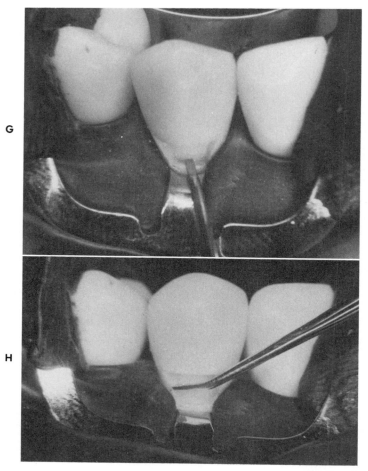

Continued.

Fig. 15-5, cont'd. G, Undercutting the gingival wall for retention with the monangle hoe. **H,** Monangle hoe is used to smooth the proximal cavity walls.

The mesial and distal walls are prepared with the end cutters of the No. 34 bur; they are placed to the same depth. The wall will extend to just inside the dentinoenamel junction, which usually can be judged by the bur.

The axial wall, which is located in the dentin, is then established with the end cutters. The curvature is somewhat flatter than the external surface of the tooth so as to increase the box form of the preparation. The wall is smoothed as much as possible with the bur and the line angles are located at this time.

The side cutter is then used to plane and establish the occlusal wall. The margin is placed in an immune area and the internal wall is prepared so that it meets the axial wall. The bur should not undercut the wall because this will cause a gold shadow in the enamel next to the restoration.

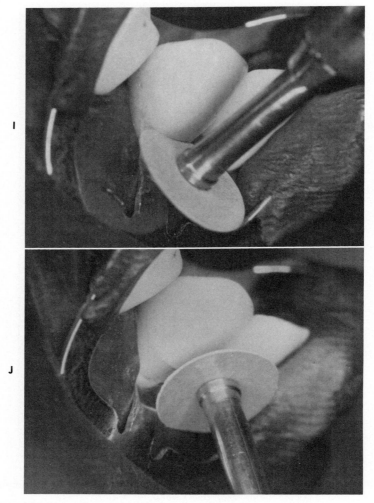

Fig. 15-5, cont'd. I, Finishing the occlusal wall with the disk. **J,** Smoothing the external enamel near the cavosurface margin.

3. The No. 15 Wedelstaedt chisel (medium width) is used to obtain the final outline form. The final extension is produced and the wall angulations are established with this instrument. All angles in the preparation are 90 degrees with the exception of the gingival wall, which is undercut for retention. The cavosurface and the internal line angles are 90 degrees to produce a definite resistance form and sharp cavosurface detail. The mesial and distal cutting edges of the chisel are pushed into the corners and down the walls to develop the internal architecture.

The last application of the Wedelstaedt chisel is for polishing the axial wall.

Small light strokes are employed to remove the bur marks and depressions from the dentin. A polished and slightly curved axial wall will result.

Much time is saved with the proper application of the No. 34 bur and the Wedelstaedt chisel. These instruments produce the outline and resistance form, and the remaining instrumentation is for cavity refinement.

4. The monangle hoe (No. 8-4-10) or a similar instrument is used to smooth the mesial and distal walls and set the angulation of the gingival wall. This procedure establishes the final line angles on the proximal aspects and places the undercut retention in the preparation. The hoe is used with a chopping motion on the gingival wall, but delicate pressure is used for smoothing the mesial and distal walls.

5. The angle formers (No. 2½-7½-9, right and left) are used to angulate the corners of the preparation and to place the point angles in the dentin. The angle formers are used as a hoe and chisel to form the four corners of the trapezoid, which is also the shape of the instrument. This produces the necessary retention form and finishes the internal portion of the preparation.

6. The cavosurface is smoothed to remove the unsupported enamel. Most of the enamel will be located on the occlusal margin and thus should be given special consideration. A No. 000 cuttlefish disk (⅝ inch) is placed in the small mandrel and rotated against the occlusal enamel wall. The disk is then turned and pulled lightly across the enamel surface at the cavosurface margin to smooth the tooth structure. This removes the depressions and superficial voids from the marginal area and decreases the scalloping in the finished margin.

The final cavosurface is smoothed with a freshly sharpened Wedelstaedt chisel. The instrument is used with light delicate strokes to remove the weak areas missed by the disk. Successful application of the cutting edge of the chisel caused Ferrier to state that "the gold foil preparation bevels itself." This completes the preparation, and the tooth structure should be thoroughly cleaned at this time.

The retention form of the preparation is adjusted for the type of starter or core gold that is used. The retention forms should be minimal because undercuts weaken the tooth and produce shadows in the enamel. Gold foil does not require excessive undercuts, but it does demand sharp retention forms to hold the restoration while it is being started. As with the other types of restorative materials, most retention is obtained from the interlocking of the material and the angulation of the walls. Following are the various retention forms used (Fig. 15-6).

For *noncohesive cylinders* the gingival wall is undercut in its entire length. This is the only resistance to dislodgment in the preparation. The walls are kept definite and smooth for the placement of the cylinders. For mat and powdered gold, undercutting the gingival floor provides adequate retention in an average size preparation. If the preparation is enlarged, some supplemental retention is gained by placing undercuts at the incisal or occlusal point angles, which will

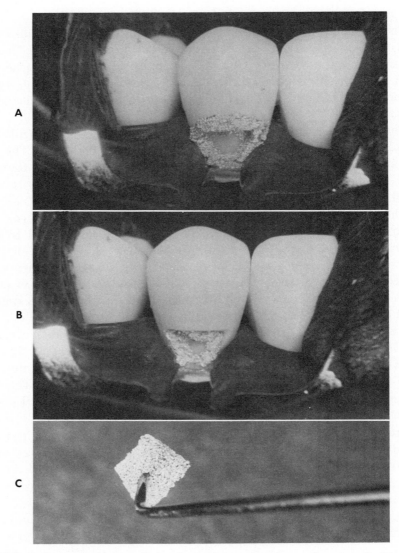

Fig. 15-6. A, Four noncohesive cylinders in position to start the condensation. **B,** Small cohesive pellets used to start condensation. **C,** A piece of mat gold the same size as the cavity preparation is used for the axial wall. **D,** Mat gold in place and readied for condensation, burnishing, and cohesion with regular cohesive veneer.

D

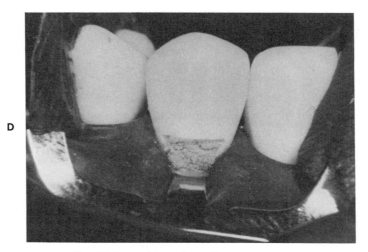

Fig. 15-6, cont'd. For legend see opposite page.

provide ample retention. Mat and powdered gold are placed by hand pressure. The undercuts are useful in stabilizing the material while pressure is being applied.

Bases and liners are useful for the gold foil restoration. Axial penetrations should be filled in with calcium hydroxide or zinc phosphate cement to the recommended location of the axial wall. This protects the pulp tissue and reduces thermal conductivity.

Cavity varnish should be applied following the cleaning of the preparation. Two applications of varnish deposit a thin organic residue on the tooth structure. This is helpful in reducing postoperative sensitivity by improving the seal of the restoration. The varnish should be used routinely. When it dries the gold placement can be initiated.

•   •   •

In summary, characteristics of the Ferrier Class V gold foil restorations are as follows:

1. The basic form of the Ferrier Class V gold foil restoration is a trapezoid shape, with the widest part being the occlusal or incisal wall. The outline can be altered to suit the individual tooth, the lesion, or the esthetic problem. Ideally, the only margin visible after the restoration is completed is the occlusal margin; all the others are covered with gingival tissue.
2. The occlusal and gingival walls are parallel to the labial jaw of the No. 212 clamp and the occlusal plane of the posterior teeth.
3. The mesial and distal walls are parallel to the proximal surfaces of the tooth being restored.

4. The axial wall is slightly convex and is placed with the other retention forms 0.5 mm. inside the dentinoenamel junction.
5. A space of 0.5 mm. of cementum is left between the cervical wall and jaw of the clamp. This space permits access for finishing the margin and vision for condensing the gold.
6. The occlusal cavosurface enamel, like other preparations for gold foil, is only slightly beveled to produce the nearly perfect smooth surface and to minimize the display of gold by forming a neat outline. The minimal bevel is needed to reduce the friable enamel that would fracture during condensation and finishing.

Pit cavities

The small pits that occur on the buccal surfaces of mandibular molars, lingual surfaces of maxillary molars, and lingual surfaces of maxillary lateral incisors are restored with a small circular outline. The caries and susceptible enamel are removed with a small round bur, and the round outline and square axial walls are made with the fissure bur. The outline is kept small because these surfaces are readily cleaned by natural factors. The preparation is completed by placing two small undercuts in the dentin, and a small but definite bevel is placed on the cavosurface with a small fissure bur.

The small lesion is conducive to the use of regular cohesive gold. There is not room enough for the combination techniques, and the small circular preparations are quickly condensed with the monangles and finished in the conventional manner. The same small and confined cavity preparation is used for the incisal edge and cusp tip defects that are restored with the direct golds.

GOLD INSERTION

The size of the cavity must be determined in order to select the type of gold that will be used to build the restoration. Different types of gold are available that reduce the building time and facilitate placing the gold into the tooth. Special methods are used to condense the core and starter golds, making access a factor in the selection. The walls of the restoration and surface are covered with regular or noncohesive gold. The center of the restoration, which is relatively unimportant for adaptation and marginal integrity, is filled with mat or powdered gold; this is called the combination technique. Some operators prefer to build the entire restoration with No. 4 cohesive gold.

The golds commonly selected for the Class V restoration are as follows:

Regular cohesive or powdered gold	Small lesions
Mat gold	Medium-large lesions
Powdered gold	Medium-large lesions
Noncohesive cylinders	Medium-large lesions
Laminated gold	Surface veneer for any lesion

Most dentists have one or two restorative combinations that they use most

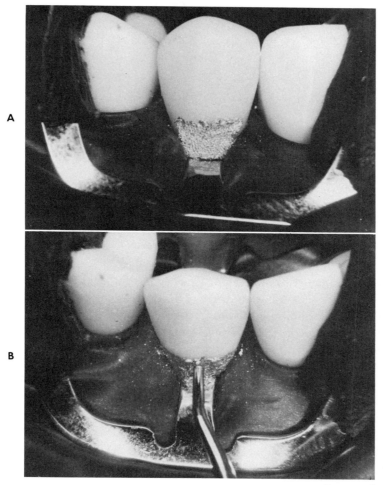

Continued.

Fig. 15-7. A, Concave gold shelf encourages good cavity wall adaptation. **B,** Small monangle condenser is used to build the contour of the restoration. **C,** Foot condenser is used to adapt the gold over the cavosurface margin.

often. It is not necessary to use all the materials, but it is advisable to select a procedure that works rapidly and efficiently. The use of noncohesive cylinders and regular cohesive gold should be mastered first to develop the skills for condensation and finishing.

Regular cohesive gold. The rules for condensation of gold foil, particularly the lines of force and intensity, are applicable to this material. The retention forms are all filled and then condensed to form a ring around the internal line angles. The distal wall is then adapted with the pellets until the cavosurface is covered by a thickness of two pellets of gold. All four of the walls are banked,

C

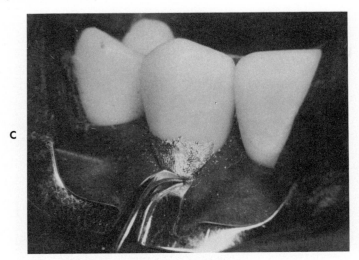

Fig. 15-7, cont'd. For legend see p. 467.

using the small monangle condenser to form a building shelf. The lines of force of the condenser are applied at an angle of 45 degrees to the axial wall in order to bisect the surrounding cavity walls. Also the pressure on the condenser is directed at right angles to the building shelf. The cavity walls are all banked, the margins covered, and the center or axial wall remains as a depression.

The pellets are then condensed into the central concavity with a small foot condenser or the same monangle condenser (Fig. 15-7). The lines of force are maintained perpendicular to the building shelf, and this produces the adaptation of the gold to the cavity wall. When the concavity is filled, the contour in the gingival third of the restoration is developed. The surface of the restoration, including the gold over the marginal areas, is then recondensed for the final hardening; the resultant layer facilitates burnishing the restoration.

Uniform stepping and adequate forces must be used on all the inserted pellets. The desired hardness is then developed. When the clamp is stabilized, the tooth will not be damaged by movement or condensing forces. If mobility is observed during condensation, the tooth should be stabilized with the index finger of the free hand.

The final surface addition of the regular cohesive gold and the condensation procedures are used for all Class V restorations. This type of gold produces an excellent margin and surface. The final surface is slightly overcontoured for the relationship that is expected in the restoration.

Mat gold. The combination technique is widely used for ease in starting and building the gold. The material is hand condensed into the preparation. Large convex condensers are used and an extensive amount of hand pressure is needed for satisfactory adaptation. The gold must be forced into the undercut point angles and hardened before it is locked in the preparation.

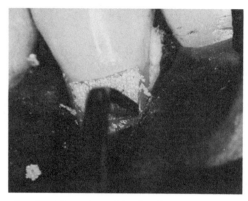

Fig. 15-8. Powdered gold condensed by hand pressure with a parallelogram.

A trapezoidal piece of mat gold, the same size as the axial wall of the preparation, is cut from the sandwich. It is inserted into the cavity in one piece. The large convex condensers are used with rocking forces in the center of the mass. The piece of mat gold is "ironed out" with this motion to all the line angles of the preparation. The last condensation can be done with a small monangle and hand mallet to drive the gold into the point angles. The entire surface of the mat gold is burnished to allow cohesion with the other material that is added.

The surrounding walls are then banked with regular cohesive pellets to cover the margins, as was previously discussed. The central depression is observed for size. In large restorations another portion of mat gold can be added and condensed in the same manner. If this is not necessary, the depression is filled in the same way by maintaining the shelf and adapting the gold with the proper lines of force for the contour.

Powdered gold. This material is condensed in approximately the same way as mat gold. The density in the powdered pellet is greater, which means that more force and attention are necessary to ensure adaptation. The building is faster because of the density, but bridging can occur if the forces are not controlled. The material is forced into the retention forms with the condensers that were designed for this purpose (Fig. 15-8).

Two or three of the encapsulated pellets are placed on the axial wall to cover the area. The pieces are condensed until the axial wall is hardened. The gold in the retention forms is then hardened with extensive forces by rocking the condenser to bisect the retention areas. This surface must also be condensed until it appears burnished to make sure there is cohesion of the gold.

The walls are covered and the restoration is completed in the same manner as the mat gold. Some operators restore the entire area with powdered gold. Other operators prefer to veneer the surface with regular cohesive gold.

Noncohesive cylinders. The technique for noncohesive cylinders is different from the other procedures and offers additional advantages. The cylinders are placed on the four walls to facilitate starting the restoration. The noncohesive gold is also softer and is located on the cavosurface to permit a more rapid and exacting margin. Naturally the buildup and restoration time are shortened by using the cylinders.

Four cylinders are placed in the preparation by adjusting the length to fit snugly into each wall. Two rectangular condensers designed by Ferrier are used to place each cylinder on the wall. The condensers confine one half of the width of the cylinder to the wall and the remaining half is tamped down over the external enamel. The cylinders are wedged into place and adapted uniformly to the walls with these instruments.

The center of the preparation is filled with the large ⅛ or 1/16 pellets of No. 4 gold. These pellets push the cylinders against the wall to produce excellent adaptation. The axial wall is covered to support the cylinders and then the walls are banked with the cohesive pellets. This locks the cylinders in place and tightly adapts them over the cavosurface. The building shelf and surface condensation are accomplished by the same method previously discussed.

This technique complements the properties of the restoration. The rapid buildup, good adaptation, and ease of finishing have inspired the experienced dentist to use this method more than any other.

•   •   •

The combination techniques make the Class V gold restoration versatile and interesting. No technique should be used that sacrifices the qualities of the restoration. The rules of condensation and finishing should be followed in detail if adequate adaptation, contour, and marginal relationship are to be attained. As long as all the requirements are met, the operator can select whichever technique is efficient for him.

The gold is inserted so that the form is similar to the expected in the finished restoration. This can only be accomplished by uniformly controlled condensation. The excess gold provides material that is used in the finishing and polishing procedure.

FINISHING

Three factors are to be accomplished during the finishing procedure.

Development of the contour of the restoration. The Class V restoration replaces the protective contour in the cervical third of the tooth. As discussed previously, this contour protects the gingival tissue from food impaction. In some restorations it is necessary to overbuild the contour in order to produce additional protection against an undesirable tissue relationship.

Smoothing of the surface layer. The metallic gold surface must be hardened and smoothed to promote tissue health. The surface is polished to enable the gingival tissue to react as though it were resting on sound enamel. A smooth surface discourages tarnish and corrosion of the gold.

Refinement of the margin of the restoration. The margin of the restoration is critical to adequate sealing and good esthetics. The gold is elongated during the filing to directly interlock the metal to the tooth. The gold foil restoration provides the finest margin in dentistry and it can only be produced by careful management of the restoration and the tooth.

Dental restorations are not considered finished until they are polished. Because the tooth is stabilized, ideal conditions for polishing are present after the insertion of the gold. The area is dry and all the margins are observable. The finishing procedures requires more time than the other phases of placing the restoration. There are a number of critical steps that must be fulfilled. The instrumentation demands controlled and forceful hand movements. Skill in finishing depends on control of the forces.

Finishing is accomplished in a sequential manner. The surface of the metal is gradually prepared, with most of the time being consumed by the filing. The instruments are confined to the surface of the gold to avoid damage to the tooth structure. The forces are directed from the gold to the tooth in order to elongate the gold and protect the enamel. The hand finishing produces the thin, hard surface layer characteristic of direct gold restorations.

Burnishing. The voids on the surface of the restoration are closed and hardened with a small round burnisher (Fig. 15-9). Much force is needed on the instrument, which indicates that the tooth should be stabilized with the free index finger during the process. The entire surface of the restoration is pressed downward as if air were being pushed out of the metal.

The gold will develop a bright burnished appearance. Surface sinking in local areas is indicative of voids in the restoration. At this point the depressions should be filled in with small pellets of gold and burnished once again to produce contour in the restoration. The burnishing hardens the surface of the gold and conditions the metal for filing. The hardness keeps the gold from flaking after a number of years of service.

Filing. A number of files can be used for this procedure. As previously mentioned, this is the most important aspect of the finishing phase (Fig. 15-10). The files can be obtained in different shapes and sizes. The blades are arranged to produce push- and pull-cut instruments. The type of file used depends on the size and access of the lesion and the personal preference of the dentist. In filing, the forces are also directed from the gold to the tooth to develop and protect the marginal gold.

Filing is one of the last procedures in completing the restoration. The surface, the contour, and the margin are established during the filing procedure.

To expedite the filing a number of special burnishers and knives have been developed that are sometimes needed when a gross surplus contour is dis-

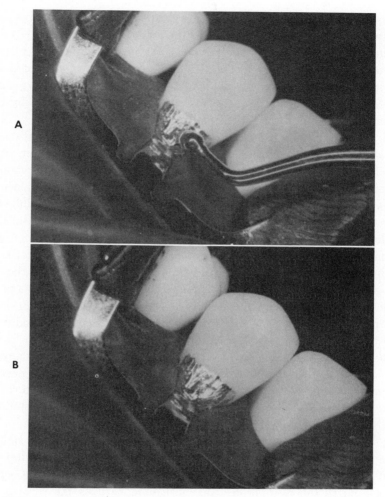

Fig. 15-9. A, Burnishing the condensed gold with excessive hand pressure. **B,** Burnished surface ready for filing.

covered. After using instruments such as the Spratley burnisher and Jones knife, the surface is filed again for smoothness. Very little will need to be done to the restoration if the proper filing procedure has been used. When rotary instruments are used to remove excess gold and develop contour, the result is a less desirable gold surface and tooth abrasion.

The Rhein and rectangular designs are commonly selected for filing. They have push- and pull-cut blades and are selected by the type of access produced. In order to develop a smooth and uniformly contoured surface, filing pressure is lessened as the desired contour evolves.

Disking. The No. 000 cuttlefish disk (⅜ inch) is used in a small straight

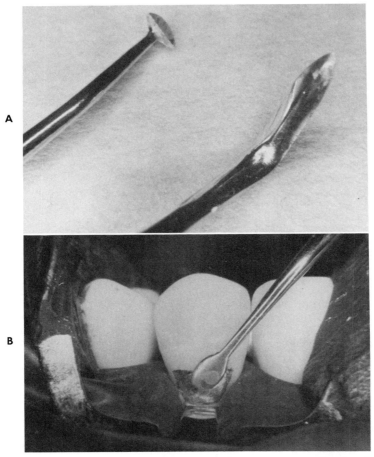

A

B

Continued.

Fig. 15-10. A, Jones knife and Spratley burnisher are helpful in finishing the Class V restoration. **B,** Round file on the surface of the gold. **C,** Rectangular file is used to refine the occlusal margin of the restoration. **D,** Proximal margins are refined while the rubber dam is retracted with the plastic instrument. **E,** Filing is completed and the restoration is ready for the disking procedure.

mandrel that has been previously adjusted (Fig. 15-11). The screw head is rounded to permit closer apposition of the disk to the surface of the metal. The dome shape is produced by grinding off the corners of the screw head with a heatless stone and then smoothing the surface with a rubber abrasive. Occasionally the mandrel screw should be lubricated to allow a tight application of the disk in the mandrel head. This prevents slippage on the surface of the gold restoration.

Slow speeds and a lubricant (Vaseline) minimize temperature rises and prevent the disk from wrapping up the rubber dam. The disk is continually moved over the surface of the restoration in an occlusal direction. The smoothing

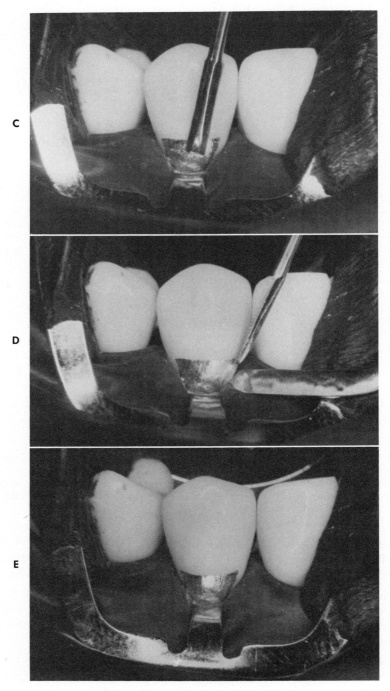

C

D

E

Fig. 15-10, cont'd. For legend see p. 473.

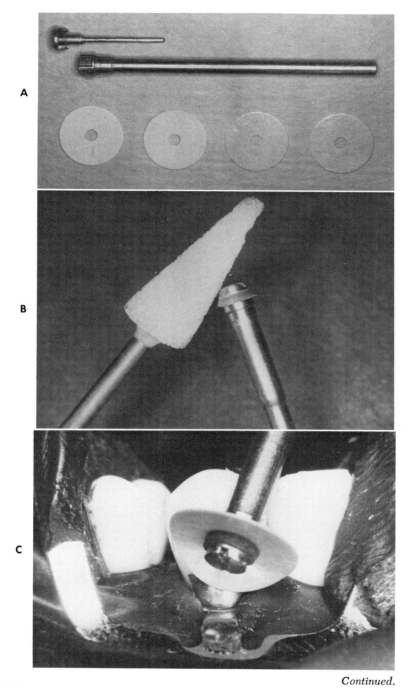

Continued.

Fig. 15-11. A, Snap-on mandrel and small No. 000 cuttlefish disks are used for the disking procedure. **B,** Rounding the head of the small mandrel to better approximate the gold surface. **C,** Light strokes are applied with a disk lubricated with Vaseline. **D,** View of the disk from above to make sure that the abrasive is confined to the gold surface. (**B** courtesy Bruce B. Smith.)

D

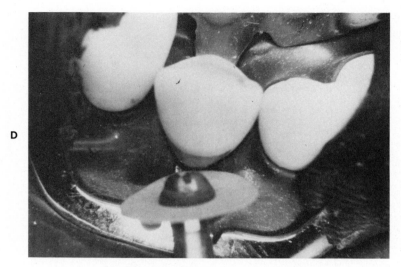

Fig. 15-11, cont'd. For legend see p. 475.

is preferably accomplished with only one or two disks. The disks should be confined to the surface of the gold.

Polishing. The surface luster of the restoration is produced by polishing (Fig. 15-12). A soft black rubber cup is used in a straight mandrel. Different types of abrasives are employed to shine the surface. The initial abrasive can be silica, pumice, or corundum powder. The final luster is produced with metallic oxides. Usually tin and aluminum oxides are preferred.

The powders should be used in a dry form. Caution is exercised at all times to keep the disk and abrasive on the surface of the metal. The cementum in particular can be abraded with the rubber cup, producing a sensitive tooth and a nidus for bacteria.

The cup should be moved gradually over the entire surface with light pressure. Only minimal polishing is needed, and inspection should be made between each application of the cup to see if a smooth and lustrous surface has developed.

Polishing completes the finishing procedure, and a final inspection of the restoration is made. Compressed air is used to clean the debris from the edge of the rubber dam and the embrasures. Cotton moistened with water is sometimes needed if a wet abrasive has been used. The surface, contour, margin, and adjacent tooth structure are closely inspected with magnifying loupes for the last time.

The rubber dam is removed quickly, taking care not to scratch the surface of the gold. The forceps is engaged in the clamp grooves and the buccal jaw is taken off the cementum. The clamp is slowly rotated over the tooth, leaving the lingual jaw seated. As soon as the restoration is cleared the clamp is further

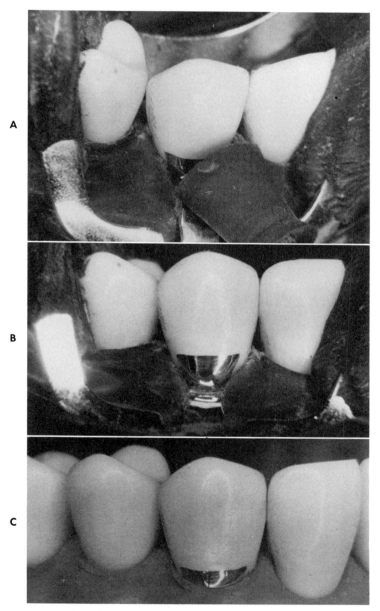

Fig. 15-12. A, The soft rubber cup is used to polish the surface with powder compounds. The cementum must not be touched with the cup. **B,** Completed Class V restoration. **C,** Artificial gingiva covering the bottom of the restoration.

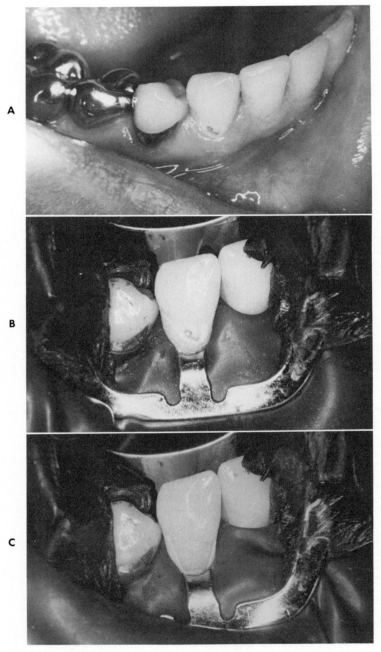

Fig. 15-13. A, Note the lesion on the labial surface of the cuspid. **B,** Surgical field and extent of the caries. **C,** Cavity preparation.

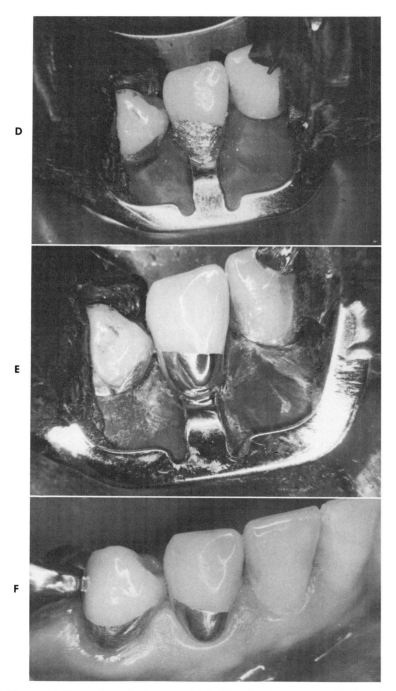

Fig. 15-13, cont'd. D, Condensed cohesive gold. **E,** Completed restoration. **F,** Clinical appearance of restoration a few weeks after placement.

separated and lifted from the tooth. Slippage will not occur in removing the clamp if the grooves have been adequately deepened with the No. 558 bur.

The rubber dam is then stretched and the septal rubber is cut with the curved scissors. The lingual side of the dam is pushed to pull the cut rubber ends through the embrasures. The teeth are cleared and any remaining clamps are removed at this time.

The side of the retainer toward the operator is unfastened and the corner of the rubber dam is pulled to remove the entire apparatus from the patient. The rubber dam napkin still remains on the face and is used to clean the patient's lips and cheeks of debris. The excess protective ointment that was placed before the dam was applied should also be removed.

The restoration and the surrounding area are inspected. The tissue is dried with the air syringe and then illuminated. If small pieces of compound or abrasive remain in the gingival sulcus, they are removed with an explorer. The tissue is swabbed with an antiseptic solution and the patient is given a mirror to inspect the restoration. Postoperative instructions are given at this time to allay any of the patient's apprehensions and to facilitate repair of the tissue with saline rinses and periodic massage.

The Class V direct gold restoration provides long-term service (Fig. 15-13). The quality of the restoration justifies the discipline and dedication required by the dentist. The selection of gold for cervical lesions is increasing, making the study of the recommended procedures well worth the time. In addition to providing a permanent restoration, the training and experience gained from applying the rubber dam and refining the tooth structure and gold will result in greater skills in other areas of operative dentistry.

ADDITIONAL READINGS

Brass, G. A.: Gingival retraction for Class V restorations, J. Prosth. Dent. **15**:1109, 1965.

Dilts, W. W., and Wittwer, J. W.: A surgical technique for tissue control with Class V restorations, J. Am. Acad. Gold Foil Operators **14**:71, 1971.

Drucker, H., and Wolcott, R. B.: Gingival tissue management with Class V restorations, J. Am. Acad. Gold Foil Operators **13**:34, 1970.

Ellsperman, G. A.: Fundamental procedures in gold foil operations, J. Prosth. Dent. **8**:1019, 1958.

Ferrier, W. I.: Gold foil operations, Seattle, 1959, University of Washington Press.

Gilmore, H. W.: Methods of pulp protection for gold foil procedures, J. Am. Acad. Gold Foil Operations **9**:16, 1966.

Hodson, J. T.: Microstructure of gold foil and mat gold, Dent. Progr. **2**:59, 1961.

Hollenback, G. M.: The why and the wherefore of laminated cohesive gold, J. Alabama Dent. Assoc. **47**:17, 1963.

Ingraham, R., Koser, J. R., and Quint, H.: An atlas of gold foil and rubber dam procedures, Buena Park, Calif., 1961, Uni-Tro College Press.

Koser, J. R., and Ingraham, R.: Mat gold foil with a veneer cohesive gold foil surface for Class V restorations, J.A.D.A. **52**:714, 1956.

Myers, L. E.: Filling a Class V cavity with combination mat and cohesive gold foil, J. Prosth. Dent. **7**:254, 1957.

Neilson, J. W.: A periodontist's restorative reflections, J. Am. Acad. Gold Foil Operators 4:37, 1961.

Ogilvie, A. L.: Vital factors interrelating periodontology and restorative dentistry, J. Am. Acad. Gold Foil Operators 4:15, 1961.

Oman, C. R.: Techniques and materials for the management of gingival cavities, J.A.D.A. 34:151, 1947.

Ostlund, L. E.: Restorative dentistry and periodontal health, J. Am. Acad. Gold Foil Operators 4:8, 1961.

Smith, B. B.: Broader concepts of gold foil, J. Prosth. Dent. 6:563, 1956.

Spratley, D. A.: Technical procedures in gold foil and their relation to periodontia, J. Am. Acad. Gold Foil Operators 4:30, 1961.

Stebner, C. M.: The Class V cavity—its treatment with gold foil, J. Am. Acad. Gold Foil Operators 2:79, 1959.

Stebner, C. M.: Economy of sound fundamentals in operative dentistry, J.A.D.A. 49:294, 1954.

Stibbs, G. D.: Appraisal of the gold foil restoration, J. Am. Acad. Gold Foil Operators 2:20, 1959.

Wolcott, R. B., and Vernetti, J. P.: Sintered gold alloy for direct restorations, J. Prosth. Dent. 25:662, 1971.

chapter 16

Proximal direct gold restorations

The proximal restoration has broad application in the field of operative dentistry. The direct gold restoration is advocated because the mesial-distal diameter of the tooth is maintained and the contour that is developed serves to protect supporting tissues. The gold material will not change appreciably in dimension, wear at the margin, or dissolve on the surface; therefore, this restoration achieves the same degree of permanency as the Class V gold restoration. The proximal direct gold restoration lasts as long as the tooth; a number of clinical records indicate that more than one-half century of service has been provided by this type of restoration.

The outline form of the proximal preparation is designed to develop a harmonious union with the tooth in order to hide the objectionable gold color. In posterior teeth the direct golds often prove to be more esthetic than amalgam and gold casting. This also applies to restoration of the proximal surface of bicuspids and the mesial surface of first molars because the direct gold restoration can be placed in a smaller preparation and finished more exactly in order to conceal the metal in the interproximal space. The conservative outline form, the elimination of the laboratory fee, and the exacting procedure encourages the experienced dentist to use direct gold whenever possible. The more that is known about the gold restoration, the more often it is selected over the cast inlay.

The proximal direct gold restoration is indicated in incipient caries on the mesial or distal surface of the tooth. Both the anterior and posterior teeth are first attacked by proximal caries immediately below the contact areas. When the lesions are first detected, the areas should be restored with cohesive gold if the dentition is healthy and the patient desires the service. In the typical lesion where direct golds are used the enamel is penetrated but there is only a slight lateral spread of caries at the dentinoenamel junction. As an operator gains experience in placing cohesive gold, he is more inclined to offer this service. The many lesions that are suitable for the procedures outlined in this chapter will become more apparent with experience in spite of the impressive reduction in smooth surface caries in fluoridated areas.

Amalgam discolors tooth structure. The material is capable of causing "black bicuspids" by ion migration and shadowing. The discoloration can be reduced with cavity varnish, but the possibility of discoloration has caused many dentists to advocate the use of gold materials for restoration of bicuspid teeth. Gold materials cannot be advocated for all patients, but whenever the oral condition and dentition of the patient merit the service, the Class II direct gold restoration should be used to enhance or support esthetics. As previously discussed, the Class III lesion is most commonly restored with direct gold. When the interproximal surface is recontoured and the restoration is surrounded by sound tooth structure, the area approximates the condition of normal tooth structure. Many ouline forms have been used in an effort to minimize the undesirable gold color. Although research has not proved the merit of using one particular outline in preference to another, the existing methods have been refined and changed during the last 75 years in order to improve esthetics. The purpose of all labial outline forms is to produce harmony with the tooth structure while providing access for placing the gold (Fig. 16-1). The lingual surface is also critical in that extension must be regulated in order to prepare the cavity and to maintain adequate tooth structure for condensation of the gold.

The Class IV direct gold restoration is used when there is no direct stress on the incisal angle. The cohesive metal will chip and fracture from direct shear stresses. The Class IV restoration is indicated for cuspids and bulbous lateral and central incisors. These restorations do not commonly require replacement of the incisal edge when stress is a problem. Although this technique should be familiar to most dentists, it is not frequently used. Most lesions involving the loss of the incisal angle have a weak, undermined labial plate, and restoration will necessitate a greater display of gold. Therefore, the full-coverage unit or the resin veneer inlay should be considered. Cast gold inlays are advocated when the replaced surfaces function in incisal guidance or other excursive movements of the mandible.

Many factors are involved in the selection of materials for the restoration of the proximal surface. In selecting direct gold materials, the wise operator takes care that the limitations do not exceed the merits of the technique. Despite the physical properties of gold that make for a permanent restoration, the surface hardness permits an attritional wearing much like the enamel surface on the contact area. The rigorous proximal restoration techniques require dedication and skill. If patient welfare is to be the prime consideration in the dental practice, the proximal gold restoration should become an integral part of the service offered by the dentist.

Separation has been described in an earlier chapter but will be mentioned here because it is an important adjunct to the proximal gold procedure. Mechanical devices are chiefly employed to separate and stabilize the teeth being

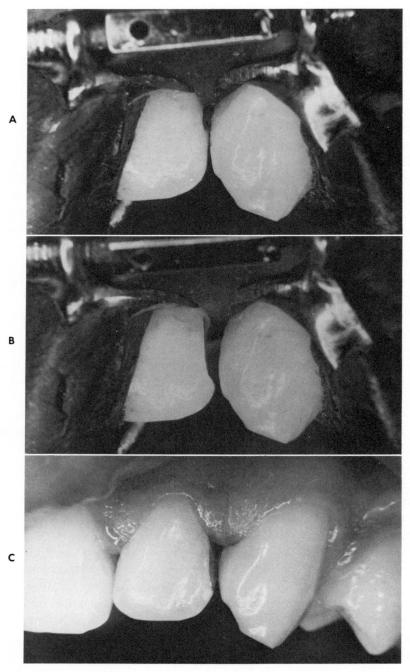

Fig. 16-1. A, Carious lesion on the distal surface of the lateral incisor. **B,** Prepared cavity as advocated by Ferrier for esthetics. **C,** Completed Class III cohesive gold restoration.

restored. Occasionally separators are used to provide access to the preparation so that only a limited amount of the labial wall need be removed. Recently many small instruments have been specifically designed for use in small preparations. Stabilization of the teeth with separators to resist the forces of condensation is a major need in small preparations. When the teeth are engaged and blocked with compound, the forces developed in placing the gold are absorbed by the entire asembly, not by the individual preparation. When such support is utilized, the gold placement is an atraumatic procedure.

Ferrier separators are desiged to fit all types of interproximal spaces. There are six separators to a set and they lend themselves well to the embrasures they are desiged to fit. These are traction-type separators that have a double bow to cover adjacent teeth on both sides of the restoration. When compound is used, five or six teeth are commonly splinted together for stability. Because of the increased distribution offered, the Ferrier separators are preferred by most operators.

With the advent of powdered gold, which requires an excessive amount of hand pressure with various lines of force for condensation, a new type of stabilization for the proximal gold restoration was developed. A quick-curing acrylic die is employed as a matrix to stabilize the teeth. The material forms a splint on the labial and lingual surfaces of the incisors to support the matrix and wedge. The acrylic splint becomes a finger rest and the prepared tooth is not unduly displaced when heavy pressures are applied.

The stability afforded by separators and acrylic materials for the numerous proximal techniques must be considered before beginning the treatment because the type of gold material and preparation dictates which stabilizing method is employed. The mechanical factors as well as the rules for reshaping or applying the stabilizing device are important considerations in the proximal gold restoration. Direct gold procedures are often blamed when inadequate stabilization and traumatic applications of mechanical devices are actually the factors responsible for tooth damage.

CLASS II RESTORATIONS

The development of new gold compounds has increased the use of gold materials in the Class II restoration. Cavity preparations in the bicuspids differ slightly with each material. The same general concepts apply to mesial preparations in the first molars as in bicuspids. Although some preparations do not require occlusal extension, it is included to cover the procedure for the Class I restoration.

The occlusal outline form employs a sweeping curve resembling a butterfly, but it is more conservative than most preparations. The cavosurface margin is located on immune enamel, but the outline form appears to be more constricted. When direct gold material is used in the treatment of small lesions, only conservative extension is necessary. Excellent vision is required to locate the immune boundary, and it is helpful to wear loupes during the cutting.

Ferrier advocated some modifications for the occlusal restoration that have proved beneficial. According to his method, the dovetail is ended with a sharper, more boxlike outline that displays straight lines and corners, making it possible to use noncohesive cylinders in this area because wedging between the walls is simplified. The corners facilitate finishing in that the location of the margins is simplified and also because regular soft cohesive golds are better condensed into a cavity with angles.

The Ferrier outline form is advocated for the occlusal portion except when powdered gold is employed. The square walls are flared in areas where the enamel makes an abrupt turn. The flared walls in the dovetails and groove extremities make excellent wall angulations to direct the lines of force. The same rules govern the Class I preparation except that two dovetails are located in the outline form. This sharp constricted outline form is employed for gold restorations because the preparation is intracoronal and as much tooth structure as possible should be preserved. Bulk is not needed because the gold is resistant and strong on the margins.

The preparation for powdered gold employs the same general extension on the occlusal surface except that the sharp corners are not prescribed. Condensation necessitates removal of all small, sharp corners because it is difficult to force powdered gold into these areas. The powdered gold restoration requires rounded dovetail and groove extremities and bulky retention forms. As with the Ferrier outline, the enamel margin is located on the cusp planes. With the exception of a cavosurface bevel, the technique for the Class II powdered gold preparation is similar to that used for the modern amalgam preparation.

Instrumentation

The instruments are small and comparable to those used for amalgam restorations (Fig. 16-2). The lesion or deepest pit is penetrated with the No. ½ or No. 1 round bur. The No. 34 inverted cone bur is used to completely excise the uncoalesced occlusal primary groove. The No. 700 bur produces the final extension and cavosurface margin, which is carefully extended to rest on smooth enamel. The small, tapered fissure bur is used because the cutting must be delicate and accurate; the angulation of the bur can be used to flare the walls with little effort. The air turbine handpiece is helpful but must be accurately controlled because of the small dimension allowed for error in the preparation.

Retention is placed in the groove extremities by lateral forms in the dentin with the No. 33½ inverted cone bur. The walls are smoothed and the cavosurface is slightly beveled with small monangles and Wedelstaedt chisels. The instruments must be checked before each preparation is begun because they must be sharp in order to remove the small pieces of fragile enamel.

The proximal portion of the restoration is less extended than the outline

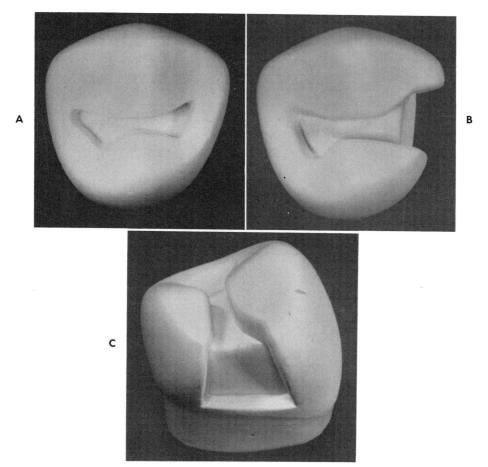

Fig. 16-2. A, Occlusal Class I direct gold cavity preparation. Observe the narrow isthmus, sharp dovetails, and flared enamel walls. **B,** Class II direct gold cavity preparation. Observe the minimal extension and reverse curve on the mesial-buccal wall of the proximal preparation. **C,** Side view of the Class II preparation, showing the required slope of the pulpal wall and the square, definite proximal preparation.

form for amalgam restorations. The walls must not be in contact with the adjacent teeth, but they are more confined to assist condensation by backing the gold in the contact area. The margins are still cleansable, but they are inconspicuous. The gingival floor usually extends to a position within the gingival sulcus. Heavy rubber dam adequately reflects or depresses the gingival tissue to simplify access to the gingival wall location.

The proximal outline form has undercut walls, making this area appear as an inverted truncated cone. This design is produced by uniformly extending the buccal wall until it becomes perpendicular to the cervical wall. Because of the larger embrasure, the lingual wall is slightly undercut to produce most of the retentive qualities. As in the Class III preparation, long, full wall bevels are used in the proximal cavosurface margin. The proximal portion is constricted above the contact area to reduce the amount of finishing necessary in the marginal ridge.

The retention forms are modified according to the type of gold that is selected. Soft cohesive gold is placed in sharp line angles that resemble convenience points. These are made with angle formers and marginal trimmers and are located in the dentin. The undercuts for powdered gold are rounded and are placed with the No. 33½ or No. 699 inverted cone bur. The bur is placed in the gingival-axial buccal and lingual point angles and is slowly withdrawn as the occlusal surface is approached. The forms must not be grossly undercut because this weakens the covering enamel. The widest area in the retention forms is at the gingival wall, making dislodgment of the gold impossible. Noncohesive cylinders merely require a square cervical wall for the Class II restoration.

A special preparation was designed by Ferrier for the mesial suface of first bicuspids. It involves only the proximal surface and can be used more frequently in the mandibular arch. Occlusal forces are negligible, if not absent, on this marginal ridge, and the occlusal grooves in the first bicuspids are often well coalesced. The single proximal boxlike preparation is produced by the method previously discussed. This preparation should be used whenever possible because it is the most conservative of the Class II preparations. Because of

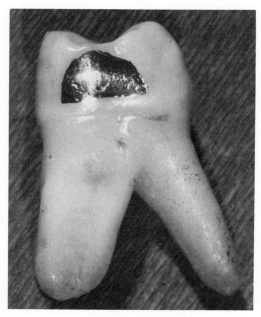

Fig. 16-3. Conservative Jeffery preparation for the mesial surface of the first molar. (Courtesy Mrs. Alexander W. Jeffery.)

occlusal stresses and the enamel formation, this restoration is not often used posterior to the mesial surface of first bicuspids.

Jeffery preparation

Jeffery advocated a single-surface preparation for small accessible lesions on the mesial surface of first molars (Fig. 16-3). The preparation is a small, slightly undercut box made to preserve the marginal ridge. Although use of this preparation is limited, the value of the technique is worthy of discussion. These areas are restored when the second deciduous molar is lost, exposing the mesial surface of the first molar. Occlusal caries or poorly coalesced grooves often necessitate excision of the occlusal surface to produce a two-surface restoration, but the Jeffery preparation can also be used.

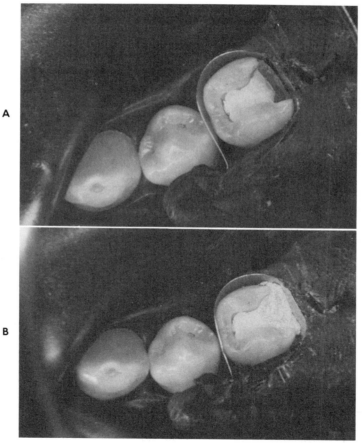

Continued.

Fig. 16-4. A, Class II regular cohesive gold preparation with an intermediary zinc phosphate cement base. **B,** Proximal preparation filled with gold.

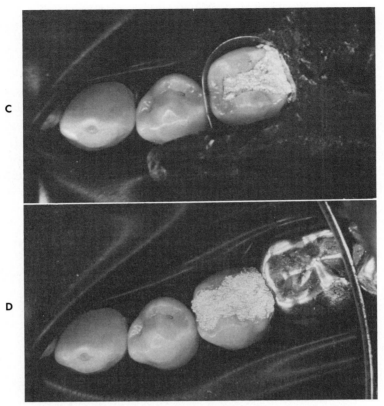

Fig. 16-4, cont'd. C, Pulpal wall covered with gold and united to the proximal portion. **D,** Overfilling the Class II preparation with regular cohesive gold.

Gold insertion

The proximal portion of the preparation is first condensed, beginning in the deepest portion on the cervical wall (Fig. 16-4). Regular cohesive gold can be placed with or without a matrix; the choice depends on experience and personal preference. The powdered gold inlay requires an anatomic matrix locked in with acrylic. The proximal portion should be condensed level to the pulpal wall before any gold is placed in the occlusal portion.

The cervical wall is covered to adapt the gold over the entire wall. Three to four noncohesive cylinders are used to rapidly cover the wall. Regular cohesive pellets are added to lock in the soft cylinders and build up the proximal form. A small monangle condenser is used to fill the retentive corners and is stepped back and forth across the seated gold until all the metal is hardened. The buccal and lingual walls are banked with the monangle to cover the cavosurface margins. If access is limited, a parallelogram can be used. A concave surface is developed with the same angulation and condensers until the gold is slightly above

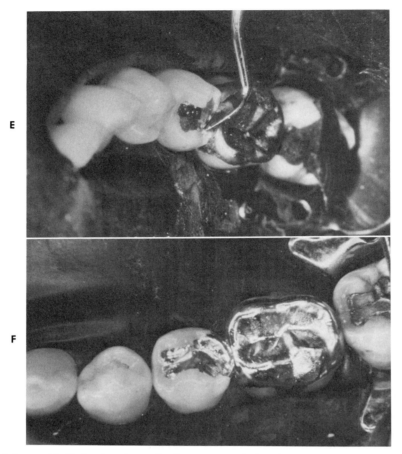

Fig. 16-4, cont'd. E, Carving the occlusal anatomy with the cleoid carver. **F,** Completed regular cohesive gold restoration.

the pulpal wall. The gold will support the matrix and be firm for cohesion of the occlusal gold.

The occlusal surface is then condensed in a systematic manner. The small monangle points are used to fill in the retentive undercuts in the grooves and dovetails. A gold shelf is started and a flat surface is developed against which the forces are directed. Before many pellets are added, all the line angles are filled and made to join with the proximal gold. The pulpal wall is covered and the entire surface is condensed with the monangle to adapt the gold.

A concave shelf is established on the occlusal surface. This angulation prevents bridging and facilitates placing the lines of force. The monangle condenser is used to build the surface by uniformly stepping the gold. All the margins are covered and the area adjacent to the matrix band is brought up to the necessary height for the marginal ridge. The contour of the occlusal surface is finished by

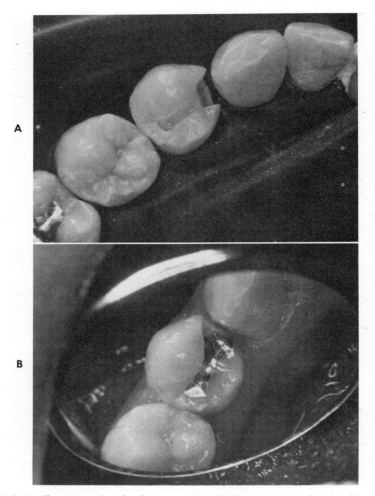

Fig. 16-5. A, Class II powdered gold preparation. **B,** Completed powdered gold restoration.

developing the cusp planes and contours around the grooves in the condensed gold. The planned contour will minimize the amount of gold needed and will reduce the time of the operation.

The occlusal gold surface is uniformly hardened with small monangle condensers. The gold will become closely compacted, preparing the surface for hardening and burnishing procedures. The final contour of the condensed gold should be similar to that of the completed restoration and should include excess metal for finishing.

The condensation of powdered gold is similar to cohesive gold, but special instruments are required (Fig. 16-5). Hand pressure with mechanical condensing aids can be used to adapt and harden powdered gold. The pressure is applied

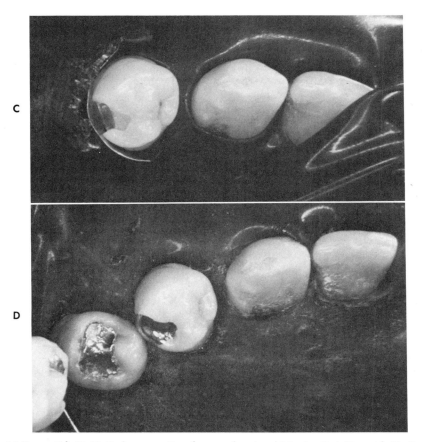

Fig. 16-5, cont'd. C, Limited preparation for powdered gold in the first bicuspid. **D,** Completed Class II powdered gold restoration.

with a forceful rocking and scrubbing motion toward the walls and retentions and is always directed toward the inside of the preparation. Powdered gold also requires a concave shelf and gingival wall covering. The pellets are placed on the preparation and then the cohesive sheaths are ruptured. The loose gold is pressed against the wall to produce the concave building shelf, which minimizes bridging of the surface.

Care must be taken to slowly build the restoration after the proximal portion is filled. The occlusal insertion is rapid because of the higher density of the powdered gold pellet. The application of greater pressures and the rapid building process suggest that the techniques of using regular cohesive gold should first be mastered in order to develop proficiency for condensing powdered gold. The finished surface should appear to have the same color, contour, and hardness as the regular cohesive gold.

The force needed to condense powdered gold necessitates the use of an anatomically contoured matrix stabilized with acrylic die in Class II restorations. The method of matrix construction is similar to that of the amalgam restoration. Brass T band matrix strips or regular strip matrix (0.001 inch thick) is contoured with pliers and wedged against the cervical wall. The band and wedge are covered with the acrylic die and held during polymerization to lock them in the embrasures. While the acrylic is yet moldable, the matrix is forcibly burnished toward the contact and away from the proximal margins to help provide a slight excess of gold at the margins for finishing purposes. The acrylic die is needed to stabilize the matrix and tooth for building the successful Class II powdered gold restoration. The assembly can be quickly removed with a periodontal scaler following condensation.

Finishing

Occlusal gold is burnished by applying heavy pressures with a small ball-shaped instrument. The metal is rubbed until it shines, indicating that the surface is adequately hardened for application of other instruments. Large pieces of flash can now be removed with the cleoid carver. The edge of the metal is then reburnished.

The matrix band is removed in order to inspect the proximal surface. If the margins are soft and poorly adapted, more gold must be added before the blade burnishers are used to push the metal against the tooth. The surface is then hardened with the burnisher to develop the same texture as the occlusal gold. The buccal and lingual proximal margins must be examined to make certain that they are in apposition with the tooth.

When all margins are closed, the surface is hardened, any excess contour is removed, and the restoration is finished by filing and cutting. Small round files are used to wear down the surface and remove as much excess metal as possible. The discoid carver is then applied to the occlusal surface in much the same manner as the amalgam restoration. The carver is pulled from the gold toward the tooth to find the margin and shape the anatomy. The surface can then be smoothed rapidly with rotary abrasives. The occlusal surface of the gold restoration can be carved with a sharp instrument.

After the surface is burnished, small cuttlefish sandpaper disks and rubber wheels are used to locate and smooth the proximal margins. If large flashes exist, the margins must be filed again. Separators are sometimes applied in order to pass a finishing strip between the contact areas to smooth the blocked metal.

Regular rotary speeds are used to revolve the small disks on the occlusal surface and to round and contour the marginal ridge. To avoid temperature elevations the disks are moved lightly down the cusp planes and rotated to polish the carved grooves. A smooth surface is produced when the disks are carefully used. The rubber wheels must be pointed numerous times to develop an edge that will reach the grooves.

To complete the restoration, luster is produced on the surface by applying silica and whiting with a soft rubber cup. The highly shined surface is dried with air and cleaned with the explorer so that the dentist can check the margins and contour. The patient can also inspect the restoration before the rubber dam is removed.

The finishing of powdered gold utilizes a similar technique. Hand-working the surface of the restoration, such as burnishing, filing, or partial cutting with a cleoid-discoid carver, produces the best surface. Sharp gold knives are useful in shaping parts of the proximal portion of the restoration. There will be times when rotary instruments will be needed to expedite the procedure, and it is advisable to use small plug finishing burs or small stones. The burs are revolved slowly from metal toward the margin. Following the burs or stones, the surface again should be heavily burnished. The metal is pinched off at the cavosurface margin and the desired contour is gradually shaped. After removal of the rubber dam the occlusion is examined for premature contacts and any necessary adjustments are made. The occurrence of premature contacts will be the exception rather than the rule because most of the functioning tooth structure has been preserved in the conservative outline form.

The Class II direct gold restoration is a refined operative service that is not much more difficult than the amalgam restoration. Indications for the use of a particular type of gold and the recommended design of the cavity preparation will differ with each situation. The benefits of the restoration present a challenge to the operator to master the variations in procedure.

CLASS III DIRECT GOLD RESTORATIONS

The anterior proximal gold restoration has been the subject of more discussion than any other operative service. This restorative procedure has been used in state board examinations and clinical training in all parts of the country because it requires more skill and discipline than most restorations. As a result of the pressures during examination and training, many dentists are adverse to using this restoration. However, because of the potential for long-term service, this is still a valid restoration.

Initially gold foil was the only material suitable for Class III lesions because plastics had not been developed and the use of silicate cements was not broadly accepted. The mechanics of inserting the gold was mastered by most dentists within a short time because the material was commonly used. At this time the display of gold was not as disagreeable to the patient because it was the only method to save the damaged tooth. The development of tooth-colored compounds caused many dentists and patients to disregard the advantages of gold restorations. The newer compounds have a shorter clinical life than the gold restoration, but they are often used because of easier techniques. Specific problems are identified with the cavity preparation in incisors. Access to the preparation can be provided by proper instrumentation, separation, and cavity design.

The unique problem is the small amount of retention and resistance form available for maintaining esthetics and health of the pulp. The Class III preparations have sharp, small retentions placed in the dentin at strategic locations around the labial and lingual enamel walls. The labial wall is prepared to conceal the gold and the lingual wall is made to provide access for condensation and preparing the internal structures.

The pulp size and the amount of available dentin discourage the use of direct gold in the proximal surfaces of teeth in young and adolescent patients. The remaining dentin thickness between the pulp and restoration must provide protection for the tooth. The axial wall is ideally placed 0.5 mm. within the dentinoenamel junction to provide room for the convenience points. In the newly erupted tooth this depth may result in a pulp exposure; therefore, the tooth must be allowed to develop until secondary dentin fills in the pulp chamber for protection.

This problem is more acute on the lateral incisor because the tooth is much smaller. Precautions such as close observation of radiographs in young patients are necessary to be certain of adequate dentin support and thickness.

A controversial aspect of the Class III preparation is the selection of the outline form. It is commonly agreed that the labial margin should be inconspicuous, but the concepts have not been summarized or compared in any one publication for the beginning student. The original Class III outline form by Black has been modified in many geographic areas and in some instances within an individual state. The student is advised to master one specific design and instrumentation before making a comparison of the other possible variations. The desired esthetics narrows the selection of the outline.

In the original Black outline a curved wall is used, the reverse of the proximal surface contour. The extension is greatest in the middle third of the tooth, which was believed to be the most esthetic. The labial line is called "Hogarth's curve." The access produced with this form is now considered to be more than is actually required for gold insertion. The access is in the middle of the outline and not where it should be located to form the gingival portion of the preparation. However, this outline form is still used in some areas. This preparation should only be used with tooth-colored restorations and then only for replacing large defective fillings.

Under the influence of Wedelstaedt, G. V. Black started numerous study clubs throughout the Midwest. The principles and nomenclature originally corresponded to Black's method of preparation, but many of the clubs soon developed their own particular outline forms and methods of instrumentation.

The first contribution of significance was made by Woodbury. The study club that developed the Woodbury Class III preparation and the specifically designed cutting instruments for the system is still quite active today. The Woodbury preparation is made to parallel the axial line of the tooth. This preparation has exacting dimensions, resulting in a more refined restoration. Another innovation was the concave axial wall and curved gingival wall that stimulated many departures from the original Black design.

Harry True, who also received his training in the Middle West, became Woodbury's student and extensively taught his modifications. True developed the inconspicuous preparation, which in some ways can be considered an extension of the Woodbury design. True's preparation has limited application because the outline form actually extends past the angle of the tooth, producing a Class IV restoration. A carious lesion rarely undermines the enamel in such a configuration that makes the use of this preparation feasible. For an incipient proximal lesion the design would require the cutting away of much sound tooth structure for the sake of esthetics. True's outstanding contribution to direct gold procedures was outlining the methodology of placing the restoration for both the dentist and the assistant. Cabinet arrangement, instrumentation, and noninterfering separators were all excellent refinements. The True outline form is curved to the same extent and direction of the tooth. This innovation caused a reevaluation of the method of teaching gold restorative procedures and motivated many clinicians to attempt to develop esthetic outline forms.

During the 1920's Wedelstaedt and Searl began teaching postgraduate courses in the Pacific Northwest. In Seattle they met and worked with Ferrier. Within a few years Ferrier assumed leadership of the study clubs. Ferrier's technique became the key to the modern outline form. The concepts he advocated have survived through the years and are the most esthetic outlines available for gold restorations. The Ferrier preparation blends with the tooth contour and hides the restoration. Ferrier's concepts are just beginning to be appreciated in many areas of the country. Because of his influence, various preparations were advocated, instruments were designed to prepare the teeth and insert the gold, and stable and effective separators were produced.

The Ferrier cavity preparation displays less gold because it blends with the contour of the tooth being restored (Fig. 16-6). The Class III labial outline form is made to parallel the calcification lobe of the surface on which the restoration is being placed. The lines are straight on bulbous teeth but have an incisal turn on flat proximal surfaces. The labial margin is located just outside the embrasure in order to reflect light from the restoration (Fig. 16-7). If this is not done, the metal appears shadowed and dark in the interproximal space. The labial margin ends below the gingival tissue and joins the cervical wall to be protected.

The lingual wall has an incisal turn but is directed toward the gingival in a straight line to provide access for the hand instruments in forming the lingual portion of the preparation. Ferrier designed the preparation to end in a lingual-gingival shoulder, a technique he considered to be his most important contribution to dentistry. The shoulder can be accurately condensed when the monangle point is used for building the cervical wall and gold shelf (Fig. 16-8).

Definite dimensions are placed in the Ferrier preparation. A double wall is placed in the inside dentin portion and is obtuse with the axial wall. The gingi-

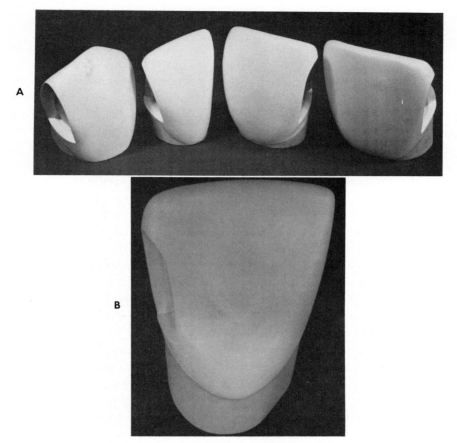

Fig. 16-6. A, Plaster models of several anterior teeth to demonstrate the Ferrier outline form. **B,** Ferrier outline form for lingual preparation.

val wall is slightly acute with the axial wall because a small undercut is formed for locking in the restoration, a technique similar to the Class V preparation for noncohesive gold cylinders. The definite wall dimensions and the flare in the axial wall produce extra resistance, and with the boxed incisal retention form they secure the restoration.

A "carryover" from other preparations is the beveled enamel margin. The margins have long, full wall bevels that prevent scalloped enamel and an uneven appearance in the restoration. Hence in direct gold restorations, long full wall bevels are used on all the margins that are placed in enamel. The cementum margin is slightly beveled, but it is confined to prevent flashes of metal and difficulties in smoothing and polishing (Fig. 16-9).

The Ferrier method is still basic to the modern practice of dentistry. The techniques of preparation and gold placement can be performed without diffi-

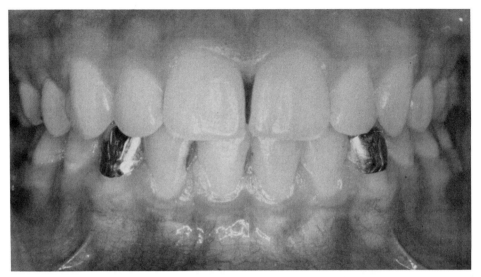

Fig. 16-7. Two Class III restorations with esthetic outline forms on the mesial surfaces of the maxillary central incisors.

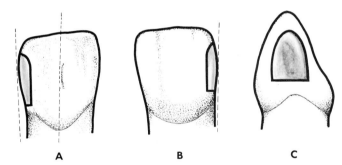

A   B   C

Fig. 16-8. Ferrier design Class III gold foil restoration. **A,** Lingual view; **B,** labial extension; **C,** proximal orientation.

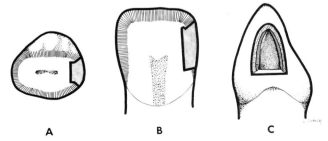

A   B   C

Fig. 16-9. Ferrier Class III gold foil preparation. **A,** Cross section demonstrating the resistance walls and the flared walls to the cavosurface. **B,** Labiolingual cross section depicting the inclination of the gingival and incisal walls. **C,** Proximal view depicting the labial and lingual flares, the precisely developed resistance walls, and the location for gingival and incisal retention.

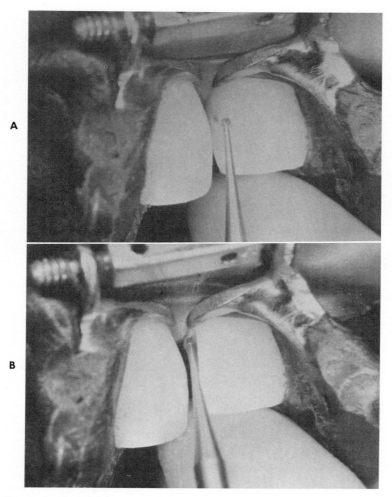

Fig. 16-10. A, Small round bur is used for gaining access to caries and undermining a portion of the enamel. **B,** Inverted cone bur is used for squaring the cervical wall. Side cutters are also used to plane the labial and lingual walls.

culty once the mechanics are understood. When the ability to conceal the gold is developed, evaluations of other procedures can be made.

Instrumentation

A study of the literature reveals that instrumentation for Class III preparations for direct gold restorations falls into a similar pattern. Mastery of the basic instrumentation, with the exception of a few special instruments, will result in the ability to prepare any of the designs. Only the essential instruments are listed because a minimal number of instruments should be employed (Fig. 16-10).

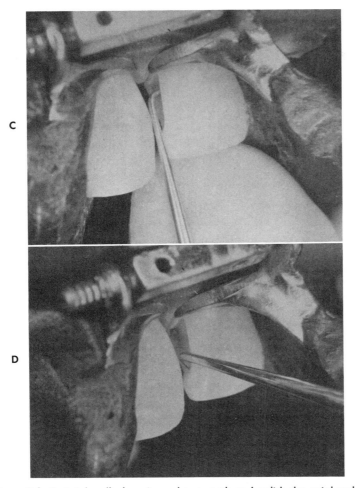

Fig. 16-10, cont'd. C, Axial wall plane is used to smooth and polish the axial wall. **D,** Bibeveled hatchet is used to cut the dentin in order to create the incisal retention form.

1. The straight handpiece and burs are used because the long shank enables better cavity approach. Because only a small amount of tooth structure is removed, the regular speeds (2,000 to 3,000 rpm) are used.

The No. ½ round or bilevel drill is used to perforate the undermined labial enamel. The bur penetrates to the dentin and is pushed laterally to undermine the labial and lingual enamel. The cutting is done slowly to avoid excessive axial depth. The entire involved area is undermined after locating the caries and pushing the bur under the enamel.

The small, thin Wedelstaedt chisel is then used to fracture unsupported enamel and produce the rough outline form. The labial and lingual enamel is cleaned to develop access for the extension.

2. The No. 33½ inverted cone bur in the straight handpiece is used to extend, square, and flare the walls of the preparation. The end cutters square the gingival wall and the side cutters of the bur establish the labial and lingual wall of the preparation. The lingual side of the preparation is prepared from a lingual approach and the labial portion is reduced by a direct approach.

The cavity outline is finished with the same small Wedelstaedt chisel and small monangle hoes.

3. Retention forms are started with a spear point or No. ¼ round bur. The convenience points are placed in the cervical corners and are triangulated to produce sharp corners in the dentin.

The incisal point angle is the largest of the undercuts and is started with the No. ½ round bur and refined with the bibeveled hatchet. The incisal retention is squared and made into box form to receive a bulk of gold to absorb the stresses produced by the lower incisors.

The convenience points are squared and pointed with small angle formers and monangles. This results in three divergent point angles directed away from the pulp and undercut to retain the gold. Excessive cutting of the retentions does not aid in locking the restoration but only serves to weaken the overlying enamel. The retentions are pointed to facilitate wedging of the first pellets and building of the triangular bars that support the restoration.

4. Finishing the walls of the Class III preparation is similar to the other movements. A sharp Wedelstaedt chisel is used to smooth the enamel walls. In some cases the small monangle should be used to reach the cervical walls or the line angles where this structure meets the labial and lingual walls.

All preparations should be finished by using the axial wall plane. This small hoe is pulled across the axial wall to smooth the dentin. The internal double wall is produced with the small monangles and angle formers. Ferrier's publications may be consulted for specific applications. Gold placement should not be initiated until the cavity preparation is clean and flawless.

Gold insertion

The Class III preparations require the use of regular cohesive gold. The intensity of the blow, lines of force, and uniform stepping are extremely critical in these preparations. The placement of gold is complicated by the intact incisal enamel, indicating a condensation procedure with a labial and lingual approach. Black divided Class III gold placement into starting, establishing the building shelf, building the contour, turning the incisal point angle, and labial completion. His rules are used with minor modifications for all Class III preparations. The application of special condensers and devices has been advocated, but the lines of force and the building shelf require the same general approach for all procedures in order to provide access.

1. A small monangle condenser is used to condense the initial pellet in the lingual-gingival point angle. The forces are directed to trisect the point angle

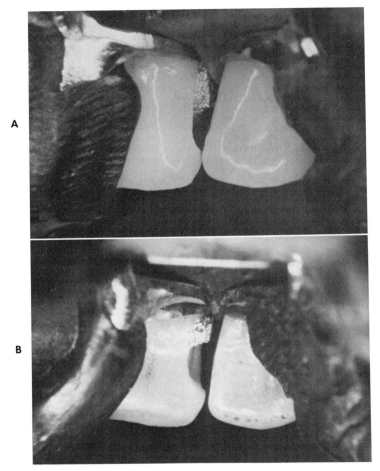

Fig. 16-11. A, Labial view of the gold shelf advocated by Black. **B,** Lingual view of the gold shelf advocated by Black.

and completely fill the convenience point. The condenser is placed through the labial opening.

A few pellets are added in the gingival-axial line angle and condensed to form a bar across the gingival wall. A pellet is then added in the labial-gingival convenience point and the same condenser is used to harden the gold through the lingual opening. If access is limited, the bayonet condenser can be stepped around the labial plate to impact the gold in the labial convenience point. This is done until the convenience points are filled and joined by a thickness of two pellets of gold over the cervical wall.

2. The monangle condenser is used to form the building shelf (Fig. 16-11). The gingival wall is fully covered to produce a gold shelf. The angulation of the ledge should enable the monangle to impact the surface at right angles. The

lines of force should be directed 45 degrees to the axial wall. The shelf is maintained until two thirds of the cervical preparation is filled. Care must be taken to cover and adapt the labial and lingual margins as the shelf progresses or the margins will be blocked out and impossible to reach after most of the contour is developed.

The foot condenser is sometimes used for building the restoration because the angulation of the nib is useful in maintaining the shelf. The foot is applied to adapt the lingual-cervical portion of the restoration if it cannot be reached with the monangle condenser. The building shelf is maintained at right angles to the lines of force in the angulation suggested, with all the forces directed toward the inside of the tooth.

3. Making the turn and filling in the incisal point angle are done in steps. The lingual line angle and surface are closed with the small monangle. The incisal retention form is filled with the bayonet from the labial opening. When the incisal retention form hardens, the concavity is obliterated with the small monangle or foot condenser. At this time the lingual surface is closed, the incisal retention form is united to the restoration, and the incisal wall and part of the labial wall are covered.

4. Developing full contour is now possible because only a small concavity and a portion of the labial margin are present. The convex or monangle condenser is used to direct the forces inside the preparation. The labial wall is built to have a uniform but surplus contour for finishing.

5. The surface hardening or "aftercondensation" is accomplished with the foot condenser by placing the toe into the embrasure and applying force toward the axial wall. The foot is then stepped over the entire labial surface to minimize voids and to improve adaptation of the cavosurface margin.

Special condensers should be used only if they facilitate placing the gold. They are sometimes helpful for rotated and poorly aligned teeth.

Finishing

The procedure for finishing is generally the same as described in Chapter 15. Rotary instruments are not used except to form the concavities on the lingual surface. The contour is produced with files, burnishers, and knives. Finishing strips are used to locate the margin and to smooth the surface. The recommended procedure is as follows:

1. A small round or blade burnisher is used to harden the surface. The pressures are directed toward the axial wall so as not to disturb the marginal seal. The metal is rubbed vigorously until it appears burnished and intact.

2. Hand files, preferably those with rectangular push-cut and pull-cut designs, are used to wear down the metal and locate the margin. If the gold is excessive and cannot be reached in the gingival embrasure, it should be cut out with the gold knife in order to shorten the procedure. The filing can also be done with the small round Jeffery file or any other instrument that can be moved

in and out of the embrasure to produce a smooth surface and exacting margin.

Most of the finishing is done at this time. Special designs of push-cut and pull-cut files, knives, and burnishers can be selected if they prove efficient for the individual. With the exception of smoothing the surface, the restoration is now completed unless the lingual opening is wider than usual. If the entire marginal ridge has been replaced, it is necessary to place a concavity in the lingual surface with a discoid carver. Minimum extension will prevent the need for concavities on the lingual surface.

3. The surface is then smoothed and luster is produced with finishing strips. The long strips are preferred and are used in an order of descending abrasiveness. The garnet abrasives are inserted first and pulled from the lingual to the labial surface. The separator may need to be opened to permit the passing of the first strip. As soon as the first strip is moved through the embrasure, the separator is removed in order to control the strip and confine it to the restoraion. The grits are gradually reduced by using light pressures with compressed air to prevent trauma. The plain linen strip is used last in order to pick up gold particles from the surface of the restoration so that the embedded gold rubs against the restoration to produce a natural satin finish. The Class III regular cohesive gold restoration will produce the best polished surface. The smooth metal will shine but will not be noticeable to the casual observer.

This method can be used effectively to marginate and polish the Class III cohesive gold restoration. The finished restoration will be a clear yellow color, indicating that the gold has not been abused during polishing.

SPECIAL PROXIMAL DIRECT GOLD RESTORATIONS
Class III powdered gold restoration

The new encapsulated powdered gold has done much to encourage the dentist to offer the direct gold operative service. The dense pellets require well-controlled procedures, but once mastered, an excellent service can be produced. The Class III powdered gold restoration requires a special preparation because of the density of the material and the condensation method.

The retentions and angles are rounded to facilitate adaptation of the gold. The tooth is normally penetrated from the lingual using a No. ½ bur with high speed. Following the penetration the bulk of the hard tissue removal is done with a No. 69 bur. Care is taken to avoid overcutting on the lingual or toward the labial. Ideally, the labial margin should be positioned labial to the contact area to help produce a reliable metal margin. The greatest precaution is taken to be sure that the lingual incisal turn is properly done (Fig. 16-12). Following the bulk removal, the Jeffery instruments are used to define the preparation with proper walls and line angles. If extension allows, a curved chisel is used from the labial direction.

Angle formers designed by Jeffery and an offset bayonet angle former are the key instruments for the preparation (Fig. 16-13). Condensers are specifically

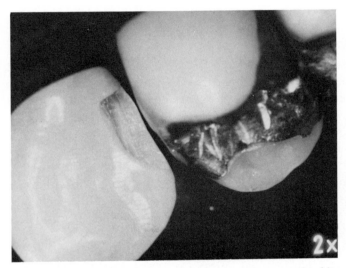

Fig. 16-12. Completed direct powdered gold preparation showing style of lingual turn.

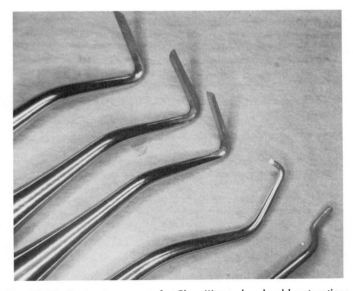

Fig. 16-13. Cutting instruments for Class III powdered gold restorations.

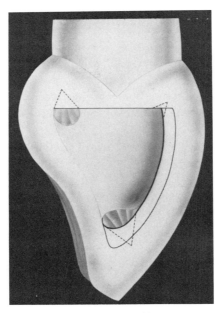

Fig. 16-14. Completed model of direct powdered gold preparation emphasizing walls and retention.

designed to allow condensation of powdered gold in the proximal restoration. Instruments required to prepare and place this restoration are available from Chico Dental Specialties, Chico, California, and American Instrument Company of Missoula, Montana. These instruments should be acquired before attempting this restoration.

The cavity preparation for incisors can be made by either of two methods: the labial enamel wall may be preserved or removed. Whenever possible the enamel wall should be left intact and a lingual box formed with an exaggerated incisal turn. The broad lingual opening aids in inserting the powdered pellets. Two major retention forms are utilized, one at the incisal portion of the preparation and the other at the lingual-gingival wall (Fig. 16-14). A supplemental retention of smaller magnitude is often placed at the labial-gingival margin. The retentions at the incisal and lingual margins are initiated by a No. ½ or No. ¼ bur, which cuts the bulk required and refined by a hand instrument. The incisal retention proceeds in an incisal, axial, and labial direction and is refined by an incisal angle former. Care must be exercised to maintain adequate bulk for connecting the actual retention with the body of the restoration. The lingual-gingival retention is placed primarily in a gingival direction, and it is defined by using a bayonet angle former. The labial-gingival retention is placed in a labial direction by the action of a Jeffery angle former. It is an extension of the gingival-axial line angle and is sharply instrumented. In contrast, the other two retentions will be rounded and bulkier in style.

If the labial wall cannot be preserved, it is opened with a straight labial outline that parallels the calcification lobe in an area that can be reached for finishing (Fig. 16-15). This preparation has an incisal turn, and an extra retention form is added on the labial-cervical wall, which is rounded like the others. The labial outline is designed for esthetics; in most cases the Ferrier lines can be used. The inside of the preparation is quite large and is more retentive than the forms for cohesive gold. Smooth cavity margins with a small bevel promote finishing.

When the labial margin terminates toward the labial surface, some operators may prefer to place an acrylic matrix that will function as an aid to condensation. This is an optional feature, and as operators gain condensing experience it is used very little. The cavity preparation is filled with warm gutta-percha and smoothed into the approximate contour of the completed restoration. A mix of quick-setting acrylic die is made and a splint is placed over the labial and lingual surfaces of the anterior teeth. Only a small opening remains on the lingual surface of the prepared tooth and in the embrasure area. If flashes of acrylic block the cavity, the material can be removed with a sharp gold knife before it completely hardens. The gutta-percha is removed and the cavity is blocked out and stabilized for insertion of the gold. When separation is necessary, a wood wedge is contoured and moistened, placed below the cervical wall to move the teeth, and incorporated into the matrix where it remains during insertion of the gold.

Hand condensation is employed for powdered gold. Two or three small pellets are placed on the gingival floor and lightly condensed with a curved condenser. Following this, a bayonet condenser is used to firmly anchor the gold into the gingival retention, beginning with the labial and proceeding to the lingual-gingival portion. Next, the gingival margin is secured wth a parallelogram style condenser that is used with a firm rocking motion. The condensation moves up the labial wall and into the incisal retention with an incisal condenser point to avoid bridging of the gold. Whenever possible, a palm grasp is employed to produce condensing pressure.

Each pellet is broken apart before condensing and positioned to produce a uniform contour as the restoration develops. At all times the margins are overcontoured with gold to provide adequate material for finishing. Force is applied with a rocking motion while the condenser is held with a palm grasp. The pellet is strain hardened and blocking out is prevented with the development of heavy forces and movements of the condenser. The margins are overlapped and adapted with this method and surplus contour is developed on the proximal and lingual surfaces.

Finishing of a Class III powdered gold restoration calls for some of the same procedures as employed for the Class V restorations. The preferred method calls for a maximum amount of hand working with metal instruments to workharden the surface. Cleoid-discoid carvers, files, gold knives, and burnishers or

Text continued on p. 515.

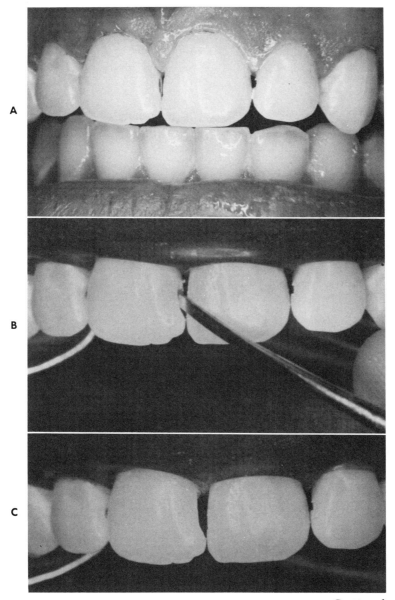

Continued.

Fig. 16-15. A, Carious lesion on the mesial surface of the right maxillary incisor. **B,** Undermined enamel is removed with the small Wedelstaedt chisel. The rough labial outline is established. **C,** Labial outline form.

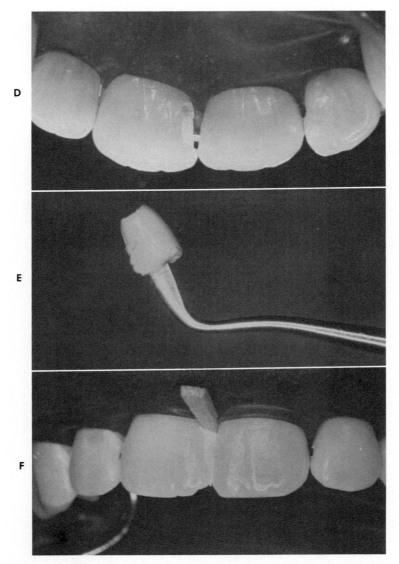

Fig. 16-15, cont'd. D, Lingual outline form and lingual-cervical point angle. **E,** Warmed gutta-percha for insertion into the preparation. **F,** Wood wedge is used for separation. The cavity preparation is packed with gutta-percha and smoothed.

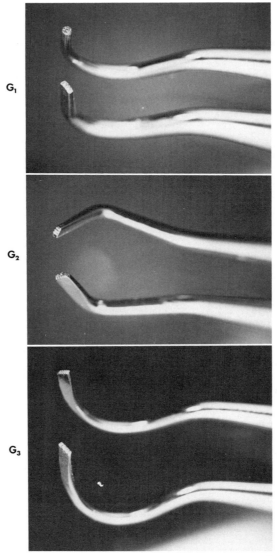

Continued.

Fig. 16-15, cont'd. G, Hand condensers used to condense Class III direct powdered gold restorations.

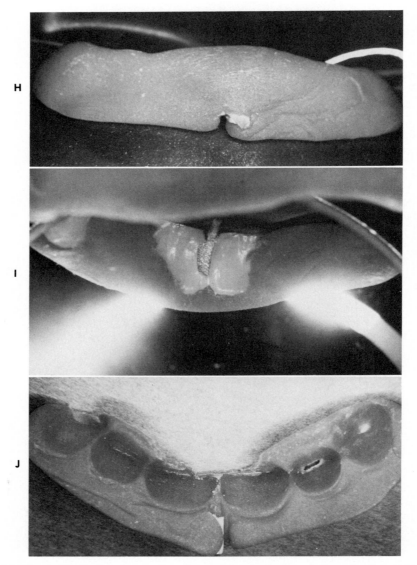

Fig. 16-15, cont'd. H, Anterior acrylic splint and matrix. **I,** Lingual view of splint and opening. The first portion of the powdered gold has been condensed. **J,** Removed acrylic splint.

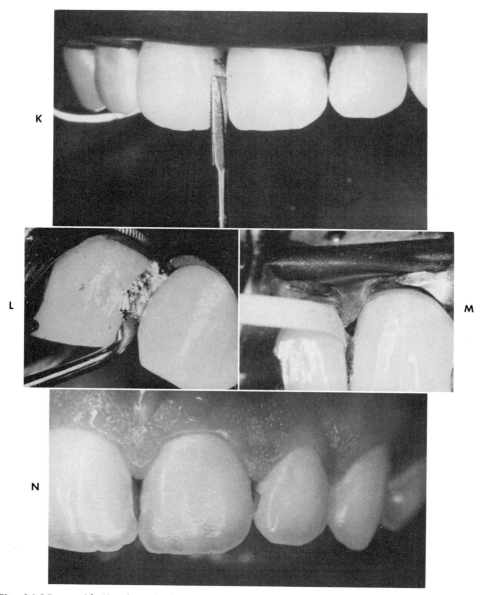

Fig. 16-15, cont'd. K, Filing the labial portion of the restoration. **L,** A cleoid-discoid used to remove excess gold and to harden surface. **M,** An 18 inch narrow fine linen strip used for finishing a Class III direct gold restoration. **N,** Clinical appearance of the restoration.

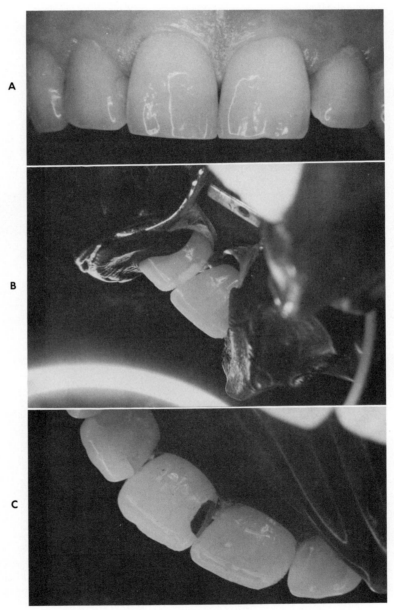

Fig. 16-16. A, Class III powdered gold preparation with the labial enamel wall intact. **B,** Lingual view of the preparation with the separator in place for stability. **C,** Finished powdered gold restoration that is invisible from the labial aspect.

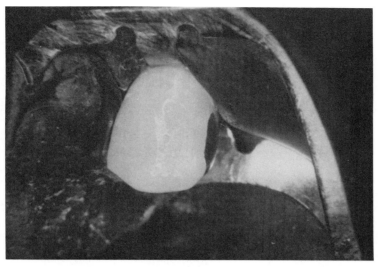

Fig. 16-17. Powdered gold restoration on the distal surface of the cuspid that is a partial denture guiding plane.

finishers are to be used to produce optimum surface hardness. As far as possible, these same instruments are very effective for contouring the lingual portions of the restorations.

Subsequent to burnishing and contouring, it is recommended that a Ferrier separator be placed and blocked into place with stick compound. Separation is slowly activated so as to allow a thin swager to enter between the condensed gold and the adjacent tooth. Then fine and extrafine grit 18-inch strips should be used to produce final contour and finish. There must be a stream of air utilized while strips are passed over the surface of the restoration (Fig. 16-16).

Skilled operators can build Class III powdered gold restorations in shorter periods of time than when using regular cohesive gold. Special instruments, different types of hand pressures, and experience are all necessary to obtain optimum results. The powdered gold can be veneered with regular soft cohesive gold, especially if poor adaptation is discovered on the labial wall after the matrix is removed. A $\frac{1}{64}$ cohesive gold pellet is placed in the void. Sometimes the powdered gold restoration is placed from a lingual approach in silicate designed box preparations. It takes only a few minutes, and the use of gold has many advantages over the cement restoration (Fig. 16-17).

Jeffery lingual approach technique

Alexander Jeffery, a dedicated student and teacher, refined some of the concepts advocated by Ferrier. Jeffery developed the lingual approach for Class III cohesive gold restorations, which further concealed the labial margin. The procedure is used successfully in incipient cavities and selected cases. The experi-

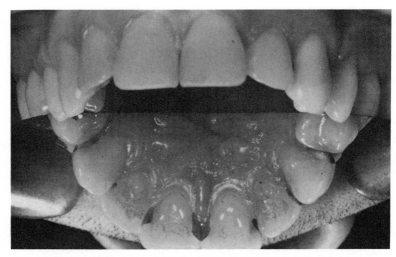

Fig. 16-18. Cohesive gold restorations placed from the lingual approach using the Jeffery instrumentation. (Courtesy Mrs. Alexander W. Jeffery.)

enced operator uses this preparation for incisors in well-cared-for dentitions. Jeffery also modified the Ferrier No. 1 separator and designed hand instruments and condensers for the lingual approach technique. When the Jeffery lingual approach can be used to produce cohesive gold restorations, there is no visible labial exposure (Fig. 16-18).

The procedure is similar to that outlined by Ferrier. All instrumentation is accomplished from the lingual surface. Regular cohesive gold pellets are used in a box preparation with three retention forms and an intact labial wall. Hand malleting is employed in the usual method, but the condensers designed by Jeffery are used. To grasp the modifications advocated by Jeffery takes time, but the service is unexcelled and the restoration is completely hidden. The off-angle chisels and hatchets designed for the lingual approach are employed for the Class III powdered gold restorations.

A number of inconspicuous preparations have resulted from the development of the lingual approach method. The preparation advocated by Ingraham is useful and is similar to that used for powdered gold. The labial wall is left intact, and retention and resistance are produced by a two-dimensional, undercut, square preparation. Mat gold is used to wedge an extra pliable cohesive gold cylinder against the labial wall. Regular cohesive pellets are inserted in the remainder of the cavity. The restoration can be built quickly and is invisible from the labial surface. Many variations of this method have been advocated. Any procedure is acceptable if the labial enamel wall is not damaged during the preparation because it is needed to afford resistance for placing the initial increments of gold.

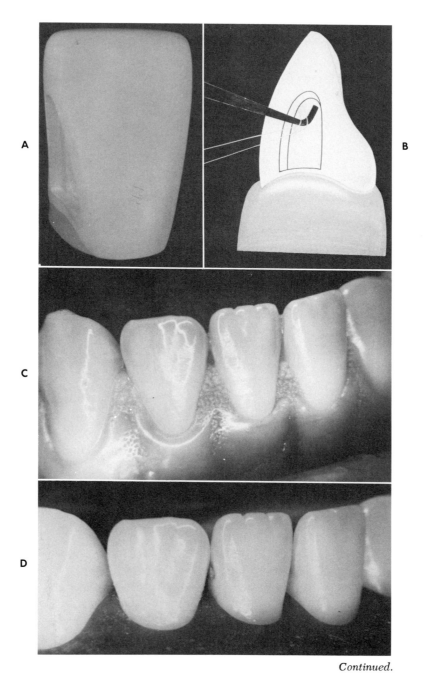

Continued.

Fig. 16-19. A, Labial view of Ferrier Class III preparation for the lower incisor. **B,** Side view of mandibular Class III cavity preparation. **C,** Carious lesion on the distal surface of the right mandibular central incisor. **D,** Surgical field and carious lesion.

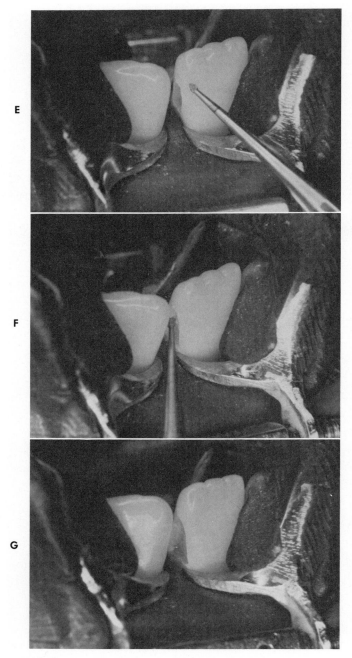

E

F

G

Fig. 16-19, cont'd. E, Caries removal and access are produced with the small round bur. **F,** Lingual wall and outline form are established with the No. 33½ inverted cone bur. **G,** Completed cavity preparation.

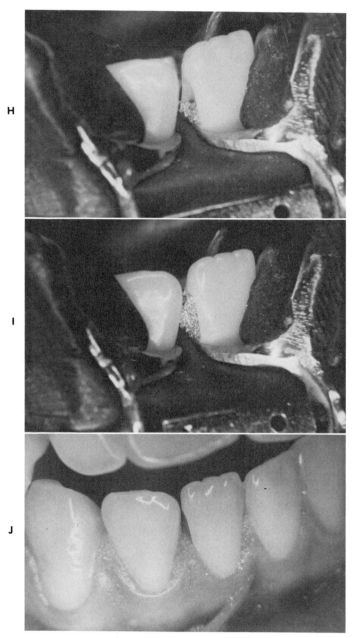

Fig. 16-19, cont'd. H, Cervical retention forms and gingival wall are filled with regular cohesive gold. **I,** The lingual wall is banked with gold. **J,** Clinical appearance of Class III restoration.

Restoration of mandibular incisor

Some of the most difficult restorations in operative dentistry are those in the lower incisor. This small tooth creates unique problems because of its brittle incisal edge. Proximal caries is not as prevalent in lower incisors as in other teeth, and the lesions can usually be detected in the incipient stage. When the angle of the tooth is lost, it becomes necessary to cross the incisal edge for retention if inlays are used. Tooth appearance and protection of the pulp are the main considerations in extensive restorations; therefore, it is quite advantageous to detect or prevent caries in the mandibular incisors. Retention of the lower incisors as well as cuspids is essential to avoid full prosthodontic replacement.

Restoration of the lower incisors can be accomplished either with cohesive gold or powdered gold because of the small cavity and thin enamel plates (Fig. 16-19). When the lesion is small and the lingual wall is intact, gold can be selected for lower incisors. The Ferrier outline is used for esthetics and not much access is needed because of the wide labial embrasure. If the outline parallels the calcification lobe and is placed behind the line angle of the incisor, it will be well concealed.

The techniques for cavity preparation and placement of the gold are simple. Since the lingual wall is intact, a four-walled preparation is produced that supports the incisal edge. The placement of gold is similar to that for the occlusal restoration, and the finishing procedure is similar to that used for the proximal cohesive gold restoration. The small cavity preparation and the excellent access it provides shorten the time needed.

As with other Class III restorations, the preparation is entered with the small round bur and chisel. The cavity form is established with the No. 33½ bur in the straight handpiece. The same general movements are used and care must be taken to smooth the intact lingual wall with the end cutters of the bur. The smoothing of the preparation and establishing of retention forms are done in the usual manner with hand instruments. A box preparation is established with the same degree of smoothness, using the Ferrier outline form. Three small, sharp point angles and the flat axial wall serve to retain the cohesive gold.

The gold is placed by filling the lingual-gingival convenience form and then covering the lingual wall. When the incisal point angle is filled, the insertion is finished by covering the axial wall and eventually locking in the restoration by condensing the gingival-labial convenience form. The gold is placed in the deepest concavity in the center of the restoration and the building is continued until the labial wall is evenly contoured.

The restoration is finished by strain hardening the gold and polishing the metal against the tooth. Contour, margins, and smoothness are developed rapidly because the restoration is quite small. A separator is used as an optional aid throughout the preparation and insertion procedures to avoid possible damage to the small root and supporting tissues. When the restoration is polished and

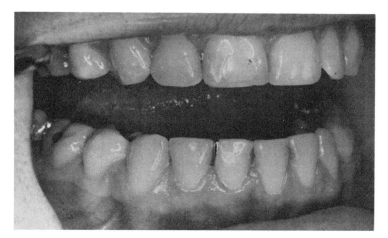

Fig. 16-20. Clinical appearance of Class IV restoration.

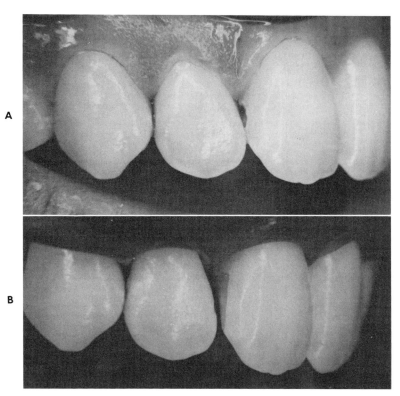

Fig. 16-21. A, Lesion on the distal surface of the central incisor. **B,** Concealed, esthetic restoration will last for many years.

the rubber dam is removed, it will be difficult to see the restoration because it blends so well with the tooth structure (Fig. 16-20).

• • •

The proximal direct gold restoration is a valuable service (Fig. 16-21). The primary considerations are the outline form, esthetics, and convenience of preparing the tooth and inserting the gold. Diagnosis and selection of the lesion are important because incipient caries is best suited for the procedure. The operator is not limited in the selection of a preparation or the type of gold. The development of new gold materials, efficient methods of cavity preparation, and preventive fluoride measures have limited the size of lesions. Direct gold restoration of the proximal surface is a practical and ideal service.

ADDITIONAL READINGS

Blackwell, R. E.: Black's operative dentistry, ed. 9, Milwaukee, 1955, Medico-Dental Publishing Co., vol. 2.

Brinker, H. A.: Gold foil—can we afford to do without it? J. Am. Acad. Gold Foil Operators 15:25, 1972.

Butter, A. B., Green, R. O., and Simon, W. J.: The proximal gold foil filling involving the incisal angle, J.A.D.A. 30:1853, 1943.

Ferrier, W. I.: Gold foil operations, Seattle, 1959, University of Washington Press.

Ferrier, W. I.: Use of gold foil in general practice, J.A.D.A. 28:691, 1941.

Going, R. E.: Pin-retained gold foil, J. Am. Dent. Assoc. 78:323, 1969.

Green, R. O., Pattridge, M. O., and Simon, W. J.: Variations in the proximal cavity for a gold foil filling, J.A.D.A. 30:643, 1943.

Green, R. O., and Simon, W. J.: The proximal gold foil filling, J.A.D.A. 29:559, 1942.

Ingraham, R.: The application of sound biomechanical principles in the design of inlay, amalgam, and gold foil restorations, J.A.D.A. 40:402, 1950.

Ingraham, R., Koser, J. R., and Quint, H.: An atlas of gold foil and rubber dam procedures, Buena Park, Calif., 1961, Uni-Tro College Press.

Jeffery, A. W.: Gold foil filling: description of special technic, J.A.D.A. 34:593, 1947.

Jeffery, A. W.: Invisible Class III gold foil restorations, J.A.D.A. 54:1, 1957.

Jones, E. M.: Treatment of initial caries in anterior teeth with gold foil, J.A.D.A. 25:532, 1939.

Kramer, W. S.: Gold foil in pedodontics, J. Am. Acad. Gold Foil Operators 2:58, 1960.

Lund, M. R., and Baum, L.: Powdered gold for the Class III restoration, J. S. Calif. Dent. Assoc. 33:262, 1965.

Nolen, J. H.: A different approach to the proximoincisal gold foil restoration, J. Am. Acad. Gold Foil Operators 1:18, 1958.

Nolen, J. H.: The use of the iridioplatinum pin in the Class IV gold foil, J. Am. Acad. Gold Foil Operators 11:48, 1968.

Seymour, J. G.: Instant orthodontia for aesthetic gold foil restorations, J. Am. Acad. Gold Foil Operators 13:69, 1970.

Smith, B. B.: A permanent and esthetic anterior restoration, J.A.D.A. 40:326, 1950.

Smith, E. G., Hodson, J. T., and Stibbs, G. D.: A study of the compaction of pure gold into retention holes, convenience points and point angles in Class III cavity preparations, J. Am. Acad. Gold Foil Operators 15:12, 1972.

Stebner, C. M.: The Class III compacted gold foil restoration, J. Am. Acad. Gold Foil Operators 10:17, 1967.

Stibbs, G. D.: Gold foil, J. Canad. Dent. Assoc. 13:155, 1947.

True, H. A.: Inconspicuous Class III gold foil restorations, J.A.D.A. 30:1352, 1943.

Woodbury, C. E.: The making and filling of cavities in the proximal surface of the front teeth with gold foil, Council Bluffs, Iowa, 1929. (Published by the author.)

chapter 17

Cast gold restorations

The cast gold restoration has been a challenge to the dental profession for many years.[1] The properties of gold are conducive to mold casting; therefore, it is possible to form restorations with desirable contours. There are many reasons for selecting the gold casting for the restoration, and there are several acceptable techniques for fabricating the restoration. The procedure involves an accurate cavity preparation, an impression and wax pattern, and the investment material to develop a mold to receive the molten gold. Fabrication of the gold casting requires many materials and technical considerations.

If the indirect method is used to make the impression for the inlay, a number of factors must first be regulated. Possibilities for error are obvious if the impression is taken with materials that distort after removal from the teeth, if the Hydrocal used for the die and models expands upon setting, if the wax patterns shaped for the casting distort, if the investment mold expands during heating, or if the gold casting shrinks while it is cooling. These are five changes in the original dimension that could alter the accuracy of the finished casting. Many studies have been conducted concerning each of these aspects.[2] A perfect fit of the casting has not as yet been developed, but numerous present-day fabrication methods produce a casting that will cover all the margins of the cavity preparation and minimize the thickness of the cement lines necessary to hold the restoration in place. The resultant technique must result in a casting that completely covers the marginal area with gold.

The advent of the ultraspeed air turbine has caused many dentists to reevaluate the techniques for making gold castings. The rapid tooth reduction possible with these speeds has encouraged quadrant treatments with indirect fabrication. A number of teeth are prepared in the quadrant, full-arch impressions are taken, models are made that can be accurately articulated, and a number of castings are made in the laboratory. This has encouraged the development of new temporary materials and initiated studies concerning the management and displacement of gingival tissue. The many research projects and the renewed interest have stimulated many postgraduate courses and study clubs to improve the cast gold restoration.

The direct method is a quick and useful procedure for producing the small gold inlay. The wax pattern is carved in the cavity preparation after tooth reduction is completed. Problems of intraoral carving are alleviated by establishing a dry field and by using magnification. The wax pattern is adapted inside the cavity form and carved to the desired contour. Excellent margins and fit are produced, indicating that the direct method should be used for small restorations. However, the gingival areas and occlusal relationship are not as accurately reproduced in the wax as in the indirect method. Well-fitting gold castings that have accessible surfaces in the outline form can be produced by the direct method.

The interest in research has extended to gnathologic procedures, resulting in more realistic approaches to reconstruction treatment.[3] Studies of the neuromusculature and the determinants of occlusion are helpful. New concepts in tooth morphology have resulted in cone-waxing techniques for multiple patterns and have aided in accurately articulating the carvings and the resultant castings. The improvement in articulators and dental materials has made reconstruction easier for the practicing dentist. The total mouth concept has been influential in producing a more suitable and functional inlay.

One notable property of the cast gold inlay is that the metal will not tarnish or corrode in the oral cavity. The ductility of gold makes it possible to move the metal toward the die or tooth to produce an excellent margin that will not break down after years of service. Thin layers and knife edges on the casting that can be fitted to bevels, chamfers, and other finish lines are helpful in this regard. This thin margin on the casting is used to contact the remaining tooth structure in order to rebuild and strengthen the individual tooth and to facilitate finishing the gold to the tooth.

Gold castings can be adjusted and polished to desirable contours. The occlusal surface is restored with ideal functional relationships, and proximal contours can be developed to protect the supporting tissues. With the exception of very soft alloys, the gold surface will not measurably change after it is placed into function. With careful manipulation little detail will be lost from the original wax pattern to the finished inlay.

A disadvantage of the cast gold inlay is the cementing medium necessary to secure the restoration to tooth structure. Zinc phosphate cement, which is susceptible to dissolution in the oral fluids, is commonly used as the luting agent (Fig. 17-1). Several dilute organic acids are present in the diet and plaque that rapidly dissolve the cement and leave the margin and cavity wall open for secondary caries.[4] Recurrent caries is a problem when patients fail to follow good hygienic and dietary practices. Therefore, patient education is an important aspect of this service because of the time and expense required to fabricate the cast restoration.

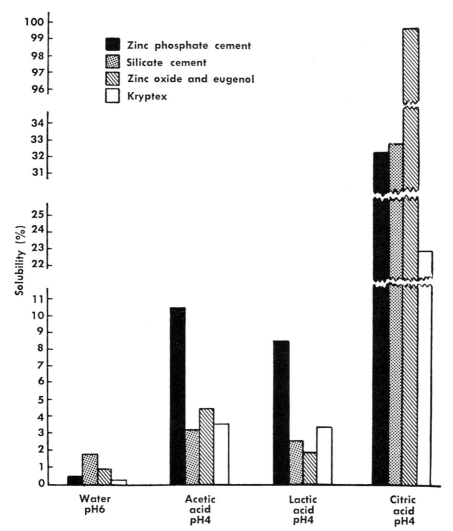

Fig. 17-1. Solubility of cementing materials in several types of acids that are found in the oral cavity in a 7-day period. (From Skinner, E. W., and Phillips, R. W.: The science of dental materials, ed. 5, Philadelphia, 1960, W. B. Saunders Co.)

The dentist should explain the mechanism of caries that undermines the casting and advise the patient in regard to protecting the service. The additional time and number of appointments involved are pointed out to the patient so that he is aware of the higher fee necessary for the service. Cooperation of the patient is needed throughout the treatment because of the exacting nature of the tooth preparations, impression procedures, and registrations for the articulator or die technique and the time necessary for fitting and cementing the finished casting. This increase in time and expense necessitates an excellent rapport between the patient and the dentist. Patient education is directed to include the advantages of sound dental health and the service that is received with the cast gold restoration. A patient who is not interested in his dental health should not receive this type of restorative service.

The fabrication of multiple inlays is often assigned to the laboratory technician. Although this sometimes increases the cost of the casting, the dentist is free to spend more time in the operatory. Accurate hydrocolloid and rubber materials and adjustable aticulators that can be aligned to simulate the movements of the mandible are instrumental in producing exacting guides. The castings are then constructed in the laboratory according to the records taken by the dentist.

INDICATIONS FOR CAST GOLD RESTORATIONS

Because of the specific properties of the gold casting, there are distinct indications for selecting the restorative material.[5]

Restoration of large carious lesions or traumatic conditions. Gold castings are used to restore large carious lesions or traumatic conditions that involve an extensive amount of tooth structure. Generally the larger the lesion the greater the indication for the cast gold inlay. More stresses will be placed on the metal in large restorations, creating a need for proper design in the cavity form. The surfaces of the restoration are shaped to permit desirable function and to support the remaining tooth structure. Large lesions associated with secondary caries involvement around amalgam restorations, cusp fractures, and other traumatic conditions indicate restoration of the tooth with cast gold inlays. Replacement of large surfaces with other materials, including pin-retained amalgam, result in breakdown and fracture. The gold casting is the only material with the necessary strength to rebuild large areas of the tooth for full application of masticatory stresses. Better functional relationships can sometimes be obtained with the casting than was present with the original tooth. Gold castings can be made to resist wear for the entire lifetime of the patient.

Correction of periodontal problems. The casting is used to physiologically restore the contact area by forming ideal embrasures, marginal ridges, and the actual area of contact. The proximal surface is restored ideally according to the existing tooth anatomy to prevent food impaction, maintain the proper tooth diameter, and prevent damage of the gingival tissue and supporting structures. Periodontal problems are prevented by replacing protective contours and building a firm relationship with the adjacent tooth.

Restoration or creation of ideal occlusion. Centric contacts and pathways can be created in the gold surface to restore or create ideal occlusal relationships by covering the cusps or using large occlusal outline forms. Accurate adjustments in the wax pattern and gold casting allow the development of good holding fossae and contacting cusps in order to create desirable and atraumatic masticatory conditions. Unlike other materials, gold does not abrade and will remain functional indefinitely. Balancing relationships with horizontal stresses cause wear patterns to develop on the gold that have a burnished appearance and a shape similar to the facets on enamel. The gold casting must not only fit the tooth but must also harmonize with the functional range of movements of the mandible.

Improvement of esthetics. Esthetics are improved with the gold inlay because the cavity outline form can be made to have straight and exacting margins that will blend with the tooth if given the proper contour. Some dentists have advocated the exclusive use of gold inlays in the bicuspids and mesial surfaces of the first molars to keep the teeth from discoloring. Ion migration is responsible for tooth discoloration in the amalgam restoration. Even though cavity varnish partially blocks the silver and tin ions that are moved by galvanic currents, discoloration can still occur in silver amalgam restorations. The gold inlay is an esthetic restoration even when the cusps are capped, provided that the outline form has been handled conservatively. Tarnish and corrosion of the gold inlay are occasionally observed when the material is placed in contact with a dissimilar metal such as amalgam in the same tooth. This is not considered a serious problem because it is not a common practice. Castings that reflect rather than absorb light are esthetic restorations.

Multiple castings. Inlays are indicated when numerous other castings have been placed. The gold casting can be used to restore new caries when it is necessary to avoid contact with dissimilar metals. This requires the conservative preparation for incipient lesions in bicuspid teeth. If tooth morphology is favorable, the powdered gold restoration is occasionally used, but still this material has limitations when access is inadequate. Small inlays are also permanent because of the exacting margin that is produced. The margin would be as effective as with direct golds if a cement liner were not always required for the casting.

Permanent restorations. The casting provides a more permanent restoration. Occasionally patients with low caries susceptibility develop pit and fissure defects. The inlay can be used when extension is necessary to make the large outline form. The superior marginal strength will provide many years of service for the patient who has good dental health. The control of acid in the oral cavity will help to produce a more permanent restoration.

Restoration of areas of stress. Castings are used in areas of excessive stress or in prosthetic abutment teeth. This applies to fixed and removable prosthetic appliances, to terminal teeth in the arch, and to the angles or the anterior teeth. Gold castings are also used to replace the working cusps and marginal ridges that function in the mastication of food and teeth that curtail the mandibular range of movements. Whenever possible a gold that wears comparable to tooth structure should be selected to prevent traumatic relationships after many years of service.

As with other procedures, the dentist will become well acquainted with these indications. Successes and failures of clinical restorations aid the dentist in determining when castings are useful. In some situations only the gold casting should be used if the patient is able to afford the service.

CASE DIAGNOSIS AND WORKING RECORDS

The additional time and skill on the part of the dentist merits a thorough study and examination of the conditions. The patient is questioned to determine the nature of the complaint and symptoms and to acquire a record of the medical history. The patient's motivation and confidence can be determined during the examination. The tooth or area to be restored is examined thoroughly to determine the gingival health and the quality of the patient's toothbrushing. The amount of remaining tooth structure, the demand for esthetics, the amount of caries, the degree of fracture, and the form of existing restorations are noted.

Diagnostic casts serve as a useful and usually necessary guide for designing the cast restoration. These study models are mounted on an adjustable articular to determine the mandibular movements and to what extent the range of motion will influence the restoration design. The upper diagnostic cast is mounted with a facebow transfer to standardize the position of the upper cast to the articulator. The lower cast is mounted by a centric record in the desired jaw relationship before the lateral records are taken for setting the articulator.[6]

The procedure to be followed is described in Chapter 2 in the discussion of occlusal analysis. Right and left interocclusal records are used to set the condylar guidance and Bennett components on the articulator. The models can then be moved to determine premature or traumatic occlusal contacts and the relationship of the anterior teeth. It can be determined whether the castings should be limited to the immediate problem, whether some of the traumatic contacts should be removed by shaping the natural teeth, or whether an additional plan should be presented for preserving the natural dentition.

The diagnostic casts are used later for making impression trays and are saved as the preoperative models. The size of the tooth defect or existing restoration can be penciled on the stone and the proposed cavity form can be shown to the patient. The models will help point out the need for the specific treatment as well as aid in establishing an organized treatment plan.

The articulated models are used to determine what jaw relationship is indicated for the patient. The use of two bites—one in the acquired maximum interdigitation, which is called centric occlusion, and one in centric relation, which is the most retruded position of the mandible—is used to determine the amount of discrepancy that is present between anatomical and functional jaw relationship.[7] The acquired position is usually selected because it is the most common jaw relationship; a change in position usually results in altering many natural tooth surfaces.

The centric relation record is taken with the condyles in the most posterior, upper, and middle position of the glenoid fossa. The bites are taken with wax; the teeth are not allowed to contact because of the deflection that would result in the mandible. This position, called the hinge axis, is where pure rotation occurs around the horizontal condylar plane.

This axis is used for reconstruction because it is the only position of the mandible that can be statically reproduced, and it is from this point that all jaw movements are started. To allow maximum interdigitation of the teeth in centric relation the premature contacts must be removed from the occlusal surfaces of the posterior teeth. This equilibration is necessary before reconstruction is started but is usually not needed when only a few cast restorations are made. The two interocclusal records are helpful in determining the amount of error and the degree of interdigitation in the occlusion. The greater the number of castings being constructed, the more important is the use of hinge axis. The nearer the tooth interdigitation is to centric relation, the fewer problems in the joints, musculature, and teeth.

In most cases the diagnostic casts will dictate that the restorations be made in the maximum interdigitation position. It is usually anterior to centric relation by 1 to 2 mm. and is the method to use unless all the quadrants are being restored with castings. In such cases pantographing, use of the fully adjustable articulator, and the full gnathologic approach to treatment should be considered.

The interdigitation record is taken by guiding the patient to normal closure. The right and left lateral interocclusal records are taken to set the Bennett guide and condylar inclination. The readings on the articulator are recorded and all future casts can be mounted by using only the facebow transfers and centric record. The articulator readings should be recorded for each patient and are reproducible.

Some techniques do not require full-arch models or an adjustable articulator. However, developing accurate function and tooth morphology is more difficult and more adjustments must be made when the casting is cemented.

CAVITY PREPARATION

Black's principles for inlay preparations are strongly advocated, with some modifications (Fig. 17-2). The preparation is more extended and has a wider outline form than the amalgam preparation.[8] The boxlike form is reduced in size because resistance is not as important. The surrounding cavity walls are tapered to facilitate removal of the pattern and seating of the casting. Generally bulk is not present in the inlay preparation; therefore, the walls are more tapered and flared. The conservative approach involves a shallow surface extension and coverage with limited depth in the intracoronal mortise form. These factors rely on the strength of the gold and reduce caries susceptibility at the margins.

Characteristics of inlay preparations in posterior teeth

1. Extension is greater than with the amalgam preparation and there is a wider and more visible outline form. When the tooth structure is weak, particularly when thin remaining cusps are present, the casting grasps the enamel and

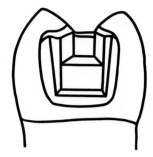

Fig. 17-2. Black's Class II inlay preparation. Note the bulk in the preparation, taper of the internal walls, and cavosurface bevel.

the entire occlusal surface is replaced. The proximal margins are opened to allow disking of the buccolingual margins, making the margin closer to the line angles. This places all the margins in self-cleansing areas and helps to prevent plaque formation or caries on the edge of the restoration. The cervical wall is located below healthy gingival tissue and out of contact with the adjacent tooth, and it is not extended farther than the amalgam preparation or beyond the cemento-enamel junction.

2. The axial-pulpal depth of the preparation is limited when compared to the amalgam restoration because bulk is not necessary to resist fracture. The resistance form of the inlay is produced by smooth, full-length walls with definite internal line angles. The walls are placed just inside the dentinoenamel junction, but width of the mortise form is not critical. Thickness in the gold casting is needed only to prevent spread or distortion of the metal from occlusal forces.

3. The retention form is developed from dovetails, the taper of the walls, and postholes. Grooves are sometimes used as well as cusp capping and surface reduction for retention of large castings. The amount of wall taper and surface coverage appear to be the critical factors for retaining the casting.

4. The cavosurface margin of the preparation should be beveled where the tooth approaches a right angle. This creates bulk on the edge of the tooth structure, which is helpful in waxing the pattern and finishing the casting to maintain the seal of the restoration. The good margin is enhanced by the bevel and reduces the amount of the cement liner that will be exposed to oral fluids (Fig. 17-3).

The air turbine handpiece alleviates much of the work associated with tooth reduction and has encouraged multiple restorations in the quadrant procedure. Black's sequence of instrumentation was originally advocated, using the tapered fissure burs for tapering the enamel walls. Because of the widespread acceptance of the turbine, this instrumentation will also be described. Time is saved in multiple preparations because the cutting point does not require replacement until the task has been completed for all the teeth. The quadrant procedure should only be used by the experienced operator because many landmarks are lost when

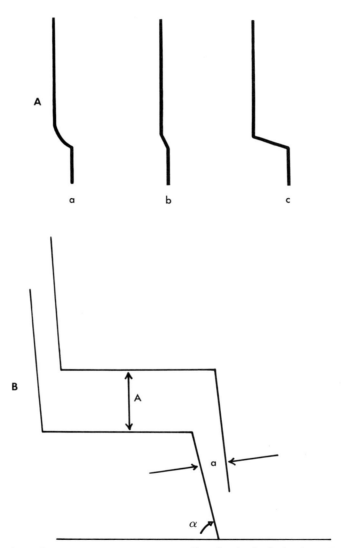

Fig. 17-3. A, A variety of preparation terminations. *a,* Chamfer finish; *b,* feather edge or slight bevel; *c,* shoulder finish. **B,** The influence of a bevel. *A,* Distance between crown and tooth vertically; *a,* space between side of tooth and internal part of casting. Bevels cause this distance to decrease. (**B** adapted from Rosner, D.: J. Prosth. Dent. **13:**1160, 1963.)

an extensive amount of tooth structure is removed. Black's instrumentation follows a similar sequence of bur application, from inverted cone to tapered fissure burs.[8]

Instrumentation for Class II inlay preparations

The surgical field is established and the teeth are examined to determine the amount of extension needed in the preparation. The proximal contact size and embrasure form are noted as well as the area in which the cervical wall will be terminated. The outline form should be ascertained before any reduction is started.

Regular-speed No. 34 inverted cone bur. The regular-speed No. 34 inverted cone bur in the contra-angle handpiece is used to penetrate the occlusal caries and extend the primary grooves to the width and depth of the bur. The rough occlusal outline form is produced by undermining the enamel or pulling the bur up from the dentin floor. The isthmus will usually be one third or more of the intercuspal distance because of the larger lesion.

The proximal portion of the preparation is formed by moving the No. 34 end cutter back and forth on the enamel when an undermined surface is present. In incipient lesions a welling technique in the dentin with the No. ½ round bur is used to undermine the enamel to enable fracture of the proximal enamel with hand instruments. The rough dimensions of the proximal outline form are made with the end and side cutters of the inverted cone bur.

No. 701 tapered fissure bur. The No. 701 tapered fissure bur is used in a contra-angle handpiece to establish and flare the cavity walls and the internal line angles. Not much cutting will be needed if the inverted cone has been properly applied. The occlusal portion is smoothed and then the bur is used to angulate the proximal area. The end and side cutters are applied while the bur is slowly revolved to permit vision and accurate extension.

If the air turbine handpiece is used to produce the outline form, the small tapered fissure bur (No. 699 or No. 700) is selected in order to regulate surface temperatures. The occlusal portion is opened first, and then the small bur tip is used to open the proximal portion in the same manner as with regular speeds. The cutting should be done with an intermittent 4 to 6 ounce load on the handpiece. The entire outline form and cavity depth are produced with the same bur. Cautious application and excellent vision are needed to prevent overcutting the tooth.

This completes the "roughing out" portion; all subsequent steps involve finishing of the cavity form.

Wedelstaedt or binangle chisels. Wedelstaedt or binangle chisels are used to cleave the buccal and lingual proximal enamel walls (Fig. 17-4). The walls are adequately opened to allow access for disking the buccal and lingual walls of the proximal preparation. The chisels are placed by the marginal ridge and thrust toward the axial wall. The cavosurface margin is placed just inside the

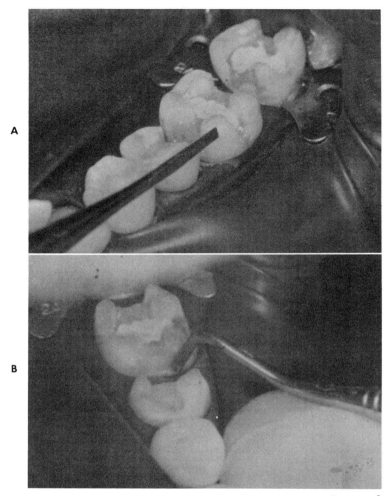

Continued.

Fig. 17-4. A, Smoothing the reduced tooth structure and finish lines with the chisel. **B,** Placing the proximal bulk for the "box line" resistance form with the enamel hatchet.

line angle in a tapered but straight line toward the gingival tissue. Mesial and distal cutting edges of the chisel make it possible to reach both the buccal and lingual walls.

Enamel hatchets. Enamel hatchets are used to remove the proximal dentin and make the box form. The hatchet is rotated slightly to cut the dentin portion of the buccal and lingual wall and form a mortise form with uniform width and sharp angles. The blade of the hatchet is pulled across the cervical wall to smooth and form the two point angles in the gingival corners.

Sandpaper disks. The ⅜ or ½ inch cuttlefish sandpaper disks are used in the contra-angle mandrel to smooth the buccal and lingual walls of the proximal

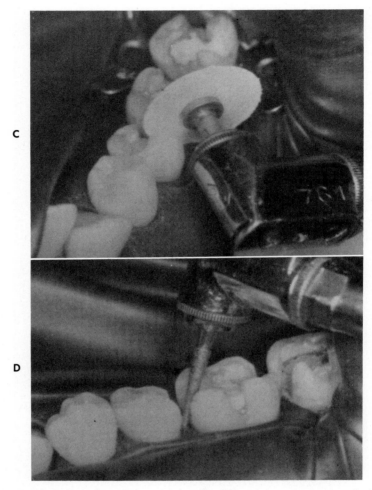

C

D

Fig. 17-4, cont'd. C, Smoothing the proximal walls of the cavity preparation with the sandpaper disk. The smooth margin facilitates waxing and polishing the inlay. **D,** Smoothing the cervical cavosurface bevel with the thin, tapered diamond. The same diamond is used for smoothing the other cavity walls, cusp cappings, and bevels.

preparation. The disk and an abrasive are used to produce the desired amount of smoothness and angulation on all the walls.

Margin trimmers. Margin trimmers are used to bevel the cervical margin. The right and left instruments are used for each cervical bevel by placing the cutting edge on the tooth structure and dragging the blade to the buccal and lingual walls. Light pressure must be used to avoid slipping out of the preparation. The bevel is uniformly placed the full length of the cervical cavosurface margin.

Small flame-shaped diamond burs are useful for forming the cervical bevel. They are placed on the margin and revolved slowly to form the accurate bevel.

Inadequate vision may complicate this procedure, and in most cases the cervical bevel is smoothed with hand instruments following application of the diamond instrument. The cervical bevel is made 45 degrees to the cervical wall.

Flame-shaped and tapered diamond burs or the No. 700 fissure bur. These burs are used to form the occlusal cavosurface bevel. A small, thin reduction is made where the margin is sharp or approximates a right angle. This area is confined to the grooves and dovetails. Sometimes in the large outline form the margin on the cusp planes cannot be accurately beveled because of the obtuse angle. The small tip of the diamond bur is revolved slowly to produce the bevel, which should also be made 45 degrees to the enamel surface.

If the cusps have been reduced for capping procedures, the surfaces are smoothed with the diamond bur at this time. The reduction includes contra bevels in the enamel that must be smoothed before the impression is taken. Smoothing is accomplished by slowing turning the bur and using light pressure. Any other bevels that are needed are placed at this time. This might be in surface extensions such as steps or chamfered areas.

Wedelstaedt chisel. A sharp Wedelstaedt chisel is used for the final smoothing of all the margins. Delicate, short strokes will remove small pieces of enamel, especially those in the corners that are missed by the diamond bur. The preparation is completed by polishing the prepared tissue with prophylactic paste.

•   •   •

The amount of taper in the cavity walls influences the retention of the casting. Less interference and marginal closure are associated with the highly tapered wall, but this is not entirely desirable. In this situation the casting is more likely to be displaced from the tooth. The surrounding walls should be tapered 8 to 12 degrees to give resistance and retention to the restoration. This will negate the use of many accessory retention forms such as posts and grooves, and in turn it is less complicated to develop a well-adapted casting.

The slice preparation has been advocated for quadrant work because the proximal outline form is rapidly developed. This is done by slicing the proximal surface through the middle of the marginal ridge with a disk after the occlusal area has been prepared.[9] The proximal caries is removed and retention is gained by a groove in the axial wall dentin. The axial groove retention is made into a box when the size of the lesion is extensive.

The popularity of the slice preparation has declined because its application is limited to small proximal lesions. The multiple uses of the disk encourage slipshod procedures. Because the cervical wall is curved, the preparation is not considered to be as protected from caries as the conventional Black preparation.

The indications for cusp capping and protection must be thoroughly understood (Fig. 17-5). One great advantage of the cast gold inlay is the ability to cover and rebuild weak portions of the tooth. Thin remaining cusps should be reduced and protected by gold. The isthmus dimension used for a weak cusp is

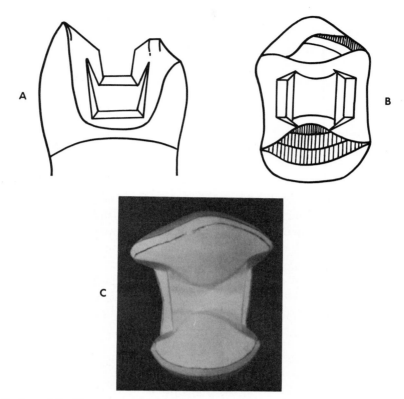

Fig. 17-5. A and **B,** Illustrations showing the extent and angulation of cusp capping on the bicuspid tooth. **C,** Occlusal view of capped cusps.

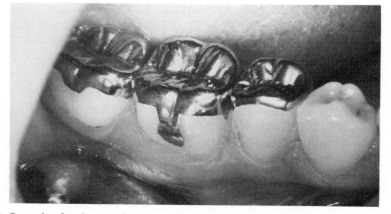

Fig. 17-6. Example of reductions for the working cusps in inlays. Note the cohesive gold restoration in the buccal pit of the first molar.

Table 17-1. Force required to fracture teeth with M.O.D. cavities of different design*

Tooth prepared for	Average force required (arbitrary units)†	
	Filled	Unfilled
Amalgam	90	89
Gold inlay	96	92
Gold inlay with cusp protection	192	87

*From Vale, W. A.: Irish Dent. Rev. 2:33, 1956.
†The figures represent an average of not less than six tests.

when the isthmus on the occlusal surface is wider than one third of the inter-cuspal distance.[11] This creates a short cusp plane. If the cusp is one that functions (a working cusp), it should be protected by capping.

The working cusps are the lingual surfaces of the maxillary teeth and the buccal surfaces of the mandibular posterior teeth, and these areas are reduced the most (Fig. 17-6). The cusp is reduced in two planes in the same contour of the original surfaces, which creates the contra bevel. The outside or contra bevel is made one third or less the thickness of the inside bevel. This enables the casting to grasp the tooth to prevent fracture. The contra bevel of the maxillary teeth, especially in bicuspids, is kept shorter than this when esthetics is necessary so that only a thin line of gold will show on the finished casting. The reduction is made to produce a clearance of 1 mm. in all dimensions to allow proper thickness of the casting.

The reduction of the nonworking cusps, which are the buccal surfaces of the maxillary teeth and lingual surfaces of the mandibular teeth, follows a similar pattern. The inside reduction is greatest and should also allow a clearance of 1 mm. The contra bevel on the maxillary bicuspids is kept very thin or may be omitted when the display of metal would be objectionable. No problem results if contact of the tooth is not possible in the eccentric jaw movements.

The outline form of the capping should be slightly rounded and follow the same general lines of the cusp arms. The esthetic bevel is uniform in thickness and is smoothed to develop a straight edge on the casting. The smooth, exacting margin and proper contour cause the gold to be reflected so that the casting is less noticeable. Wherever the tooth appears to be weak, the cusps should be covered by the gold casting.

The instrumentation described represents a minimum number of instruments and procedures for making the acceptable Class II preparation. Other instruments can be used to produce the preparation if they are considered to be more helpful. The time spent in perfecting the preparation will produce rewards when fabricating and placing the gold casting. For this reason the preparation is considered the most important aspect of the technique, as is true of the other restorations. Only the Class II preparation is explained at this time because it is the most common design used with multiple indirect procedures. Modifications of the Class II preparation are made for surface coverage and steps when necessary, which involves a chamfer finish line similar to the full-coverage concept. The entire outline form should be located on smooth enamel.

INDIRECT METHOD OF CAST CONSTRUCTION
Gingival displacement

Prior to taking the impression of the cavity preparations the gingival tissues that abut the cervical finishing lines or bevels must be displaced.[12] Many methods may be used for exposing the cervical margins of the tooth. Gingival displacement is done prior to taking the impression so that all the margins of the tooth that must be placed on the restoration will be recorded. The elastic impression materials are not rigid enough to move the tissue from the tooth, making displacement necessary. The delicate tissue must be handled carefully and the retracting cord and drug, which are placed in the free gingival margin to temporarily move the tissue, must be properly selected to avoid tissue damage.

Conservative methods

The technique of placing the cord in the crevice, the type of cord employed, and the nature of the chemical used for displacement affect the gingival tissue. In most techniques a string is used in the gingival crevice to physically and sometimes chemically remove the gingiva from the cavity margin. The gingival crevice is normally only 2 mm. and it must be treated with caution or the tissue will be damaged. The available displacement materials as well as the problems associated with each in displacing the tissue are presented for evaluation. The method that is selected should allow proper recovery of the tissue and should not produce any untoward effects on the patient.

Materials and contact time for tissue displacement are as follows:
1. Heavyweight rubber dam
2. Plain cotton thread commercially available—10 minutes
3. String saturated with 1:1,000 epinephrine (for noncardiac patients)—10 minutes
4. String saturated with 100% alum solution—10 minutes
5. String saturated with 5% aluminum chloride solution—10 minutes
6. String saturated with ferric subsulfate (Monsel's solution)—3 minutes
7. String saturated with 20% tannic acid—10 minutes
8. String saturated with 8% zinc chloride (bitartrate)—3 minutes
9. String saturated with 4% levo-epinephrine with 9% potassium alum—10 minutes

The contact time of the string varies with the type of chemical used. Some solutions act as astringents and caustics if left in contact with the tissue for lengthy periods. Correct timing is important, and if not observed, can prove detrimental when taking the impression. Superficial necrosis occurs from chemical trauma, which results in loss of tissue and exposure of the cavity margin after the casting is cemented.

Gingival retraction has been simplified by the development of new heavy-weight rubber dams. The retraction produced actually compresses the tissue. Rubber dam retraction is more advantageous for tooth reduction, but it can also be used when taking the impression. The clamp is blocked out with wax to prevent withdrawal, and ideal impressions are obtained when the preparations are clean and dry. Full-arch models cannot be obtained with the rubber dam in place, but the procedure is useful in cases that are not extensive or with the direct inlay.

Different types of string have been advocated for use in the gingival crevice. Plain cotton thread, unwaxed floss, and cord the size of a 20 gauge needle are the most commonly used.[13] A number of instruments are used to gently place the strings in the crevice and in contact with the gingival tissue. The technique should not cause hemorrhage or laceration of the gingival attachment. A soft-textured thread will facilitate placement with the instrument.

The solutions may be placed on the strings after they are seated in the crevice or the strings may be saturated with the solution and dried before application. Some operators use combinations of chemicals for retraction by applying one solution to the string prior to application and applying another solution after the string has been placed in the crevice. A combination of alum and aluminum chloride is acceptable.

Research has indicated that measurable amounts of trauma occur with conservative retraction procedures. Harrison[14] states that the least amount of damage occurs in the gingival epithelium of dogs when strings treated with 1:1,000 epinephrine, 100% alum, styptic pencil, and 5% aluminum chloride are used. These chemicals caused irritation and a subsequent loss of only 0.1 mm. of gingival tissue within a few days. Harrison cautioned against the use of zinc chloride. Applications of 8% zinc chloride solutions resulted in severe necrosis and pus formation that did not heal for 60 days.

Drug application is further limited when the dangers of epinephrine are considered. A string, 1 inch long, saturated with 8% epinephrine contains fifteen times the recommended safe dosage of the drug. Although it is unlikely that complete absorption will occur, there is clinical evidence of adverse reactions in cardiac patients. The problem becomes more acute in the full-coverage preparation because more epinephrine will be absorbed.

Clinical application of the previous data has been studied in monkeys.[15] The animals' blood pressures were monitored during the introduction of the string saturated with epinephrine, and an elevation of normal blood pressure to 200/180 occurred. According to these data, the use of epinephrine is contraindicated in cardiac patients or when capillary beds have been exposed during cavity preparation, such as occurs in the deep finishing line in a full-coverage

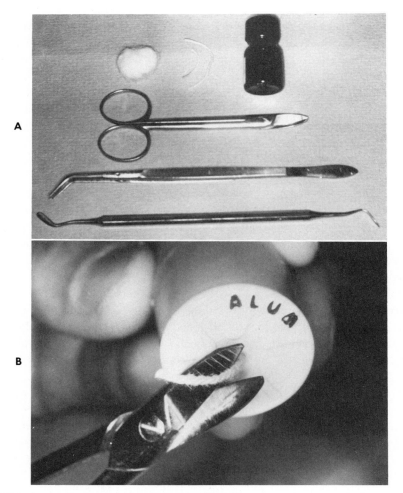

Fig. 17-7. A, Armamentarium for gingival retraction: cotton, alum string, solution, and string placement instruments. **B,** The desired length of alum string is cut from the dispenser.

preparation. Other solutions should be selected that are effective in retraction but do not cause systemic reactions.

Many types of instruments are used to place the strings in the gingival crevice (Fig. 17-7). Specially manufactured designs or adjusted cement instruments that have blades parallel to and at right angles to the shaft enable the operator to reach all four surfaces of the tooth for seating the string. The blade used to tuck the string should be small and blunt and should preferably have a square working end to avoid tearing the tissue. The string is placed in the crevice and gently tamped and rolled to the bottom to rest on the gingival attachment. Pressure and the medicament on the string will result in collapse of vessels and displacement of the tissue.

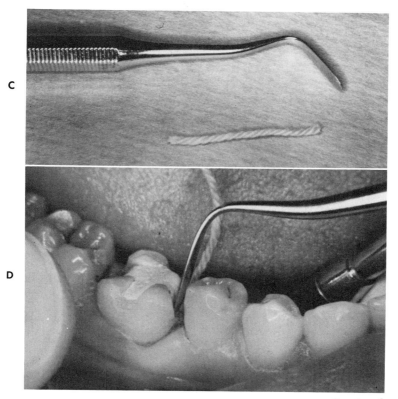

C

D

Continued.

Fig. 17-7, cont'd. C, Blunt instrument for string placement and length of string commonly used for the interproximal surface of a molar tooth. **D,** The alum string is placed between the free gingival margin and the tooth surface.

The string is cut to reach around the proximal surface, past the buccal and lingual line angle. The dimension of the bottom of the crevice is the measurement used because this is where the string must rest. This area must be thoroughly dried and protected throughout the impression procedure. Saliva must be controlled with cotton rolls and the ejector because it will dilute the medicament and cause inadequate retraction. This length of string is used to cause partial displacement of the papilla that serves to hold the free margin against the tooth. Inadequate displacement occurs when an incorrect length of cord is used.

When the string is in place, the aluminum chloride solution is applied to the crevice with the beaks of the cotton pliers. The solution is allowed to saturate the string and contact the tissue. Small pledgets of cotton are tamped into the interproximal space to prevent dilution or movement of the medication. The contact of the drug is timed from the saturation of the last string to ensure full utilization and optimum retraction.

The string must be removed carefully in order not to induce bleeding. The

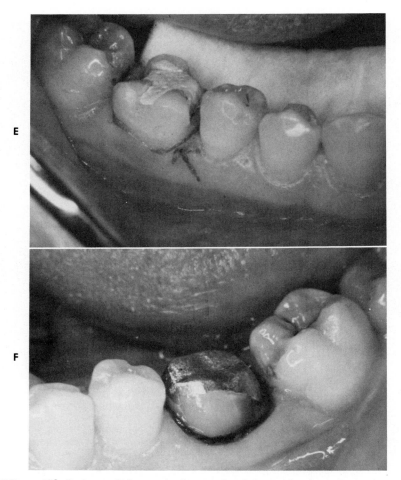

Fig. 17-7, cont'd. E, Arrow indicates the line angle of the tooth where the string must be extended for effective retraction of gingival tissue in this area. **F,** The string is in place for a full-coverage preparation.

cotton is removed and the end of the string is grasped with the cotton pliers. Slow, gentle removal will leave the crevice open and allow full vision of the beveled margin. If the preparation needs adjusting, it should be done quickly at this time. The finished field is gently dried with the air syringe just before injection of the impression material. If the entire finish line can be observed before taking the impression, it may be left in place to avoid seepage that occurs with removal.

Problems associated with tissue displacement are as follows:
1. Laceration of the tissue during cavity preparation
2. Inadequate control of hemorrhage

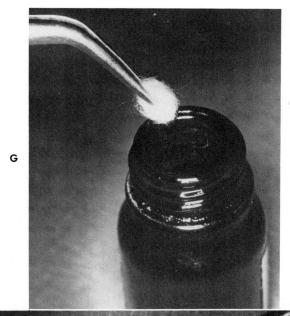

G

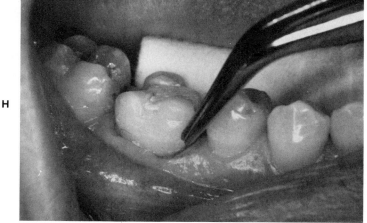

H

Continued.

Fig. 17-7, cont'd. G, Solution is sometimes applied with small pledgets of cotton. **H,** Solution may also be placed on the string with cotton pliers. The string must be saturated.

3. Debris left in the preparation because the area was not completely dried
4. Irreversible tissue damage cause by prolonged contact of the displacement string (chemical and nonchemical) with the gingival sulcus
5. Alteration of the periodontal attachment when the cavity preparation is extended too far in the gingival sulcus
6. Lack of knowledge and understanding of the use of chemicals and tissue reaction

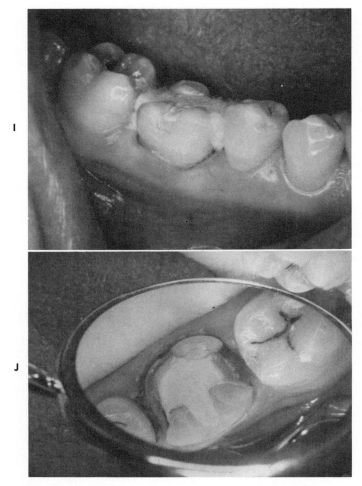

Fig. 17-7, cont'd. I, Saturated strings are covered with absorbent cotton and left undisturbed for 5 to 10 minutes. **J,** Gingival tissue displaced from the cervical margins of the cavity preparation.

Radical methods

A. Surgery
   1. Knife
   2. Electric cautery
   3. Electrocoagulation
   4. Cold cautery

B. Chemical cautery
   1. Zinc chloride (40%)
   2. Sodium sulfide
   3. Potassium hydroxide
   4. Negatan solution

Radical procedures are occasionally justified to expose the cervical cavo-surface margin. Such procedures can also be used to remove inflamed and diseased tissue. Chemical cautery with the use of caustic drugs should not be considered for gingival displacement because it produces irritation and necrosis.

When electrosurgery is used, the dentist must have a thorough knowledge of the principles involved and understand the use of the instrument. This is essential to minimize tissue destruction and encourage healing after surgery. Different electrosurgery techniques are used for fulguration or coagulation (hemostasis). It is thought that the high-frequency current desiccates the tissue but does not actually produce a cutting action. Desiccation is accomplished by placing the needle on the tissue, while fulguration is produced by a spark-gap between the needle and the tissue. Coagulation is caused by a bipolar current with a two-pronged needle inserted into the tissue; this is the most severe procedure for removing tissue.

Electrodes are employed with electrosurgery. A high-frequency alternating current creates a density charge on the surface of the epithelium. Desiccation produces only superficial coagulation necrosis that subsequently sloughs and heals. These instruments produce a trough around the tooth that is related to the size of the electrode and the number of applications of the instrument tip.

Research with electrocoagulation has been enlightening in regard to the healing rate involved.[16] It was demonstrated in dogs that the gingival tissue completely recovered within a week. The reduction of tissue height was found to be less than that experienced with conservative retraction procedures. The data indicate that controlled electrosurgery is a valuable and relatively atraumatic procedure as compared to other radical procedures. Sound electrosurgical technique is not considered to be a radical procedure.

If surgery is employed preparatory to making an impression, it is essential that the accepted principles of sound periodontal procedures be followed to ensure proper healing and to produce the desired tissue morphology.

Management of the gingival tissue is important in making the inlay. Minimal trauma will result in a properly contoured tissue that fully covers the cervical margins of the restoration. Unless hyperplastic tissue is present, conservative management is the method of choice.

To make cast restorations by the indirect method an accurate elastic impression material must be used. Models are obtained from the molds on which the inlays are made. This technique is called the indirect method because fabrication of the casting is accomplished on the model.

Impression materials

At this time three impression materials are considered to be accurate enough for the indirect method. These are mercaptan and silicone rubbers and the reversible hydrocolloid materials. The first two materials are similarly manipulated, making it possible to describe and classify them as synthetic rubbers. A syringe must be used for placing all three materials inside the preparation to minimize discrepancies and air entrapment. Therefore, it is necessary to understand the syringe and tray material before a successful impression can be made.

The criteria for selecting an impression material are the accuracy obtainable, ease of manipulation, and cleanliness of the technique. The set material must be tough but must also be elastic so that it will not tear upon removal from the preparation. However, not all of these properties are possible with any one material; selection is based on personal preference. The accuracy obtained with either the synthetic rubbers or reversible hydrocolloid is acceptable. Manipulation of the materials is explained separately.

Synthetic rubbers

The mercaptan and silicone materials are dispensed as pastes. There are two tubes, one for the syringe and one for the tray. The setting times are regulated to enable individual manipulation. Thorough mixing and correct timing are required for polymerization of the rubber. Some products use only one material for the syringe and tray portions.

The factors influencing the accuracy of the synthetic rubbers are as follows[17-19]:

1. The pastes must be thoroughly mixed. The rubber is spread on the mixing pad with spatulas to produce a uniform color; no streaks should be present in the mix.

2. A minimum thickness of material is used between the tray and the cavity preparations. The thickness of the material should be less than 2 mm., which indicates that a custom-made acrylic tray be used for each impression.

3. Adequate time should be allowed for polymerization to minimize dimensional change after removal of the impression. At least 12 minutes is required from the beginning of the mix to allow 8 minutes of curing time on the teeth. The master die should be poured within 30 minutes after removal of the impression to minimize the amount of distortion caused by continued polymerization and the collapse of bubbles in the rubber material.

Acrylic tray construction. Only the custom-made acrylic tray ensures a small, uniform thickness of impression material (Fig. 17-8). The optimum thickness of the layer should be less than 2 mm., and this is regulated with the tray. A special tray model is made from an alginate impression or a diagnostic cast of the teeth. The mucobuccal fold is the boundary for taking the impression, building the tray, and trimming the models. This standardizes each individual case. The bases for the models are needed only for strength. The teeth can be more easily reached when large bases are not placed on the models.

The model is trimmed and dried and the tray is constructed prior to the appointment for the preparations and impressions. One layer of baseplate wax is placed over the teeth and to the fold of the soft tissue areas. If undercuts are present in the flanges, they are blocked out with additional pieces of wax. When the wax has cooled, holes are cut to expose the occlusal surface of the posterior

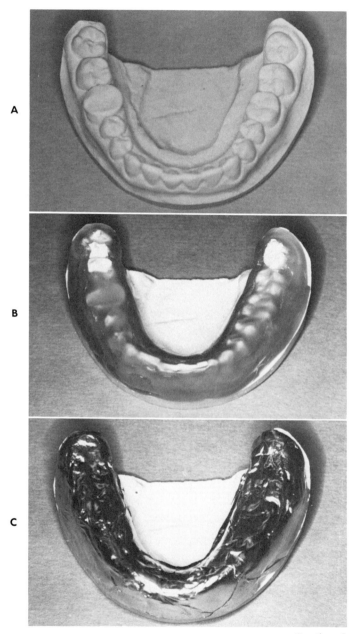

Continued.

Fig. 17-8. A, Tray model or diagnostic cast to construct the impression tray using Thiokol and silicone impression materials. **B,** One layer of wax is applied to the model for minimum and uniform thickness. The model is exposed in the anterior and posterior areas to produce stops for the impression tray. **C,** Layer of tinfoil over the wax serves as a separation medium for the acrylic tray.

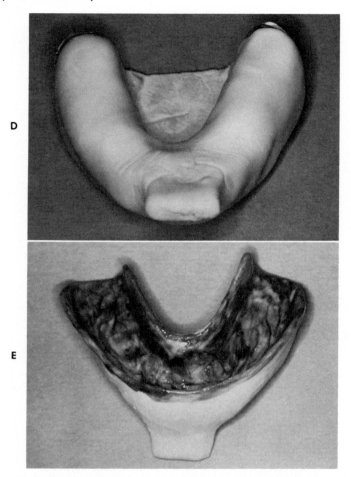

Fig. 17-8, cont'd. D, Molded acrylic tray. **E,** Appearance of custom-made tray after it has been removed, trimmed and smoothed on the borders, and painted with rubber adhesive cement.

teeth on each side and one anterior tooth. These will serve as stops and prevent the tray from being seated too far down over the preparations. Some dentists prefer to use asbestos for the model liner, but uniform thickness is difficult with this material.

A layer of tinfoil is placed over the wax and trimmed at the borders. The quick-setting tray acrylic is mixed and molded to shape over the tinfoil by lubricating the fingers with Vaseline. The acrylic is then placed over the tinfoil and spread to form a tray ⅛ inch thick. The borders are placed down into the fold to make round, smooth edges on the tray similar to the border of an artificial denture. A tray handle of suitable size is placed over the incisors in the midline and the model is left undisturbed for 5 minutes to allow the acrylic to cure.

The tray is removed from the model while the wax is still warm from the exothermic curing reaction of the acrylic. The wax will stick to the model, promoting easy removal of the acrylic. The tray is smoothed and rounded with an arbor band on the lathe and then is finished with a large acrylic stone inserted in the handpiece. All round projections and the borders are smoothed to prevent trauma of the soft tissue when the impression tray is seated. The inside of the tray is coated with liquid rubber adhesive cement and the tray is stored on the model until the inlay appointment. Accurate tray construction eliminates the need for a trial fitting and numerous chairside adjustments. Preliminary finishing and coating can be done at odd times so that the office schedule will not be disrupted.

Dispensing. The two pastes for the syringe and the tray material are dispensed on the slab by the assistant while the gingival retraction strings are being placed (Fig. 17-9). Equal lengths of the catalysts and base are placed on the stiff paper mixing pad. The syringe material is dispensed in 3 inch lengths and the tray material is dispensed in 8 inch lengths. The pastes are placed apart on the slab to prevent contact and contamination prior to the mixing procedure.

Mixing. A tough, resistant paper pad is used for the mixing surface. A number of spatulas have been designed for the mixing procedure; the preferred design has a straight and sharp edge. The catalyst material is lifted off the pad with the spatula and placed on the base material. Force is exerted to thoroughly mix the two materials with the flat side of the spatula. Thorough mixing results in a uniform paste. When the material runs over the slab, it is scooped up with the sharp edge of the spatula and incorporated back into the mix. No streaks of either the catalyst or the base material should appear in the mix.

The light-bodied and the regular or heavy-bodied tray material are spatulated the same way. Thorough mixing of both materials is necessary for a uniform and complete setting reaction. The light-bodied syringe material is mixed first and then loaded into the syringe used for injecting the rubber. The tray material is mixed last and placed in the tray. The setting reaction of the syringe material is prolonged so that adequate working time is allowed for manipulating the rubber, injecting the material, and seating the tray. The dental assistant may aid in performing the various tasks of manipulation.

Loading the syringe. The rubber syringe has a barrel, a plastic tip, and a snugly fitting plunger (Fig. 17-10). The plastic tip can be cut to produce the desired amount of opening for the injection and is small enough to fit into the smallest of outline and retention forms. There are two methods of loading the syringe with the light-bodied material. The process is messy, and the loading method should be selected according to the convenience and cleanliness of the equipment.

Cone loading. A paper cone is made out of 5½ × 7 inch stiff paper. The paper is folded over until a point is formed and a pocket is present in which to place the mixed rubber. The paper is opened and placed on the work surface until the mixing is started.

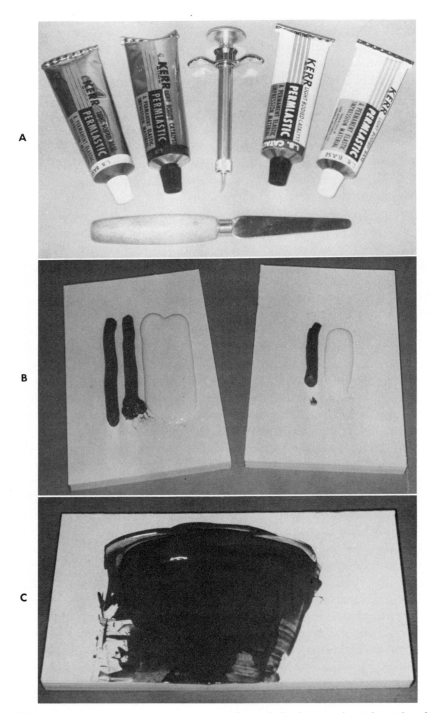

Fig. 17-9. A, Impression materials: syringe, spatula, and the base and catalyst tubes for both the syringe and base material. **B,** Thiokol dispensed on the mixing pads. Note equal lengths of the base and catalyst materials. **C,** Mixed rubber base showing homogeneous color and absence of streaks in the material that is characteristic of an adequate mix.

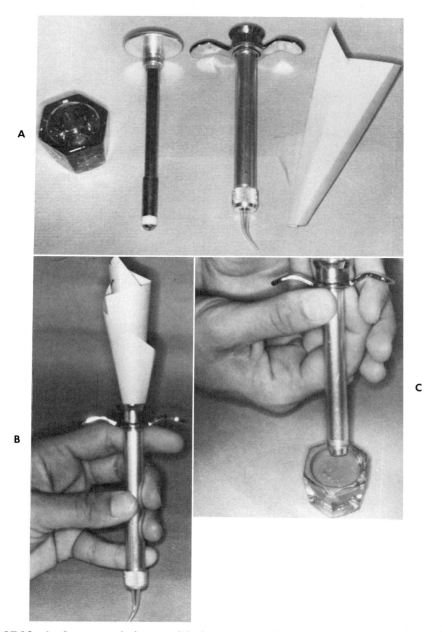

Fig. 17-10. A, Syringe and dappen dish for aspiration loading and the paper funnel for loading the syringe. **B,** Mixed syringe material is placed inside the paper cone and forced into the syringe barrel for the cone-loading technique. **C,** Aspiration loading is accomplished by placing the syringe in the dappen dish and withdrawing the plunger.

The mixed syringe material is placed inside the paper, which is refolded to form a cone. The small cone tip is placed at the base of the syringe barrel and the rubber is forced into the container. The cone is removed and discarded. The plunger is slowly seated until the rubber fills the plastic tip and the syringe is then placed on the bracket table.

Aspiration loading. This method produces more soiling but seems to be the easiest way of loading the syringe. The mixed light-bodied syringe rubber is placed in a dappen dish. The plastic tip is removed from the barrel and the nose of the syringe is placed down into the mix. The handle and plunger are slowly withdrawn to pull the rubber into the syringe. When the bulk of the material is loaded, the barrel tip is wiped with a tissue and the plastic tip is reapplied.

Careful mixing and slow loading with steady pressure will minimize air entrapment in the syringe material.

Taking the impression. The preparations are dried as previously described to facilitate duplication of the cavity details. The syringe is held in a pen grasp, with the point on the most distal wall of the cavity preparation. The rubber is slowly ejected to fill in the cavity detail by moving toward the anterior of the preparation. The gingival tissue is pushed aside with the plastic tip and the rubber is injected into the free space to copy the cervical bevels. When the floor of the preparation is covered, the material is then ejected to envelop the entire tooth (Fig. 17-11).

The slow anterior movement to gradually fill the preparation and cover each tooth will prevent bubbles and discrepancies in the impression. The injecting continues until all the preparations are covered. If some syringe material remains, it can be used to fill in the occlusal surfaces of adjacent teeth.

The loaded tray is seated firmly on the teeth. The tray is seated slowly and vibrated just before the stops are reached. Measures must be taken to prevent the injected material from becoming coated with saliva because this can result in poor bonding of the two rubber materials and produce distortion in the reproduction.

The tray is held firmly with the thumb and index finger of each hand. The saliva ejector can be placed into the sublingual space if swallowing is difficult. The tray is held in its seated position for at least 10 minutes from the beginning of the mix, at which time the rubber is tested with a blunt instrument to see if it will recoil. If a depression results, the impression must be held in place until the test indicates that the material is cured.

Removal of the tray is sometimes difficult because of the toughness of the cured rubber. Removal is best accomplished with a quick snap in a line parallel to the long axis of the teeth. The thumbs or index fingers are placed on the border of the tray in the bicuspid areas. This position develops more leverage, and a quicker removal is possible than by using the tray handle.

The impression is inspected and then washed with tap water. If water con-

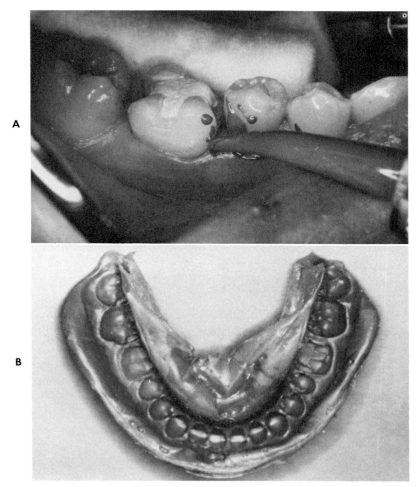

Continued.

Fig. 17-11. A, Injection is started inside the gingival crevice and the entire cavity preparation is eventually covered. **B,** Complete-arch Thiokol impression that is poured twice, first for the dies and then for the working model for articulation. **C,** Impression showing detail of the cervical finishing line.

tacts the acrylic tray, dimensional change can occur. The soft tissues are inspected and the impression is dried and stored in air while preparations are made to form the models.

The rubber materials are gaining popularity because of the ease in making the full-arch model. The tray is simple to make, and the impression for the complete arch is no more difficult to accomplish than a partial impression. The complete model is helpful in developing the wax pattern because occlusal relationships are more accurately determined when more interdigitation can be observed. For this reason rubber impression materials are used extensively by gnathologists

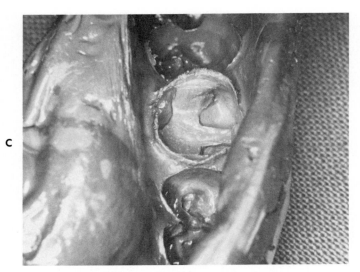

C

Fig. 17-11, cont'd. For legend see p. 553.

for reconstruction procedures. The full impression is helpful in guiding the laboratory technician in making the gold casting. A reduction in chairside adjustments when the casting is cemented makes it an obvious advantage.

The ability to make multiple models from one impression is another advantage of the synthetic rubbers. It is possible to pour the impression twice and obtain the working dies and the master model (Fig. 17-12). The working die is used for final refinements in the wax patterns before investing, so the first impression made is used for the dies. Upon separation of the dies, which entails pouring only the part of the impression where the prepared teeth are located, the working models can be poured. The loss in accuracy from the first to second model is equal to what would have occurred if the impression were left standing in the storage environment.[17] The rubber material is rough and does not tear; since only one impression of the prepared teeth should be made, this durability is a great asset.

The toughness of the rubber materials makes it possible to limit the extension on the proximal walls of some cavity preparations. The hydrocolloid materials will tear if bulk is not present in this location. Limitation of the outline form to minimize the display of gold in the bicuspids is therefore possible with the rubber material.

Reversible hydrocolloid

Hydrocolloid has been popular for 30 years and was used extensively before the development of rubber materials because it was the only elastic material that possessed the accuracy for making inlays with the completely indirect method.[20] The main ingredient of hydrocolloid is agar, a thermoplastic material.

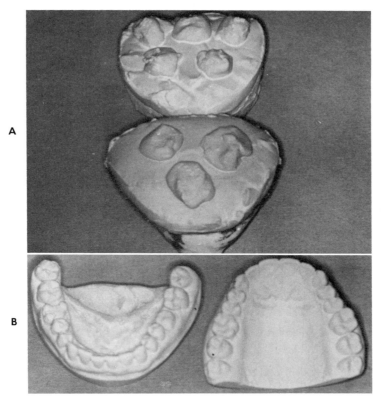

Fig. 17-12. A, Two models with nodules placed on the base to interlock with the mounting stone for the articulator. **B,** Two working models trimmed to the mucobuccal fold and suitable for articulator mounting.

The gel is reversible, which is caused by heating and cooling the material. The technique for taking the impression differs from that used for the rubber materials, and many details must be accurately followed. A syringe and tray material are used in stock impression trays that are cooled by the circulation of water while they are seated over the teeth. The sharp detail of the stone die is similar to that obtained with the rubber materials. There are a number of reasons for selecting reversible hydrocolloid.

The factors influencing the accuracy of reversible hydrocolloid are as follows[21]:

1. The greater the bulk of material present between the tray and the tooth, the better the accuracy of the model. For this reason bulky stock trays are used for taking the impression; the opposite is true of the synthetic rubber materials.

2. Slow, regular cooling of the impression will enhance accuracy. Tap water at 70° F. is used for the entire cooling for the best results and com-

fort to the patient. If cold water is circulated through the tray, stress develops and distorts the gel. The stress is relieved when the impression is removed, resulting in an inaccurate model.

3. Movement of the tray in the mouth, as with the other materials, is to be avoided because of the viscosity of the hydrocolloid. Any movement during gelation ruins the impression procedure. Stability is aided by modeling compound stops in the corners of the tray.

4. The impression must be poured immediately upon removal of the tray from the mouth. The dimensional change that results if the impression is allowed to stand 15 minutes is sufficient to produce an inaccurate model. This includes the time during which the impression is placed in 2% potassium sulfate to harden the stone.

The equipment required for reversible hydrocolloid is costly, but the initial cost is soon equalized because this impression material is less expensive than synthetic rubber. An advantage of using the reversible hydrocolloid technique is that manipulation is less difficult because the unit conditions the material for taking the impression.

Reversible hydrocolloid comes in tubes for use in the impression tray and in small cylinders for the syringes. The materials in the two tubes are identical but are different colors and packed to fit the specific need. Union of the two materials must occur in the impression or else distortion may occur. The injection procedure, like that for synthetic rubber, decreases the chance of air entrapment in the impression. The presence of air in the impression will result in failure to reproduce cavity detail.

The three water compartments on the unit are used for boiling, storing, and tempering the reversible hydrocolloid. The tubes and the loaded syringes must be boiled for at least 15 minutes. The water must cover the tops of the tubes so that the enclosed material will change from a gel into a sol. Inadequate boiling produces a granular mass, which if used in the impression, will result in stress and distortion. It is more convenient to boil the hydrocolloid at the beginning of the day in order not to interfere with the patient schedule. The boiling should be periodically observed to make certain that the water covers the tubes at all times.

The storage bath is in the center of the unit and the water is kept at 140° F. The bath is large enough to store a number of tubes and syringes until they are needed for the impression. The temperature of the water must be warm enough to maintain the sol condition. Problems can occur from prolonged storage. If the material is stored throughout an entire day, distortion may be caused by partial gelling. Many dentists prefer to boil the hydrocolloid for each half-day period.

The tempering bath is used to reduce the temperature of the tray material before it is placed in the mouth. The length of the tempering varies according to the temperature of the bath. If the tempering bath is 105° to 115° F., the filled tray is left from 5 to 15 minutes. The tubes are taken from the storage bath to fill the tray, which is placed in the water prior to removal of the gingival strings. When the tray is taken from the tempering bath, the water-soaked surface layer is removed with a spatula to obtain good union of the injected material on the teeth. Tempering is critical for patient comfort and for producing a satisfactory consistency of the tray material. At this time gelation has usually been initiated, giving the reversible hydrocolloid body.

Many stock impression trays come with the unit; others can be purchased in specific sizes as they are needed. The large trays have a rim lock to allow bulk and dislodgment of the material. A small tube encircles the border and body of the tray for circulating water to cool the impression in the mouth. A small rubber tube is connected to the tray and attached to the water outlet or cuspidor for circulation. Because the temperature changes required to transform the sol to a gel can be uncomfortable to the patient, it is advisable to anesthetize the prepared teeth.

The large trays are movable and unstable in the mouth. To prevent movement during the impression procedure, compound stops are placed in the posterior borders and another stop is placed over the anterior teeth. The compound is warmed and placed in the tray at the time of tray selection. The high-fusing black compound is used to prevent softening in the tempering bath. The impression is then placed into the stops. The tray is again stabilized with the thumbs and index fingers. The dental assistant slowly turns on the water and cooling is continued for a minimum of 5 minutes. The hydrocolloid technique requires two workers for passing and handling the impression material and the component parts.

The patient and tray are stabilized all during the cooling period. The gelation is tested with a blunt instrument and the tray is then removed with a snap in a line parallel to the long axis of the prepared teeth to minimize distortion and tearing of the material.

The syringes used for this technique are available with each type of unit. Like anesthetic syringes, they vary in design to facilitate grasping the instrument and injecting the material. The inside bore of the barrel is approximately the same so as not to limit the type of syringe material employed. The needles range in size from 10 to 14 gauge, which is large enough to allow passage of the material. Rubber bands are used to hold down the plunger after the syringes are loaded and placed into the boiling bath. The syringes remain in the storage bath until they are used for injection of the material. The syringes are coated with rubber to prevent tissue burns and should be wrapped in a towel to prevent irritation to the patient's lip during injection.

The storage media for hydrocolloid has beeen studied; the best environment is an atmosphere of 100% humidity. Hydrocolloid is best controlled with this medium because it tends to gain or lose water readily, which is referred to as imbibition and syneresis. If the impression is stored for periods longer than

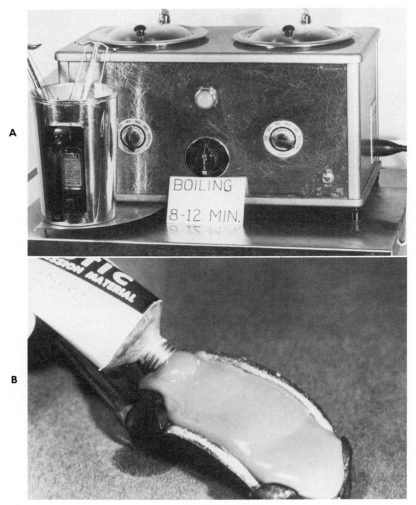

Fig. 17-13. A, Reversible hydrocolloid unit. The syringes are in the boiling compartment. The storage and tempering baths are on top of the unit. **B,** Tray material being loaded into the stock tray manufactured for water circulation and cooling. Upon removal from the tempering bath the water-soaked layer is removed from the surface of the material. (Courtesy Dr. Fredrick Hohlt.)

15 minutes, distortion is inevitable. It is preferable to pour the impression before the temporary restorations are inserted.

To obtain a superior stone surface on the model the reversible hydrocolloid is placed in a 2% solution of potassium sulfate. This solution penetrates the surface of the impression and acts as an accelerator for hardening the hydrocolloid. The impression is left in the potassium sulfate for only 5 minutes because only the surface needs to be coated. The poured impression should not

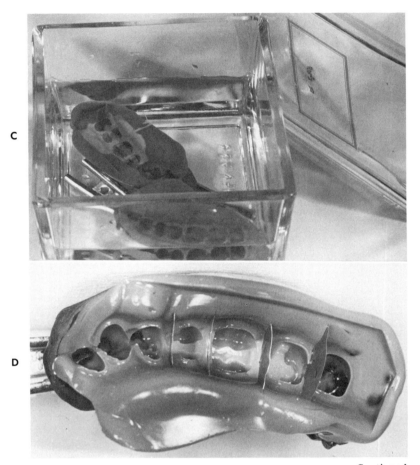

C

D

Continued.

Fig. 17-13, cont'd. C, The impressions are placed in 2% potassium sulfate to accelerate the setting of the poured Hydrocal and produce an exacting model. **D,** Metal inserts are sometimes placed in the impression to assist in making the dies. Note the light-colored syringe material in the copied teeth. (Courtesy Dr. Fredrick Hohlt.)

be separated for 1 hour in order to allow adequate hardening of the stone. The model will have a smooth surface and sharp details if the correct technique has been used.

The procedure for using reversible hydrocolloid is as follows (Fig. 17-13):

1. The syringe and tray material are boiled a minimum of 15 minutes. The tray material is in tubes; the loaded syringes must be kept covered with boiling water the entire time.
2. The two materials are placed in the storage bath for 1 hour prior to taking the impression.
3. The gingival tissue is retracted in the conventional manner, the impression tray selected, and the compound stops placed in the tray for stability.

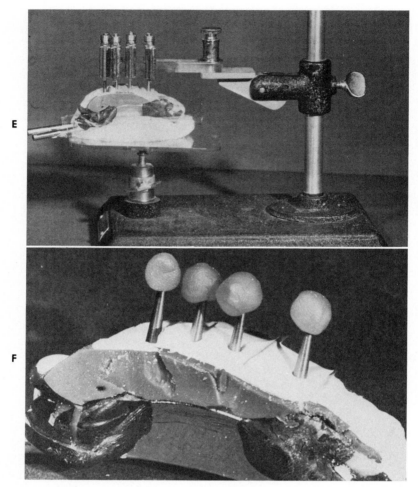

Fig. 17-13, cont'd. E, A paralleling device for placing dowel pins that serve as handles and holders for the dies. **F,** Dowel pins are inserted and tipped with wax prior to pouring the model base. The dies can then be removed on the articulated model.

4. The tray is loaded and placed in the tempering bath for 5 to 15 minutes.
5. The syringe material is injected after the gingival strings are removed and the preparations are dried.
6. The filled tray is taken from the tempering bath, the water-soaked layer of material removed, and the tray seated.
7. The water is circulated through the tray for a minimum of 5 minutes to produce the gel.
8. The tray is removed from the mouth with a snap parallel to the long axis of the teeth.
9. The impression is placed in 2% potassium sulfate for 5 minutes and the

models made in the conventional manner. The hydrocolloid impression must be poured within 15 minutes from the time it is removed from the teeth.

Reversible hydrocolloid produces an accurate model with good surface detail. The main advantage is the ease of preparing the material with the conditioning unit. The procedure is cleaner than that for the synthetic rubbers and the hydrocolloid has a pleasing odor and appearance. The dental assistant must be trained to share the responsibility of the technique. Because the conditioning unit is usually not located in the operatory, the assistant can bring the syringe and tray to the operatory at the time they are needed. The assistant can aid in numerous ways to make the impression procedure less difficult for both the dentist and the patient.

The reversible hydrocolloid impression can be poured only one time; therefore, a number of removable dies have been designed to facilitate the procedure. The impressions are poured into keying devices or dowel pins are used for the removable dies.[22] This makes it possible to articulate the model and manipulate the individual die in the hand because it can be separated from the model. The removable dies are less trouble than taking two impressions, which is thought to impair the material.

Reversible hydrocolloid is acceptable for the indirect method of making inlays. Accuracy is the primary factor in selecting an impression material, but there are secondary factors that may require employing different methods for the completely indirect technique.

Model fabrication and articulator procedure

The finished models that are placed on the articulator will closely reproduce the location and movement of the prepared teeth. The gold casting must not only be made to fit the tooth but it must also function properly in the range of mandibular movements. The more thorough the use of the articulator, the better the function of the castings. For the individual casting or the quadrant restoration the use of full-arch models, facebow transfer, interocclusal wax bites, and a set articulator is strongly advocated. Setting the articulator can be done quickly in the office or it can be delegated to a laboratory technician. The procedure for making the casting should not be selected for convenience to the operator but rather for the quality of the service.

The teeth in the opposite arch are reproduced with irreversible hydrocolloid, or alginate impression material, in the same way the diagnostic casts were produced. The tray is selected that best fits the mucobuccal fold and the lower lingual flanges. The trays are tried for fit before taking the opposing impressions. The difference in setting time of the alginate is explained to the patient.

The alginate material is mixed according to the manufacturer's directions to develop a thick, smooth consistency. Using the recommended water and powder ratio, the water at 70° F., ensures proper consistency and setting time. The material is mixed with the spatula against the side of the bowl for 1 minute to reduce air entrapment and is then loaded into the tray in small increments. The last portion of alginate in the bowl is picked up with the index finger, the teeth are dried, and the material is wiped into all the occlusal surfaces. The tray is seated and held in position for 2 minutes after the first sign of gelation. To control dimensional change, only distilled water is used to mix alginate material.

The alginate impression is removed with a snap in a direction parallel to the long axis of the teeth. The opposing impression is also poured with the same Hydrocal to develop a hard and accurate model. The base is formed and trimmed the same as the master model for uniformity and neatness.

Model fabrication

Hydrocal, a dental stone, is used to make all the dies and models in the procedure because the material is more accurate. These stones are harder, have less setting expansion, have lower water-powder ratios, and are usually quicker setting.[23] The hardness and low dimensional change are the reasons for selecting the material. The dental stones expand only 0.6% to 0.25% upon setting, and they are usually colored to facilitate better examination of the margins and detail on the die surface. Many kinds of dental stone are available and they should be selected to produce the desired color and hardness of the finished model.

The stone is mixed with a vacuum unit according to the recommended water-powder ratio. The setting expansion is thus regulated and less air is incorporated in the mix, minimizing voids in the model surface. A thick, creamy consistency is developed and the 4-minute working time allows adequate time to pour and base the impression. Stardardization of the mix results by using accurate ratios, and manipulation and pouring will be improved by being able to predict the consistency. This procedure can be performed by the assistant if meticulous detail is used to make the models. Failure to produce an acceptable model necessitates another impression or an additional pour, which produces a more distorted model.

The working dies are poured first because they require the greatest degree of accuracy. When synthetic rubber is used, the material is poured to the height of the tray border and allowed to set. This thickness is necessary to develop the die handle for holding the object during waxing. When reversible hydrocolloid is used, the whole impression is poured and the dowel pins or keying devices are inserted in the base. Nearly perfect copies of the preparation are made by avoiding the entrapment of air and producing a dense mix of stone.

A small mix of stone is used for making the dies. It may also be necessary to pour the opposing impression at this time. The stone is picked up in small increments with a cement spatula and vibrated into the corner of the mold. The bottom of the individual tooth mold is covered and then completely filled before the adjacent tooth mold is filled.

The impression tray is held on the vibrator with the same angulation and the stone is added in the same place. If the preparation is extremely small, the stone can be initially placed with a small sable brush or wax spatula. The dry, clean rubber base impression has a high surface tension that complicates pouring the occlusal surfaces and small crevices. The use of small increments and vibration helps to prevent discrepancies. The die pour is allowed to set for 1 hour before it is separated from the impression. This amount of time is necessary to develop hardness and prevent breakage upon removal. The impression can be placed on the laboratory bench during the setting period because the synthetic rubber does not require a special storage media.

The master model is poured after the dies are separated. If small pieces of stone or debris are present in the rubber mold, it should be cleaned with water and dried before the material is poured. An adequate amount of stone is mixed for the teeth and base of the model. The material should be weighed or may be obtained in packaged form to reduce waste. Only a 1 inch thickness of stone is placed on top of the border because additional space will be needed for the mounting stone for the articulator. A few small nodules are placed on the base of the models to lock them to the mounting stone.

The impression is slowly filled with dental stone in the manner previously described. The stone is added at one posterior border of the impression and the flow is continued until the impression is filled to the border. Again small increments, steady vibration, and one angulation of the tray are used. For the lower models a wet towel or wax is placed in the sublingual space to prevent blocking out the lingual surfaces of the lower teeth. This helps to base the lower model by holding back the mixed stone. The initial set gives the residual material in the bowl stiffness, which assists in putting the base on the model. The same thickness of 1 inch and three nodules are placed for the upper and lower cast. The bulk will prevent breakage and assist locking the model to the mounting ring on the articulator.

The models are allowed to set for 1 hour before separation. Then the stone is removed gradually to avoid breaking the teeth. The models are shaped on the model trimmer back to the depth of the mucobuccal fold, where all impressions and models end and where the trimming is stopped. The mold base is slightly beveled to reduce the diameter of the mounting stone in order to better observe the teeth on the model. The base of the model is slightly flattened and smoothed for the articulator mounting.

Die trimming. The original dies are used for the final waxing, at which time the adaptation and perfection at the margins are attained (Fig. 17-14). The die is also used for polishing the casting, making it necessary to trim and shape each die to specification. The cervical margins of the die are trimmed to uncover the finish line that produces access for waxing and polishing. A handle is then formed at the base of preparation to hold the die during the manipulation of the wax pattern.

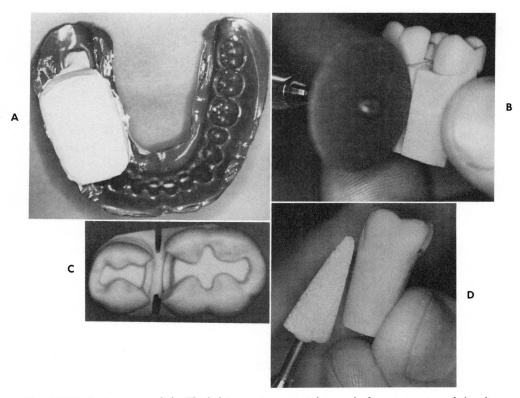

Fig. 17-14. A, First pour of the Thiokol impression material is made for construction of the dies. **B,** The dies are sectioned with a separating disk. **C,** View showing the extent of the disk cutting to separate the dies. The plaster knife is used to split the model apart. **D,** Acrylic stone is employed to make the long, tapered handle for the die.

Prior to trimming the poured dies the stone surface is saturated with die lubricant to prevent dissolving and coating of the die with the water in the trimmer. A model is then shaped on the trimmer to block out the dies into a tapered model in anticipation of the handle. A separating disk or ribbon saw is used to separate each die through the interproximal surface. When they are single units, the beveled margins are uncovered by cutting away the excess stone with a sharp scapel or binangle chisel. Any small bubbles present in the corners are removed at this time.

The handle of the die is formed by tapering the stone to make the widest portion the cervical dimension of the tooth below the finish line. The handle should be at least 1 inch long in order to firmly grasp the die. Reduction of the die handle is done with an arbor band on the lathe and then finished with a large acrylic stone in the handpiece. This produces the smooth finish and taper necessary for the die handle. An air coolant or dust evacuator is helpful while making the handle in order to reduce laboratory contamination.

The completed die should be washed and cleaned with a sable brush and die lubricant. The die is placed in cotton for protection until the wax is added for the pattern.

Recommendations for controlling the accuracy and surface detail of models include the following:

1. The stone and alginate are mixed only with distilled water. Tap water additives produce significant dimensional change.
2. The proper water-powder ratio is employed. This is accomplished only by weighing the stone to the gram and dispensing the water with a pipette.
3. Vacuum mixing is used for all gypsum products that will be used for models.
4. Slurry water is used for wetting the cast prior to trimming to prevent etching the model with the tap water used as a trimming lubricant. Slurry water is made by storing old models in distilled water for 48 hours. Slurry water is used also to mix with the stone for mounting the models on the articulator. A quick set and low dimensional change results.

Articulator procedure

The selection of an articulator depends upon the difficulty of the adjustments and the measurements that can be transferred from the patient to the device. A fully adjustable instrument, used for gnathologic procedures, can reproduce the complete range of mandibular movements of the patient. Cemented aluminum clutches are placed on the upper and lower teeth, the hinge axis is located, and the movements of the jaw are pantographed. The main advantage of this articulator is that the Bennett movement, or "side shift," of the mandible can be traced and reproduced on the articulator. The instrument is then set to a curved path, which is the actual contour of the temporomandibular joint.

The regular construction of castings does not require an articulator with this degree of sophistication. A semiadjustable articulator that copies the border movements is most often used.[24] The facebow transfer and the records produce order in the procedure and provide an adequate number of movements so that only a few chairside adjustments need to be made. The hinge axis closure for relating the casts is not often necessary and the castings are built where maximum interdigitation is experienced by the patient.

Many articulators can be used to furnish the guiding factors of condylar inclination and lateral limit of the side shift. These are the guiding factors of the glenoid fossa and, together with the incisal guidance of the anterior teeth, are used to determine the occlusal relationship of the casting. These measurements are set on the articulator with interocclusal records. In Fig. 17-15 the procedure is illustrated using the Quick Mount Whip Mix articulator. The guiding factors are on the upper member, making it an "arcon" articulator. The design facilitates using the interocclusal records.

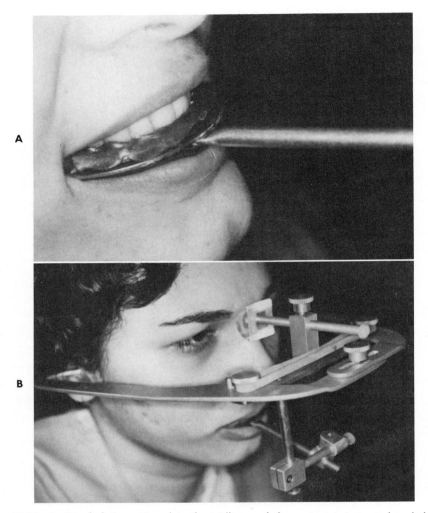

Fig. 17-15. A, Bite fork is positioned in the midline and the patient is instructed to hold it securely. **B,** The facebow and nasion guide are attached to the bite fork for the purpose of mounting the upper model. The facebow is also seated in the external auditory meatus.

Facebow transfer. The facebow transfer is taken to transfer the opening and closing axis of the patient to the articulator. A third reference point is used, which is the infraorbital foramen or nasion. Gnathologists use a tattoo mark 2¼ inches from the incisal edge of the cuspid. This standardizes the vertical height of the upper cast to the upper member of the articulator.

The facebow transfer permits additional models to be mounted to the articulator without changing any of the settings or taking any eccentric interocclusal records.[25] The upper cast is held in position by the bite fork to assist mounting

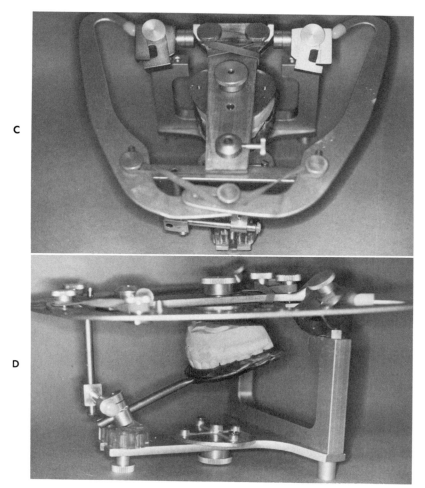

C

D

Continued.

Fig. 17-15, cont'd. C, The facebow and bite fork are attached to the articulator for mounting. **D,** The upper model is seated in the bite fork prior to the attachment of the cast to the upper member of the articulator.

the cast to the upper articulator member. The time required for the transfer is a matter of seconds and it gives the model mounting a starting point.

Bite registration. The relationship for closure of the jaws is recorded in wax by the indentations of the teeth. The difference in centric occlusion and centric relation has been previously discussed. The jaw relationship needed should be determined and the centric bite made at this place of contact. The patient is given a number of opportunities for closing in the selected position to lessen the chance of erroneous recordings.

The wax-bite wafer, which has been specifically designed, is placed over the maxillary teeth. The patient is instructed to close in the same position in the

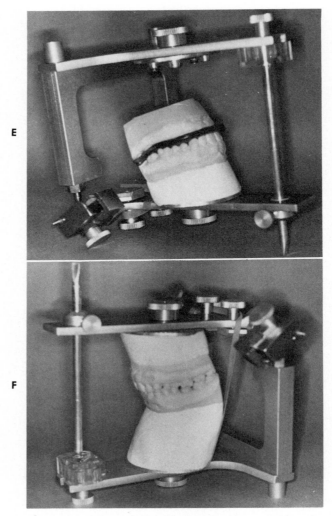

Fig. 17-15, cont'd. E, The articulator is inverted, the centric bite is placed, and the lower model is seated. The guide pin is opened 2 mm. and the lower model is attached to the articulator. **F,** Working casts are mounted for construction of gold castings.

warm or soft wax. Only the points of the cusp tips are recorded because full closure results in deflection of the mandible. As soon as the depressions are made in the satisfactory location, the mandible is opened and the wax is removed. If the accuracy is doubtful, the bite is reinserted and the biting relationship is retested and finalized with zinc oxide–eugenol paste.

The lateral border movements are then taken with right and left interocclusal records. The patient is instructed to close end to end on the cuspids on one side at a time. Only small indentations are made in the wax. A guide to relate the models in the same position on the articulator is all that is necessary.

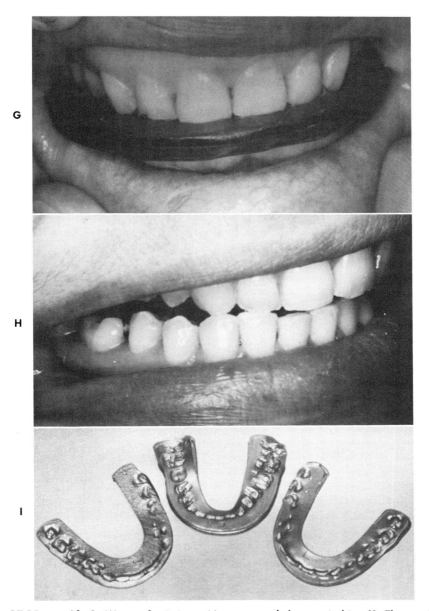

Fig. 17-15, cont'd. G, Wax wafer is in position to record the centric bite. **H,** The cuspids are end to end, which is the relationship for the right and left lateral checkbites for the interocclusal records. **I,** The centric bite (center) is used to mount the lower cast. The right and left lateral checkbites are used to set the articulator.

Two bites are obtained, one for the right and left sides, and are used to set the two guiding factors on the articulator. A protrusive bite is used for setting the condylar guidance and lateral wax bites for determining the Bennett movement with some articulators. In most procedures the protrusive reading is not used on the articulator and all the waxing is done to the resultant condylar guidance and Bennett shift measurement.

The procedure used to take records and adjust the articulator are listed (Fig. 17-15):

1. The facebow transfer is taken and the upper model is mounted. The vertical adjustments are arbitrarily set at 30 degrees and the Bennett adjustments are set at 10 degrees to prevent slipping of the upper member of the articulator during mounting.
2. The centric record is taken and the lower cast is related to the upper cast and mounted to the lower member of the articulator.
3. The right and left eccentric interocclusal records are taken.
4. The guiding factors on the articulator are adjusted. The right wax record is placed between the models and the left joint, which is the translating joint, is adjusted. The vertical and horizontal plates are loosened and turned until they contact the surface of the condylar ball.
5. The left record is placed between the models and the right joint of the articulator is adjusted and set in the same manner.
6. The models are moved to see if the articulator is working and all the parts are stable. The incisal guide plate can also be set to prevent wear of the anterior teeth on the models.
7. The readings on the articulator are recorded on a card and placed in the patient's record. The readings can also be used later, making it necessary to take only a facebow transfer and centric bite to set the articulator.

The articulator should be examined to see that all the fittings are secure. The movements are duplicated to determine whether proper clearance has been given to the preparations and the approximate locations of the functioning parts of the wax pattern. Many articulators will duplicate the movements that are taken with interocclusal records. The wax pattern produced will be more functional and less traumatic to justify using an articulator.

Other methods can be used to make the casting in which the articulation is sacrificed and fewer teeth are included. If used by the experienced operator, it is difficult to distinguish what method has been employed. The modifications might be useful with small inlays but not multiple procedures. If good articulation is absent when producing the wax pattern, more chairside adjustment must be made before cementation. The techniques are described for evaluation.

Articulated partial-arch models

This procedure is nearly as accurate as when an adjustable articulator is used. The articulators for partial-arch models are usually not adjustable and can be employed only for opening and closing the casts. Only the centric contacts can be accurately restored but with experience some small castings can be handled with this method.

The arch containing the cavity preparation is poured in a die "keying bar" so that it can be removed and sectioned. The removable die is used to make the wax pattern in the same manner as the reversible hydrocolloid. Many castings are made with this method, but because duplicate movements are not possible with the articulators, more chairside adjustments are necessary.

The indirect techniques favor the use of the full-arch articulated models. The student should first master this technique, which is not really involved once the advantages are realized, before attempting any variation of the fabrication technique. The possibilities for accuracy should be learned and observed while studying the movement of the mandible and its potential for function and trauma. More accuracy and function of the casting and a reduction in intraoral adjustments are the reasons for using accurately articulated full-arch models.

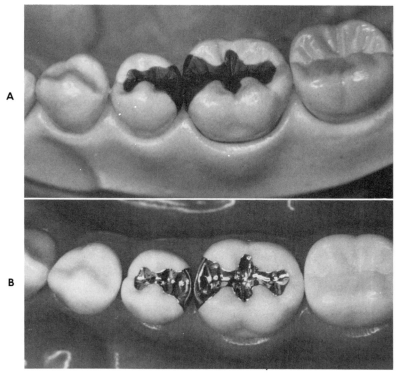

Fig. 17-16. A, Two wax patterns for intracoronal inlays. Margination and carving of the wax produce a well-fitting casting. **B,** Completed castings showing the recovery of the exacting relationships on the gold surfaces.

Fabrication of the wax pattern

The wax pattern is made on the articulated model and the die with the contour and precision needed in the casting (Fig. 17-16). The wax pattern is then invested, removed from the mold by high temperatures, and cast in the selected gold alloy. The wax carving is exacting in all aspects because the casting can be no better than the pattern that is invested.

Inlay wax is quite soft and pliable and melts at 120° F. The main ingredient is paraffin wax, which keeps the material soft and produces the flow.[26] The inlay wax is colored to simplify examination of the margins on the stone, and the pattern can be adjusted a number of ways to produce a desirable occlusion with the models. The pattern is delicate, and if not handled properly, distortion occurs when the wax is added to the die or while it is being invested, producing a poorly fitting inlay. Careful manipulation of the wax will prevent this.

Internal stress in the pattern is a potential hazard. The following methods help to control stress and produce an acceptable wax pattern.[27,28]

1. The wax should be adapted to the die with as high a dry heat as possible. Water baths will cause the wax constituents and fillers to be removed in the water heater, thereby changing the properties of the wax.
2. The wax should be tightly adapted and held under pressure in the die until it cools. Surface contraction that occurs with cooling is controlled by pressure from the fingers.
3. Patching and pooling of the wax should be avoided unless it is necessary when shaping the pattern. This is considered to cause stresses to accumulate in the pattern.

The wax should be of sufficient quality to allow development of a highly shined, smooth surface in addition to creating a clean mold for the casting. The residue in the mold is regulated by the A.D.A. Bureau of Standards specification of 0.1% residue at 500° C.

The waxes differ according to color, amount of shrinkage upon cooling, degree of hardness, and carving properties. Selection is based upon individual preference, the ease of manipulation, and production of the casting.

Regular pattern formation. The trimmed dies are lubricated several times to prevent the wax from sticking to the surface, and the excess liquid is removed with absorbent cotton. The melted inlay wax is carried to the working die, where the original and final adaption is accomplished. Cotton pliers are used to pick up the wax, and when the die is contacted, the molten wax is allowed to spread across the surface of the Hydrocal. The wax is then pressed with the thumb and index finger while it is cooling. The entire pattern is filled in this manner, making sure to cover all the margins.

The wax is carved to the desired margin and shape for the restoration (Fig. 17-17). The pattern is removed from the die and placed on the working model. The proximal contacts are carved first, then the buccolingual contour is established if the preparation has capped cusps. The cusp tips and fossae are made

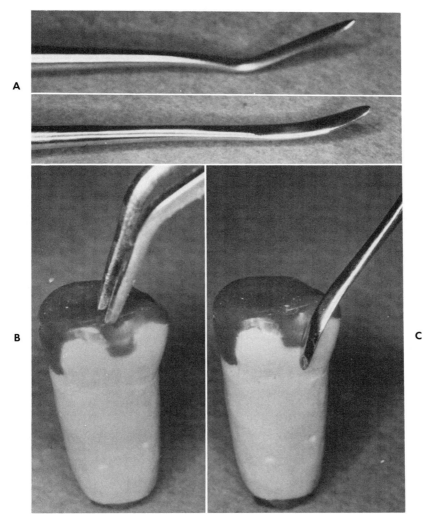

Fig. 17-17. A, Two Darby carvers that are useful in forming the wax pattern. **B,** Cotton pliers are used to add wax to the lubricated die. The wax is carried between the beaks of the pliers. **C,** The wax is carefully carved from the pattern toward the stone surface to avoid abrasion of the die.

to articulate with the teeth in the opposing arch. The working cusps, which are the buccal cusps of the lower teeth and the lingual cusps of the upper teeth, are made to contact opposing fossa or marginal ridges in centric occlusion.

The occlusal contacts should be determined in centric position. An even distribution of forces, with the cusps centered in the fossae, is considered to produce the best function. The articulator is then moved to make certain the cusps on the pattern do not interfere with the teeth in the eccentric movements of the mandible. All the function that is possible at this time is placed

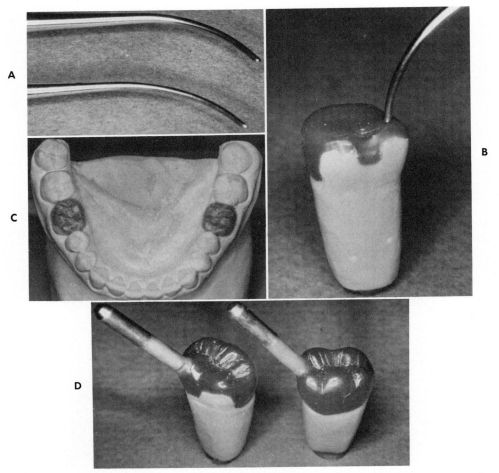

Fig. 17-18. A, Two P.K.T. waxing instruments that are used to aid the flow of the wax onto the pattern. **B,** Position of the P.K.T. instrument to form a cone for the cusp on the wax pattern. **C,** Zinc stearate powder on the articulated wax patterns shows the abrasion contacts. **D,** Attachment of the sprue pins to the wax patterns.

in the pattern by making good contacting surfaces. Occlusal contacts are observed by abraded areas on the wax; these can be deepened and reformed with the carving instruments if necessary.

The roughly carved pattern is transferred back to the individual die. At this point the pattern requires only marginal adaptation, smoothing, and additional wax on the proximal surfaces. The seated pattern is warmed and readapted around the margins with a blunt instrument. The necessary wax is added and final anatomic adjustments are made. The surface of the pattern is polished with a nylon cloth or cotton warmed with water to develop the final smooth surface.

Cone-waxing method. For multiple castings, especially in gnathologic procedures, a cone-waxing technique has been devised by Everitt Payne.[13] This technique is also useful in forming the individual wax pattern once the cone method is learned. Small cones of inlay wax are first placed on the prepared models to serve as cusps, which are useful when determining the occlusal pathways. The cone method has been modified to serve different concepts of articulation and has resulted in wide usage and the design of special instruments for applying the wax.

The special instruments designed by Peter K. Thomas are referred to as the P.K.T. set (Fig. 17-18). The set includes a group of four double-ended instruments that aid the flow of wax on the models and are also used to carve the wax. There are four working points for flowing, which is primarily the way the pattern is produced. The waxing is a "buildup" technique to gradually place the anatomic function in the pattern, which is contrary to the "carve down" method using a block of wax inside the preparation.

The initial application of wax is made on the working die by placing a thin layer on the inside of the preparation. When making a series of patterns, the thin shells are transferred to the articulated models. The small cones are first placed where the working cusps in the upper and lower arch are to be located. The nonworking cusp are then added, and the articulator movements are made to see that no collision occurs and that ample room is present to properly contour the pattern to function. When this is satisfactory, the buccal and lingual contours and the marginal and triangular ridges are waxed to add the components of the occlusal surface. The last portion of the anatomy to be placed is the fossa, at which time the tripoded centric contacts are placed in the wax (Fig. 17-19).

The contacts are analyzed by placing zinc stearate powder on the wax and moving the articulator through the routine patterns. The contacting areas are detected as burnished spots on the wax, and the areas are directly changed by moving the cusp and the fossa individually or together in opposing patterns to obtain ideal conditions. The zinc stearate is applied with a brush and is easily removed on the completed pattern. Small accumulations of the powder will not produce a rough surface on the casting because it is burned out with the inlay wax.

When all the anatomy and adjustments are completed on the patterns, they are transferred back to the dies. The margins are first readapted, then the contact areas are filled to develop the ideal interproximal relationship. The final smoothing and carving are done with the P.K.T. instruments, taking care not to change the occlusal morphology before the sprue pins are attached for investment procedures. Because there is more detail in the occlusal surface, it will probably not be possible to obtain the smoothness acquired with the regular wax pattern.

The cone-waxing method has been altered for different occlusal concepts. The cones can be placed to develop a cusp ridge or cusp fossa relationship

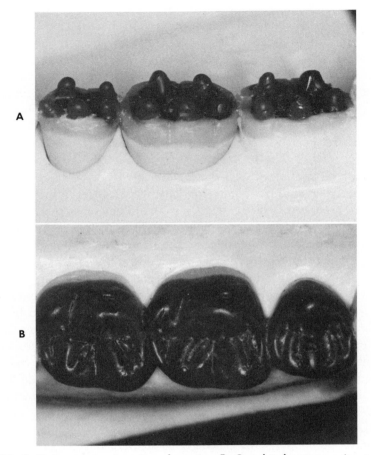

Fig. 17-19. A, Cone wax step in pattern formation. **B,** Completed patterns using a cone waxing method.

when two arches of patterns are being made. The cusp ridge is commonly developed when a few patterns are being made, as compared to the fossa relationship for the full-arch pattern. The cusp ridge is considered to be a 1:2 tooth relationship, which allows more tooth movement than the 1:1 relationship of the cusp fossa waxing. Regardless of the method, the cones are always added first, and then variations are made in the degree for which the other components of the occlusal anatomy are added.

The cone method is helpful for the multiple procedure and is particularly useful in teaching the relationship that must exist for the individual pattern. The knowledge gained from the cone method is beneficial for forming the individual pattern. The requirements for the wax pattern are the same, regardless of the method used for fabrication. The working parts, smooth surface, and exacting margin must be present on the pattern. The casting can be no better

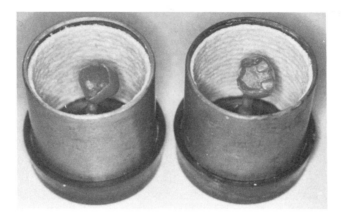

Fig. 17-20. Relationship of the wax patterns, sprue former, and inlay rings. The asbestos liner is ⅛ inch from the end of the ring and the wax patterns are ¼ inch from the end of the investment ring.

than the wax pattern that is invested, which becomes the mold for the gold alloy.

Investing

The wax pattern is surrounded by an investment that hardens and forms the mold in which the casting is made (Fig. 17-20). The investing procedure is directed to preserve the detail of the pattern and to avoid distortion of the wax while it is being invested. The investment is selected on the basis of available expansion to accommodate for the shrinkage that occurs when the gold alloy solidifies.[29] There are several techniques and materials available for investing. The description of one workable system for the student and the more experienced operator is given; however, other methods may be used to produce acceptable results. It is not possible to discuss all the investment procedures in detail here, but a text on dental materials can be consulted to evaluate all the investment compensating techniques. An investment should be selected to provide the necessary expansion, casting density, and surface detail for the restoration.

Spruing. A pin is attached to the wax pattern to provide the sprue way for the molten gold during the casting.[30] The sprue pin holds the wax pattern on the sprue base and regulates its position in the inlay ring. The pin should be made of a metal that will not rust, or it may be made of plastic to prevent the possibility of mold roughness and contamination. In order to admit the gold into the mold the sprue should not be smaller than 12 gauge. If a smaller sprue is used, the gold first freezes in this area, causing shrinkage porosity in the casting. Only in small thin patterns such as the lingual pin-retained inlay or pinledge can a smaller sprue pin be used to prevent distortion of this type of

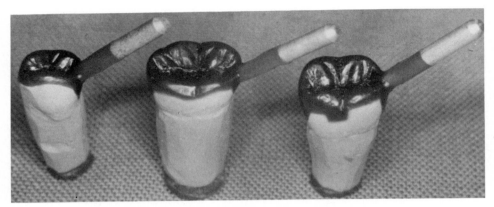

Fig. 17-21. Sprue pin attachments for the patterns in a quadrant restoration.

wax pattern. The 12 gauge sprue is large enough to eliminate the use of wax reservoirs to combat shrinkage porosity.

The sprue pin should be attached in the heaviest part of the pattern so that it will not interfere with the functioning cusps or fossa (Fig. 17-21). The pin is placed at an angle to the surface and is pointed toward the thinnest areas of the wax pattern. When the sprue pin is attached, caution must be exercised not to overheat the pattern because contraction will occur in the carving when it cools. A small bead of wax can be added to the surface to lessen the possibility of damage while attaching the pin.

The pin is heated in a flame and attached to the pattern while it is on the die. When the surface has melted, both objects are stabilized until the surface has cooled. The pin is then secured with additional wax to form a right-angle joint where it meets the surface. When the second application of wax has cooled, the pin is used to pull the pattern off the die and place it in the sprue base. The pin is attached to the base with extra wax to form a curved relationship so that no sharp corners will fracture and be carried into the mold by the force of the gold.

Ideal locations to attach the sprue pin are the marginal ridges of posterior teeth or incisal corners of anterior teeth. The buccal and lingual surfaces next to the cusp tips are used in large restorations. It is seldom necessary to use an accessory or double sprue in small castings. In full-coverage preparations with veneers an accessory sprue can be attached to the thin area to prevent early solidification in this area, but this is seldom necessary with inlays.

Selection of investment. The investments are selected according to the amount of expansion needed in the mold. The casting should exhibit a snug fit under finger pressure, as previously described, and the expansion should vary according to the length and angulation of the cavity walls. The long cavity wall that is nearly parallel requires more expansion than the tapered preparation.

The greater the number of walls and the larger the restoration, the more expansion will probably be needed in the investment.

The shrinkage of gold has been studied in relation to the size and type of casting.[31,32] The accepted shrinkage is 1.25%, and the mold expansion is regulated above or below this amount. The precisioned preparation that is nearly parallel is more difficult to fit with the casting, but this should not discourage proper cavity design.

Casting investments are made of a refractory silica material and a gypsum binder. There are a number of additives for controlling the setting time and surface of the mold to develop a smooth, sharp casting. The investment is mixed using a precise water-powder ratio, which is instrumental in regulating the setting expansion and hardness of the material.

The investment is expanded in a number of ways. All the materials have a regular setting expansion of 0.3%, which is helpful in producing a larger mold. If the fresh mix is placed in contact with water during setting, a hygroscopic expansion can be produced that has been measured at two to three times the setting expansion. If the investments are heated, a thermal expansion of 0.8% to 1.4% can be produced at certain temperatures, depending on the composition of the material. These expansion methods have produced a large selection of investments. The problem is to select an investment that produces enough expansion.

The silica component of the investment produces the expansion. Silica is available in many forms, with quartz, tridomite, and cristobalite being used in the dental investments. The quartz will expand 0.8%, and the cristobalite can attain a 1.4% expansion. One technique utilizes a combination of two materials called cristobalite and control powder to produce mixes of varying expansion.[33] Dimension is produced by thermal expansion of the mold when the investment is heated to a temperature of 1,200° F. before making the casting.

The vacuum investing method eliminates many of the variables and reduces the number of casting failures. A constant water-powder ratio produces the dense surface for the sharp casting and minimizes the entrapment of air bubbles on the surface of the wax pattern. Wetting solutions reduce surface tension on the wax but are not required for making a smooth casting when vacuum mixing is used. Only distilled water is used with investments to control the dimensional change.

In hygroscopic expansion, compensating techniques that place water in contact with the investment to cause mold expansion are used.[34] The casting rings are immersed in a controlled temperature water bath or the water is added in a rubber container on the top of the ring. Following the timed setting reaction the sprue pin is removed and thermal techniques are used for casting the gold at reduced temperatures. Some compounds have varied expansion by changing the water-powder ratio; these compounds are reported to be acceptable.

The casting ring and the asbestos liner are other variables in the dimensional change that occurs inside the mold. The ends of the ring permit more expansion to occur than the limited sides. The asbestos liner is used to allow the investment to expand in the ring. The soft liner provides room for thermal expansion in the ring in addition to enhancing hygroscopic expansion where the liner touches the investment. The degree of change can be increased by using more than one liner, but this is not necessary with the proper selection of other expansion methods. There will always be a need to evaluate investments because of the changes that occur with the materials producing expansion.

Divestment procedures. Divestment is a commercially available material* that functions both as a die and as an investing material. Using material of this type, it is possible to develop a wax pattern and to leave it on its die for purpose of investing. Many patterns receive some damage or distortion, no matter how slight, in the process of investing.

Divestment is a refractory material, that involves a powder and a special liquid containing a concentrated colloidal suspension of silica. There has been work done to establish that the material has a good capacity for clinical reliability.[35] Reliable clinical results are obtained when using 14 to 16 ml. of liquid for 50 grams of powder.

The setting time and consistency will vary, depending on the powder-liquid ratio, the rate, and the time for spatulation. The time needed to achieve the hardness required for laboratory activity with a model will vary from 30 to 90 minutes. The hardness values are less than that for improved stone but effective if the powder-liquid ratio used produces a heavy mixture.

For making impressions polysulfide or silicone rubber is most conveniently and most effectively used with Divestment. Hydrocolloid also may be used for impression, but special instructions, which are supplied by the manufacturers, are essential.

The impression tray must be rigid and is made from tray-forming acrylic. There must be adequate clearance between the teeth and the tray to prevent breaking the model upon separation and to allow the setting expansion of the model material. Divestment possesses a high setting expansion and low thermal expansion, which is the reverse of most materials used for this purpose.

For consistency, the material should be mixed under vacuum with a slow-speed mixer. The material does not flow as easily as a water base material, so special care must be observed when pouring the models. A suggestion is to use a camel's hairbrush or a blunt instrument to be sure all the details of the preparation are secured, thus avoiding the formation of bubbles. It is best to allow at least 45 minutes before separating the model from the impression. A special precaution should be observed with a polysulfide rubber impression, in that prolonged contact with Divestment will cause an adherence that makes it difficult to separate the model. To avoid this problem, polysulfide impressions

---

*Whip-Mix Corporation, Louisville, Kentucky.

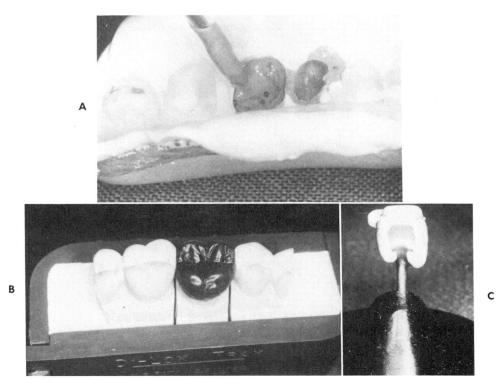

Fig. 17-22. **A,** Silicone impression being filled with Divestment by aid of a brush. **B,** Routine wax-up of a Divestment die. **C,** Divestment die and wax pattern mounted on a sprue former. (From Lund, M. R., and Shryock, E. F.: J. Prosth. Dent. **18:**253, 1967.)

should be separated within 3 hours. Silicone materials do not have this problem. To prevent the problem of adherence, the surface of the impression may be sprayed with a releasing agent that will allow easy release if the model is in contact beyond 3 hours. An aerosol dry lubriant spray by DuPont, "Slip-Spray," or similar materials available at a hardware store will relieve this problem.

The die is prepared in the same manner as for die stone. If a saw blade is used, it becomes dull much quicker because of the high silica content. After the die is separated and trimmed with a small brush, it is covered with one or two thin coats of "Whip-Mix Separator No. 2" to within 0.5 mm. of the margins. This material is a suspension of mica and functions as a shim between the casting and the model. It will produce the same effect as would acid etching or electrical stripping.

During waxing, the essential precaution is to prevent the wax from extending beyond the margins; for even though this wax is carved back, it will invite a thin flash of metal upon casting (Fig. 17-22). Since the die and the pattern are sprued as a unit, the only concern is to secure proper support with the sprue attachment.

It is not required to line the casting ring with asbestos, but instead, a generous film of Vaseline is used to coat the internal aspect of the ring. A mixture of 16 ml. of liquid to 50 grams of Divestment powder is used to invest the pattern, and it is allowed to set 30 to 45 minutes before burnout.

Divestment should be burned out at 1,250° F. for 1 hour and, following the casting, bench cooled. Then the mass is removed from the ring, which should not be difficult unless the ring is deformed. The casting is recovered in a conventional manner.

This technique is particularly advantageous for fabrication of castings involving miniature parallel pins. A popular pinlay technique embodies the use of nylon bristles as part of the total wax pattern. Technical problems and easy distortion occur if this type of a pattern is removed from a die. The use of Divestment significantly simplifies the procedures required to produce casting with multiple pins.

Investment procedure. A thermal expansion investment is advocated because research and clinical observations support the effectiveness of this method.

1. The 12 gauge sprue pin is attached to the wax pattern and waxed to a right-angle joint. The pattern is removed with the pin and inverted in the sprue base so that it is ¼ inch from the end of the ring.
2. One layer of asbestos is placed on the inside of the ring ⅛ inch short of the ends. This allows room for the thermal expansion liner. The unlined portion of the ring keeps the investment from falling during the casting process.
3. The ring is placed over the top of the sprue base and sealed to develop a vacuum and stabilize the ring.
4. The investment is weighed on a commercial scale and mixed in the bowl. The water is measured with a graduate cylinder and placed on top of the powder. The mixture is hand mixed momentarily to develop consistency.
5. There are several acceptable types of vacuum units. The unit is turned on to check the effectiveness of the air tube and the ladle is attached to the bowl. The vacuum is developed by placing the tube in the opening and the powder mix is made to develop an ideal investing consistency. The drive shaft of the ladle is disengaged and the bowl is inverted to slowly vibrate the mix into the ring.
6. After the vacuum is broken the filled ring is removed and placed on the laboratory shelf for 1 hour before the heating procedure is started.

The vacuum investing procedure can be done with less strain because bubbles or surface irregularities rarely occur on the pattern. A reliable estimate of the fit of the casting is possible when the behavior of the investment material is known (Fig. 17-23).

The pattern can be invested by hand when vacuum apparatus is not available. The pattern is sprued in the conventional manner and attached to the

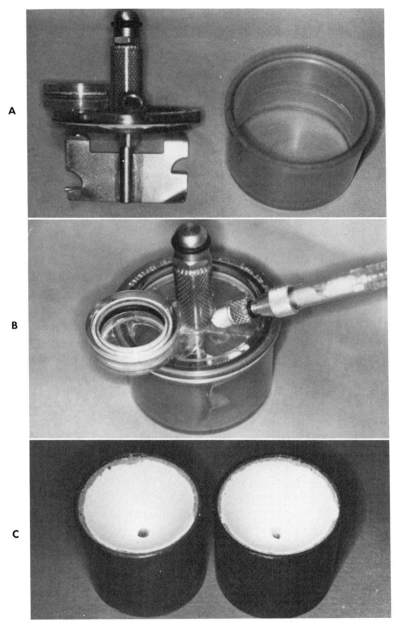

Fig. 17-23. A, Ladle and mixing bowl used to invest the wax pattern. **B,** Assembled mixing bowl with the vacuum tube attached. The open circle is for the casting ring and wax pattern. The power for mixing is applied to the rubber washer and post that turns the ladle. **C,** The investment mold after setting and with the sprue pins removed. The patterns are prepared for the burnout procedure. (**A** courtesy Whip Mix Corp., Louisville, Ky.)

sprue base. A small amount of wetting agent is painted on the pattern to reduce surface tension. The same investment is used but 1 ml. more water is added than in vacuum investing to enhance painting of the pattern. A small sable brush is used to paint the pattern until it is completely covered with the investment. The remainder of the investment is vibrated into the ring into which the sprue base and painted pattern are inverted. The investment is allowed to set for the prescribed time. The disadvantages of the hand method are that the surface is rougher and the investment mold is weaker.

The casting ring is prepared for the burnout procedure a minimum of 1 hour after investing. The sprue base is removed and the rim of material next to the ring is trimmed to eliminate small fragments that might break and fall into the mold. The sprue pin is then heated and gently removed in order not to break the sides of the sprue way. The opening is inspected and the rings are wiped clean with a damp towel and stored until casting.

Casting procedures. The casting procedure includes the burnout for wax elimination, expansion of the investment, and placement of the gold into the mold. Improper management of the gold or the investment material in this phase of fabrication can produce insufficient castings. The casting is made when the gold freezes in the mold and is removed to be cleaned for the polishing.

Gold selection is not a problem because only types I and II can be used to make individual castings.[26] These golds are classified by the Bureau of Standards as soft and medium alloys, and both are sufficient for the individual casting. Type I, with a Brinell hardness number of 40 to 75, is indicated for small castings with limited stress. Type II, with a Brinell hardness number of 70 to 100, is indicated for the complex restoration and cusp capping. Type II is the most commonly used gold in operative dentistry.

These alloys have melting ranges of 1,700° to 1,920° F. and are ductile. The percentage elongations are 20% to 30%, meaning that the gold can be manipulated to place the beveled casting margin next to the tooth structure. Because most of the casting alloy is gold, the restoration will resist tarnish and corrosion. The two types of gold have different melting and finishing characteristics and colors. The soft type I gold is easier to work and polish.

The inlay rings for the thermal expansion investments are heated slowly to 1,200° F. in preparation for the casting. The oven should have a pyrometer to register the temperature of the burnout and prevent too rapid or too much heating of the rings. The procedure is started by setting the oven on low for 20 minutes and then on medium for 45 minutes to reach the casting temperature. A rapid or excessive burnout causes flaking and cracking of the mold and produces porosity and fins on the casting. A pyrometer is necessary because ovens will vary in heating time. The color of the sprue was formerly used to gauge the temperature, but this method is now impractical in the busy office.

The casting temperature of 1,200° F. is above the compensating curve for cristobalite investment. The casting must be made within 2 minutes to stay within the expansion time because cooling is accompanied by contraction. The residual carbon gas from the wax pattern is removed at this temperature to prevent damage to the gold. The remaining gases are pushed through the thin ¼ inch layer of the investment out the end of the casting ring. Some hygroscopic expansion techniques have lower casting temperatures.

A gas torch is used to melt the gold. The flame is regulated so that it has an inner cone that develops a reducing atmosphere around the metal. This avoids burning out the base metal zinc, which acts as an oxide scavenger for the casting. The inner cone of the flame is kept on the metal at all times to quickly melt the gold in the proper atmosphere.

The gold is placed in the bottom of the crucible in such a position that the color of the melted surface can be observed. The melting is accomplished with the addition of a borax and boric acid flux to prevent oxidation. The gold is heated until it has a bright orange color. The casting is made when the slag or oxides disappear from the surface, when the proper color is attained, and when the gold appears to be spinning. In order that the gold can be cleaned during the casting procedure, one-half new gold is added for each restoration.

Different kinds of casting golds should not be mixed especially those containing solder, because the melting range will be changed or a eutectic metal will be formed. An incomplete casting results when the gold freezes too quickly after it enters the mold with the eutectic metal.

The sequence to be followed in casting is as follows:

1. The rings are placed in the oven for the prescribed time to obtain a gradual expansion until the temperature reaches 1,200° F. The castings are heated at this temperature for 15 minutes to make certain that the mold is fully prepared and contains no residue.
2. The residual gold from previous castings is premelted to form a button and reduced with flux. The casting machine, which is usually the centrifugal type, is turned four times on the spring to ensure adequate pressure.
3. The melted button and the new gold are placed in the crucible, which is still warm from the preheating. The oven, borax flux, and the carrying tongs should all be within reach because the flame must be kept on the melted gold at all times.
4. The gold is heated in the reducing portion of the gas flame until it becomes a bright orange color and has a "spinning" appearance.
5. The casting ring is placed in the cradle of the casting machine and the crucible is moved up and locked to the end of the ring with the sprue way. The flame is kept on the gold at all times to keep the gold molten.
6. The casting arm is released to force the liquid gold into the mold. The arm of the centrifugal casting machine must be left alone until the spinning stops because injury may result from the revolving metal.
7. The rings are removed from the cradle of the casting machine, and when

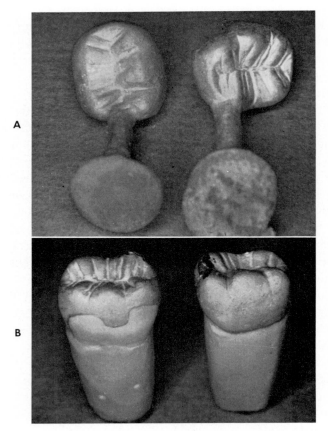

Fig. 17-24. A, Raw castings after removal from the investment mold and pickling of the metal. **B,** Gold sprues are removed and the castings are placed on the dies and evaluated for fit.

the sprue button is darkened, it is dropped in the water. This aids in breaking up the surrounding investment from the gold casting.

8. The castings are recovered and scrubbed with a hard-bristle toothbrush and water to remove all the investment particles.

The surface oxides are then removed from the surface of the casting. This procedure is called "pickling" and is accomplished with hydrochloric or sulfuric acid and equal parts of water. There are commercial preparations that make excellent pickling solutions that can also be used to reduce the corrosiveness of other metal objects in the office, especially that caused by hydrochloric acid.

The castings are placed in a glass beaker or porcelain dish and the pickling solution is poured to cover the metal (Fig. 17-24). The solution is heated slowly to prevent boiling. When the oxides are cleaned from the surface, the color of the gold will change. The castings are removed from the pickling solution and thoroughly washed in water. Then the sprue button is removed and polishing is initiated.

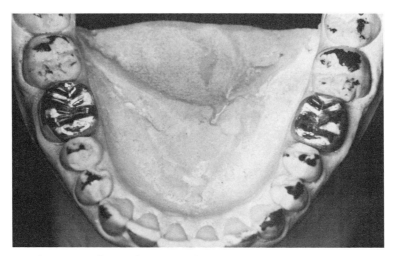

Fig. 17-25. Preliminary occlusal adjustments of the castings made on the articulator to lessen the time required for intraoral adjustments.

Electric casting units are helpful in multiple procedures. The gold is heated in a muffle in a reducing atmosphere. The temperature inside the muffle is regulated by a resistance dial. The electric unit standardizes the casting procedure and the use of the torch is eliminated.

Improper spruing, investing, or casting result in casting failures because of occluded gas porosity, shrinkage porosity, and incomplete margins.[36] These defects make the castings inadequate; a text on dental materials should be consulted for specific problems. Inherent subsurface porosity has been discussed with the accepted casting procedures.

Finishing

The rough casting requires some refining before it can be tried on the prepared tooth, corrected, and finally polished for cementation (Fig. 17-25). The sprue should be quickly removed with cutters or a separating disk, taking care not to distort the casting. The surface where the sprue pin was attached is smoothed back to the curvature that existed in the pattern. Fitting the die, polishing the margin, and dressing down the surface of the casting can be initiated after sprue removal.

The polishing procedure is directed to place the edge of the casting in contact with the tooth. In the process the final occlusal morphology, as determined by interocclusal adjustment, is obtained and the surface is polished. The final contours are made on the surfaces and the gold is polished to protect the gingival tissue and to make the casting resistant to tarnish and corrosion. This is all done with finishing burs, stones, and other abrasives in an order of descending abrasiveness. The surface abrasion caused by the agents produces luster and smoothness of the polished layer.

There are many different abrasives available, and caution must be exercised not to reduce the size and type of the abrasive too rapidly because the smoothing must be completed before it can be polished. On the contrary, excessive polishing of the casting occurs with harsh abrasives. The polishing procedure is divided between preliminary die working and making the adjustments to the patient.

Die working. The rough castings are placed on the die and seated with minimal pressure. Any roughnesses or projections on the inside of the casting that prevent seating should be removed with a sharp round bur. The fit can be determined at this time. No relationship can be used that does not allow full seating and covering of the margins of the die with the gold. The gold can be elongated, but not to the extent that it will close a margin that is visibly short. The casting should fit the walls of the preparation snugly, but excessive pressures cannot be used to seat the casting. A tight relationship will fracture the die or tooth and the casting must be remade.

Stripping of the casting has been advocated to remove part of the inside wall to allow for the thickness of the cement liner. The gold is removed by a deplating stripping unit or by placing the casting in a solution of aqua regia. The margins and surface of the inlay are coated with wax before contacting the solution because loss of metal in these areas would destroy the casting. Routine use of stripping results in loose castings, and it should not be used to improve the marginal fit. The process of stripping is helpful in the parallel pin casting because of the accuracy of the long posts. In some cases the stripping unit can be used to produce a better marginal relationship in large castings that have limited taper, but it is employed as a terminal effort for the extratight casting. The fit of the casting is regulated by the proportions of the investment powders.

The margins of the seated casting are smoothed on the die with fine cuttlefish sandpaper disks in a straight mandrel. A ½ or ⅜ inch disk is used to reach the sharp curvatures and depressions. All surface roughness, scalloped areas of flash, and porosity are reduced to a smooth knife edge for the margin. The disk is moved slowly and is confined to the gold to prevent abrasion of the stone surface. The same procedure is used for polishing the margins with the crocus disk. The metal will be highly polished from the iron oxide on the paper disk. This completes the margin polish because the gold is thin and it will be quickly abraded to produce an open casting.

The proximal surfaces and large portions of the buccolingual surfaces are smoothed with the large cuttlefish sandpaper disks. The contact areas are smoothed down to the fine grit and the remaining excess is used for the intraoral adjustment. The disks are applied lightly to smooth parts of the occlusal surface and areas around the cusp tips.

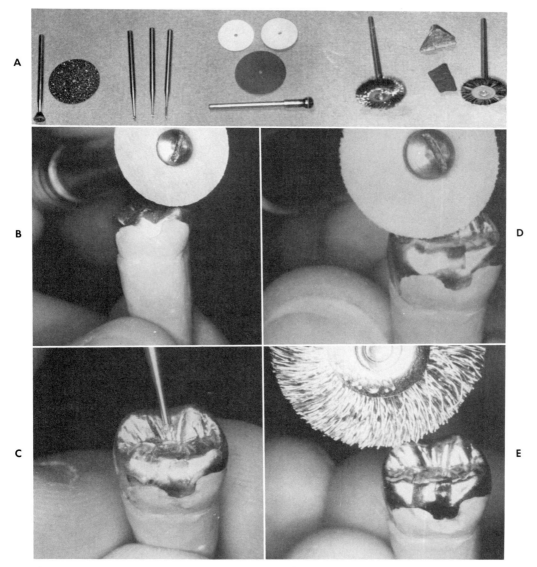

Fig. 17-26. A, Armamentarium for polishing the gold casting: stones, burs, disks, mandrel, wire brush, and soft brush with tripoli and rouge. **B,** Fine cuttlefish sandpaper disk for smoothing the surface and margins. **C,** Burs are used to refine and polish the grooves by removing the oxides. **D,** The soft rubber abrasive wheel is applied to the surfaces to smooth the metal. **E,** The gold surface is burnished with the wire brush in preparation for the wax abrasives.

The rough surface oxides are cleaned out of the occlusal grooves. The length and the occlusal design placed in the wax pattern are followed. The bur is not used to trench the gold but only to remove the roughness inherent with the casting process.

The entire occlusal surface is burnished with a steel wire brush mounted on a straight mandrel. The bristles of the brush will clean the occlusal surface and make the gold appear burnished and polished. The roughness will be rapidly removed, but caution must be exercised so as not to remove the occlusal form.

All these procedures can be accomplished in the laboratory and should be completed before the appointment. The fit is checked on the stone die and the surfaces are smoothed to a degree necessary for the occlusal adjustments. A higher polish than this should not be produced because the casting is adjusted once again intraorally and is then completely polished (Fig. 17-26).

Fitting the casting. Most properly made castings are found to be high in occlusion when fitted in the cavity preparation. This is caused by the wax expansion and last-minute pooling or adjustment of the pattern before investing. The finding results in more interocclusal adjustment than is usually expected. The cementation appointment involves removal of the temporary restorations, trial-and-error fitting of the casting to the tooth, and grinding of the inlay on the die for the final shape.

The castings are seated in the preparation and articulating ribbon is inserted between the inlay and the involved teeth. The patient is asked to move the mandible in the directions that have been copied on the articulator to mark the castings where contacts are made with the opposing teeth. Premature contacts and uneven stress distributions are observed as heavy markings on the gold surface. The castings are removed and all the adjustments are made while holding them in the hand to minimize trauma to the tooth. With careful manipulation of the casting, the patient will not have to be anesthetized, making a more accurate adjustment of the casting possible.

The casting is remounted on the articulator to refine the occlusion. This is helpful and is certainly indicated for all cases but is done mainly when extensive alteration has been made in the occlusal plane. Remounting involves placing the cast units back on the articulator and making the adjustments with the opposing model. The overall refinement is directed by the surfaces of the new models and the settings of the articulator. Remounting is routine for all reconstruction procedures.

The castings are placed back on the teeth after the interproximal adjustments are made. An impression is made of the occlusal surface with a rigid material such as quick-curing acrylic die and then covered by an alginate or rubber base impression. The impression is removed, the castings are lubricated and placed in the impression, and the stone is vibrated into the mold. The model will have the castings attached in the same relationship that existed in the mouth. A new centric bite and facebow transfer are taken to remount the models and the castings. The refinement of the gold is done on the model with sharp burs, as otherwise would have been done by hand adjustment.

Remounting refines extensive castings. It should not be limited to prosthetic appliances. Even if terminal chairside adjustments need to be made, the overall effects of remounting will enhance the accuracy of the restoration. Theoretically the casting will be more efficient in mastication and have fewer traumatic relationships with the opposing teeth.

The adjustments made on the prepared teeth for the cementation appointment fall into a regular sequence. The steps should be followed closely for finishing the restoration.

1. The temporary restorations are taken out and the small particles of cement are removed with a sharp explorer. The gingival tissue and the preparation are examined to determine the condition of the tooth before spraying the preparation and the area with 3% hydrogen peroxide. The patient is instructed to rinse with warm water to remove all debris. Pumicing the preparations is helpful to remove the debris.

2. The interproximal contact on the casting is adjusted to enable the unit to be seated. Large stones, or preferably a separating disk in the straight mandrel, are used to quickly dress down the proximal surface. An ideal contact area and embrasure form are developed with the disk. There should be a rigid relationship between the teeth; the relationship can be determined by using dental floss on the interproximal surfaces. Negative areas can be soldered, but this is discouraged because warpage can be produced in the casting. Overreduction is prevented by gradually smoothing and shaping the proximal surface with the stone or disk.

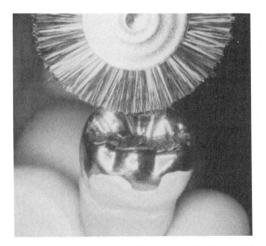

Fig. 17-27. Final surface luster is produced on the gold with the soft brush charged with wax abrasives and jeweler's rouge.

3. The marginal fit of the casting is determined when the inlay is fully seated. The quadrant is isolated with cotton rolls and the teeth are dried and examined with loupes, mirror, and explorer. Slight discrepancies can be corrected with gold files and ⅜ inch fine cuttlefish disks. The disk must be confined to the gold to avoid abrasion of the tooth structure.

4. After the marginal fit is assessed the occlusal adjustments are made on the casting. This is best accomplished by cutting the surface with a bur. The eccentric movements are made by the mandible to mark the castings with articulating paper. The adjustments are made slowly in order to develop the centric contacts and to eliminate the eccentric contacts. This requires that working and idling grooves be cut between the cusp tips to enable the two occlusal surfaces to "just miss" when entering and leaving centric relationship. The balancing factors are removed whenever possible in order to eliminate wear facets, tooth fracture, and periodontal breakdown caused by the horizontal application of force. The centric contact should form a "tripod" relationship between the cusp and fossa.

5. The initial contacts of the casting to the tooth should be disclosed to produce a better fit. The contacts are determined by coating the inside of the casting with a dye, wax, or pumice. They are then relieved with a bur and the process is continued until the casting is fully seated into the cavity preparation.

6. The adjusted casting is then smoothed on the die, which is used as a handle for stability. Only the adjusted surfaces will require extensive finishing because the margins and most of the gold were initially smoothed. The same abrasives are used in an order of descending abrasiveness to gradually polish the surface. Cuttlefish sandpaper, from coarse to fine, and then Burlew rubber wheels are applied to all the areas. This is followed by light application of the wire brush on the occlusal surface to produce a smooth, burnished appearance on all surfaces of the casting and to clean out the grooves and fossae.

7. The casting is polished with wax abrasives and iron oxide to develop a passive layer on the gold with a high luster. The tripoli abrasive is applied with a soft brush wheel in order to blend the polishing agent into all the concave areas (Fig. 17-27). The polishing should not be excessive, nor should the margins be touched with the tripoli abrasive because the surface relationship will be changed. The abrasive is removed with soap and water before the iron oxide is used. Iron oxide is referred to as jeweler's rouge, and only a small amount of surface contact is needed with the polishing brush to produce the high luster. This process should not be done if the occlusal contour is changed. Often the steel brush is the last polishing done on the occlusal surface.

The castings are scrubbed with soap and warm water to remove all traces of the abrasive. They are then placed on the teeth and examined for proper fit and occlusal relationship. The casting should feel smooth to the patient, and the union of metal and tooth should be undetectable. When these criteria have been fulfilled, cementation can be initiated.

The polished inlay is luted to the tooth with zinc phosphate cement. This material is selected for its physical properties. There are disadvantages of solubility, acidity, and film thickness, but no other cement better satisfies the conditions for securing the castings in the preparation.[37] Research with zinc oxide–eugenol and polycarboxylate cements is encouraging, but until certain properties are improved, the materials should not be routinely used for the cementation of a permanent casting. The type of cementing medium is critical for prolonged life of the gold casting. The patient must observe certain hygienic and dietary rules to prevent dissolution of the liner between the casting and the tooth.

A radiographic analysis is made of the castings before they are cemented to determine the cervical adaption of the restoration. In taking the bitewing radiograph, the angle for the film should parallel the cervical wall. This area normally rests below the gingival tissue and it is impossible to accurately observe or determine the cervical relationship using only the explorer. If the cervical margin is open on the radiograph, the impression must be retaken because the casting was previously smoothed to the die in this area. An open cervical margin does not often occur if the casting fits the tooth with a minimum of adjustments during the initial fitting procedure.

The rubber dam is applied because a dry tooth surface facilitates cleaning of the tooth structure and application of the cavity varnish liner.[38] The adjusted No. W8A clamp is used to retain the dam and expose the margins on the tooth distal to the one receiving the inlay. The clamp produces deflection of the gingival tissue and has broad application on the molar teeth.

The surgical field is sprayed with 3% hydrogen peroxide to remove debris and sediment. The preparations are rinsed with water and the area is dried with warm air and small pieces of absorbent cotton. Two applications of cavity varnish are applied to the walls of the cavity preparation and allowed to dry. The teeth are now ready to receive the castings.

A retarded mix of zinc phosphate cement is made because it allows time for a thorough technique. This will also enable an adequate amount of powder to be incorporated and will permit the desired consistency to be produced. Extra powder reduces the solubility of the cement, but too thick a mix must not be produced because full seating of the casting will be prevented. The technique described will produce a desirable cement for placing the casting (Fig. 17-28). To save time the assistant can perform the mixing procedure while the preparations are being cleaned with peroxide.

The slab is first chilled and then wiped until moisture condensation no longer appears on the slab. The temperature of the slab will be just above the dew point and is the lowest that can be used. The liquid cement is placed in the center of the slab. Approximately 5 drops are used for a large casting. The powder is placed on the right corner of the slab if the operator is right-handed, and a small pinch of powder is placed in the liquid to retard the set. After a few minutes the mixing procedure can be initiated.

The mix is produced slowly by incorporating small portions of powder into

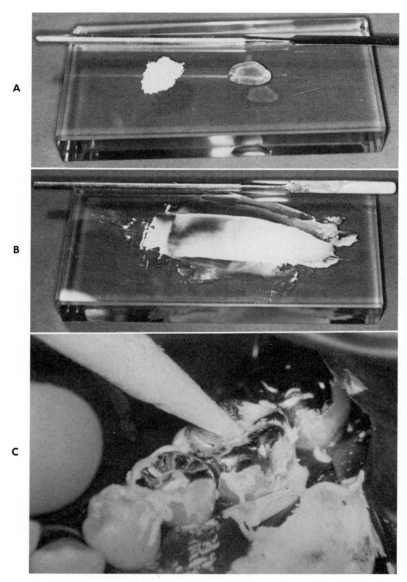

Fig. 17-28. A, The clean slab is chilled prior to mixing for cementation of the casting. **B,** The cement is mixed to a creamy consistency for luting the casting. **C,** Castings are held under pressure with the sharpened orangewood stick. A dry tooth surface and application of pressure are essential for cementation.

the liquid on a large area of the slab. The flat blade of the spatula is used to blend in the powder; slow movements will also retard the setting reaction. The spatulation is continued until the mix develops a thick, creamy consistency but still has a surface sheen. A thicker mix will not allow the casting to be fully seated into the cavity preparation.

The mixed cement is placed uniformly on the inside of the casting, and care is taken not to cover the external surface. The walls should be entirely covered. With small restorations the cement can be loaded inside the preparation instead of on the casting. A forceful amount of pressure will be needed to fully seat the casting in the tooth.

The coated casting is placed on the tooth and forcefully seated parallel with the insertion path. A sharpened orangewood stick is placed in the central fossa or on the incisal edge and forced down manually. Force is exerted several times to express the cement outside the cavity form, and the apposition of the casting is checked by wiping the wet cement off the margin with the index finger. When the casting is fully seated, the patient is instructed to bite forcefully on the orangewood stick and the casting for 5 minutes. Since there is a steady application of forces, the patient's head should be stabilized at all times.

The use of the mallet for seating inlays is not encouraged. Prolonged pressure applied with the orangewood stick is more effective than the impact of the mallet, and in most molar teeth the malleting forces cannot be directed along the insertion path. Injury of the soft tissue occurs when the mallet causes the stick to skip off the casting. For these reasons only the steady application of pressure should be used to seat the finished casting. While the cement is setting the margins of the gold casting are forcefully pushed down to the tooth with a burnishing instrument. This assures adaptation and a fine margin.

The hardened cement is removed from the teeth and the casting with the sharp explorer. No attempt should be made to insert the explorer point between the metal and the tooth because the casting can be lifted off the tooth. The largest pieces are removed grossly and the portion adhering to the margin is removed with the side of the explorer point by moving from the gold toward the tooth. Nothing should be used that will scratch the gold surface, such as the explorer tip.

The gingival embrasure is then tested with the explorer. The point is used like a scaler to remove the excess cement over the cervical margin in order to prevent gingival irritation. Dental floss is passed on the bias between the teeth to remove cement fragments and to smooth the proximal surface of the gold. The entire areas is cleaned with a sponge moistened with alcohol or water, and the rubber dam is then removed.

The quadrant containing the new restorations is sprayed with peroxide, and the patient is instructed to rinse with water. Final inspection is made by drying the restored teeth with air and testing the occlusal function. The patient is then allowed to observe the casting with a hand mirror and the comfort of the new

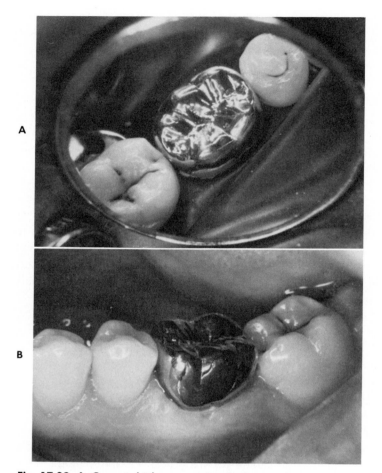

Fig. 17-29. A, Cemented inlay restoration. **B,** Cemented crown restoration.

restorations is assessed (Fig. 17-29). This completes the procedure of making the cast gold inlay. The indirect technique requires attention to detail in each of the aspects of construction. Proper design and fabrication of the inlay results in many years of service in the well-cared-for dentition. All the possible measures for accuracy of the casting must be utilized to produce a long-lasting restoration.

DIRECT METHOD OF CAST CONSTRUCTION

The direct method is a useful but sometimes overlooked procedure for making an inlay. This method is accomplished by placing wax directly in the preparation and shaping the pattern on the tooth. It was widely used before the development of accurate elastic impression materials, and dentists using the method were skillful and understood the problems of fitting the gold to the tooth. A number of techniques have been advocated for using the direct fabrication method. This procedure is used primarily for making small castings in the anterior and bicuspid teeth, and for this reason the preparations used in these areas will be discussed here.

The advantages of the direct method are as follows:

1. When compared to the indirect method, the time required to construct the inlay is shorter and the technique requires less material. Only two appointments are needed: one for preparing the tooth and carving the pattern and the another for seating the casting.

2. Less expense is involved; therefore, the patient can obtain the service for a lower fee. With the exception of waxing and casting the pattern, the laboratory procedure and technician fee are eliminated.

3. The fit of the inlay and marginal relationship appear to be better because the pattern is taken directly on the tooth. Distortions are prevented by careful manipulation of the pattern; only the investment and the gold material will undergo dimensional change in the finished restoration. Finishing of the casting on the tooth produces a good marginal relationship.

Anterior cast gold restorations

Whenever possible the direct method should be used to make the anterior casting. The preparation is accessible and a good surgical field will make the wax pattern as accurate as if a die were being used. The same quality can be achieved for small two- or three-surface bicuspid inlays and some mesial exposures on the first molars. When the preparation is extensive and includes several accessory retention forms, the indirect method is selected to make the inlay.

The casting is primarily used in anterior teeth to replace the lost angle. The incisors are noted for having large pulps in relation to the amount of tooth structure, which complicates the location of retention forms for the casting. When a display of gold is objectionable, the labial portion of the casting is removed and a veneer of resin is used to improve esthetics. Retention and esthetics are paramount, and the only material strong enough to resist stress on the incisal edge is the gold inlay or the full-coverage restoration.

The use of nylon pins has improved esthetics by making it possible to use a more limited outline form. The pins are used to produce nontapering posts on the inlay that accurately fit the postholes in the dentin. The parallel pin technique for bridges and splints requires the nylon pin kit. This procedure is explained separately.

Anterior inlay preparations have basic patterns that are altered according to the type of damage in the individual tooth. The preparations are classified according to the type of retention employed to secure the casting. Variables for selecting the preparation are the size of the caries or the trauma, the thickness and length of the tooth, and the functional relationship with the opposing arch, which is the incisal guidance.

Basic designs

Groove and post design. The most commonly used and retentive anterior inlay is the groove and post design. The rule is to have only one axial groove and one post placed as far apart as possible in the preparation. The groove is made parallel to the incisal two thirds of the tooth and is located on the axial wall. If necessary, the groove itself can be made to end in a posthole. A posthole is also located in the dentin on the incisal edge where the calcification lobes join to replace the biting edge of the tooth in gold. For auxiliary retention a posthole can be placed on the lingual-gingival corner of the preparation. The important retention forms are the axial groove and incisal posthole.

The groove and post preparation can be a two- or three-surface replacement, with or without coverage of the lingual surface. If the mesial-incisal-distal surfaces are restored, two grooves are used on the axial dentin that end in postholes. The path of withdrawal is toward the incisal surface.

The outline form of the casting is made to be esthetic by keeping the margin behind the line angle and in the embrasure. The proximal surfaces are straight to improve appearance and the incisal gold is usually concealed. On the mesial surfaces the use of a resin veneer for the inlay should be considered if the margin is past the line angle.

The retention can be additionally increased by covering the lingual surface. This is done when the tooth is short and extensive damage has occurred on the axial wall. Even more retention is produced by placing ledges and postholes on the lingual surface similar to those used for bridge retainers (Fig. 17-30). Whenever the surface area is limited in the labial outline form, additional retention must be gained on the lingual surface. Increased retention is used when a veneer is employed because some stability in the casting is lost when the metal is removed for the plastic.

Lingual lock design. The lingual lock preparation is sometimes employed for esthetics. The incisal surface is not reduced because retention is gained by a

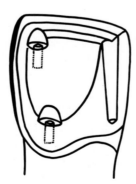

Fig. 17-30. Lingual preparation involving a proximal groove and two lingual pins.

dovetail lock on the lingual surface. Esthetics is improved by showing only a thin line of gold on the proximal surface that is being restored. The pattern removal is toward the lingual surface. All patterns must be waxed directly.

The lingual lock design has many disadvantages and is not commonly used because the restorations are frequently dislodged. The retention in the lock is not effective and forces on the incisal corner cause it to be displaced. The lingual lock design cannot be used on a short or thin tooth or when there is a minimum of horizontal overlap of the incisors because the casting will produce shadowing on the labial surface or will be displaced by incisal stresses.

Design utilizing the root chamber for retention. The endodontically treated tooth can be restored with an inlay by utilizing the root chamber for retention. The canal filling is removed from the crown and the top portion of the chamber up the conical space, with the withdrawal path being toward the incisal surface.

This design is not often used for a restoration because the full-coverage restoration has better application. The remaining incisal and labial enamel becomes discolored and the fit of such a large casting is difficult. The preferred technique is to make a cast core that fills in the top portion of the root chamber and forms an ideal crown preparation. The full-coverage porcelain and gold or jacket crown is made to fit over the prepared tooth stump.

• • •

The direct method for small bicuspids is discussed because it is a departure from the regular inlay design. The lesions are usually incipient, with the direct method dictating that a conservative outline form be used. The value of limited cavity width has been discussed in relation to amalgam restorations and the same rules apply to the direct inlay. In the lower bicuspid teeth with the diminutive lingual cusp the isthmus can be limited to one third or less of the intercuspal distance. A small degree of taper and a short bevel are used on the occlusal surface, and the regular proximal design is used to produce the cavity form. The patterns can be carved quickly because many anatomic guides are present on the occlusal enamel. A minimum of occlusal adjustments is needed because the conservative outline form is confined to the groove area.

Instrumentation

The instrumentation is similar for all the anterior inlay preparations (Fig. 17-31). Disks and tapered burs are used to place the inclination for making the casting. The outline forms are similar and straight but tapered cavity walls are employed to avoid undercuts.[39]

1. The separating disk or thin diamond disk in the straight mandrel is used to slice the proximal surface where the lesion is located. To avoid pulp damage the slowly revolving disk is sloped to the lingual surface and made to parallel the marginal ridge. The cutting is started on the incisal surface and the disk is moved

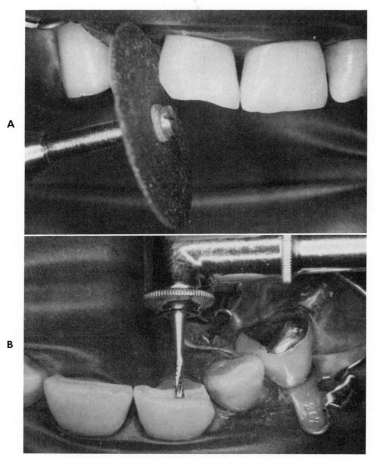

Fig. 17-31. A, The initial disk cut is slanted lingually to establish an esthetic outline, lingual margin, and cervical chamfer. **B,** Placing the incisal step with the carbide fissure bur.

in a gingival direction. One movement of the disk establishes the labial outline, the lingual wall, and the gingival wall. Overcutting is avoided by proper slanting of the disk.

2. The small wheel stone in the straight mandrel is used to reduce the incisal edge. The reduction is accomplished at the expense of the lingual surface to develop thickness in the casting that will support the incisal edge. Less gold will be displayed this way and the labial surface is only smoothed for a short bevel. The incisal-lingual reduction is made only to uncover the dentin tissue for the ledge and posthole.

3. A No. 701 carbide bur in the straight handpiece is held parallel to the long axis of the tooth and the axial wall is tapered and smoothed. The end cutters of the bur form a small cervical shelf. Any undercuts in the proximal

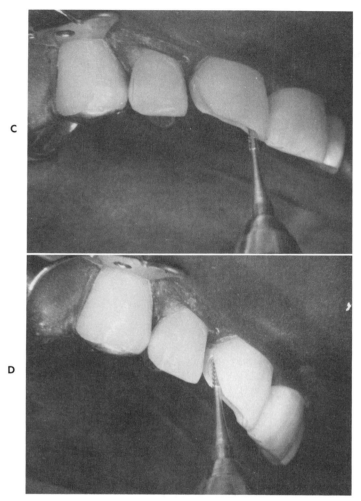

Fig. 17-31, cont'd. C, Incisal posthole is placed with the No. 700 tapered fissure bur. **D,** The proximal groove and posthole are placed with the No. 700 tapered fissure bur.

walls are removed at this time. If necessary, a small inverted cone bur can be used to refine the incisal edge.

4. A No. 699 or No. 700 bur in the straight handpiece is held parallel to the incisal two thirds of the labial plate, and the grooves are placed in the axial wall at a depth of one half the diameter of the bur. If postholes are desired at the bottom of the grooves, they are placed at this time. If it is a two-surface restoration, the incisal retention is placed following the groove and they are made parallel and to a depth of 1 mm. The grooves and postholes are cut slowly in the dentin, using an air coolant, to produce the ideal depth and angulation.

5. The Wedelstaedt or binangle chisel is used to sharpen the line angles and

to smooth the walls and margins of the preparation. Delicate strokes are used to remove the brittle tooth structure.

The lingual lock preparation is made with a similar instrumentation. The disk is used to form the opening with the same depth and angulation. The lock is prepared in the middle third of the lingual surface with the No. 701 bur in the contra-angle handpiece. All the walls of the lock are made to taper for the lingual removal of the pattern. The margin of the lock is extended to opposite junctions of the calcification lobes and made to rest on smooth enamel at the base of the marginal ridge. The lock should have bulk to prevent the casting from bending and distorting during fabrication.

The other retentive factor for the lingual lock preparation is a No. 700 bur groove in the cervical axial line angle. The groove is made to parallel the path of withdrawel. When a thick tooth is being restored, the groove can end in a small posthole in the labial enamel plate. Refinement of the preparation is done with a slowly revolving bur or a mounted stone and the conventional chisel.

Application of the lingual lock inlay is limited because of poor retentive factors, but when the proper conditions prevail, the preparation can be used to produce an esthetic restoration.

Pattern formation

The waxing procedure should be explained to the patient to prevent anxiety when the use of warm instruments is noted in carving the pattern. The patient's head is reclined, the rubber dam is checked and readjusted if necessary, and the unit light is directed on the prepared tooth. The preparation and the neighboring teeth are lubricated with a brush and gently dried with air to leave only a thin film of solution. For the anterior teeth, wax placement and waxing will be simplified when the patient's head is held posterior to the normal position. When working on the bicuspids, the chair position should be adjusted for the operator's comfort.

Two methods are available to place the inlay wax into the preparation.

Open method. The open method is the method of choice for small restorations. The inlay wax is softened in the flame until a point is formed on the end of the stick. The point is removed, placed on an explorer, and heated until the surface glistens while the point is held. The heated cone is forced into the preparation parallel to the path of insertion and held under pressure until the wax cools. The pattern is then readapted with a warm instrument, preferably an old explorer, to copy the post, groove, and imprint of the cavity wall. The wax pattern is again held under pressure to avoid contraction from the tooth and then carved to develop the surface dimensions, contours, and margins with the preferred carving instruments.

Closed method. The closed method is used to confine the wax for carving the posterior pattern. A matrix band and retainer are adjusted in dimension and festooned to fit the tooth accurately but loosely. The wax stick is heated in the flame and compressed in the fingers to be packed into the band. The wax is then reheated and forcefully placed around the prepared tooth while the thumb or index finger pushes the wax into the preparation. The wax is held to allow cooling and the flash is removed on the occlusal surface before readapting the cavity walls with a carving instrument. When the wax has cooled, the assembly is removed and the band is discarded. The pattern is reinserted and carved to form.

The carved pattern should be smoothed and adapted at the margins while using magnifying loupes. The surface is highly polished with small pieces of silk or cotton moistened with warm water. The polishing procedure on the gold is shortened by proper fabrication of the wax pattern.

Spruing

If the pattern is accessible, the sprue pin can often be attached while the wax is on the tooth. Distortion is prevented by attaching the sprue to the thickest incisal corner and pointing it toward the thin margins. The wax additions to the sprue pin are made at this time and cooling is allowed to control the dimensional change in the wax. If the pattern cannot be reached, it should be removed and the pin placed while holding the pattern in the palm of the hand.

Finishing

The rough casting is cleaned and placed on the tooth after the inside surfaces have been inspected for roughness and the sprue pin has been removed. To avoid tooth fracture the casting is carefully seated until the margins oppose the tooth structure. This cannot be done until the proximal surfaces are adjusted, and this results in numerous attempts while the contact area is slowly reduced and shaped with the disk. When the margins are approved, the occlusal relationships are tested with articulating paper and the functional contours placed in the gold with the burs. All excursive movements and centric contacts are adjusted to create an atraumatic inlay.

The polishing procedure is all that remains. Because with the direct method the tooth is refined, the rubber dam must be applied and the casting seated and held under pressure. The ⅜ inch sandpaper and crocus disks are used to smooth the margins down against the enamel surface. Gold files are useful for pulling the gold toward tooth structure. The surface is then polished with sandpaper and Burlew wheels. The wax abrasives are applied while the castings are held in the hand. The castings are cleaned with surgical soap and water while varnish is applied to the tooth.

A mix of zinc phosphate cement is made and the casting is thoroughly coated (Fig. 17-32). The inlay is placed on the tooth and held under pressure until the cement hardens. The flash and loose fragments of cement are removed with a sharp explorer and a 2×2 inch alcohol sponge. If necessary, the cemented casting is then polished with silica and whiting to develop surface luster. All debris is removed for final inspection of the inlay before the rubber dam is

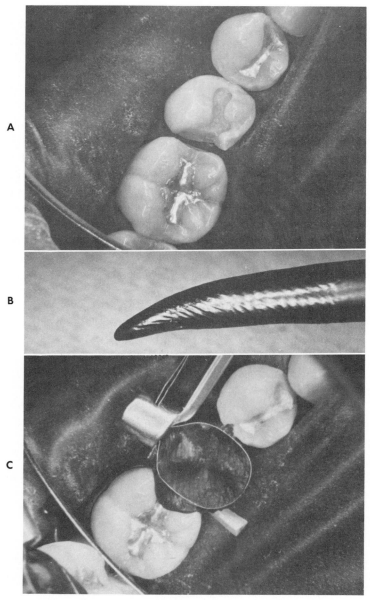

A

B

C

Fig. 17-32. A, Cavity preparation for an inlay on the distal surface of the second bicuspid. **B,** Inlay wax is softened and pointed for placement in the prepared cavity form. **C,** Inlay wax is seated inside the matrix band and cavity preparation.

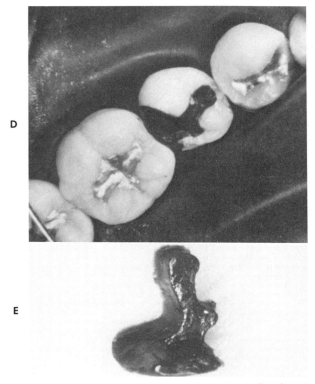

D

E

Continued.

Fig. 17-32, cont'd. D, Completed wax pattern. **E,** The pattern is removed for analysis of adaptation of the wax to the cavity wall.

removed. The patient may then observe the casting. The rubber dam is removed and the relationship of the casting with the range of mandibular movements is examined.

If a plastic veneer is used in the labial wall, the gold is cut back but not to include the proximal retentive groove. The casting is cemented and then under-cut with a small inverted cone bur. Sulfinic acid plastic is inserted using the brush method and is finished with the conventional instruments. The reduction in time and improvement in fit merit the use of the direct technique for making the small accessible cast restoration.

PIN CASTINGS

A recent improvement in the design of restorations and castings is the nylon pin technique devised by E. David Shooshan (Fig. 17-33). It has been widely used in splinting and bridge abutments and is sometimes called the parallel pin procedure. The use of small nontaper pins makes it possible to increase the re-tention of the gold casting. The advantage of this technique is that it is possible

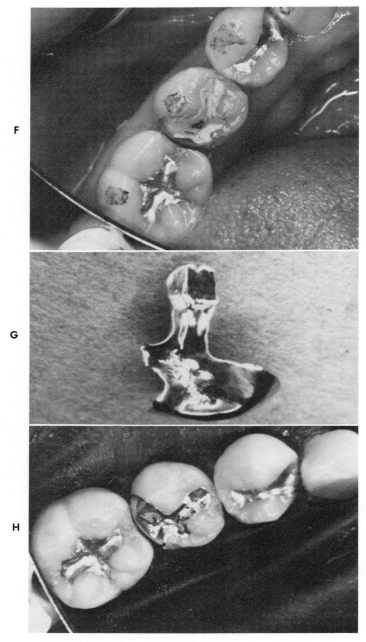

Fig. 17-32, cont'd. F, The seated casting with the markings for occlusal adjustment. **G,** Polished casting prior to cementation. **H,** Completed inlay carved directly on the second bicuspid.

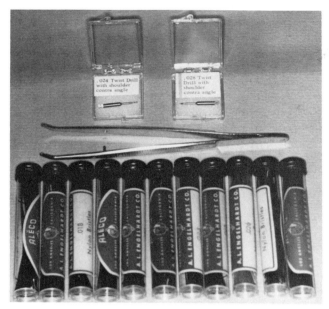

Fig. 17-33. Nylon pin armamentarium for retentive gold castings. (Courtesy Englehardt Products.)

to limit the outline form and labial exposure of gold and still make a restoration capable of supporting the incisal edge or retaining the bridge without being dislodged from the tooth. Shooshan introduced the pins as an adjunct to the pinledge preparation.[39]

Armamentarium

A kit has been manufactured for the casting pin procedure. The acceptance of this type underpinning has been partly a result of the ease in using the components of the kit.

1. Spirec burs (twist drills) with diameters of 0.024 and 0.028 inch are used for making the postholes in the dentin. The cutting edges are 3 mm. in length.
2. Nylon bristles are used to form the wax pattern and stabilize the temporary restoration. They range in size from 0.020 to 0.028 inch in diameter. The bristle sizes are increased by 0.001 inch to give an assortment for the two bur sizes.
3. Grooved cotton pliers are used to manipulate the pins in and out of the postholes. Holding the nylon pin is simplified by making a flat nail head on the end that fits into the groove of the pliers.
4. A single-edge razor blade is used to cut the nylon bristles to the desired length.
5. The round, curved end of a No. 7 wax spatula is used to flatten the head

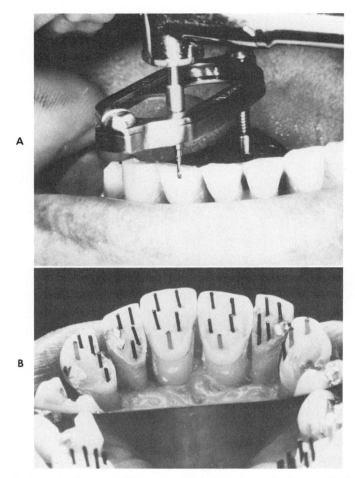

Fig. 17-34. A, Loma Linda paralleling device in position for multiple pins. **B,** Pin holes drilled and nylon bristles in place.

of the bristle so that it can be retained in the impression or wax pattern. The spatula is placed in the flame and then on the end of the bristle to develop the flattened end. Many commercial pin kits are available that work in a similiar manner. When multiple pins and splints are used, a paralleling device is necessary (Fig. 17-34).

The pin technique is useful in many ways but is primarily advantageous for refining the technique of making the posts on castings. Before the armamentarium was devised it was nearly impossible to inject an elastic impression material into a posthole of the size used for anterior teeth and to obtain an accurate impression. When made properly, the castings accurately reproduce the nontapering pin on the gold casting.

Formerly, in order to increase the retention for anterior castings, surface extension was advocated to include the proximal surface for boxing or grooves. Extension can now be confined because of the support given by the "underpinning." The posts are placed from 1.5 to 2.5 mm. in the lingual dentin of the incisors for the support. Thus castings can be made with limited outline forms to improve esthetics for the restoration of the angle or the retention of the bridge. Multiple, lingual parallel pin restorations have been advocated for splinting periodontally involved anterior teeth.

The pins are used in operative dentistry for Class IV inlay restorations that have the labial gold removed for masking purposes. The labial "cut out" of the casting is undercut and restored with a sulfinic acid catalyst resin to improve the appearance of the tooth. Gold removal on the labial surface also eliminates part of the casting opposing the cavity wall, which seriously decreases the retention of the regular casting. The pin technique is used for retention, and two or three well-placed posts will support the casting without covering the entire lingual surface of the incisor.

The construction of regular anterior inlays can be made with less lingual surface coverage. Like the pinledge, the inlay casting is made without covering the entire incisal edge of thick or bulky teeth. Nylon pins have been advocated for the restoration of incisal cusp tips such as abraded cuspids to increase the incisal guiding factors of the tooth. If this retention is adequate to withstand the forces of cuspid protection, the technique can be used with success almost anywhere in the oral cavity. The greater ease of producing the gold posts with nylon pins than with the conventional technique should be considered.

Procedure

The steps involved in the nylon pin technique will be described.

1. The outline form of the restoration is made with minimal extension. The lingual surface or the area to receive the pins is reduced to expose the dentin.

2. The posthole is made by entering the dentin with a No. ½ round bur. The twist drill is inserted in the depression and the posthole is cut to the desired depth. The No. 028 drill is used for large teeth and the No. 024 drill is used for the lower incisors and upper lateral incisors. The postholes are made one after the other by slowly revolving the bur. This enables the proper depth and angulation of the postholes to be judged and aligned with the other parts of the preparation.

3. The cavity is finished with hand instruments, and small ledges or indentations are made around the postholes to give bulk to the gold in these areas. The next smallest size bristle, ½ inch in length, is placed in the posthole and flattened on the end.

4. The elastic impression is taken in the conventional manner, being sure to meticulously inject the material around the pins.

5. The model is made with Densite and the bristles are slowly removed with cotton pliers after the trimming and die formation have been done.

6. The next smallest size nylon bristle is placed in the stone model and adjusted to project out 2 mm. This post is used for the wax pattern and will be 0.002 inch smaller than the twist drill. The pattern bristle is flattened and the wax is adapted and carved to the desired contour and marginal relationship.

7. The pattern is invested and cast in a conventional manner and is polished like other castings.

8. The casting is seated in the preparation by first excising the lip of the posthole with a No. 1 round bur. This removes the dentin for the discrepancy that usually occurs around the base of the pin. Some dentists have advocated an electrolytic stripping of the inside of the casting. The bur method is preferred because the stripping method may produce an undersized casting and ruin the posts. Occasionally the No. 1 round bur is used to countersink the postholes if the surface roughness of the cast post prevents complete seating.

9. The casting is placed on the tooth and checked at the margins. If additional filing or disking is needed, it should be done at this time. If the labial wall is to be cut out for the resin, it is reduced with a fissure bur in the air turbine handpiece. The gold is removed back to the proximal groove to provide a veneer of resin 1 mm. thick. The casting is undercut with a small inverted cone bur to assist retention of the plastic (Fig. 17-35).

10. The casting is then luted to the tooth with a regular mix of zinc phos-

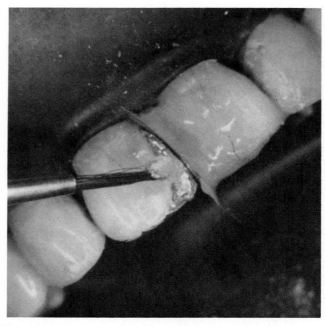

Fig. 17-35. Sulfinic catalyst resin is placed with the brush method to veneer the pin-retained casting.

phate cement under the rubber dam. The cement is placed in the postholes with the Lentulo spiral and the inside of the casting is coffered to be seated and held under pressure for 5 minutes.

11. The cement is cleaned from the tooth and resin is added by the brush method and is shaped with the No. 4 round bur and gold knife. The entire restoration is polished with silica and whiting with the soft white rubber cup.

The nylon pins can also be used to make accurate posts for posterior castings. The procedure is helpful in restoring brittle endodontically treated bicuspid teeth. The pins should never be used as a substitute for the principles for cavity preparation. They merely complement the design afforded by accurately angulated smooth walls and margins.

The nylon pins are helpful in making a more accurately retained casting. The use of the armamentarium makes it possible to limit the outline form in some cases to produce a more esthetic restoration. The other advantage in using the pins is the simplicity of the technique.

•   •   •

The principles and some of the accepted methods for producing the cast gold restoration have been presented. The superior qualities of the gold margin and surface contour are obtained by an increase in time and cost of the restoration. The techniques are all directed toward conserving or supporting tooth structure and producing a casting that minimizes thickness of the cement liner. Meticulous attention to detail is needed for all aspects of preparing the tooth and fabricating the inlay. If the oral cavity is properly maintained by thorough cleaning and a reasonable diet, the gold casting should last for the clinical life of the tooth.

REFERENCES

1. Hollenback, G. M.: A brief history of the cast restoration, J. S. Calif. Dent. Assoc. 30:8, 1962.
2. Hollenback, G. M.: Science and technic of the cast restoration, St. Louis, 1964, The C. V. Mosby Co.
3. Stuart, C. E., and Stallard, H.: Diagnosis and treatment of occlusal relations of the teeth, Texas Dent. J. 75:430, 1957.
4. Norman, R. D., Swartz, M. L., and Phillips, R W: Studies on the solubility of certain dental materials, J. Dent. Res. 36:977, 1957.
5. Thom, L. W.: Indication, cavity preparation, and wax manipulation in the cast gold inlay process, Minneapolis Dist. Dent. J. 22:9, 1938.
6. Johnston, J. F., Phillips, R. W., and Dykema, R.: Modern practice in crown and bridge prosthodontics, ed. 3, Philadelphia, 1971, W. B. Saunders Co.
7. Ramfjord, S. P., and Ash, M. M.: Occlusion, ed. 2, Philadelphia, 1971, W. B. Saunders Co.
8. Blackwell, R. C.: Black's operative dentistry, ed. 9, Milwaukee, 1955, Medico-Dental Publishing Co., vol. 2.
9. Simon, W. J.: Clinical operative dentistry, Philadelphia, 1956, W. B. Saunders Co.
10. Vale, W. A.: Cavity preparation and further thoughts on high speed, Brit. Dent. J. 107:333, 1959.
11. Thompson, M. J.: Exposing of the cavity margin for hydrocolloid impressions, J. S. Calif. Dent. Assoc. 19:17, 1951.

12. Bassett, R. W., Ingraham, R., and Koser, J. R.: An atlas of cast gold procedures, Buena Park, Calif., 1964, Uni-Tro College Press.
13. Harrison, J. D.: Effect of retraction materials on the gingival sulcus epithelium, J. Prosth. Dent. 11:514, 1961.
14. Stark, M., and others: The effect of topically applied epinephrine on blood pressure and pulse rate, paper presented at the International Association for Dental Research, March 26, 1966, Bal Harbour, Fla.
15. Oringer, M. J.: Electrosurgery in dentistry, Philadelphia, 1962, W. B. Saunders Co.
16. Phillips, R. W., and Schnell, R. J.: The use of rubber impression materials, Pract. Dent. Monographs, May, 1962, pp. 3-32.
17. Phillips, R. W.: Physical properties and manipulation of rubber impression materials, J.A.D.A. 59:454, 1959.
18. Gilmore, H. W., Schnell, R. J., and Phillips, R. W.: Factors influencing the accuracy of silicone impression materials, J. Prosth. Dent. 9:30, 1959.
19. Sears, A. W.: Hydrocolloid impression technique for inlays and fixed bridges, Dent. Digest 43:230, 1937.
20. Phillips, R. W., and Ito, B. Y.: Factors influencing the accuracy of reversible hydrocolloid impressions, J.A.D.A. 43:1, 1951.
21. Hohlt, F. A., and Phillips, R. W.: Evaluation of various methods employed for constructing working dies from hydrocolloid impressions, J. Prosth. Dent. 6:87, 1956.
22. Toreskog, S., Phillips, R. W., and Schnell, R. J.: Properties of die materials, a comparative study, J. Prosth. Dent. 16:119, 1966.
23. Moulton, G. H.: Transfer records in crown and bridge prosthetics. In Goldman, H. M., Forrest, S. P., Byrd, D. L., and McDonald, R. E., editors: Current therapy in dentistry, St. Louis, 1964, The C. V. Mosby Co., chap. 9.
24. Pavone, B.: Oral rehabilitation and occlusion, San Francisco, 1965, San Francisco School of Dentistry Medical Center, University of California, vol. 2.
25. Skinner, E., and Phillips, R. W.: The science of dental materials, Philadelphia, 1960, W. B. Saunders Co.
26. Phillips, R. W., and Biggs, D. W.: Distortion of wax patterns as influenced by storage time, storage temperature, and temperature of wax manipulation, J.A.D.A. 41:28, 1950.
27. Hollenback, G. M.: A study of the behavior of pattern wax, J. S. Calif. Dent. Assoc. 27:298, 1959.
28. Hollenback, G. M.: A report on the comparative accuracy of three methods commonly used in the production of dental castings, J. S. Calif. Dent. Assoc. 30:249, 1962.
29. Hollenback, G. M.: Simple technique for accurate castings: new and original method of vacuum investing, J.A.D.A. 36:391, 1948.
30. Coleman, R. L.: Physical properties of dental materials, National Bureau of Standards, Research Paper No. 32, Washington, D. C., 1928, U. S. Government Printing Office.
31. Hollenback, G. M., and Skinner, E. W.: Shrinkage during castings of gold and gold alloys, J.A.D.A. 33:1391, 1946.
32. Phillips, D. W.: Present day precision inlay investing and casting technique, J.A.D.A. 24:1470, 1937.
33. Ryge, G., and Fairhurst, C. W.: Hygroscopic expansion, J. Dent. Res. 35:498, 1956.
34. Leinfelder, K. F., Fairhurst, C. W., and Ryge, G.: Porosities in dental gold castings. II. Effects of mold temperature, sprue size and dimension of wax pattern, J.A.D.A. 67:816, 1963.
35. Bales, D. J.: An evaluation of castings made to refractory dies, M.S.D. thesis, Indianapolis, 1972, Indiana University School of Dentistry.
36. Norman, R. D., Swartz, M. L., and Phillips, R. W.: Additional studies on the solubility of certain dental materials, J. Dent. Res. 30:1928, 1959.
37. Stibbs, G. D.: Operative procedure for gold inlays, J. Prosth. Dent. 3:267, 1953.
38. Boyd, D. A.: Sophomore manual for operative dentistry, Indianapolis, 1966, Indiana University School of Dentistry.
39. Shooshan, E. D.: A pinledge casting technique—its application in periodontal splinting, Dent. Clin. N. Am., Mar., 1960, pp. 189-206.

ADDITIONAL READINGS

Arbo, M. A.: A simple technique for castings with pin retention, Dent. Clin. N. Am., Jan., 1970, p. 19.

Baum, L., and Contino, R. M.: Ten years of experience with cast pin restorations, Dent. Clin. N. Am., Jan., 1970, p. 81.

Courtade, G. L.: Methods for pin splinting the lower anterior teeth, Dent. Clin. N. Am., 1970, p. 3.

Lund, M. R., and Shryock, E. F.: Castings made directly to refractory dies, J. Prosth. Dent. 18:251, 1967.

Rosner, D.: Function placement and reproduction of bevels for gold castings, J. Prosth Dent. 13:1160, 1963.

chapter 18

Ceramic restorations

COLOR

The esthetic considerations measuring success and acceptability in many segments of restorative dentistry weigh especially heavily when considering ceramics. Successful ceramics depends on the ability of the operator to create an esthetic restoration by beginning with some selected and refined materials and then forming them into a pleasing cosmetic result. A key feature to successful ceramics is understanding the influence of color. It is important for a dentist to be able to interpret and distinguish how apparently small differences will influence accuracy and patient appreciation, which are part of the criteria for success. The dentist must be very concerned with detail when attempting to establish a desirable appearance for a restoration.

The word "color" is a general term referring to the effects of light waves striking the retina of the eye. The gradation of color is called "hue." Hue is the characteristic that allows us to distinguish between colors; when we speak of red, green, yellow, blue, these are specifically different hues. Often the words "color" and "hue" are used interchangeably, but very often "color" is used to include hue plus other modifications.

After a hue is identified, one may wish to define its intensity or strength; the characteristic that does this is "chroma." An example would be the hue called pink, which is in effect a low chroma red.

The other feature needed to complete the cycle is termed "value." Value is the amount of gray or white included in a color system, and this is what gives us lightness or darkness. Value has a high and low range. Of the features mentioned, value is by far the most important dimension in dental restorations. This is what makes the restoration appear natural or artificial in the mouth. When observing natural dentition, we may see variations in hues and yet it will appear natural; but if the value varies, the results are not as esthetic. Value is what gives the appearance of vitality.

The higher the value, or the more toward white, the more noticeable is the brilliance of the restoration. If the value is too high, the restoration will appear unnatural and its value should be reduced. If the value is too low, emphasizing the gray, the restoration will appear dull or devital. This is difficult to modify. It is much easier to reduce value than to increase it.

Shade selection and laboratory prescription

One of the most significant aspects of the ceramic restoration involves the directions given to the ceramist. He must receive as complete a picture as possible to help produce an esthetic restoration.

The dentist should secure several available ceramic shade guides to aid in shade selection. Included should be the Lumin Vacuum* shade guide, since more selection may be made from it than from any other currently available guide. The selection should be made under the best possible conditions. The most reliable lighting to use is daylight; the northern exposure is ideal. Many times there will be only an artificial light source, and there are now available fluorescent lights color-corrected for daylight that work very well. It is also best if the ceramist has good quality lighting. The unit or operating light should not be used during shade selection.

Shade selection should not be influenced by bright and distracting environmental colors such as a bright or multicolored wall. The patient's towel should not be a bright color. Lipstick should not be excessive, since it and brightly colored clothing may also influence the selection.

The tooth to be matched should be free of metal restorations to avoid this distracting influence. It may be necessary to relate to an adjacent or opposite tooth for reliability.

Several shade tabs that appear to relate reasonably well should be quickly selected and then eliminated one by one to arrive at the proper selection. The guide and the tooth should be moistened when making a selection.

Validation of the shade should be made by quick glances. One should not stare at the tooth and tab since color fatigue takes place quickly, causing a shift in the shade impression. The initial view is likely to be the most accurate. The shade should be observed at close range and at arm's length; it is also helpful to have an assistant check from several feet away. Some dentists may be color-blind and may need to train and depend upon an assistant to confirm a shade.

The patient should not be actively involved in selection of shades, since he does not have the background and training necessary to accurately make the proper selection. There are times when the patient can be shown what has been selected, though when this is done it is sometimes best to show first a tab that is not quite acceptable so that the patient may see the difference.

For some difficult color matching problems it is necessary to divide the tooth into three shade areas and consider each part individually. When neces-

---

*Available from Unitek Corporation, Monrovia, California.

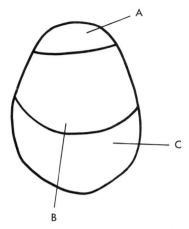

Fig. 18-1. A suggestion of a diagram to indicate to the ceramist the color scheme of a tooth. **A,** Gingival areas; **B,** midportion of tooth; **C,** incisal segment.

sary a separate shade may be designated for the gingival middle and incisal areas.

All information that will be of help to a ceramist must be accurately recorded on the prescription blank. The prescription should be made in duplicate for purpose of record and reference. The directions must be specific. Diagrams may be used to help the ceramist visualize the requirements; this includes check lines and stain areas (Fig. 18-1).

In addition to a detailed prescription, the ceramist should also receive adequate models to serve as guides. This may include an original study model as well as a wax corrected model. It is important when planning treatment for a patient requiring several ceramic crowns to give consideration to tooth position and alignment. When modification of the given alignment is advisable, it is good procedure to produce those changes on a working study model so that both the operator and the patient will have an idea as to expected result. This also becomes a valuable aid for the ceramist.

PORCELAIN FOR ESTHETICS

It has been traditional that those doing operative dentistry are concerned with the stability of the restorations being placed. Dependable restorations will reliably maintain the teeth in their best functioning position, which includes their occlusal and tissue relationships.

The esthetic features of restorations are continually of interest, but they often have had secondary importance because of materials limitations. In recent years, patients have become concerned and explicit in their expectations for acceptable esthetic results in their dental treatment. For this reason, patients are becoming more resistant to metallic restorations in locations where appearance is a sensitive concern. So among the available types of restorations, ceramics is used more and more to satisfy the demands for esthetics.

The major advantages of fused porcelain are its lifelike appearance and low conductivity to thermal change. Properly glazed porcelain is compatible with gingival tissue and is not subject to color change.

The disadvantage with ceramics is the difficulty of producing margins that are as acceptable as those possible with other materials. Any adjustment of ceramic margins in the mouth is done at the expense of the ceramic finish, so it is hoped the restoration can be accurately processed and placed without adjustment. The disparity between tooth and ceramic material may cause a clinical difficulty with the cementing material, with a possible cement line.

CLASS V PORCELAIN INLAY

There has been greater utilization of fused porcelain for inlays since the development of high heat refractory investments. Previously it was mandatory to use a platinum matrix for processing the porcelain. It requires expert manipulation of the platinum foil to minimize the potential space between the completed restoration and margins of the preparation, and the possibility of wrinkles in the platinum would exaggerate any discrepancy. The high heat investment allowed for elimination of the platinum matrix and improved the marginal accuracy. It is relatively easy to manipulate the porcelain, and its condensation occurs more readily as moisture passes through it and into the investment, producing a high density porcelain.

For an investment to function properly it must be able to withstand the processing temperature without deterioration. The essential ingredients are a form of silica, a bonding agent of gypsum, and a stable pigment material—for example, ferrous oxide—to allow a contrasting color while condensing the porcelain. The particle size must be fine to permit smooth adherence to mold walls.

Fused porcelain will be used most frequently as an inlay for Class V lesions. Other common options for that location include amalgam, resin, gold foil, and gold inlay. The least acceptable esthetic results are obtained by amalgam. The technical procedures with gold discourage its use, and the esthetic values are questioned. A resin product is often used, since it is convenient and esthetic. Unfortunately it becomes misused, since it requires adherence to exacting procedures for success. It is not entirely color stable with the passing of time and abrades easily. So it is possible that a porcelain inlay is the best option when considering esthetics and stability.

Shade selection

The initial consideration when planning a porcelain inlay is selection of shade. The most appropate shade guide is the "New Hue" guide, which includes several of the low and medium fusing porcelains. Since the problem is located in the gingival third of the tooth, shade selection is not as critical as for an entire tooth surface.

Each time a bottle of porcelain powder is purchased, a color tab should be processed for verification of its actual color, and, if convenient, that can function as a shade tab. When actually selecting the shade, the operatory should have as much daylight as possible. The shade tab and the tooth in question should be moistened. The process of elimination is often used to arrive at the desired shade. Color fatigue takes place rapidly, so observations should be done in a fleeting manner to minimize this fatigue. If using a conventional shade tab, the middle portion of the tab should be used for a reliable color selection.

Preparation

The Class V porcelain inlay does not follow a rigid style, location, or outline pattern. Its dimensions are governed by the extent of caries, abrasion faults, or previous defective restoration. Because of the location of these defects, the gingival margin will usually be positioned below the level of the free gingiva. The essential criterion is that the extension must include any weakness in the existing enamel structure or the extent of abrasion and erosion.

The preparation is similar to a gold inlay. The major difference with porcelain is the need to avoid sharp angles in outline form. It must not be specifically round, since this would create a difficulty of orientation during cementation. The walls of the preparation must diverge slightly from the pulpal wall. There should be no undermined enamel remaining and there must be no beveling of the cavosurface. If the preparations are small, the pulpal walls should remain flat; larger preparations should be slightly convex (Fig. 18-2).

The depth of the preparation must be greater than that for amalgam or gold foil. The retention of a porcelain inlay depends on proper depth and on gingival and incisal walls that are nearly parallel but that diverge enough to allow placement of the inlay. Porcelain is not as tolerant of deviations in preparations as gold.

When the high-speed handpiece is used, a No. 70 bur is the best choice to outline the preparation and supply the proper angulation to the walls. If slow speed is used, a No. 701 bur is effective to finalize the outline and direction of the walls.

The need for hand instrumentation is minimal. A curved chisel is used to plane the various walls and a hoe is utilized for smoothing the pulpal wall.

The impression tray may be very simple. A segment of a plastic bur box will perform very well for a single or two adjacent preparations. The tray must be rigid. If there are several preparations involved, it is best to make a costume tray of acrylic. The tray should cover the labial surface and be painted with the adhesive required for a polysulfide or silicone rubber material.

When required, gingival retraction is accomplished to make the margin accessible. One of several chemically impregnated strings properly placed will achieve this.

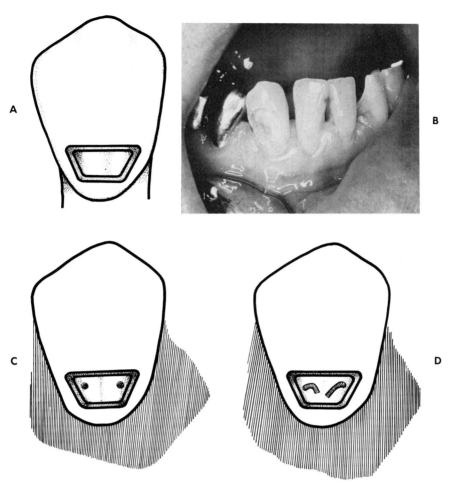

Fig. 18-2. A, Diagram for Class V porcelain inlay preparation. **B,** Preparation for Class V porcelain inlay. **C,** When retention is questionable, a 0.024 inch drill is used to drill pin holes to a minimum depth of 1.5 mm. **D,** The pins used for added retention may be P.G.P. wire (J. M. Ney Co., Bloomfield, Conn.) or they may be cast from a plastic bristle of a palladium gold alloy. **(B** from Health Information Systems: Dentistry for the '70's, New York, 1971.)

An impression syringe with a small plastic tip is used to obtain a rubber impression of a Class V inlay preparation. The amount of impression material required will be small, but it must be well mixed to ensure proper polymerization. Care is taken while extruding the material into the preparation to be sure there is not any air trapped near the walls or margins of the preparation. This problem is more crucial with porcelain than with gold. The tray is then positioned over the tooth and impression material (Fig. 18-3). An additional precaution should be to limit the impression material exclusively to the labial surface. If the proximal embrasures are open, it is best to block them with wax

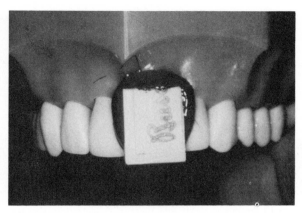

Fig. 18-3. An impression tray in position over polysulfide rubber. (From Kinzer, R.: J. Prosth. Dent. **14**:980, 1964.)

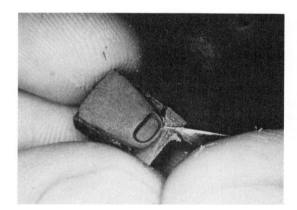

Fig. 18-4. A porcelain investment die trimmed to size. (From Health Information Systems: Dentistry for the '70's, New York, 1971.)

to prevent impression material from forming a lock on the lingual surface of the teeth. It is necessary to remove the impression in a facial direction. Conventional zinc oxide–eugenol preparations may be used for temporary restorations, though the removal may be inconvenient. Dura-Seal, by Reliance Company, is useful for this purpose, since it remains soft and is easily removed.

Laboratory procedures

The impression is boxed with wax to keep it small. A porcelain inlay investment is used to fill the impression. Loma Linda Porcelain Inlay Investment is preweighed for convenience. The mixture as recommended is thin to help prevent formation of bubbles, which is critical in so small an area.

It is best to separate the inlay die in an hour's time to allow for ease in

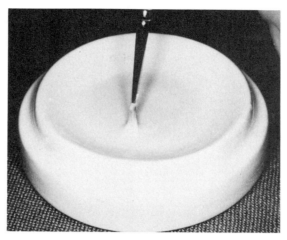

Fig. 18-5. A creamy thickness of porcelain and distilled water for use with a porcelain inlay. (From Health Information Systems: Dentistry for the '70's, New York, 1971.)

trimming the model. The model must also be trimmed to reduce it to a size small enough for handling in the oven (Fig. 18-4). After separating the die from the impression, the impression is repoured into an improved stone, which will provide a model on which the completed inlay may be tried.

The investment model must be prefired in the porcelain oven at the proper temperature. This reduces impurities that may be present and removes the moisture in the binder.

The equipment needed for baking will be small sable brushes 000 to 00000, a segment of a razor blade mounted in a wooden handle, absorbent tissue paper, two porcelain dishes for water and porcelain, distilled water in a squeeze bottle, and a porcelain spatula to help with vibration. Low fusing porcelain is used (for example, Ceramco 1600) that matches the middle third of the "New Hue" shade guide. The porcelain oven need not be expensive, since it does not require a high fusing muffle.

Baking the inlay. Before adding porcelain, the model is soaked with distilled water. The porcelain is mixed to a creamy texture to allow adaptation to cavity details (Fig. 18-5) and added with the brush to avoid damage to margins. The underside of the model is blotted with tissue as the porcelain is added. For the initial baking, the preparation is filled even with the margins, not beyond them (Fig. 18-6). This is accomplished by washing a small sable brush and carefully removing any porcelain that may extend onto the surface of the tooth. Moisture is removed repeatedly and blotted to ensure good condensation. Vibration will also help ensure condensation. Before the porcelain dries, it is scored with the razor blade to create four sections. This controls the shrinkage of the porcelain and prevents it from easily pulling away from the margins.

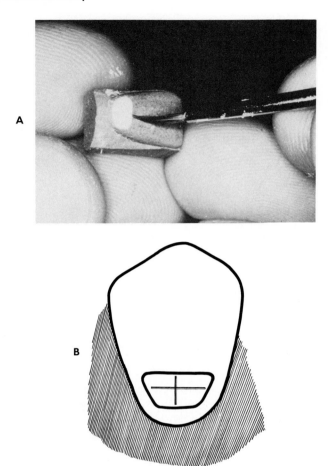

Fig. 18-6. A, A moistened sable brush used to clear porcelain from the die surface. **B,** Scoring the porcelain with a razor blade prior to first baking. (**A** from Health Information Systems: Dentistry for the '70's, New York, 1971.)

The oven is preheated to 1,000° F. and the model is placed inside close to the open door, or barely inside the muffle, for 5 minutes, to allow for drying of the model and porcelain. The door is closed and the temperature increased to 1,625° F. at 100° per minute, after which the model is removed and cooled. The shrinkage of the porcelain will be apparent, but since the additional volume of porcelain will be small, further shrinkage will not be readily noticed.

In preparation for the second baking, the model is saturated with distilled water. Wet porcelain is again added with a brush and the surface is slightly overcontoured. Condensation is accomplished by systematic blotting with tissue paper. After adding the porcelain the margins are carefully cleared. The model is dried slowly and placed into the oven following the same procedure as before.

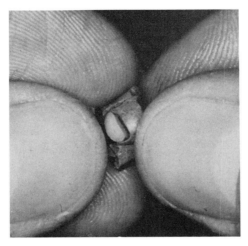

Fig. 18-7. Separating the completed inlay from the die. (From Kinzer, R.: J. Prosth. Dent. **14:** 980, 1964.)

If required for contour, the addition of porcelain is repeated a third time. When the temperature of 1,625° F. is reached again, it is held for 1 or 2 minutes to glaze the surface and then the porcelain is cooled. The baking process should be accomplished in as few times as possible to prevent overcuring of the porcelain.

Separating the inlay from the investment is best done over a bowl of water, since the inlay is small and easy to lose. The investment is separated by hand pressure (Fig. 18-7). A coarse toothbrush is helpful in scrubbing the investment from the inlay. If additional effort is required, small mounted stones or unmounted sandpaper disks may be used to hand rub the investment from the inlay. Metal instruments should not be used since they will leave gray marks on the porcelain. An ultrasonic cleaner is also helpful for removing investment.

If any porcelain excess appears at the periphery of the inlay, it may be reduced by a handheld mounted stone or sandpaper disk.

To check the inlay, the walls of the preparation in the stone model are penciled. The inlay is luted to the end of an instrument and inserted into the penciled preparation (Fig. 18-8). Any discrepancies present will leave a mark on the inlay, and they may be reduced by a small mounted stone. This completes the inlay.

Cementation

A suggested cementing medium would be the Justi-Resin cement or a silica phosphate "Floro Thin," by S. S. White. The resin cement polymerizes very rapidly, so the working time is very short. Regardless of which cementing medium is used, it is mixed and placed into the preparation, and the inlay,

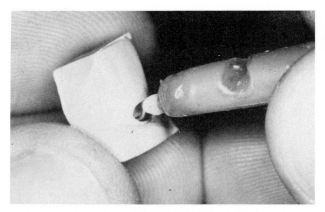

Fig. 18-8. Seating the porcelain inlay into the penciled stone die. (From Health Information Systems: Dentistry for the '70's, New York, 1971.)

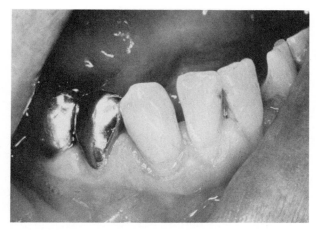

Fig. 18-9. A cemented Class V porcelain inlay on cuspid. (From Health Information Systems: Dentistry for the '70's, New York, 1971.)

which is attached to a plastic instrument, is seated. An orangewood stick used with a vibratory action helps to position the inlay and extrude the excess cement. After setting, the excess cement is removed. However, if a resin is used the excess should be cleared away immediately.

In the event that a margin must be adjusted, a small white gem stone may be used lightly at that portion of the margin. A small felt or leather wheel impregnated by levigated aluminum is helpful in polishing places where the glaze has been disturbed. The esthetic results with this restoration should be satisfactory to the patient and the operator (Fig. 18-9).

Before forwarding the master cast with the preparation to the laboratory, the die margins should be inspected. If there is a question as to the designation of those margins, the dentist should trim the die to accurately locate the margins, for it is his responsibility to forward reliable information to those who provide technical help.

PORCELAIN BONDED TO METAL RESTORATIONS

Historically, many who have requested dental treatment have been concerned with the appearance of their restorations. This concern is expressed most often regarding the anterior teeth. For many years the dental profession was unable to satisfy this esthetic concern. However, recent developments have improved the dentist's ability to meet some of the esthetic needs, and patients now can expect to obtain cosmetic satisfaction from their dental restorations.

As long as the problem is confined to a single surface of the anterior teeth, there are options utilizing silicate, unfilled resins, composites, and direct gold that may effectively restore the defect and retain desirable esthetics. (However, some of these materials do not remain visually acceptable over a long period of time.)

When the problem becomes enlarged or if the incisal angle is involved, it is desirable to use a casting to maintain form and function. Often this does not offer desirable esthetics. Traditionally, when the problem exceeds the single surface the porcelain jacket crown is employed. This produces the most predictable and desirable esthetic result.

Pulpal and gingival anatomy

Of great concern during diagnosis is the proximity of the pulpal anatomy. The radiographic interpretation is important to ascertain the location of the pulpal horns. If these horns extend widely to the mesial and distal surfaces, it decreases the possibility of using a bonded restoration. If the pulpal chamber extends toward the labial direction, the crown preparation may cause near or possible exposures; this is more noticeable with teeth that have a pronounced incisal curvature. If treatment is essential in spite of an undesirable pulpal location, it may be best to treat the tooth endodontically before proceeding. This is a reason why this restoration is attempted on young people with reservations.

The age of the patient should also be considered in regard to the location of the labial margin. Through the teenage years the clinical crown becomes more exposed, with the free gingiva tending to settle in an apical direction. Because of this shift it is difficult to place the labial margin to an esthetic advantage and expect this relationship to the gingiva to remain static. The parameters for success with a porcelain crown are limited. The porcelain always requires an adequate and even bulk throughout the restoration, and on many teeth this is not possible. Where occlusal forces are excessive, porcelain does not have the needed physical properties for success, since it is brittle and does not perform well under tensile and shear stress. Thus short clinical crowns and heavy occlusal forces reduce the possibilities for success with porcelain jacket crowns. An alternate method for full-crown coverage utilizes a heat cured resin material. This would either be in the form of a complete resin crown or a metal casting with a resin veneer. A major disadvantage to this material is that it does not have adequate wear resistance while in the mouth, and frequently the color stability is not adequate.

The ability to bond porcelain to metal creates a greater versatility for using ceramics as an esthetic solution for several types of problems. With the porcelain bonded to a metal base, the incidence of ceramic fracture is reduced. It is then possible to use this where a porcelain jacket would be a great risk. This allows free use of the restoration with destroyed incisal angles, accidental fractures, esthetic problems because of caries, and discoloration as a result of endodontics. It also allows for an orthodontic result with teeth that may be slightly malaligned. Since the preparation does not require any more lingual reduction than does a gold casting, it allows for more possibilities in developing retentive requirements.

The dentist must be very specific in selecting shades for a bonded restoration, since there is no possibility of modifying the shade after its completion, which is one of the advantages of the porcelain jacket crown.

Preparation of maxillary central incisor

To facilitate the preparation of a bonded crown, the operatory should be arranged as conveniently as possible. The reduction calls for use of high-speed instrumentation. The efficient use of auxiliary personnel minimizes the time required for the procedure and is less taxing on the operator.

The patient will require anesthesia for the reduction procedures. Any time high-speed reduction takes place with diamond instruments, an adequate water coolant should be utilized. This is helpful in maintaining control over the pulpal environment. It is also important in maintaining the cutting efficiency of the diamond instrument since the water functions as a lubricant. An additional advantage is that the water spray and subsequent evacuation tend to suppress the odor caused by debris and the effects of tooth reduction.

It is not possible to relate a specific diamond instrument to a specific procedure unless the discussion involves a single manufacturer of that instrument. At this time nomenclature of diamonds is indicated by the various manufacturers. A numbering system does exist for diamonds but currently it is not routinely employed.

Incisal reduction. An initial guide cut is made into the incisal edge of the tooth enamel to establish the depth of the necessary reduction, or removal of the enamel. This cut may be made either with a small wheel or a bullet-nosed tapered diamond stone (Fig. 18-10). It is best to do a cut to quickly determine the amount required for removal, for if the reduction takes place gradually over

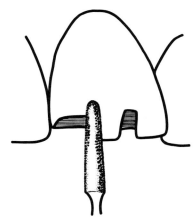

Fig. 18-10. Incisal guide cut and reduction with a diamond instrument.

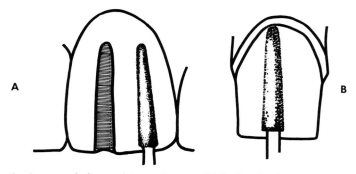

Fig. 18-11. A, A tapered diamond is used to establish the depth of reduction for the facial surface. **B,** A tapered bullet nosed diamond is used to accomplish most of the labial and interproximal reduction.

the incisal edge it is easy to lose orientation and to remove excessive tooth structure. At least a 2 mm. reduction of incisal enamel is needed to allow room to develop the restoration. When the length of clinical crown allows, it is helpful to reduce the incisal enamel beyond 2 mm. to provide leeway for developing the cosmetic appearance. After the incisal guide cut is made, the enamel is reduced to the level of the guide.

Labial reduction. Removal of the labial enamel follows the format for incisal reduction. The initial or guide cut is made with a tapered bullet-nosed diamond stone. The cut is made in the central portion of the labial surface near the gingival level by depressing the instrument to the level of the contemplated completed preparation (Fig. 18-11). It is good to keep in mind that once the labial depth is established, the incisal curvature of the tooth may require that the diamond be utilized at a different angle at the incisal portion to maintain depth uniformity. This guide cut may be done at the same time as the incisal cut or subsequent to it. The diamond stone used should be selected on the basis of tooth size and ease of handling. The minimal axial depth required to accommodate the casting and the porcelain is 1.5 mm.; this will assure adequate thickness of porcelain needed for esthetics.

The gingival boundary is marked by a heavy and definite chamfer, which in most cases will be made by the diamond stone.

The labial reduction is then made. During the early stages the finish line is carried to the gingival boundary, with final location to be established later. This labial reduction is carried into the embrasure area and the normal contact area. (This assumes the tooth has a normal position in the arch form.) The heavy chamfer must develop in this manner to allow proper thickness of porcelain for esthetics.

Interproximal reduction. For this step a thin tapered diamond stone is used to avoid abrading the adjacent tooth and to avoid overcutting the preparation (Fig. 18-12). The interproximal finish line terminates part way into the free gingival sulcus. The interproximal walls are tapered to develop proper resistance form for the restoration.

Lingual reduction. The same diamond stone used in the interproximal reduction may be used to reduce and position the lingual margins, or a slightly larger diameter diamond instrument may be used to produce the marginal finish. The tooth is reduced to allow replacement of the enamel by metal without overcontouring the restoration. While not considered mandatory for all cases, the margin will usually terminate in the gingival sulcus with a penetration of 0.5 to 1 mm. The degree of chamfer would be the same as for a three-fourths crown restoration. There must be a definable margin, and the metal must have adequate rigidity to prevent flexion of the restoration. When possible the lingual margin should surround the cingulum, leaving as much of the cingulum as possible for good resistance form.

The lingual fossa and part of the cingulum are reduced to allow for thickness of metal and, if space exists, for a partial overlay of porcelain (Fig. 18-13). Where function is not involved, the minimum reduction would be 0.5 mm.; where occlusal contact does take place, it should be 1 mm. The cingulum should retain as much of its height as possible. Cingulum reduction may be made by a small wheel diamond, though an egg shaped instrument that will produce proper reduction where needed is preferred. This instrument is not as likely to leave ridges in the preparation as the wheel diamond.

Labial chamfer. The preparation is almost complete. There remains only the final location of the labial margin and finishing of the tooth (Fig. 18-13).

The labial margin is located at the level of the gingival tissue. The objective now is to position the labial margin into the gingival sulcus. The preferred depth is half the distance into a healthy sulcus, which will be 0.5 to 1 mm. This should be done in such a way as to cause minimal distress to the gingival tissue. A

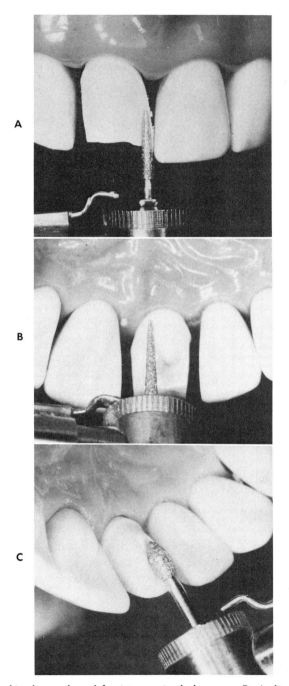

Fig. 18-12. A, A thin diamond used for interproximal clearance. **B,** A diamond instrument used to produce the lingual finish line. **C,** A diamond instrument effective for lingual reduction.

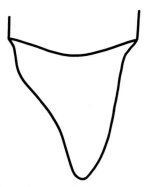

Fig. 18-13. Completed preparation contrasting the labial and lingual reduction.

bullet-nosed diamond stone must be selected that will stay within the confines of the chamfer area and properly locate this chamfer below tissue level.

A suggested method for protecting the tissue is for the assistant to use a flat blade instrument and, by segments, depress or reflect the tissue while the margin is brought to its proper location. Another method of displacing the tissue to give some space for the instruments is to use tissue retraction cord.

The tissue contour must function as a guide as the preparation proceeds toward the interproximal area. Unless caution is exercised, it is easy to over-depress the margin at the interproximal location. At times the labial margin is used as a depth guide for the interproximal margin, which results in damage to tissue and serious problems in properly restoring the interproximal portion of the preparation.

Finish of preparation. Personal preference will determine the degree of smoothness required of the finished prepared tooth. Part of this may be achieved by using finishing burs to remove the effects of the diamond instruments. Sandpaper and cuttle disks are also useful in producing a smooth surface (Fig. 18-14).

A regular excavator can be used to smooth the labial chamfer area by employing the cutting end on the preparation. The side of the excavator may be used to smooth the labial and interproximal portions of the preparation.

The degree of smoothness required will be based on personal preferences. If the prepared tooth is too smooth, cementation effectiveness may be lost. The tooth should not be left in a completely roughened condition, but the degree of smoothness may vary.

The prepared tooth is now available for any impression. The procedures for making the impression are discussed in Chapter 17.

The dentist then arranges that his ceramist has the best possible models and information from which to fabricate a desirable restoration. If a dentist elects to do his own laboratory work, he is referred to technical bulletins or a crown and bridge text.

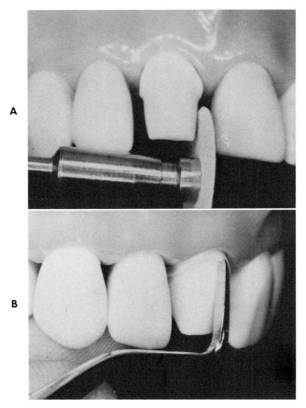

Fig. 18-14. A, A sandpaper disk used to smooth the preparation. **B,** An excavator used to smooth the chamfer portion of the preparation.

Temporary restoration

If the prepared tooth is in the anterior segment of the mouth, careful attention must be given to the temporary restoration. An alginate impression may be taken prior to beginning any reduction. The impression should be stable when again it is positioned in the mouth, and it is kept moist in a paper towel until needed.

An acrylic material designed for making temporary restorations is mixed to a thick, creamy consistency and placed into the alginate impression where needed. The acrylic, at this texture, will have a shiny surface; when the shine disappears the impression is positioned accurately in the mouth. A segment of the material is held in the hand to determine the rate of reaction. The cool moisture in the impression will cause a delay in setting. When it is determined that the acrylic is firm but not yet set, the alginate impression is withdrawn, leaving the acrylic on the tooth.

As the temporary restoration becomes firm, it should be partially removed

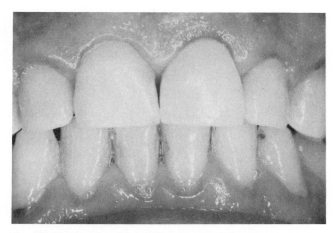

Fig. 18-15. Completed bonded restoration following cementation.

from the tooth to assure withdrawal and then reseated. When polymerization is completed, the restoration is adjusted to the tooth. The most significant part is the relationship of the margins and the comfort for occlusion. The margins should be adapted to have adequate coverage but should avoid surface roughness and overhangs. If the temporary restoration is irritating, it may cause gingival distress with possible recession of the gingiva.

If required, additional acrylic may be added to provide proper form. It may be necessary to adjust the form by using disks or burs. The surface should be smooth, to avoid irritating the gingival tissue or tongue.

The color selected for the temporary restoration should not be a perfect match with the adjacent teeth, since it may predispose to problems if the final restoration is that well matched.

The temporary restoration is cemented with a material that will allow for ease of removal when desired. This may include mixing Vaseline with zinc oxide–eugenol or using materials employed for periodontal packs. There are also commercial materials used for temporary cementation. The gingival crevice must be checked for excess cement and occlusion verified before the patient is dismissed.

Cementation of restoration

Most patients will need anesthesia when the temporary restoration is removed. After removal of the temporary restoration, all the cement must also be carefully cleaned away. The permanent restoration is then fitted to its proper place. It may be necessary to make adjustments at contacts or to make slight variations in morphology to make the restoration appear natural. This may require that the restoration be reglazed. If the adjustment is on the lingual portion or is not of great consequence, the restoration may be refined using a fine heatless stone and then abrasive rubber wheels for a smooth surface, followed by polishing using levigated alumina. The margins must check out and be reliable. The contour of the restoration at the gingiva must not impinge upon the gingival tissue (Fig. 18-15).

Cementation is accomplished in the same manner as for routine castings. The selection of a cement will vary depending upon the preference of the operator. A final check should be made to see that the contacts and the gingival crevice are free of excess cement.

ADDITIONAL READINGS

Ceramco Color System, Ceramco Equipment Corporation, Long Island City, New York.

Johnston, J. F., Mumford, G., and Dykema, R. W.: Modern practice in dental ceramics, Philadelphia, 1967, W. B. Saunders Co.

Johnston, J. F., Phillips, R. W., and Dykema, R. W.: Modern practice in crown and bridge prosthodontics, Philadelphia, 1971, W. B. Saunders Co.

Kinzer, R. L.: Porcelain inlays fabricated with a new high heat refractory investment, J. Prosth. Dent. 14:980, 1964.

Kinzer, R. L., Bonlie, D., and Mertz, K.: Preliminary report: high heat investments in constructing porcelain restorations, J. S. Calif. Dent. Assoc. 30:314, 1962.

Lund, M. R.: Esthetics as influenced by porcelain bonded to gold alloy restorations, New York, 1972, Health Information Systems.

Lund, M. R.: Present day techniques for the porcelain inlay, New York, 1972, Health Information Systems.

Myerson, R. L., and Dogon, I. L.: The rate of the porcelain inlay in restorative dentistry, Bioceramics Engineering in Medicine, Symposium No. 2 (part 2), pp. 405-441, 1972.

Shell, J. S., and Nielsen, J. P.: Study of the bond between gold alloys and porcelain, J. Dent. Res. 41:1424, 1962.

Warnick, M. E., and Morrison, K. N.: Indirect technique for making porcelain inlays, J. Prosth. Dent. 11:948, 1961.

chapter 19

Maintenance of the teeth and practical preventive measures

Dental health depends on the care given by the office team, patient, and health agencies. It in turn affects the general health status of the individual. Restorative and periodontic treatment must be supplemented with daily care by the patient and periodic visits to the dentist. Frequent toothbrushing and regular dental appointments every 6 months or 1 year help preserve the natural dentition. Good patient hygiene and preventive dental care create optimal conditions for the teeth.

The term "preventive dentistry" is often used to mean only early detection and prophylactic measures for eliminating dental caries. The term actually encompasses the entire area of dentistry that is devoted to the prevention of injury or disease to the teeth and related structures. In its proper context, preventive dentistry becomes a concept or philosophy that involves oral cancer, cavity preparation, prosthetic replacements, diet analysis, community programs, and any other program that can eliminate or minimize dental problems.[1] Preventive concepts are used in the areas of diagnosis and treatment. The preventive methods for supporting restorative treatment are presented in this chapter.

The literature reporting preventive measures has been extensive, and as a result there has been a significant reduction in many types of dental diseases.[2] Although it appears that the clean tooth does not decay, this is only part of the program. The influence of the diet at various ages is not clearly established; although the fluorides, phosphates, and other measures reduce the incidence of caries, the problem is not completely eliminated. To survey the literature and advocate a specific procedure for prevention of caries and maintenance of the teeth that would include all conditions is impossible. However, it is possible to offer suggestions and make general statements on how to achieve good oral hygiene.

It is accepted that dental caries begins on an external tooth surface. The following equation is presented as an aid in understanding the complex nature of the problem.[3]

Microorganisms + Suitable media = Harmful products
Harmful products + Susceptible surface = Dental caries

A number of factors influence each variable, creating a myriad of physiologic, biochemical, developmental, bacteriologic, and dietary problems in reducing dental caries.

To promote dental health one is advised to employ the hygienic principles of cleanliness. Whether there is caries reduction or not, toothbrushing improves the appearance of the periodontium and the teeth, reduces unpleasant odors and tastes, and removes some of the media that contribute to caries.[4] For these reasons cleaning the teeth is advocated as a caries-control measure. Hygienic measures should be used to keep the teeth clean and free of foodstuff, plaque, and stain. The methods used to accomplish this are described as home care measures or oral physiotherapy.[5] Hygiene is advocated as an adjunct to fluoride treatment to create the best possible oral environment.[6]

HOME CARE PROCEDURES

To maintain oral hygiene the patient must use home care procedures regularly. The most important aspect of oral hygiene is to keep the teeth clean by brushing and rinsing following consumption of food. The foodstuffs should be removed before bacterial enzymes form acid on tooth surfaces that subsequently decalcifies the enamel.

Devices used to clean the teeth are manual and electric toothbrushes, interdental stimulators, and dental floss or dental tape. Tissue health is maintained by removing the causes of disease; these devices can be used in a number of ways for this purpose.

Toothbrushing

The teeth are cleaned by brushing with bristles that contain an abrasive. Only the accessible tooth surfaces can be brushed; they include the buccal or labial and lingual, the occlusal, and a portion of the proximal surface.

The aims of toothbrushing are listed as follows[4]:

1. It should remove all food debris, accumulations of microorganisms, and recently deposited, uncalcified supragingival calculus from the teeth.
2. It should dislodge collections of food, debris, and accumulations of microorganisms from the interproximal spaces below the contact areas and between the teeth.
3. It should gently massage the gingival tissues to promote a good blood supply and adequate keratinization of epithelium.
4. It should not irritate or lacerate the gingival tissues.

The design of the toothbrush naturally influences the effectiveness of the cleaning. The type of bristles, their arrangement, and the size of the brush head influence the contact that is made with the tooth surfaces. The differences in design are notable, sometimes causing patients to become confused when purchasing a toothbrush. The problems of obtaining and standardizing natural bristles have led to increased use of plastic bristles. The stiffness of the plastic bristles is graded by the diameter of the fiber. The brush selected should not produce excessive gingival massage.

The acceptable brush has a semirigid handle 6 inches long with a head 1 inch long.[4] The size of this brush head does not prevent placing it in various positions in the oral cavity, so it is effective in getting the bristles to the teeth. The use of the toothbrush varies. Commonly, the Bass and Roll techniques are taught with the soft-rounded bristle brush. (A description of these techniques may be found in periodontic textbooks.) Brochures should be obtained to reinforce the oral hygiene procedures presented to the patient.[7,8] Most hygiene programs include use of the toothbrush, dental floss, and rinsing. The brochure is retained by the patient for periodic review and should contain recommendations to combat the specific cleaning problems evident with the patient.

A study including 470 young individuals for 46 months showed that practice of effective oral hygiene improved the health of the supporting tissues.[9] Plaque and hard deposit scores with less loss of epithelial attachment were found in the groups that received instruction in toothbrushing and preventive treatments.

The toothbrush must be charged with some type of abrasive before the enamel surface can be cleaned effectively. There are a number of dentifrices available that are effective for cleaning; some have therapeutic value, which will be mentioned later in the chapter. The abrasives in dentifrices are calcium phosphate or calcium carbonate; these should not severely abrade the tooth.[10] The toothpastes are recommended for regular care because they are not considered as traumatic as the powders. Occasionally tooth powders can be used to improve the appearance of the teeth if staining is a problem.

Electric toothbrushes. Recently many automatically powered toothbrushes have been manufactured and are being used for home care measures. They have been evaluated in many studies, and like other areas of oral hygiene, the results are conflicting. There are points to be considered before they are prescribed for individual patients. Studies have shown that automatic toothbrushes are not harmful and that they can be used to promote the health of the gingival tissue and to clean the teeth.[11-12]

The Council on Dental Therapeutics of the American Dental Association has stated that "the brushes for these devices will require many of the same general characteristics that are desirable for the hand toothbrush such as durability, inexpensiveness, ability to be readily cleaned and aerated."[13] Bristle specifications and the shape of the brush should be adapted to the motion and power characteristics of each individual toothbrush. The Council also stated that "it is of the opinion that these devices must be evaluated individually."

The Council on Dental Therapeutics has recognized automatic toothbrushes as having the potential for producing superior oral hygiene.[13] They are quick to point out, however, that it is still recognized that the regular brush, when manipulated properly, is an effective cleaning device. In cases where limited mental ability or manual skill prevents proper brushing, the automatic devices should prove valuable.

The studies have not proved whether the automatic toothbrushes have any therapeutic value. Studies have been reported in which the devices caused a reduction in gingival inflammation, and other reports have shown that differences in hand brushing and electric brushing are not evident in dentally oriented subjects. It is recognized that hand and automatically powered toothbrushing are valuable in keeping the teeth clean and stimulating the soft oral tissue. One of these procedures must be used by the patient to remove food particles following meals. The convenience and attraction of electric toothbrushes should not be overlooked in considering them for children.

Dental floss

Plain dental floss or tape that is not coated with wax is helpful in cleaning the interproximal surfaces of the teeth, which cannot be reached with the toothbrush. The floss is a small silk or cotton thread that is placed between the proximal surface contact areas and below the gingival tissue to polish the enamel and remove food debris. The technique is done cautiously so as not to injure the tissue or the attachment. Dental floss is used at the end of each day to remove all material that brushing and oral rinsing have missed.

A 10 to 12 inch length of dental floss is wrapped around the index finger of each hand. While the patient stands in front of a mirror, he passes the dental floss slowly between the contact areas and into the embrasure between the gingiva and the tooth. The floss is taken to the bottom of the crevice and then it is slowly pulled toward the buccal or labial surface. This movement may be repeated several times on each proximal surface to remove the residual material and to polish the proximal enamel surface. The dentist uses the same procedure to remove the abrasive following prophylaxis, which is an ideal time for the technique to be demonstrated.

Dental floss should be used immediately following meals if there is a problem of food impaction. Gross accumulations of food are removed to prevent breakdown and acid formation or periodontal irritation. If food impaction persists, restoration of the proximal surfaces by building desirable contours may be advisable rather than using dental floss to correct the problem.

Proper use of dental floss is an adjunct to thorough brushing and is advocated as a routine home care measure. Dental floss is effective in cleaning around bridge abutments and pontics and the cervical margins of interproximal restorations.

Oral rinsing

Another method of cleaning the teeth is rinsing with water. Rinsing removes food debris, plaque, and bacteria after they are loosened with the toothbrush. It is also a precaution after eating when the brush cannot be used.

To rinse properly, 20 to 30 ml. of water (or a generous mouthful) is taken into the buccal or labial flanges. The water is forced through to the lingual side and returned. This procedure is repeated several times. The rinsing is done on both sides and in the anterior segment of the mouth.

Oral rinsing is beneficial in removing semifluid carbohydrates and it is considered a caries-control and hygienic measure. The effect of a single 20 ml. water rinse on the clearance of carbohydrates from the oral cavity has been studied.[14] In this study the mouths of patients were saturated with sugar. One half of the group rinsed with 20 ml. of water and the control group did not rinse at all. The results demonstrated sugar-free saliva in the group of patients who rinsed. The value of reducing the acid potential of the oral cavity with oral rinsing indicates that the procedure be used after toothbrushing and all meals as an adjunct to the other practices.

Interdental stimulators

Some patients need massage and stimulation of the interdental papillae. This is done with rubber stimulators and small wood pieces. This procedure is often advocated for the patient who has had periodontal surgery and has a larger tissue space open below the contact areas. The stimulators are pushed through the small opening numerous times to massage the soft tissue and to assist in plaque removal. This procedure is not a regular home care practice but is often prescribed by the periodontist for the patient who needs this type of stimulation.

OFFICE PROPHYLAXIS

The dentist does much to preserve the dentition and restorations by thorough and regular dental prophylaxis. This is done in the dental office on a regular basis by using the recall system. The patient should periodically receive a thorough scaling and polishing of the teeth. In addition this provides an opportunity to give an oral examination, take the necessary radiographs, update the individual medical record, give preventive treatments, and check the effectiveness of the patient's home care techniques.

The scaling procedure removes calcific deposits and food debris that serve as local periodontal irritants. Removal of calcium and plaque must be done in the dental office since the deposits form in areas that cannot be reached or observed by the patient. The time interval for this procedure is determined by the rate of calculus formation. Most patients are given appointments on a 6 month basis; however, some form deposits sooner and should be treated more frequently. For patients with exceptionally clean mouths a 1 year recall schedule is employed. The prophylaxis serves to support the efforts of the patient by removing stain and deposits that are missed in home care procedures. Restorative dentistry should not be done at the recall appointment and the patient should not leave the office with stain and calcium deposits on the teeth.

The oral prophylaxis is done cautiously and with good judgment, being certain to remove the entire calcium deposit with the scaling instruments without lacerating the gingival tissues. The polishing and stain removal are accomplished with a soft rubber cup, a commercial abrasive, and a slow-moving dental engine. The actual technique of prophylaxis can be found in the textbooks on periodontics. There is no conclusive evidence that clean teeth prevent caries, but the regular measures taken by the dentist and the patient are considered beneficial for many other reasons.

Patient instruction

Home care instructions are explained when the treatment plan is organized and presented. The value of good oral hygiene is demonstrated to the patient by using radiographs, models, and the patient's teeth. The philosophy behind thorough oral hygiene must first be established, and then the patient usually becomes motivated to follow the instructions of the presentation. The mechanisms of caries and periodontal disease are discussed to emphasize the necessity for a thorough program of oral hygiene.

Toothbrushing methods and the use of dental floss should be demonstrated on commercial models. Pointing out the shape of the teeth and the number of susceptible surfaces emphasizes the time and attention required for each aspect of the technique. The recommended procedure should be demonstrated initially and reemphasized at each recall appointment. An examination of the oral cavity will reveal the effectiveness of the individual's efforts. In many cases a reminder and review will be needed. A program of good oral hygiene is the best way the patient can protect his investment in professional dental care.[15,16]

DIET

An often overlooked factor related to dental health is the diet or nutrition of the patient. Childhood and adolescence are critical times because the diet influences tooth formation, calcification, and growth and development. The dentist must recommend a diet that supports sound body health. He serves his patients by detecting nutritional deficiencies, regulating the refined carbohydrate intake, and seeking the advice of a physician when problems are discovered or suspected. An adequate diet does not mean that sound body nutrition is assured if the foodstuff is not absorbed and assimilated, but problems of this nature can only be found by a thorough physical examination. Sound nutrition is necessary for the growth and development of the cells, the defense mechanisms, and the energy requirements of the body.

The National Dairy Council published a *Guide to Good Eating*[17] that is endorsed by the Council on Foods and Nutrition of the American Medical Association. Foodstuffs have been placed into four categories and the number of servings advocated daily from each group specified. This dietary plan is advised for children as well as adults. The groups and servings that are considered the basic daily requirements for the individual are as follows:

Group   I   (milk)—3 or more glasses for children; 4 or more glasses for teenagers; 2 or more glasses for adults

Group   II   (meat)—2 or more servings of meat, fish, poultry, eggs, or cheese; dry beans, peas, and nuts are alternates

Group   III   (vegetables and fruits)—4 or more servings of dark green or yellow vegetables and citrus fruit or tomatoes

Group   IV   (breads and cereals)—4 or more servings of enriched or whole grain; added milk improves nutritional values

These recommendations should be followed daily for a sound nutritional diet. Specific diets for nutritional disorders, metabolic diseases, and weight problems are provided by a physician. The effect of the diet on the incidence of caries has been studied, but the relationship is not clearly understood. There is little that the dentist can do about individual food selection at mealtime to alter the incidence of dental caries. Research indicates that the calcium : phosphorus ratio can be altered with carbohydrates to reduce caries at this time the use of the diet should done only by trained personnel.[18]

The dietary caries-control measure prescribed by the dentist is the regulation of between-meal carbohydrates consumed by the patient.[19] The frequency of snacks, including the adhering, sticky refined sugars, is known to affect the incidence of caries in the patient. The evidence is overwhelming that refined carbohydrates are altered by bacterial enzymes to form acid solutions that decalcify the tooth and contribute to the development of caries. Acid formation and decalcification of the inorganic apatite crystals of enamel are thought to initiate carious lesions.

When the frequency of sugar consumption (many polysaccharide, disaccharide, and monosaccharide carbohydrates) is increased, there is also an increase in the acid that is formed in the dental plaque on the tooth surface. The pH drops rapidly and the acid production only lasts a few minutes, making the frequency of sugar consumption an important factor in assisting decalcification. When the same amount of sugar is eaten with the meal, the caries incidence is not increased. Therefore, the only substantiated dietary caries-control measure is restricting the between-meal carbohydrates. The caries rate in different countries is proportional to the per capita consumption of sugar. In this regard the less civilized a population is, the lower the incidence of caries. The literature is exhaustive on the role of sugar in dental caries. In general the intake of carbohydrates is to be avoided.

Sugars obviously are not needed for energy metabolism if a basic diet is being followed. Excessive consumption of carbohydrates causes the essential foodstuffs in the diet, mainly proteins, to be neglected, and this could be harmful. The plans that have been worked out for controlling the diet of a child and advising the parent are a ʳˢeful in guiding the adult. It is reported that the average amount of sugar coₙₛ..ed in the United States is 163 teaspoons a week, and this value is used to evaluate the intake of patients. An analysis of the diet is made, both for meals and for snacks, by recording the food that is consumed. Charts are available for converting all the servings to teaspoons of sugar. In this way, by underscoring the caries-promoting foods, the patient is advised of the undesirable foodstuffs being consumed that encourage dental decay. Snacks and beverages with sugar are converted to items that do not assist in acid production in the oral cavity. The adult can readily observe how his dietary habits are contributing to the development of dental caries. Dietary analysis is indicated for the patient with rampant caries who is interested in saving his teeth.

Carbohydrate consumption is higher for the United States than any other country. Normal metabolism requires from 25 to 40 pounds of sugar per year for the child or the adult. The per capita consumption was reported to be over twice this number. Some children may be consuming their own weight in excess sugar.[20] Excessive sugar consumption contributes to obesity and lack of appetite, which causes poor food selection during the regular meal.

Plaque has been indicted as the media in which bacteria convert sugar to acid. Plaque forms on nearly all teeth. It is composed of a mucoid matrix, bacteria, and cells or debris. The material clings tenaciously to the tooth surface and is capable of forming lower acid concentrations than are present in the foodstuff or saliva.[21] The acid solution is then held in apposition with the enamel to remove calcium ions from the apatite crystal of enamel when the pH drops below 5.0 (Fig. 19-1).

The pH of plaque has been measured and is found to produce acid quickly

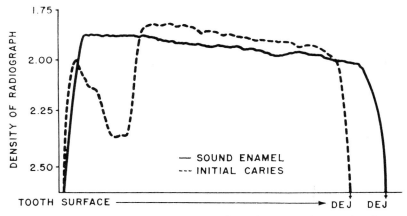

Fig. 19-1. Reduction in density of the radiograph from the external enamel surface would indicate a loss of mineral substance in the initial carious leison. (From Brudevold, F. J.: Chemical composition of the teeth in relation to caries. In Sognnaes, R. F., editor: Chemistry and prevention of dental caries, Springfield, Ill., 1962, Charles C Thomas, Publisher.)

if certain types of bacteria are present. The severity of caries is reduced by limiting the frequency and amount of carbohydrates eaten. This is true even though all plaque does not form acid. The effectiveness of plaque removal in preventing caries has not been established. Since this is not completely possible and since the plaque chemistry cannot be regulated, the acid potential of the diet must be controlled. Plaque removal for the novice should be measured with disclosing agents to assess tooth cleanliness.[22]

The decalcification potential of many foods has been determined by Bibby.[23] Different types of food were fed to clinical subjects and the amount of food adhering to the teeth was determined. This amount of food was incubated with saliva and the quantity of 0.1N acid formed in 4 hours was determined. The quantity of the food was multiplied by the quantity of the acid produced and termed the "decalcification potential." These amounts represent the cariogenicity of foodstuffs and they should be studied for the purpose of advising patients on sound eating habits.

These data would suggest that the adhesive or sticky refined carbohydrates keep acid in contact with the tooth surface for a longer period because they are not cleaned from the tooth. Knowledge of the potential danger and the method of measuring the actual intake of carbohydrates by teaspoons are useful as caries-control measures. Emphasis is placed on the elimination of carbohydrates between meals.

PREVENTIVE FACTORS

As mentioned previously, preventive dentistry is included in all aspects of the profession by the dentist who is foresighted, informed, and concerned with optimum patient treatment. This section is concerned only with the factors that are indicated in conjunction with the restorative patient.

Table 19-1. Mean numbers of DMF permanent teeth per child in continuous resident white children examined in Grand Rapids, Mich., by age, year of examination, and elapsed time since fluoridation of the community water*

Age (years)	Beginning of fluoridation (1944-1945)	After 12 years (1956)	After 13 years (1957)	After 14 years (1958)	After 15 years (1959)	Percent reduction in DMF teeth (1944-1959)
12	8.07	2.91	3.36	3.36	3.47	57.0
13	9.73	4.47	3.86	4.66	3.58	63.2
14	10.94	6.02	5.48	5.55	5.38	50.8
15	12.48	7.52	6.79	6.59	6.22	50.2
16	13.50	8.87	8.13	8.30	7.03	47.9

*From Arnold, F. A., Likins, R. C., Russell, A. L., and Scott, D. B.: Fifteenth year of the Grand Rapids fluoridation study, 253 fluoride drinking waters, Pub. No. 825, Washington, D. C., 1962, U. S. Public Health Service.

There are a number of factors that are useful in diagnosing the problems of the patient. The caries activity tests, the determination of salivary flow and viscosity, and the buffer capacity of saliva are considered useful diagnostic aids.[24] It must be remembered that these are tests and not treatments to improve the health status of the patient. These tests are used to determine the acid potential of the bacterial flora, the nature of the salivary glands, and the properties of saliva. These tests do not always have a positive correlation with caries incidence in each case. After these tests are conducted they are used to plan certain caries-control measures. Routine use of these time-consuming procedures is questionable; they are primarily utilized for extremely difficult diagnostic problems.

Fluoride materials are effective treatments for preventing or controlling dental caries. Numerous treatments have been clinically tested and proved to be of value in either reducing the caries incidence or regulating the size of the frank lesion. The value and method of using fluorides are discussed separately.

Communal fluoridation

Fluorides added to the water supply have had a significant impact on caries prevention (Tables 19-1 and 19-2). The U. S. Public Health Service gathered data in 1942 from a number of cities with natural fluorides in their water supply; the incidence of dental caries in the people residing in these areas was

Table 19-2. Dental caries prevalence in permanent teeth of continuous resident children in an area with fluoride added to the water compared with prevalence in children in an area with naturally occurring fluoridation*

Age (years)	Number examined	DMF teeth per child	Carious teeth per child†	Filled teeth per child†	Missing teeth per child
Grand Rapids, Mich., 1959 (after 15 years of fluoridation)					
12	163	3.47	0.94	2.57	0.10
13	172	3.58	1.02	2.40	0.22
14	217	5.38	1.19	3.81	0.48
15	221	6.22	1.37	4.47	0.54
16	258	7.03	1.25	5.41	0.51
Aurora, Ill., 1945 (1.2 p.p.m. naturally occurring fluoride)					
12	401	2.95	2.06	0.96	0.12
13	401	3.09	2.10	1.20	0.14
14	433	3.64	2.05	1.58	0.18
15	467	4.54	2.37	2.05	0.35
16	371	5.19	2.32	2.71	0.41

*From Arnold, F. A., Likins, R. C., Russell, A. L., and Scott, D. B.: Fifteenth year of the Grand Rapids fluoridation study, 253 fluoride drinking waters, Pub. No. 825, Washington, D. C., 1962, U.S. Public Health Service.
†A tooth both filled and carious is counted in each column.

less than in other areas.[25] In 1945, projects were started in which three cities had the fluoride content of the water supply elevated to approximately 1 part per million. The results are optimum when the fluorine is incorporated into the developing tooth. The true caries reduction cannot be predicted for a decade or longer. The chemical reaction with fluorine that strengthens the developing tooth is described by Brudevold.[26]

$$Ca_{10}(PO_4)6(OH)2 + 2F^- = Ca_{10}(PO_4)6F_2 + 2OH^-$$
Enamel hydroxyapatite + Fluoride = Fluorapatite + Hydroxyl

This reaction causes the crystalline structure of enamel to be less soluble and harder, which could contribute to the reduction in caries. According to the published data, there is approximately a 50% reduction in the number of decayed, missing, and filled tooth surfaces in patients who have resided in fluoridated areas. This appears to be the most effective method available for reducing the caries rate. It has also caused a noticeable reduction in the number of smooth surface lesions. Recent results of school fluoridation report a 39% reduction in decayed, missing, and filled teeth only after 12 years of the program.[27]

Multiple fluoride therapy

There are a number of ways the dentist can use fluorides in his practice to further reduce the caries rate or to control the size of existing enamel defects (Table 19-3). The techniques used are as follows[28]:

1. Topical application of 10% stannous fluoride for 30 seconds. This treatment places fluorine in the apatite structure but is most useful in forming tin phosphate to arrest the pre-carious lesion. The effectiveness of the topical solution is a reduction in decayed, missing, and filled tooth surfaces (DMFS) of 20% to 40%, depending on whether the water is fluoridated. The reduction is not as great in the fluoridated areas.
2. Prophylaxis with lava pumice incorporated with stannous fluoride. The solution is burnished into the enamel during the prophylaxis to form tin phosphate and to protect the sound enamel surface.
3. Fluoride-containing dentifrice. A fluoride dentifrice is used by the patient to replace the tin that is brushed or dissolved from the tooth between the regular appointments. Therapeutic dentifrices support the other two fluoride treatments for additional caries reduction.

The use of these techniques is called multiple fluoride therapy and is indicated for the adult patient who develops carious lesions (Fig. 19-2). The application of topical stannous fluoride is regulated by the number of new lesions each year. The results obtained with the fluoride treatments just described are more dramatic when used in an area with no fluorine in the water supply. A combination of all the methods of administering fluorides to the tooth causes as much as a 90% reduction in the incidence of caries when compared to a control group that has not received any form of fluorine. Multiple therapy, whenever it is necessary, is used to protect the patient and the dental restorations.

Table 19-3. DMFT and DMFS increments in subjects completing 6 months of tests*

Group†	Number of subjects	DMFT			DMFS		
		Mean‡	P	Reduction (%)	Mean‡	P	Reduction (%)
		Examiner A					
1	120	1.16 (0.155)	—	—	2.69 (0.313)	—	—
2	109	1.01 (0.141)	0.46500	12.9	2.22 (0.217)	0.21500	17.5
3	115	0.77 (0.136)	0.05700	33.6	1.42 (0.194)	0.00046	47.2
4	108	0.76 (0.131)	0.04800	34.5	1.44 (0.210)	0.00076	46.5
5	113	0.13 (0.127)	<0.00001	88.8	0.07 (0.190)	<0.00001	97.4
		Examiner B					
1	118	1.06 (0.109)	—	—	2.14 (0.219)	—	—
2	114	0.65 (0.112)	0.00850	38.7	1.28 (0.195)	0.00330	40.2
3	110	0.73 (0.093)	0.02150	31.1	1.34 (0.177)	0.00425	37.4
4	120	0.50 (0.084)	0.00003	52.8	0.86 (0.129)	<0.00001	59.8
5	129	0.25 (0.071)	<0.00001	76.4	0.49 (0.119)	<0.00001	77.1

*From Bixler, D., and Muhler, J. C.: J.A.D.A. **68**:792, 1964.
†1, control; 2, prophylaxis with SnF_2; 3, prophylaxis with SnF_2 plus SnF_2 dentifrice; 4, prophylaxis with SnF_2 plus topical SnF_2; 5, prophylaxis with SnF_2 plus topical SnF_2 plus SnF_2 dentifrice.
‡Numbers in parentheses represent the standard error of the mean.

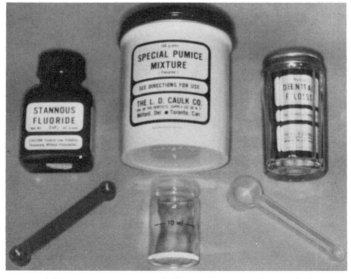

Fig. 19-2. Commercial kit containing F_2 prophylactic mixture and crystals for topical 10% solution of stannous fluoride.

Office procedure

The 10% solution of stannous fluoride is kept on the isolated teeth for only 30 seconds. At one time sodium fluoride was applied in four treatments, but this is no longer necessary. The quickness and ease of using the topical technique make it a practical office procedure. The fluorides are applied after scaling is completed at each recall appointment. The caries-active patient is treated with the topical solution every 6 months, but the routine patient needs only an annual application. If new caries is not developing, the topical solution can be omitted.

1. A thorough prophylaxis is given to remove the stain and calculus from the teeth. The patient is instructed to rinse thoroughly with water and then nonwaxed dental floss is used to remove the remaining debris from the interproximal surfaces. The patient rinses once again so that the teeth are as clean as possible.
2. The lava pumice and stannous fluoride are burnished slowly into the accessible enamel surfaces with a soft rubber cup. This places the fluoride and tin ions into the sound enamel for protection. Nonwaxed dental floss is used to carry this abrasive into the interproximal spaces to protect the enamel in these areas. The patient may then rinse.
3. The 10% fluoride solution is freshly prepared by mixing the crystals with distilled water (Fig. 19-3). The solution is stirred until the contents become cloudy and homogeneous.
4. One half of the mouth is isolated with cotton rolls by blocking the ducts of the salivary glands (Fig. 19-4). The cotton holders are used for the lower jaw, and when these are in place, the teeth are dried with the warm air syringe.
5. Two cotton applicators are used to pick up the fluoride solution, and the accessible tooth surfaces are painted and kept moist for 30 seconds (Fig. 19-5). After this is completed the patient may rinse and the procedure is repeated on the other side of the mouth.
6. Following the application the patient is instructed not to rinse for 15 minutes to give the stannous ions time to react with the phosphates in the pre-carious area.

The softened pre-carious lesions become hard and stain a light brown color. This accounts for some lesion reversals being reported in clinical studies. The tin is lost gradually and needs to be replaced to keep the areas insoluble. This is accomplished with a fluoride-containing dentifrice. The topical treatments can be stopped when the patient ceases to develop new carious lesions. If new lesions do develop, a topical booster solution should be applied to the teeth at more frequent intervals. These caries-control measures are recognized by the Council on Dental Therapeutics of the A.D.A. as being useful in reducing caries. The tin ions in the dentifrice replace the gradual loss that occurs on the tooth surface, and in adults this is found to cause a reduction in the incidence of caries.[29]

Studies have been conducted with acidulated phosphate-fluoride solutions

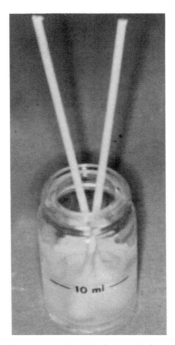

Fig. 19-3. Fresh 10% solution of stannous fluoride for topical application. All crystals are stirred into solution for the 30-second application.

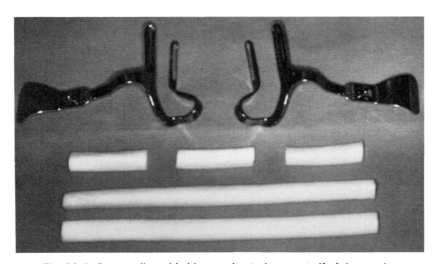

Fig. 19-4. Cotton rolls and holders used to isolate one half of the mouth.

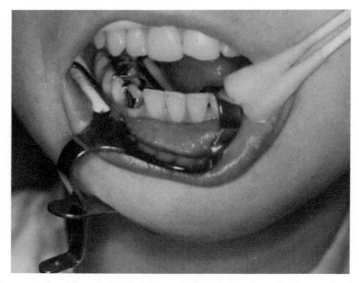

Fig. 19-5. Stannous fluoride solution being applied to isolated teeth. The teeth should be kept moistened the entire 30 seconds.

that are used in topical treatments.[30] The results are encouraging in that the fluoride uptake of enamel is enhanced by the acid solution. The fluoride in place of communal fluoridation would seem to have the same value. Topical application is reported to be helpful in reducing caries with the acidulated compounds, but additional benefits beyond the techniques presented need to be studied. In the future many other types of caries-preventive solutions will undoubtedly be evaluated for the purpose of giving the practicing dentist stronger tools for the reduction of caries.

• • •

Much progress has been made with the delivery of fluoride compounds such as gels and solutions, and the material has been incorporated into the prophylactic paste. The new growth of prevention, certainly not a new concept, has promoted the development of products. At this time the dentist must select a fluoride mechanism that is pleasing, stable, and effective for his caries-active patients. Much research still needs to be conducted concerning the delivery method of fluoride to tooth structure and concerning the control of oral disease.

Shannon[31] reported an effective method of treating root surfaces by combining stannous fluoride and an acidulated compound. Many mechanisms are available, and the experimentation should continue.

The value of the recall appointment, oral hygiene procedures, and preventive therapy is difficult to assess from a quantitative standpoint. The literature is exhaustive in these areas and well-controlled scientific studies have produced information on many of the subjects. The maintenance of the teeth is optimal only if these procedures are employed and the patient is under control. The dentist is justified in encouraging and developing programs of oral hygiene for all patients. Any preventive treatment that is reported to be helpful and that is quick and economical to the patient should be employed. Prevention should remain the first step to proper oral care.

REFERENCES

1. Sumnicht, R. W.: Preventive dentistry and dental practice, Pract. Dent. Monographs, July, 1965, pp. 1-45.
2. Fechtner, J. L., and Mallin, R. J.: 15 years of preventive dentistry in private practice, J. Am. Dent. Assoc. 84:817, 1972.
3. Hine, M. K.: Dental caries, mechanisms, and present control techniques as evaluated at the University of Michigan Workshop, St. Louis, 1948, The C. V. Mosby Co.
4. Coolidge, E. D., and Hine, M. K.: Periodontia; clinical pathology and treatment of the periodontal tissue, Philadelphia, 1954, Lea & Febiger.
5. Glickman, I.: Clinical periodontology, Philadelphia, 1964, W. B. Saunders Co.
6. Bibby, B. G.: Do we tell the truth about preventing caries? J. Dent. Child. 33:269, 1966.
7. O'Leary, T. J., and Nahers, C. L.: Instructions to supplement teaching oral hygiene, J. Periodont. 40:27, 1969.
8. Arnim, S. S.: An effective program of oral hygiene for the arrestment of dental caries and the control of periodontal disease, J. S. Calif. Dent. Assoc. 35:264, 1967.
9. Lightner, L. M., and others: Preventive periodontic treatment procedures: results over 46 months, J. Periodont. 42:555, 1971.
10. Manly, B. S.: Factors influencing tests on the abrasion of dentin by brushing with dentifrices, J. Dent. Res. 23:59, 1944.
11. Chilton, N. W., and Kutscher, A. H.: Use of an electric toothbrush by a severely handicapped man, Man. J. New Jersey Dent. Soc. 33:20, 1961.
12. Chilton, N. W., Didio, A., and Rathner, J. T.: Comparison of the clinical effectiveness of an electric and a standard toothbrush in normal individuals, J.A.D.A. 64:777, 1962.
13. Accepted dental remedies, Chicago, 1966, Council on Dental Therapeutics of the American Dental Association.
14. Lundquist, C.: Oral sugar clearance, Odont. Rev. 3:supp. 1, 1952.
15. Wheatcroft, M. G., and Arnim, S. S.: An effective program of oral hygiene the dentist can teach adolescents, Dent. Clin. N. Am. 13:373, 1969.
16. Arnim, S. S.: The effect of thorough mouth cleansing on health-case report, Periodontics 6:41, 1968.
17. A guide to good eating, Chicago, 1966, National Dairy Council.
18. Stanton, G.: A new look—diet and dental caries, J. Am. Soc. Prev. Dent. 1:34, 1971.
19. Gustafsson, B. E., and others: The effect of different levels of carbohydrate intake on caries activity in 436 individuals observed for five years, Acta Odont. Scand. 11:232, 1954.
20. Brauer, J. C., and Lindahl, R. L.: Dentistry for children, ed. 5, New York, 1964, McGraw-Hill Book Co., Inc.
21. Jenkins, N. G.: The chemistry of plaque, Ann. New York Acad. Sci. 131:786, 1965.
22. Arnim, S. S.: The use of disclosing agents for measuring tooth cleanliness, J. Periodont. 34:227, 1963.
23. Bibby, B. G.: Effect of sugar content of foodstuffs on their caries-producing potentialities, J.A.D.A. 51:293, 1955.
24. Preventive dentistry laboratory manual, Indianapolis, 1966, Indiana University School of Dentistry.
25. Arnold, F. A., Likins, R. C., Russell, A. L., and Scott, D. B.: Fifteenth year of the Grand Rapids fluoridation study, 253 fluoride drinking waters, Pub. No. 825, Washington, D. C., 1962, U. S. Public Health Service.
26. Brudevold, F.: Chemical composition of the teeth in relation to caries. In Sognnaes, R. F.,

editor: Chemistry and prevention of dental caries, Springfield, Ill., 1962, Charles C Thomas, Publisher, chap. 2.

27. Horowitz, H. S. Heifety, S. B., and Law, F. E.: Effect of school water fluoridation on dental caries: final results in Elk Lake, Pennsylvania, after 12 years, J. Am. Dent. Assoc. **84:**832, 1972.

28. Muhler, J. C.: Control of dental caries in the adult dentition, Symposium on Applied Preventive Dentistry, Columbia, 1965, University of Missouri.

29. Bixler, D., and Muhler, J. C.: Combined use of three agents containing stannous fluoride; a prophylactic paste, a solution and a dentifrice, J.A.D.A. **68:**793, 1964.

30. Brudevold, F.: Fluorides in prevention of dental caries, Dent. Clin. N. Am., July, 1962, pp. 397-409.

31. Shannon, I. L., and Wightman, J. R.: Treatment of root surfaces with a combination of acidulated phosphofluoride and stannous fluoride, J. Acad. Gen. Dent. **20:**26, 1972.

Index